DICTIONARY OF
AMERICAN
MEDICAL
BIOGRAPHY

An institution is the lengthened shadow of one man.
Emerson, *Self-Reliance*

DICTIONARY OF AMERICAN MEDICAL BIOGRAPHY

Martin Kaufman, Stuart Galishoff,
Todd L. Savitt, Editors

Joseph Carvalho III, Editorial Associate

Volume I

A-L

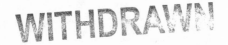

GREENWOOD PRESS

Westport, Connecticut • London, England

Library of Congress Cataloging in Publication Data
Main entry under title:

Dictionary of American medical biography.

  Bibliography: p.
  Includes index.
  1. Medicine—United States—Biography. 2. Public
health personnel—United States—Biography. 3. Healers
—United States—Biography. I. Kaufman, Martin,
1940-   . II. Galishoff, Stuart, 1940-   . III. Savitt,
Todd L., 1943-   . [DNLM: 1. Physicians—United
States—Biography. 2. History of medicine, modern—
United States. WZ 140 AA1 D5]
R153.D53   1984   610'.92'2 [B]   82-21110
ISBN 0-313-21378-X (lib. bdg.) set
ISBN 0-313-24333-6 (vol. 1)
ISBN 0-313-24334-4 (vol. 2)

Library of Congress Catalog Card Number: 82-21110
ISBN: 0-313-21378-X

First published in 1984

Greenwood Press
A division of Congressional Information Service, Inc.
88 Post Road West
Westport, Connecticut 06881

Printed in the United States of America

10 9 8 7 6 5 4 3 2 1

Contents

Preface

When we first discussed the possibility of coediting a dictionary of American medical biography, we looked at previously published works in the field. Since the last comprehensive dictionary was published in 1928, more than fifty years ago, it was apparent that a new work was in order. That dictionary, edited by Howard A. Kelly and Walter L. Burrage, represents the best resource for American medical biography to the year 1927. Since then, there has been an explosion of scientific knowledge which has changed the basis of modern clinical medicine and effected the development of new specialties and collateral fields. Therefore, we believe that a new biographical dictionary is a welcome addition to reference collections in the history of American medicine and public health. The major contribution of such a work is the inclusion of biographical sketches representing developments which occurred after the publication of Kelly and Burrage.

In addition to coverage of persons whose importance dates from the seventeenth, eighteenth, and nineteenth centuries, and the new coverage of twentieth century figures, the editors decided to include representative blacks and women whose contributions have often been overlooked in the past. We have also included groups of persons who were not necessarily physicians but who were important in the development of American medicine and public health, such as biochemists, medical educators, and hospital administrators. In order to provide geographical distribution and an insight into developments on the state and local level, we have included representative biographical sketches from each of the fifty states and the District of Columbia. Finally, this volume includes persons outside the mainstream of American medicine—health faddists, patent medicine manufacturers, unorthodox practitioners, and others whose major role was to provide alternatives to traditional medicine, and to call attention to problems that were not being adequately addressed by the orthodox approaches of the time.

With a limit of 350,000 words (which we surpassed by almost 25 percent with the permission of the publisher), the selection process was a difficult and important task. In order to maintain historical perspective, the coeditors established a cut-off date of December 31, 1976. If an important figure died after that date, he or she could not be included in this volume. We assume that persons in that category may eventually be included in new editions of this work. The editors prepared a list of well over 500 persons whose inclusion was assured by the significance of their contributions to the history of American medicine and public health. The list was then circulated to colleagues for their suggestions and recommendations. The editors are aware that, despite their best efforts, subjects who might merit inclusion in the *Dictionary of American Medical Biography* (DAMB) have been omitted. We welcome suggestions of new subjects for future editions.

After the selection process was completed, the editors set out to establish a format for the biographical sketches, a format which would provide necessary biographical information, adequate description of contributions and significance, important or representative writings of the subjects, and references. When the sketches were completed, the editors checked as much information as possible for accuracy, and added citations from other reference works to provide the reader with a guide to sources that offer fuller information. The following format was selected by the editors:

NAME OF SUBJECT (last name, first name, middle name) (date of birth, place of birth–date of death, place of death). *Occupation; Area of specialization.* Parents' names and occupations. Marital information (names of spouses, dates of marriages, number of children by each marriage). CAREER: Information including dates and positions. CONTRIBUTIONS.

WRITINGS: A maximum of five important or representative works, and where available, the location of a bibliography. REFERENCES.

In some cases, information could not be located by the contributor or the editors. The most common omissions are parents' names and occupations, spouses' names and number of children. The editors ask persons with such information to write to them so that the biographies in question can be changed in subsequent editions of the DAMB.

In order to make the information in the sketches more readily accessible, the editors have included several appendices which list the biographical subjects by various categories, and an index.

As those who have worked in teams are well aware, the success of a team depends on all the members. This work represents the combined efforts of three coeditors, an editorial associate, and as the list at the start of this volume indicates, a large number of contributors. In so vast an undertaking, involving reliance on so many persons, it was inevitable that some who initially agreed to write biographical sketches would later find that they could not fulfill their commitments. Most who assumed the responsibility of composing sketches, however, completed their assignments in good time. To them the editors are indebted for their diligence and their competence. An additional word of thanks must go to

Ronald L. Numbers of the University of Wisconsin and Edward Atwater of the University of Rochester for their critical perusal of the list of subjects to be included in the DAMB.

The editors made extensive use of the reference and interlibrary loan services at their home institution libraries. We wish to express our appreciation to the staffs of these libraries. We also want to thank Barry Murphy and the computer center of Westfield State College for their help in preparing the appendices.

Finally, the editors would like to express their appreciation to their spouses and families, who have endured much over the past four years, and who have supported them through a difficult but ultimately rewarding undertaking.

Martin Kaufman
Stuart Galishoff
Todd L. Savitt

Contributors

Paul Addis, University of Maryland

Virginia Allen, Oklahoma City, Oklahoma

Rima D. Apple, State University of New York at Stony Brook

William Barlow, Seton Hall University

Ronald E. Batt, State University of New York at Buffalo

Harold Bauman, University of Utah

William K. Beatty, Northwestern University

Irving A. Beck, Brown University

Leland V. Bell, Central State University

Whitfield J. Bell, Jr., American Philosophical Society

David W. Boilard, School of Medicine, University of North Dakota

Charles A. Bonsett, Indiana University School of Medicine

Charlotte Borst, University of Wisconsin Center for Health Sciences

John A. Breinich, Hawaii Medical Library

Patrick W. Brennen, University of South Dakota School of Medicine

Gert H. Brieger, Johns Hopkins University, Institute of the History of Medicine

Simon Rulin Bruesch, University of Tennessee Health Sciences Center

Chester R. Burns, University of Texas Medical Branch

Joseph Carvalho III, Springfield City Library

Philip Cash, Emmanuel College

James H. Cassedy, National Library of Medicine

Sandra L. Chaff, Medical College of Pennsylvania

Betty Clements, University of Iowa College of Medicine

Thomas E. Cone, Jr., Children's Hospital Medical Center (Boston, Massachusetts)

Eugene H. Conner, Louisville, Kentucky

David Laurence Cowen, Jamesburg, New Jersey

Charlotte L. Cutter, Albuquerque, New Mexico

Marc H. Dawson, Union College

Gordon B. Dodds, Portland State University

John P. Dolan (deceased), University of South Carolina

Craig Donegan, Southwest Texas State University

Virginia G. Drachman, Tufts University

John Duffy, University of Maryland

Jerome Edwards, University of Nevada, Reno

Ralph Edwards, Kingsborough Community College of the City University of New York

Samuel Eichold, College of Medicine, University of South Alabama

G. E. Erikson, Brown University

J. Worth Estes, Boston University School of Medicine

Leslie A. Falk, Meharry Medical College

Daniel M. Fox, State University of New York at Stony Brook

Stuart Galishoff, Georgia State University

Norman Gevitz, Illinois Institute of Technology

John S. Goff, Phoenix College

Gerald N. Grob, Rutgers University

E. Ashby Hammond, University of Florida

Arthur A. Hart, Idaho State Historical Society

Andrea R. C. Helms, University of Alaska

Bernice M. Hetzner, University of Nebraska Medical Center

Robert P. Hudson, University of Kansas Medical Center

Marion Hunt, Washington University

John W. Ifkovic, Westfield State College

Glen Pierce Jenkins, Cleveland Health Sciences Library

Mary Van Hulle Jones, University of Wisconsin Center for Health Sciences

Robert J. T. Joy, Uniformed Services University of the Health Sciences

Charles S. Judd, Jr., University of Hawaii School of Medicine

Martin Kaufman, Westfield State College

Elizabeth B. Keeney, University of Wisconsin Center for Health Sciences

Ramunas A. Kondratas, Smithsonian Institution

Donald Konold, Arkansas State University

Dorothy I. Lansing, Obstetrical Society of Philadelphia

Judith Walzer Leavitt, University of Wisconsin Center for Health Sciences

Susan Eyrich Lederer, University of Wisconsin Center for Health Sciences

Marshall Scott Legan, Northeast Louisiana University

Brian C. Lister, University of Maine, Farmington

Lawrence D. Longo, Loma Linda University School of Medicine

Berit Midelfort, Chicago, Illinois

Genevieve Miller, Johns Hopkins Institute of the History of Medicine

Regina Markell Morantz, University of Kansas

James Polk Morris III, University of Texas Health Science Center, Houston

Pierce C. Mullen, Montana State University

Robert L. Murphy, West Virginia University Medical Center

Kenneth R. Nodyne, West Liberty State College

Ynez Violé O'Neill, University of California, Los Angeles, School of Medicine

William J. Orr, Joslyn Art Museum, Omaha, Nebraska

Anthony Palmieri III, University of Wyoming School of Pharmacy

Steven J. Peitzman, Medical College of Pennsylvania

Martin S. Pernick, University of Michigan

Charles V. Pollack, Jr., Tulane University School of Medicine

David O. Powell, C. W. Post Center of Long Island University

Robert E. Rakel, University of Iowa, College of Medicine

Larry Remele, State Historical Society of North Dakota

Frank Bradway Rogers, Denver, Colorado

Barbara Guttman Rosenkrantz, Harvard University

Robert Rosenthal, Saint Paul, Minnesota

David Rosner, Mt. Sinai School of Medicine (Boston, Massachusetts)

Lewis Phillip Rubin, Children's Hospital Medical Center

Guillermo Cornelio Sanchez, Massachusetts General Hospital

Todd L. Savitt, East Carolina University School of Medicine

Rennie B. Schoepflin, University of Wisconsin Center for Health Sciences

Edward Shoemaker, Emory University

Dale C. Smith, Uniformed Services University of the Health Sciences

Duane R. Sneddeker, Washington University

Michael M. Sokal, Worcester Polytechnic Institute

Phinizy Spalding, University of Georgia

Elizabeth H. Thomson, Yale University School of Medicine

Lester J. Wallman, University of Vermont College of Medicine

John Harley Warner, Harvard University

Margaret Humphreys Warner, Harvard University

James Clifton Whorton, University of Washington

William H. Williams, University of Delaware

James Harvey Young, Emory University

Abbreviations

Appleton's CAB	*Appleton's Cyclopedia of American Biography*
BHM	*Bibliography of the History of Medicine*
BMFRS	*Biographical Memoirs of the Fellows of the Royal Society*
BMNAS	*Biographical Memoirs of the National Academy of Sciences*
DAB	*Dictionary of American Biography*
DSB	*Dictionary of Scientific Biography*
Index Catalogue	*Index Catalogue of the Surgeon-General's Library*
JAMA	*Journal of the American Medical Association*
JNMA	*Journal of the National Medical Association*
Kelly and Burrage	Howard A. Kelly and Walter L. Burrage, *American Medical Biographies* (1920); *Dictionary of American Medical Biographies* (1928)
Miller, *BHM*	Genevieve Miller, ed., *Bibliography of the History of Medicine of the United States and Canada, 1939-1960* (1964)
NCAB	*National Cyclopedia of American Biography*
TAMA	*Transactions of the American Medical Association*
WKW	*Wiener Klinische Wochenschrift*
WMW	*Wiener Medizinische Wochenschrift*
WWAPS	Schwartz, ed., *Who's Who Among Physicians and Surgeons* (1937)
WWCR	*Who's Who in the Colored Race*
WWICA	*Who's Who in Colored America*
ZHI	*Zeitschrift fur Hygiene und Infektionskrankheiten*

OTHER COMMON ABBREVIATIONS

Bull.	*Bulletin*
Dict.	*Dictionary*
Hist.	*History* or *Historical*
J.	*Journal*
Med.	*Medical* or *Medicine*
Q.	*Quarterly*
Rev.	*Review*
Surg.	*Surgery* or *Surgeons*
Trans.	*Transactions*

Other abbreviations follow standard practices.

DICTIONARY OF
AMERICAN
MEDICAL
BIOGRAPHY

A

ABBOTT, ANDERSON RUFFIN (April 7, 1837, Toronto, Ontario, Canada-December 29, 1913, Toronto). *Surgeon.* Son of Wilson R. and Ellen (Toyer) Abbott. Married Mary Ann Casey, 1871; five children. EDUCATION: 1856-58, Oberlin College Preparatory Department; 1861, M.B., Trinity College, University of Toronto; 1863, M.D., University of Toronto. CAREER: 1863-66, acting assistant surgeon, U.S. Army Medical Corps, stationed in Washington, D.C.; private practice: 1866-early 1890s, Toronto, Chatham, Dundas, and Oakville, Ontario, Canada; 1894-c. 1900, Chicago, Ill.; 1900-13, Toronto. CONTRIBUTIONS: One of eight black physicians appointed to Army Medical Corps during Civil War. One of Washington physicians assigned to establishing a contraband hospital out of which Freedmen's Hospital arose (1863-64). Chief executive officer of Freedmen's Hospital (1864) and director of Abbott Hospital, Freedmen's Village, Va. (1864-66). Treated many ailing freedmen at these hospitals during and after Civil War. Surgeon-in-chief, Provident Hospital, Chicago (1894-c. 1897), in absence of Daniel Hale Williams (q.v.). REFERENCES: Henry S. Robinson, "Anderson Ruffin Abbott, M.D., 1837-1913," *JNMA* 72 (1980): 713-16. Abbott's papers are in the Metropolitan Toronto Library, Toronto, Ontario, Canada.

T. Savitt

ABBOTT, MAUDE (March 18, 1869, St. Andrews East, Quebec, Canada-September 2, 1940, Montreal, Quebec, Canada). *Pathologist; Historian.* Daughter of Rev. Jeremiah and Elizabeth (Abbott) Babin but raised by maternal grandmother Mrs. William Abbott, legally assuming that surname. EDUCATION: 1890, B.A., McGill University; 1894, M.D., Bishop's College Medical School; 1894-97, postgraduate studies in London, Heidelberg, Vienna, Glasgow. CAREER: At Medical Museum, McGill: 1898-1900, assistant curator; and 1901-32, curator; 1910-23, lecturer in pathology, McGill; 1923-25, professor of pathology and director of clinical laboratories, Woman's Medical College of Pennsylvania; 1925-36, assistant professor of medical research, McGill, and member, University Clinic Staff, Royal Victoria Hospital; 1932, curator, Medical Historical Museum, McGill. CONTRIBUTIONS: Careful analysis of 1,000 cases made her "the world's authority on congenital heart disease," in the words of Paul D. White (q.v.), her work particularly furthering classification and clinical-pathological correlation. Helped found and active in the International Association of Medical Museums. While "on loan" to the Woman's Medical College of Pennsylvania, helped that school set pathology and bacteriology on a sound footing during critical days. Contributed to medical historiography of Quebec. Compiled bibliography of Sir William Osler (q.v.).

WRITINGS: *History of Medicine in the Province of Quebec* (1931); *Atlas of Congenital Cardiac Diseases* (1936); *Classified and Annotated Bibliography of Sir William Osler's Publications* (1939); numerous articles about pathology, pulmonary physiology, history, and so on. Writings listed in H. E. MacDermot, *Maude Abbott—A Memoir* (1941). REFERENCES: MacDermot, "Maude Abbott," *McGill Med. J.* 28 (1959): 127-52; Miller, *BHM*, pp. 1-2.

S. J. Peitzman

ABEL, JOHN JACOB (May 19, 1857, Cleveland, Ohio-May 26, 1938, Baltimore, Md.). *Physician; Physiological chemist; Pharmacology*. Son of George M., farmer, and Mary (Becker) Abel. Married Mary White Hinman, 1883; three children. EDUCATION: 1883, Ph.B., University of Michigan; 1883-84, postgraduate study, Johns Hopkins University; 1884-91, studied chemistry and medicine in Leipzig, Heidelberg, Würzburg, and Berlin, Germany; Strassburg, France; Berne, Switzerland; and Vienna, Austria; 1888, M.D., University of Strassburg. CAREER: 1891-93, materia medica and therapeutics faculty, University of Michigan; at Johns Hopkins Medical School: 1893-1932, pharmacology faculty; and 1932-38, director, Laboratory for Endocrine Research; 1909-32, editor, *Journal of Pharmacology and Experimental Therapeutics*. CONTRIBUTIONS: Made major discoveries about the chemical mechanisms that control the physiology of animal tissues, particularly that of the ductless glands. Extracted the first adrenal hormone, which he named "epinephrine" (1897). Later it was discovered that it was not the free hormone but a monobenzoyl derivative of epinephrine (adrenalin). Isolated insulin in crystalline form and proved that it is a protein (1927). Stressed the importance of studying the composition and structure of chemical substances as the first step in the development of a rational pharmacology. Trained many of the leading American pharmacologists of his day. Helped establish laboratory-based experimental pharmacology as an independent, university discipline. Suggested the development of an artificial kidney and developed a vividiffusion apparatus for experiments on laboratory animals (1912-13); used device to demonstrate the existence of amino acids in the blood. Was instrumental in the establishment of the *Journal of Experimental Medicine*, the *Journal of Biological Chemistry*, and the *Journal of Pharmacology and Experimental Therapeutics* and helped found the American Society of Biological Chemists and the Society for Pharmacology and Experimental Therapeutics.

WRITINGS: "On the Blood-Pressure-Raising Constituent of the Suparenal Capsule," *Bull., Johns Hopkins Hosp.* 8 (1897): 151-57 (with Albert C. Crawford); "On the Removal of Diffusible Substances from the Circulating Blood by Means of Dialysis," *Trans., Assoc. of Am. Physicians* 28 (1913): 51-54 (with L. G. Rowntree [q.v.] and B. B. Turner); "Crystalline Insulin," *Proc., Nat. Acad. of Sci.* 12 (Feb. 1926): 132-36. A bibliography is in *BMNAS* 24 (1946): 231-57. REFERENCES: *BHM* (1964-69), 7; (1970-74), 7; *DAB*, Supplement 2: 4-5; *DSB*, 1: 9-12; Miller, *BHM*, p. 2; *Who Was Who in Am.*, 1: 3.

S. Galishoff

ABELL, IRVIN (September 13, 1876, Lebanon, Marion County, Ky.-August 28, 1949, near Winnipeg, Manitoba, Canada). *Surgeon; Educator.* Son of Irvin and Sarah Silesia (Rogers) Abell. Married Caroline G. Harting, October 19, 1907; four sons. EDUCATION: 1882-89, St. Augustine's Parochial School, Lebanon; 1889-92, St. Mary's College, Marion County, B.A., 1892; 1893-94, Louisville College of Pharmacy; 1897, M.D., Louisville Medical College; 1897-98, intern, Louisville City Hospital; 1898-99, postgraduate studies, University of Berlin and University of Marburg, Germany. CAREER: 1900-8, assistant in surgery, Louisville Medical College; 1908-49, surgery faculty, University of Louisville School of Medicine; 1908-49, surgeon, Louisville City Hospital and St. Joseph's Infirmary, Louisville; president: 1925, Southern Surgical Association; 1926, Kentucky Medical Association; 1933, Southern Medical Association; 1938, American Medical Association; 1946-47, American College of Surgeons; at some time, president: American Urological Association, American Gastro-Enterological Society, Southern Surgical Congress, and Association of Military Surgeons of the United States; World War I, commander of U.S. Army Base Hospital 59; 1943-46, member, Surgical Committee, National Research Council. CONTRIBUTIONS: In two roles: as a teacher of surgery and an articulate, vigorous spokesman for the medical profession; as a member and frequent president of various national, regional, and specialty medical societies. During tenure as professor of surgery at the University of Louisville School of Medicine and chief of surgery at the Louisville City Hospital, influenced and taught numerous medical students and medical graduates pursuing advanced surgical training.

WRITINGS: No complete bibliography has been published, although many of his publications are listed in Editorial, *Southern Med. J.* 26 (1933): 77-78. Several important examples are "A Retrospect of Surgery in Kentucky," *Trans., Southern Surg. Assoc.* 38 (1925): 1-17; "Radium in the Treatment of Uterine Pathology," *Surg. Gyn. & Obst.* 46 (1928): 287-91; "Traumatic Surgery in the Curriculum of Medical Schools, " *ibid.,* 50 (1930): 327-39. REFERENCES: *NCAB*, 40: 130; obituary, *JAMA* 141 (Sept. 10, 1949): 146; *Who's Who in Am.* 19 (1936-37): 132.

E. H. Conner

ABRAMS, ALBERT (December 8, 1863, San Francisco, Calif.-January 13, 1924, San Francisco). *Physician; Internal medicine; Patent medicine.* Son of Marcus and Rachel (Leavey) Abrams. Married Jeanne Roth, 1897; Blanche

Schwabacher, 1915; no children. EDUCATION: 1882, M.D., University of Heidelberg; 1883, 1884, 1897, postgraduate courses in London, Berlin, Vienna, Paris; 1894, A.M., Portland University. CAREER: 1893-98, professor of pathology, Cooper Medical College; 1904-24, president, Emanuel Polyclinic, San Francisco; c. 1895-1905, consulting physician, diseases of the chest, Mt. Zion and French hospitals, San Francisco; gradually moved away from orthodox medicine, expounding his own electronic theory of disease. CONTRIBUTIONS: Generally regarded as one of the major practitioners of pseudoscience of this century. Discovered the "cardiac reflex of Abrams"—the change in size of the heart and aorta upon irritation of the overlying skin. Wrote two important medical texts (*Manual of Clinical Diagnosis; Diseases of the Heart*), which established his national reputation. Became increasingly eccentric (1900-10) and began to devote his studies to the "Electronic Reactions of Abrams" ("ERA")—changes in electronic vibrations measurable at the skin surface—by which he claimed he could diagnose and cure disease. Developed and sold expensive apparati, including the oscilloclast, the electrobioscope, and the biodynamometer. Traveled extensively, giving "clinical courses" in his theory of "spondylotherapy" for a substantial fee. Later expanded his methods to include long-distance diagnoses and therapy, which he could perform on a few drops of the patient's blood, on preserved tissue, or even on handwriting (all of which, claimed Abrams, exhibited the patient's vibratory rate), by means of his "dynamizer" and a system of rheostats. An investigation by *Scientific American* (1923) termed Abrams's therapy "without value," but the movement continued after Abrams's death.

WRITINGS: *Manual of Clinical Diagnosis* (1891); *Diseases of the Heart* (1900); *The Blues (Splanchnic Neurasthenia)* (1904); *Man and His Poisons* (1906); *Spondylotherapy* (1910). Writings listed in *Who Was Who in Am.*, 1: 4. REFERENCES: "Albert Abrams, A.M., M.D., LL.D., F.R.M.S.," AMA reprint of *JAMA* material on Abrams of various dates; American Medical Association Dept. of Investigation files, Chicago; David M. Bailey, "The Rise and Fall of Albert Abrams," *Okla. State J. of Med.* 71 (Jan. 1978): 15-20; *DAB*, 1: 30-31; N. Flaxman, "A Cardiac Anomaly," *Bull. Hist. Med.* 27 (1953): 252-68; *NCAB*, 19: 386; E. W. Page, "Portrait of a Quack," *Hygeia* 17 (Jan. 1939): 53-55, 92, 95; *Scientific American* series, vols. 129-31.

C. V. Pollack, Jr.

ABT, ISAAC ARTHUR (December 18, 1867, Wilmington, Ill.-November 22, 1955, Chicago, Ill.). *Physician; Pediatrics.* Son of Levi, postmaster and store owner, and Henrietta (Hart) Abt. Married Lena Rosenberg, 1897; two children. EDUCATION: 1889, completed preliminary medical course, Johns Hopkins University; 1891, M.D., Chicago Medical College (later Northwestern University Medical School); 1891-93, intern, Michael Reese Hospital (Chicago); 1893-94, studied in Vienna and Berlin. CAREER: *Post* 1894, practiced pediatrics, Chicago; diseases of children faculty: 1897-1901, Northwestern University Women's Medical School; 1902-08, Rush Medical College; 1909-42, Northwestern University

Medical School; attending or consulting physician, various Chicago hospitals; 1926-27, president, American Pediatric Society; 1930-31, co-founder and president, American Academy of Pediatrics. CONTRIBUTIONS: A founder of modern pediatrics. Administered the first diphtheria antitoxin in Chicago and was active in the movement to improve that city's milk and water supplies. Pioneered in the treatment of infantile scurvy. Believed to have been the first physician in Chicago to use incubators for premature babies and the first American physician to prescribe protein milk in the treatment of infant diarrhea. Designed and directed the construction of Sarah Morris Hospital, the first children's hospital in Chicago. Persuaded his colleagues that teething is a natural phenomenon rather than a disease. Raised the level of American pediatrics through his publications and editorial labors. For nearly 40 years (beginning in 1902), edited the *Yearbook of Pediatrics*. Edited an eight-volume encyclopedia of *Pediatrics* that brought together and made available to physicians throughout the world the most advanced developments in American pediatrics (1923-26). Edited the pediatrics volume in the Practical Medicine series. Helped establish the *American Journal for Diseases of Children* (1910).

WRITINGS: *The Baby's Food* (1917); *The Baby Doctor* (1944). REFERENCES: *BHM* (1970-74), 7; *DAB*, Supplement 5: 1-2; Miller, *BHM*, p. 2; *NCAB*, D: 223-24; *N.Y. Times*, November 24, 1955; A. H. Parmelee, "Isaac Arthur Abt (1867-1955)," in Borden S. Veeder (q.v.), ed., *Pediatric Profiles* (1957), 109-16; *Who Was Who in Am.*, 3: 12.

S. Galishoff

ADAMS, NUMA POMPILIUS GARFIELD (February 26, 1885, Delaplane, Va.-August 29, 1940, Chicago, Ill.). *Physician*. Married Osceola Marie Macarthy, 1915; one child. EDUCATION: 1911, A.B., Howard University; 1912, A.M. (chemistry), Columbia University; 1924, M.D., Rush Medical College; 1924, intern, St. Louis City Hospital No. 2 (now Homer G. Phillips Hospital). CAREER: 1912-19, chemistry faculty (chair, 1918-19), Howard University; 1925-29, private practice, Chicago; 1925-29, assistant medical director, Victory Life Insurance Company, Chicago; 1927-29, instructor in neurology and psychiatry, Provident Hospital School of Nursing, Chicago; 1929-40, dean, Howard Medical School. CONTRIBUTIONS: First black dean of an approved medical school (Howard, 1929). Despite opposition and obstructionism from within the institution, led Howard through a crucial transition period during which faculty and students improved in quality, the medical school and Freedmen's Hospital became more closely affiliated, the school's finances improved, and blacks took a strong hand in leading the school's affairs.

WRITINGS: "An Interpretation of the Significance of the Homer G. Phillips Hospital," *JNMA* 26 (1934): 13-17; "Recent Developments in Medical Education at Howard University," *Howard Univ. Bull.* 15 (1935): 1-18. Writings listed in W. Montague Cobb, *The First Negro Medical Society* (1939): 104. REFERENCES: W. Montague Cobb, "Numa

P. G. Adams, M.D., 1885-1940," *JNMA* 43 (1951): 43-52; *Who Was Who in Am.* 2: 17; *WWAPS* 1 (1938): 5.

T. Savitt

AGNEW, DAVID HAYES (November 24, 1818, Lancaster, Pa.-March 22, 1892, Philadelphia, Pa.). *Surgeon.* Son of Robert, physician, and Agnes (Noble) Agnew. Married Margaret Irwin, 1841. EDUCATION: Moscow Academy, Chester County, Pa.; Jefferson College and Delaware College; 1838, M.D., University of Pennsylvania. CAREER: 1838-43, 1846-48, general practice, Chester and Lancaster counties; and *post* 1848, Philadelphia; 1843-46, a founder of and partner in Irwin & Agnew Iron Foundry; 1852-62, bought and revived the Philadelphia School of Anatomy; 1854, surgeon, Philadelphia Hospital; 1863, surgeon, Wills Eye Hospital; 1865-84, surgeon, Pennsylvania Hospital; 1867, surgeon, Orthopedic Hospital; 1854-92, surgery faculty, University of Pennsylvania; 1889, president, Philadelphia College of Physicians. CONTRIBUTIONS: Invented splint for treatment of fractured patella. Devised splint for fracture of metacarpus (1878). Developed method for operative correction of webbed fingers (1883). Attending physician to President James Garfield when he was assassinated. One of his classes painted by Thomas Eakins.

WRITINGS: *Clinical Reports* (1859-71); *Practical Anatomy* (1867); *Treatise on the Principles and Practices of Surgery*, 3 vols. (1878-83). REFERENCES: *DAB*, 1: 124-25; John E. Kieffer, "David Hayes Agnew, 1818-1892, Master Surgeon," *Penn. Health* 1 (Nov. 1940): 27-29,33; *NCAB*, 8: 203; S. Radbill, "David Hayes Agnew, M.D., 1818-1892," *Trans., Coll. of Physicians of Phila.* 33 (1966): 252-60.

J. Carvalho

AH FONG, C. K. (October 5, 1844, Canton, China-August 19, 1927, Boise, Idaho). *Physician.* Son of Dr. Whey Fong, physician. Married twice in China; three children (two adopted). EDUCATION: Received training from his father. CAREER: 1864, arrived in America with his father, landing in San Francisco, Calif.; 1866, went to Idaho to practice among his countrymen in mining camps of Alturas County; 1889, settled in Boise, where he practiced Chinese medicine until his death. CONTRIBUTIONS: Pioneering traditional Chinese physician, serving Chinese migrants to Idaho for many years. His library and apothecary now in the collection of the Idaho State Historical Society reveal that many of his books date from the seventeenth and eighteenth centuries, and his Chinese apothecary of about 1,000 items is the largest of its kind known in the United States. Grew his own herbs in his Boise garden. REFERENCES: *Statesman* (Boise, Idaho), August 20, 1927; James H. Jawley, *History of Idaho* 3 (1920): 379.

A. A. Hart

ALBRIGHT, FULLER (January 12, 1900, Buffalo, N.Y.-December 8, 1969, Brookline, Mass.). *Physician; Endocrinology.* Son of John Joseph, financier and philanthropist, and Susan (Fuller) Albright. Married Claire Birge, 1933; two children. EDUCATION: 1921, A.B., Harvard University; 1924, M.D., Harvard

Medical School; 1924-26, medical house officer, Massachusetts General Hospital; 1926-27, research fellow in industrial medicine, Harvard Medical School; 1927-28, assistant resident in medicine, Johns Hopkins Hospital; 1928-29, studied in Vienna with Jacob Erdheim. CAREER: 1929-69, medical staff, Massachusetts General Hospital; 1930-69, medicine faculty, Harvard Medical School; stricken with Parkinson's disease while in his 30s, refused to allow the advance of the disease to interfere with his investigations, which he then pursued with even greater intensity; finally, the disease had so greatly progressed that he submitted himself to a new and untried operation (1954) that destroyed his intellect. CONTRIBUTIONS: Helped establish the study of endocrinology in America with his work on diseases of the parathyroids (1929-54). Laid the basis for the modern diagnosis and treatment of kidney stones by calling attention to their association with hyperparathyroidism (1934). Played preeminent role in bone disorders and in conditions affecting the metabolism of calcium and phosphorus generally. Made important studies of hormone-related sexual disorders (1935-54). Introduced the medical "D and C" (dilatation and curettage) (1938) and promoted the use of hormone replacement for the menopause. Advanced the diagnosis and treatment of amenorrhea, dysmenorrhea, metropathia, and testicular disorders. Among the first to suggest the use of steroid hormones to control fertility and to warn of their harmful side effects.

WRITINGS: "Studies on the Physiology of Parathyroid Glands. IV, Renal Complications of Hyperparathyroidism," *Am. J. of Med. Sci.* 187 (1934): 49 (with P. C. Baird, O. Cope, and E. Bloomberg); "Metropathia Hemorrhagica," *J. of the Maine Med. Assoc.* 29 (1938): 235; *The Parathyroid Glands and Metabolic Bone Disease* (1948). Writings listed in *BMNAS*. REFERENCES: Lloyd Axelrod, "Bones, Stones, and Hormones: The Contribution of Fuller Albright," *New England J. of Med.* 283 (1970): 964-70; *BMNAS* 48 (1976): 3-22; James Boardley and A. McGehee Harvey, *Two Centuries of American Medicine* (1976), 553-55; V. A. McKusick and F. C. Bartter, "Dedication to the Memory of Two Giants of Endocrinology," *Birth Defects* 7, no. 6 (May 1971): 1-4.

S. Galishoff

ALCOCK, NATHANIEL GRAHAM (January 18, 1881, Platteville, Wis. - December 10, 1953, Iowa City, Ia.). *Physician; Urology.* Son of James Anthony and Isabella (Graham) Alcock. Married Marjory Marshall Bates, 1913; three children. EDUCATION: 1902-3, studied with Dr. L. E. Schmidt, Yankton, S.D.; at Northwestern University: 1907, B.S.; 1908, M.S.; and 1912, M.D. CAREER: 1915-49, medicine faculty, College of Medicine, University of Iowa (1922-49, professor and head, Department of Urology); 1949-53, chief urologist, Mercy Hospital, Iowa City; 1932-33, chairman, Urology Section, American Medical Association; 1949-50, president, Iowa Medical Society. CONTRIBUTIONS: Contributed significantly to the development of urology as a subspecialty (1917-53). One of the first to understand the possibilities of transurethral surgery (1933), his operative technique revolutionized the treatment of prostatic disease, reducing the 10 to 25 percent mortality rate to less than 1 percent (1930-40).

WRITINGS: "Cases of Two-Step Nephrectomies," *J. of Urol.* 14 (1925): 239; "Frequency of Bilateral Involvement in 'Congenital' Hydronephrosis," *Trans., Am. Assoc. of Genito-Urinary Surgeons* 23 (1930): 165; "Ten Months Experience with Transurethral Prostatic Resection," *J. of Urol.* 28 (1932): 545; "Prostatic Resection and Surgical Prostatectomy," *JAMA* 101 (1933): 1355; "Prostatic Hypertrophy," *JAMA* 104 (1935): 734. REFERENCES: *JAMA* 154 (1954): 849 (obit.); *NCAB*, 47: 461; *One Hundred Years of Iowa Medicine, 1850-1950* (1950), 175; University of Iowa Archives, Iowa City, Ia.; *Who's Who in Am. Med.* (1925), 15; *Who Was Who in Am.* 3: 18.

R. E. Rakel

ALCOTT, WILLIAM ANDRUS (August 6, 1798, Wolcott, Conn.-March 29, 1859, Newton, Mass.). *Personal hygiene reformer.* Son of Obed, farmer, and Anna (Andrus) Alcott. Married Phoebe Bronson, 1836; two children. EDUCATION: district high school; 1826, M.D., Medical Institution of Yale College. CAREER: 1826-36, physician, schoolteacher, education journalist; 1836-59, lecturer and writer on personal hygiene. CONTRIBUTIONS: Directed campaign to reform the physical environment of common schools and establish student health as an important goal of education (1826-33 particularly). Leader of popular health reform movement, through which he helped establish public and professional awareness of the value of careful personal hygiene for the prevention of disease and the building of higher levels of vitality. Prodigious output as an author (nearly 100 volumes on health, education, and religion), editor (several health and education journals), and lecturer. Specific proposals for health maintenance were not widely popular, however, since vegetarianism, teetotalism, and sexual restraint were regarded by the majority as extreme self-denial. But was instrumental in the introduction of physical education into the public school curriculum.

WRITINGS: *The House I Live In* (1834); *Vegetable Diet* (1838); *Lectures on Life and Health* (1853); *The Physiology of Marriage* (1856); *Forty Years in the Wilderness of Pills and Powders* (1859). REFERENCES: *DAB*, 1: 142-43; "Dr. William A. Alcott," *Barnard's Am. J. of Ed.* 4 (1857): 629-56; Hebbel Hoff and John Fulton, "The Centenary of the First American Physiological Society Founded at Boston by William A. Alcott and Sylvester Graham," *Bull. Hist. Med.* 5 (1937): 687-734; *NCAB*, 12: 59; L. Salomon, "The Least-Remembered Alcott," *New Eng. Q.* 24 (1961): 87-93; Herbert Thoms, "William Andrus Alcott. Physician, Educator, Writer," *Bull. of the Soc. of Med. Hist., Chicago* 4 (1928): 123-30; James Whorton, " 'Christian Physiology': William Alcott's Prescription for the Millennium," *Bull. Hist. Med.* 49 (1975): 466-81.

J. Whorton

ALDRICH, CHARLES ANDERSON (March 4, 1888, Plymouth, Mass.-October 6, 1949, Rochester, Minn.). *Physician; Pediatrics.* Son of David E., businessman, and Laura Linwood (Perkins) Aldrich. Married Mary McCague, 1916; three children. EDUCATION: 1914, B.S., Northwestern University; 1915, M.D., Northwestern University Medical School; 1915-16, intern, Evanston Hospital; 1920-21, postgraduate training, New York Nursery and Children's Hospital and Boston Children's Hospital and Massachusetts General Hospital. CAREER:

1916-20, general practice with Frank H. Blatchford in Winnetka, Illinois, and X-ray work, Evanston Hospital; *post* 1921, pediatric practice including prepayment type in Chicago; various staff apppointments, Evanston Hospital and Children's Memorial Hospital in Chicago; *post* 1934, faculty, Northwestern University Medical School; 1944 to death, directed the Roch Child Health Institute at the Mayo Clinic. CONTRIBUTIONS: Spearheaded the incorporation into pediatric theory and practice of new findings from psychiatry, psychology, anthropology, with bearing on infant feeding, toilet training, sexuality, and human development. Designed a skin test to measure edema (1923, the McClure and Aldrich Test); also designed hearing test for newborn infants, based on conditioned reflex (1928). In collaboration with the AMA, brought new pediatric concepts to the public attention through articles in *Parents' Magazine* and the parent-child page of the Sunday *New York Times Magazine* (1946-48). President, American Pediatric Society (1946). Played important role in founding the American Academy of Pediatrics (1929) and was secretary (1934-44) and president (1945-47).

WRITINGS: *Cultivating the Child's Appetite* (1927); *Babies Are Human Beings* (1938, with Mary M. Aldrich); *Feeding Our Old-Fashioned Children* (1941). REFERENCES: *DAB*, Supplement 4 (1974): 7-9; *JAMA*, November 26, 1949; *Pediatrics*, December 1949; Borden S. Veeder (q.v.), ed., *Pediatric Profiles* (1957).

M. Kaufman

ALEXANDER, FRANZ GABRIEL (January 22, 1891, Budapest, Hungary - March 8, 1964, Palm Springs, Calif.). *Psychiatrist; Psychoanalyst.* Son of Bernard, philosopher and historian, and Regina (Brössler) Alexander. Married Countess Anita Venier, 1921; two children. EDUCATION: 1908, B.A., Humanistic Gymnasium, Budapest; 1913, M.D., University of Budapest; 1920-21, postgraduate work, Psychiatric Hospital, University of Berlin. CAREER: 1910-14, 1918-19, researcher, University of Budapest; 1914-18, head of bacteriological field laboratory and malaria station, Austro-Hungarian Army; 1921-30, lecturer in psychoanalysis, Institute of Psychoanalysis, Berlin; 1930, immigrated to the United States; 1938, naturalized U.S. citizen; 1938-56, taught psychology, University of Illinois; 1948-64, member, Committee on Rheumatic Diseases, National Research Council. CONTRIBUTIONS: Advanced the theory of specificity of emotional factors in different organic diseases; contributed numerous research articles on psychoanalysis and psychosomatic medicine; applied psychoanalytic principles and techniques to legal issues.

WRITINGS: *The Criminal, the Judge, and the Public* (1929, 1956, with H. Staub); *Roots of Crime* (1935, with W. Healy [q.v.]); *Psychosomatic Medicine* (1950, 1965); Fundamentals of Psychoanalysis (1948); *Dynamic Psychiatry* (1952, co-editor); *Psychoanalysis and Psychotherapy* (1956). REFERENCES: *DAB*, Supplement 7: 5-7; *NCAB*, H: 177; 52: 385; S. Pollack, "Franz Alexander's Observations on Psychiatry and Law," *Am. J. of Psychiatry* 121 (1964): 458-64.

J. Carvalho

ALEXANDER, WALTER GILBERT (December 3, 1880, Lynchburg, Va.- February 5, 1953, Orange, N.J.). *Physician; General practitioner.* Son of Royal and Amalia Henrica (Terry) Alexander. Married Lillian Hodges, 1929; no children. EDUCATION: 1899, A.B., Lincoln University (Pa.); 1903, M.D., Boston College of Physicians and Surgeons. CAREER: General practice: 1903-4, Kimball, W. Va.; and 1904-53, Orange, N.J.; 1939-47, N.J. Board of Health; 1947-53, N.J. Public Health Council. CONTRIBUTIONS: Highly respected general practitioner who also involved himself deeply in community and black affairs. Served at all levels in the National Medical Association, from state vice-president for N.J. (1906-12) to NMA president (1925-26). Co-founded the *Journal of the National Medical Association* (1909) and served as associate editor (1909-36). Organized North Jersey Medical Society (1907), a constituent society of NMA, and New Jersey State Medical Association (1939). Participated in local and state politics, sponsoring several health measures and serving on several health boards (1912-53). Elected to N.J. Assembly (1920); first black to serve as Speaker of the House (1921).

WRITINGS: Wrote many articles as associate editor of *JNMA* (1909-36). "Birth Control for the Negro . . . : A Fad or a Necessity?" *JNMA* 24 (1932): 34-39; "The Negro Health Program for New Jersey," *ibid.*, 33 (1941): 96-98. Some writings listed in Herbert M. Morais, *History of the Afro-American in Medicine* (1976). REFERENCES: W. Montague Cobb, "Walter Gilbert Alexander, M.D., 1880-1953," *JNMA* 45 (1953): 281-83; obituary, *N.Y. Times*, February 6, 1953, p. 19; "The President of the N.M.A.," *JNMA* 17 (1925): 211; *WWICA*, 7 (1950): 5.

T. Savitt

ALLEN, EDGAR (May 2, 1892, Canyon City, Colo.-February 3, 1943, New Haven, Conn.). *Physiologist and anatomist; Endocrinology.* Son of Asa, physician, and Edith (Day) Allen. Married Marion Robins Pfieffer, 1918; two children. EDUCATION: 1915, Ph.B., 1916, M.A., and 1921, Ph.D. (biology), Brown University. CAREER: 1917-19, Sanitary Corps, U.S. Army; investigator, U.S. Bureau of Fisheries: summer 1919, Woods Hole, Mass.; and summer 1922, Fairport, Ia.; 1919-23, anatomy faculty, Washington University; at University of Missouri: 1923-33, anatomy faculty; and 1930-33, dean and director of the University Hospitals; 1933-43, anatomy faculty, Yale University; president: 1941-42, American Society for the Study of Internal Secretions; and 1942-43, American Association of Anatomists. CONTRIBUTIONS: Investigated the physiology of reproduction and ovarian physiology and endocrinology. With biochemist Edward A. Doisy, discovered the existence and the effects of estrogen. Began modern study of the menstrual cycle and, with gynecologist J. P. Pratt, secured the first living ova from the human oviduct. Studied the relation of the sex hormones to cancer.

WRITINGS: "The Hormone of the Ovarian Follicle. . .," *Am. J. of Anat.* 34 (1924): 133 (with Edward A. Doisy); "The Induction of a Sexually Mature Condition in Immature Females by Injection of the Ovarian Follicular Hormone," *Am. J. of Physiol.* 69 (1924): 577-88; "The Menstrual Cycle of the Monkey, *Macacus Rhesus*. . . ," *Contributions to Embryology, Carnegie Inst. of Wash.* 19 (1927): 1-44; editor and contributor, "The Mammary Tumors and the Effects of Ovarian Follicular and Anterior Pituitary Hormones," *Am. J. of Cancer* 25 (1935): 291. A bibliography is in *Yale J. of Biol. and Med.* 17, pt. 1 (1944-45): 2-12. REFERENCES: *DAB*, Supplement 3: 6-7; *DSB*, 1: 123-24; *N.Y. Times*, February 4, 1943.

S. Galishoff

ALLEN, LYMAN (May 21, 1872, Burlington, Vt.-February 2, 1961, Burlington). *Physician; Surgeon.* Son of Charles Edwin and Ellen Cornelia (Lyman) Allen. Married Mary Cutler Torrey, 1898; three children. EDUCATION: University of Vermont: 1893, A.B.; and 1896, M.D.; 1896, 1897, house surgeon, Boston City Hospital. CAREER: 1898-1944, practiced surgery, Burlington, Vt.; at University of Vermont: 1898-1903, adjunct professor of physiology; and 1901-24, adjunct professor of surgery; 1924-44, professor of surgery and chief of surgical service, Mary Fletcher and Bishop DeGoesbriand hospitals, Burlington. CONTRIBUTIONS: One of the foremost teachers on the Vermont medical faculty. Founding member of American College of Surgeons, New England Surgical Society, and American Board of Surgery. Trustee of the University of Vermont (1944-50).

WRITINGS: "Intestinal Obstruction," *Vt. Med. Monthly* (Feb. 1908); "A Sketch of Vermont's Early Medical History," *New Eng. J. of Med.* 209 (1933): 792-98; "Head Injuries," *ibid.*, 209 (1933): 1011-14; "The Art of Medical Practice," *J. Assoc. of Am. Med. Colleges* 24 (1949): 298-304; *History of the University of Vermont College of Medicine* (1951, associate editor with W.A.B. Chapin). REFERENCES: W.A.B. Chapin, *History of the University of Vermont* (1951); M. Kaufman, *The University of Vermont College of Medicine* (1979); Univ. of Vermont Archives.

L. J. Wallman

ANDERSON, JOHN WESLEY (September 1, 1861, Lexington, Mo.-May 30, 1947, Dallas, Tex.). *Physician.* Son of Mr. Strampke (white) and unknown woman (black). Married Pearl Carina, 1929; one child. EDUCATION: 1879, Wyandotte (Kans.) High School; 1881-83, apprentice to several Wyandotte physicians; c. 1881, A.B. (?), University of Kansas; 1885, M.D., Meharry Medical School; 1886, postgraduate course, University of Michigan; 1887, D.D.S., Meharry Dental School; 1889, D.N.T. (Doctor of Natural Therapeutics), Chicago University; 1900, studied phrenology, New York City. CAREER: 1881-83, taught and served as principal of the Wyandotte High School from which he graduated; 1885-87, lecturer in anatomy and then in chemistry while a dental student; medical practice: 1885-88, Nashville; 1888-1947, Dallas. CONTRIBUTIONS: Practiced general medicine among the black, Hispanic, and white poor of Dallas for about 60 years. Donated large sums of money to many black medical and social causes and to Meharry for construction of a badly needed Anatomical Hall, dedicated in 1917 and named for him. A leading black philanthropist of his day.

REFERENCES: J. M. Brewer, *The Life of John Wesley Anderson in Verse* (1938); W. Montague Cobb, "[Dr. John Wesley Anderson]," *JNMA* 45 (1953): 442-44; oral history interview with Pearl Anderson (11/13/72), Special Collections, Fisk University Library, Nashville, Tenn.

T. Savitt

ANDERSON, WILLIAM HENRY (May 6, 1820, Norfolk, Va.-November 14, 1887, Mobile, Ala.). *Physician.* Son of Leroy Hammond and Hannah (Southgate) Anderson. Married Ann Louisa Witherspoon, 1852; two children. EDU-CATION: Early education by private tutors under his father's direction; 1841, graduated from William and Mary College; 1842, M.D., University of Virginia; 1843, resident physician, Baltimore Almshouse Hospital; later spent a year at the University of the City of New York visiting Bellevue Hospital daily with private instructor; 1846-49, studied medicine and natural history in Europe, spending a year in Paris attending the lectures of Roux, Velpeau, Jobart, Cruveilhier, Andral, Magendie, and Claude Bernard. CAREER: 1850-87, practiced medicine, Mobile; 1853-57, associated with Dr. George A. Ketchum (q.v.); 1854, 1872, president, Mobile Medical Society; 1859-61, 1868-85, dean of faculty and professor of physiology, Medical College of Alabama, Mobile; served in C.S. Army as medical purveyor of the military district commanded by Gen. Braxton Bragg; 1881, president, Alabama Medical Society. CONTRIBUTIONS: Helped organize the Medical College of Alabama (1859) and the Alabama Hospital for the Treatment of the Insane in Tuscaloosa (1861).

WRITINGS: "On the Use of Cold Water in Scarlatina Maligna," *New Orleans Med. & Surg. J.* 6 (1849-50): 193-97; "Report on the Diseases of Mobile," *Trans. Med. Assoc. State Alabama* (1850): 68-76; and idem (1854): 39-50. REFERENCES: T. M. Owen, *History of Alabama*, 4 vols. (1978); Howard Holley, *History of Medicine in Alabama* (1982).

S. Eichold

ANDERSON, WILLIAM HENRY (February 13, 1886, Dumas, Miss.-May 9, 1969, Booneville, Miss.). *Physician; Medical editor.* Son of William Walter and Mary Elizabeth (Shackelford) Anderson. Married Mildred Paulk, 1930; two children. EDUCATION: 1912, A.B., Mississippi College; 1916, B.S., University of Mississippi; 1918, M.D., Tulane University School of Medicine; postgraduate study: 1920, Tulane University School of Medicine; 1925-26, New York Hospital; and 1926, Mayo Clinic. CAREER: Began as superintendent, Hebron (Miss.) High School; mathematics teacher, Chalybeate (Miss.) High School; 1913-14, instructor, Mississippi Women's College, Hattiesburg (Miss.); 1918, began practice of medicine in Booneville, Miss.; associated with Dr. H. W. Sutherland until he opened Anderson's Clinic; at Northeast Mississippi Hospital: *post* 1918, member, Board of Directors; 1950-51, chairman of the staff; and 1918-24, house physician; 1918-retirement, private practice of medicine and surgery, Booneville; 1922-retirement, local surgeon, Gulf, Mobile, and Ohio Railroad; 1929-40, health officer, Prentiss County, Miss.; 1928-retirement, chief of staff, Anderson's Clinic; 1935-44, president, Booneville Public School Board; 1938-retirement, editor, Booneville *Independent* (weekly newspaper). CONTRIBUTIONS: Founder, editor, and publisher of the *Mississippi Doctor*, which was established at Houston, Miss., in June 1922. The *Mississippi Doctor* became the official organ of the Mississippi State Medical Association and was published for 36 years by Anderson. Became editor of the *Journal of the Mississippi State Medical Association* (1960). Co-founder of the Mississippi State Medical Association's Fifty Year Club; 1940-41, president, Mississippi State Medical Association; 1968, winner of the Mississippi State Medical Association-Robbins Award for outstanding community service by a physician.

WRITINGS: Author of numerous contributions to medical journals. REFERENCES: *American Men of Medicine*, 3d ed. (1961), 18; *Goodspeed's Biographical and Historical Memoirs of Mississippi*, II (1962), 255; Thompson, James G., *History of the Mississippi State Medical Association*, 2d ed.(1949), 118.

M. S. Legan

ANDREWS, EDMUND (April 22, 1824, Putney, Vt.-January 22, 1904, Chicago, Ill.). *Surgeon; Anesthesiology.* Married Sarah Eliza Taylor, 1853 (d.1875), five children, including Edward W. Andrews (q.v.); Mrs. Frances M. Barrett, 1877. EDUCATION: University of Michigan: 1849, B.A.; and 1852, M.A.; 1852, M.D., University of Michigan Medical School. CAREER: 1850-54, comparative anatomy faculty, University of Michigan; 1855-57, comparative anatomy faculty, Rush Medical College; 1859-1901, surgery faculty, Chicago Medical College, Northwestern University Medical School; 1860-1901, surgical staff, Mercy Hospital. CONTRIBUTIONS: Improved surgical anesthesia by developing mixture of oxygen and nitrous oxide (1868). Initiated keeping and use of surgical records during Civil War. Developed many surgical instruments and devices, for example, braces for correction of spinal curvature, appliance for trephining, and endoscope (which opened the way for modern cystoscopy). First in West to use and promote Lister's antiseptic methods (brought over after trip to England, 1867). First to perfect operation of Gasserian ganglionectomy (1893). Founder of *Peninsular Journal of Medical and Collateral Sciences* (1853). Pioneered in the use of blood transfusion in the Midwest. A founder of Michigan State Medical Society and medical department of Lind University (later, Northwestern University Medical School). Pioneer for graded medical curriculum.

WRITINGS: "The Oxygen Mixture, A New Anaesthetic Combination," *Chicago Med. Examiner* 9 (1868): 656-61; "The Relative Dangers of Anaesthesia by Chloroform and Ether—Statistics of 209,893 Cases," *ibid.*, 11 (1870): 257-66; *Rectal and Anal Surgery, with a Description of the Secret Methods of the Itinerants* (1888, with E. W. Andrews; 3rd. ed., 1892). Writings listed in *Q. Bull. Northwestern Univ. Med. School* 27 (1953): 349-52. REFERENCES: Anon., *Chicago Med. Record* 26 (1904): 111-15; *Ill. Med. J.* 146 (1974): 215-19; Manuel E. Lichtenstein and Harold Method, *Q. Bull. Northwestern Univ. Med. School* 27 (1953): 337-52; Arno B. Luckhardt, "Edmund Andrews, M.D., and His 'Oxygen Mixtures,' " *Anesth. Analg.* (Cleveland) 19 (1940): 2-11; Miller, *BHM*, p. 4.

W. K. Beatty

ANDREWS, EDWARD WYLLYS (March 25, 1856, Chicago, Ill.-January 21, 1927, Chicago). *Physician; Surgery.* Son of Edmund (q.v.), and Sarah E. (Taylor) Andrews. Married Alice S. Davis, 1890. EDUCATION: Northwestern University: 1878, A.B.; and 1881, M.A.; 1881, M.D., Chicago Medical College; 1884-85, studied at University of Vienna. CAREER: *Post* 1881, practiced surgery, Chicago; *post* 1881, surgical staff, Mercy Hospital; *post* 1883, surgery faculty, Northwestern University Medical School; surgical staff, Cook County, St. Luke's, Michael Reese, and Wesley hospitals. CONTRIBUTIONS: Greatest surgical bequest was the principle of imbrication of the flaps in hernia repairs. Introduced glass tubes for subdural drainage in hydrocephalus. Helped bring *Surgery, Gynecology and Obstetrics*, one of the world's premier surgical journals, into existence and co-founded the American College of Surgeons and the Association for Thoracic Surgery.

WRITINGS: "Imbrication or Lap Joint Method: A Plastic Operation for Hernia, " *Chicago Med. Record* 9 (Aug. 1895): 67-77; "An Improved Technique in Brain Surgery. Glass Tubes Versus Gold or Platinum for Subdural Drainage of the Lateral Ventricles in Internal Hydrocephalus," *Trans., Am. Surg. Assoc.* 29 (1911): 111-26. Wrote numerous articles on various branches of surgery and was a contributor to several well-known textbooks. REFERENCES: L. L. McArthur, "E. Wyllys Andrews," *Trans., Am. Surg. Assoc.* 45 (1927): 503-4; Mark M. Ravitch, *A Century of Surgery*, 2 vols. (1981); Mark M. Ravitch and J. M. Hitzrot, "The Operations for Inguinal Hernia," *Surgery* 48 (1960): 439-66; *Who Was Who in Am.*, 1: 25.

S. Galishoff

ANTONY, MILTON (August 7, 1789, Henry County, Va.-September 19, 1839, Augusta, Ga.). *Physician; Educator.* Son of James and Ann (Tate) Antony. Married Nancy Godwin, 1809; 11 children. EDUCATION: Apprenticeship under Joel Abbott, Monticello, Ga.; one year of lectures at the University of Pennsylvania School of Medicine. CAREER: 1822, chief organizer, Richmond County Medical Society; 1826, first to teach courses in medical education at Augusta City Hospital; founder: 1828, Medical Academy of Georgia; 1829, Medical Institute of the State of Georgia; and 1832, Medical College of Georgia (MCG); 1832-39, professor of the institutes and practice of medicine and of midwifery and diseases of women and children, MCG. CONTRIBUTIONS: In addition to being the chief founder of the Medical College of Georgia, is credited with convincing the state of Ga. to create a State Board of Medical Examiners and served as its first president (1825). The guiding spirit behind the creation of the *Southern Medical and Surgical Journal*, one of the antebellum South's best medical periodicals, and served as its first editor. Antony and Lewis D. Ford (q.v.) projected a whole series of medical reforms, including a dramatically lengthened term, which were first tried at MCG and then suggested, in a circular letter, to the most prominent medical schools in America; some experts believe the letter not only presaged the educational reforms that gradually evolved in medical circles throughout the rest of the nineteenth century, but that it also acted as a catalyst in the movement to establish a national medical association. Adept at surgery. Performed a daring operation (1821) where he excised two ribs and removed a portion of a diseased lung (reported in the *Philadelphia Journal of Medical and Physical Sciences* in 1823 and reprinted by George Fox in Ireland as late as 1893). Best remembered for his organizational abilities and by his innovative administrative and educational approaches.

WRITINGS: There were few outlets for publication in Antony's day, and Augusta's yellow-fever epidemic of 1839 cut him down in his prime. A number of his articles, however, appeared in his own *Southern Med. and Surg. J.* REFERENCES: William H. Goodrich, *The History of the Medical Department of the University of Georgia* (1928); Nancy Vashti Anthony Jacob, *Anthony Roots and Branches* (1971); Howard Kelly, *Cyclopedia of Am. Med. Biog.* 1 (1912): 27-28; Kelly and Burrage (1920), 33-34; *Memoirs of Georgia* 2 (1895): 173-75; Russell R. Moores, "Exegit Monumentum Aere Perennius," *Richmond County Hist.* 9 (1977): 10-17; William J. Northen, ed., *Men of Mark in Georgia* 2 (1906): 51-52.

                                                                          P. Spalding

APPLETON, MOSES (March 17, 1773, New Ipswich, N.H.-May 5, 1849, Waterville, Maine). *Physician; Surgeon.* Son of Isaac and Mary (Adams) Appleton. Married Ann Clark, 1801; five children. EDUCATION: 1791, graduated from Dartmouth College; taught school, Medford, Mass., for a brief period; 1793-95, Harvard Medical School, B.M., 1795; studied with Dr. John Brooks (later governor of Mass.) and after examination by a committee from the Massachusetts Medical Society received the M.D., 1796. CAREER: Settled in Waterville-Winslow area in partnership with Dr. Obadiah Williams, a successful and elderly practitioner, who soon died and left Appleton with a flourishing practice. Also became involved in real estate, distillation of whiskey, and banking. CONTRIBUTIONS: Not only served the medical needs of the area but frequently was called upon to practice dentistry, at least the extraction of teeth, and to act as an apothecary, compounding drugs for his own use and for others as well. Worked for the establishment of a U.S. Pharmacopoeia.

WRITINGS: Kept a journal that is regarded as "a unique first-hand record of the beginnings of medical education. . .and general practice in that period." REFERENCES: Frederick Hill, "Medicine in Colonial Maine," *J. of the Maine Med. Assoc.* 54, no. 2 (Feb. 1963): 27-31; Kelly and Burrage (1920); Alton S. Pope and Raymond S. Patterson, "Moses Appleton, 1800. Chronicler of Colonial Medicine," *Harvard Alumni Bull.* (Spring 1962); James Spalding, *Maine Physicians of 1820* (1928), 24-26.

                                                                          B. C. Lister

ARCHER, JOHN (May 5, 1741, Harford County, Md.-September 28, 1810, Harford County). *Physician; Educator.* Son of Thomas, Irish immigrant farmer, iron agent, planter, and storekeeper, and Elizabeth (Stevenson) Archer. Married

Catherine Harris of the family that founded Harrisburg, Pa.; ten children. ED-
UCATION: Rev. Samuel Finley's West Nottingham Academy in Cecil Co., Md.;
Princeton: 1760, A.B.; and 1763, A.M., at which point he began study for the
Presbyterian ministry, but changed to medicine after failing his examination;
1768, M.B., College of Philadelphia, where he was the "first" person to earn
a medical degree in North America after attending a series of lectures (he graduated with nine others, but was handed the first diploma). CAREER: 1767, opened
medical practice, New Castle, Del., between his second and third courses at
Philadelphia; 1769, returned to Harford County, to practice medicine in Md.
and Pa.—a practice he continued until his death despite his active role in the
American Revolution and post-Revolution politics; November 1774, a devoted
Whig, was chosen to serve on the Harford County Committee of Safety and was
involved in the war effort until 1779, when he retired due to illness; December
1774, captain of Harford County's first militia company into which he mustered
most of his own patients; January 1776, major in militia and delegate to the Md.
constitutional convention; 1777-90, a Harford County commissioner of the peace
(that is, a member of the county court); by 1783, had moved to his plantation
in Harford County, where, c. 1785, he named his home "Medical Hall" and
began teaching there; 1799, charter member, Medical and Chirurgical Faculty
of Maryland; 1800, elected as examiner, Medical and Chirurgical Faculty of
Maryland; member: 1801-7, House of Representatives; and 1802-3, Executive
Committee, Medical and Chirurgical Faculty. CONTRIBUTIONS: Archer's "Medical Hall" students established Harford County's first medical society devoted
to sharing knowledge of their medical experiments and impressions. A founder
of the Medical and Chirurgical Faculty of Maryland (1799). Introduced *Polygala
senega* (seneka snakeroot) to cure croup. REFERENCES:"John Archer, M.B.: The
First American Graduate in Medicine," *British Med. J.* 11 (Aug. 18, 1900): 452; "A
Biographical Sketch of John Archer, M.B.," *Bull. Johns Hopkins Hosp.* 10 (Aug.-Sept.
1899): 101-2, 141-47; *DAB*, 1: 340-41; Kelly and Burrage (1928), 34-35; James Mc-
Lachlan, *Princetonians, 1748-1768: A Biog. Dict.* (1976), 300-2; *NCAB*, 22: 105-6; *Who
Was Who in Am.*, Hist. Vol.: 95.

C. *Donegan*

ARMSBY, JAMES HARVEY (December 1, 1809, Sutton, Mass.-December
3, 1875, Albany, N.Y.). *Physician; Educator*. Son of Silas, farmer, and Elizabeth (Kingsbury) Armsby. Married Anna L. Hawley, 1841; Sarah Winne, 1853;
three children. EDUCATION: Worcester and Monson Academies; apprenticed to
Dr. Alden March (q.v.), Albany; 1833, M.D., Vermont Academy of Medicine.
CAREER: 1832, resident physician, Albany Cholera Hospital; 1834-38, medical
faculty, Vermont Academy of Medicine; 1839-75, medical faculty and dean,
Albany Medical School; 1849-75, medical staff, Albany Hospital; 1861, U.S.
Consul at Naples, Italy. CONTRIBUTIONS: Co-founder, with Dr. Alden March,
of the Albany Medical School and Albany Hospital.

WRITINGS: *History of Albany City Hospital* (1868). REFERENCES: William A. Benedict, *History of the Town of Sutton* (1878), 368-70; *Evening Journal* (Albany), December 3, 1875; Emerson Crosby Kelly, "Development of Medical Education in Upstate New York: The Albany Area," *N.Y. State J. of Med.* 55 (1955): 2664-68; idem, "The Doctors March to Armsby of Albany," *Bull. Hist. Med.* 30 (1956): 32-37.

D. O. Powell

ARNOLD, RICHARD DENNIS (August 19, 1808, Savannah, Ga.-July 10, 1876, Savannah). *Physician; Public health; Educator.* Son of Joseph and Eliza (Dennis) Arnold. Married Margaret Baugh Stirk; one daughter. EDUCATION: Private tutors; academy, New Brunswick, N. J.; Princeton: 1826, B.S.; and 1829, A.M.; 1830, M.D., University of Pennsylvania School of Medicine; studied medicine with W. R. Waring in Savannah; until 1832, resident, Blockley Hospital, Philadelphia; CAREER: *Post* 1832, private practice, Savannah; 1833-35, editor and one owner of the Savannah *Daily Georgian*; 1835-65, physician to Savannah Poor-House; one of the first secretaries of the AMA; helped draft its seminal "Code of Ethics" and later (1851) served as the organization's vice-president; elected to both the Georgia House and Senate; five times mayor of Savannah; pushed for registry of births and deaths in the state; an organizer, Medical Association of Georgia, and its president (1851); 1839, a founder, Georgia Historical Society; active on the Savannah Boards of Health and Education; president, Board of Water Commissioners, for 35 years; 1853, a founder, Savannah Medical College, and professor of theory and practice of medicine there; president, Georgia Medical Society, for 15 years. CONTRIBUTIONS: Pushed for the formation of local, state, and national medical associations and enjoyed considerable success in this area. An early leader in the public health movement and responsible for dramatic improvement in the cleanliness of Savannah and in improving the quality of its water supply. The city, at his urging, spent $200,000 for a new waterworks (1854). Espoused high standards for medical education, including three years study with a physician and two full-time winter courses.

WRITINGS: Wrote extensively about fevers that plagued low-country Ga. and S.C., such as dengue and yellow fever. Several of these articles appeared in the *Savannah Journal of Medicine*, which Arnold edited for a period, and the *Charleston Medical Journal. The Reciprocal Duty of Physicians and the Public toward Each Other* (1851); "Medical Education," *Savannah J. of Med.* 2 (1859-60): 54-59. REFERENCES: *DAB*, 1: 371; C. Stephen Gurr, "Richard Dennis Arnold, Savannah Physician and Unionist in the Years of Crisis, 1832-1861," *J. of the Med. Assoc. of Ga.* 59 (1970): 11-15; idem, "Social Leadership and the Medical Profession in Antebellum Georgia" (Ph.D. diss., University of Georgia, 1973); Kelly and Burrage (1920): 39; *Memoirs of Georgia* 2 (1893): 175-77; *NCAB*, 22: 424; Richard H. Shryock (q.v.), ed., *Letters of Richard D. Arnold, M.D., 1808-1876* (1929). The Arnold Papers are housed at the Perkins Library, Duke University.

P. Spalding

ASHFORD, BAILEY KELLY (September 18, 1873, Washington, D.C.-November 1, 1934, San Juan, Puerto Rico). *Physician; Tropical medicine.* Son of

Francis, professor of surgery at Georgetown University, and Isabelle Walker (Kelly) Ashford. Married Maria Asuncion Lopez, 1899; three children. EDU-CATION: 1896, M.D., Georgetown University; 1896-97, resident physician, Children's Hospital, Washington, D.C.; 1898, graduated from Army Medical School. CAREER: 1898-1917, military duty with the U.S. Army, primarily in Puerto Rico; organized the Institute of Tropical Medicine and Hygiene, Puerto Rico; 1926, when Columbia University took control of the Institute, became professor of mycology and tropical medicine; 1917, surgeon of the First Division, American Expeditionary Force; 1917, organized a field service school for medical officers at Langres; medical practice in San Juan, and head of the medical service at University Hospital, San Juan. CONTRIBUTIONS: Discovered that tropical anemia was caused by intestinal infestation by hookworm. Instrumental in the establishment of the Puerto Rico Anemia Commission which succeeded in reducing mortality from tropical anemia by one-third. Success in Puerto Rico encouraged the hookworm campaign in the southern states and the worldwide campaign under the auspices of the Rockefeller Institute. Worked on the cause of sprue which, as in the case of hookworm, resulted in substantial improvement of the quality of life in Puerto Rico and elsewhere.

WRITINGS: Numerous journal articles on tropical medicine; *A Soldier in Science* (1934). REFERENCES: *DAB*, Supplement 1: 32-33; R. Molina-Rodriguez, articles in *Bull. of the Med. Assoc. of Puerto Rico* 56 (1964): 31-50, and *Bull. of the Acad. of Arts and Sciences of Puerto Rico* 4 (1968): 367-73; *N.Y. Times*, November 2 and 3, 1934.

M. Kaufman

ATLEE, JOHN LIGHT (November 2, 1799, Lancaster, Pa.-October 1, 1885, Lancaster). *Physician*; *Obstetrical surgery*. Son of William Pitt and Sarah (Light) Atlee. Brother of Washington Lemuel Atlee (q.v.). Married Sarah Howell Franklin, 1822; three children. EDUCATION: 1815-19, studied medicine with Samuel Humes; 1820, M.D., University of Pennsylvania; 1850-52, studied medicine in Paris and Berlin. CAREER: 1820-85, practiced medicine, Lancaster; 1853-69, anatomy and physiology faculty, Franklin and Marshall College; president: 1848, Lancaster County Medical Society; 1857, Pennsylvania Medical Society; and 1882, American Medical Association; member, Pennsylvania Public School Board; trustee, State Lunatic Asylum at Harrisburg. CONTRIBUTIONS: Revived the operation of ovariotomy, which had fallen into disfavor after having been successfully performed by Ephraim McDowell (q.v.) (1809-13). Performed 78 ovariotomies (starting in 1843), with a mortality rate of 18 percent, nearly two-thirds lower than what had previously been achieved. Performed the first successful double oöphorectomy (1843). Played an active role in medical organizations. A founder and president of Lancaster County Medical Society, Pennsylvania Medical Society, and American Medical Association.

WRITINGS: *Case of Successful Peritoneal Section for Removal of Two Diseased Ovaria Complicated with Ascites* (1844); *Address Delivered Before the Medical Society of the*

State of Pennsylvania (1858). REFERENCES: *BHM* (1964-69), 17; *DAB*, 1: 413; Kelly and Burrage (1928), 43; *NCAB*, 11: 25; *Who Was Who in Am.*, Hist. Vol.: 99.

S. Galishoff

ATLEE, WASHINGTON LEMUEL (February 22, 1808, Lancaster, Pa.-September 6, 1878, Philadelphia, Pa.). *Physician; Obstetrical surgery.* Son of William Pitt and Sarah (Light) Atlee. Brother of John Light Atlee (q.v.). Married Ann Eliza Hoff, 1830; ten children. EDUCATION: 1824-27, studied medicine with his brother; 1829, M.D., Jefferson Medical College. CAREER: 1829-34, practiced medicine, Mt. Joy, Pa.; 1834-44, practiced medicine, Lancaster; c.1834-44, medical staff, Lancaster Hospital; *post* 1844, practiced medicine, Philadelphia; 1844-52, medical chemistry faculty, Medical College of Philadelphia; 1874, president, Pennsylvania State Medical Society; 1875, vice-president, American Medical Association; founder, Lancaster Conservatory of Arts and Sciences. CONTRIBUTIONS: With his brother John, established the operation for ovariotomy in the United States; is said to have performed 378 ovariotomies. Pioneered surgical removal of uterine fibroids (1853). Was active in medical organizations at the county, state, and national levels. A founder of the American Gynecological Society.

WRITINGS: "A Table of All the Known Operations of Ovariotomy from 1701-1851," *TAMA* 4 (1851): 286-314; *The Surgical Treatment of Certain Fibrous Tumours of the Uterus* (1853); "Case of Successful Operation for Vesico-Vaginal Fistula," *Am. J. of the Med. Sci.*, n.s., 39 (1860): 67-82; *General and Differential Diagnosis of Ovarian Tumors with Specific Reference to the Operation of Ovariotomy* (1872). REFERENCES: William B. Atkinson, *Physicians and Surgeons of the U.S.* (1878), 560-62; *BHM* (1964-69), 17; *DAB*, 1: 414-15; Kelly and Burrage (1928), 43-44; Miller, *BHM*, p. 5; *Who Was Who in Am.*, Hist. Vol.: 99.

S. Galishoff

ATWATER, WILBUR OLIN (May 3, 1844, Johnsburg, N.Y.-September 22, 1907, Middletown, Conn.). *Agricultural chemist; Nutrition.* Son of William, Methodist clergyman, and Eliza (Barnes) Atwater. Married Marcia Woodard, 1874; two children. EDUCATION: 1865, A.B., Wesleyan College; 1869, Ph.D., Yale University; 1869-71, studied at the universities of Leipzig and Berlin. CAREER: 1871-72, chemistry faculty, East Tennessee University (now University of Tennessee); 1872-73, chemistry faculty, Maine State College (now University of Maine); 1873-1907, chemistry faculty, Wesleyan College; director: 1875-77, Connecticut Agricultural Experiment Station; and 1887-1902, Storrs Experiment Station; 1888-91, founder and director, Office of Experiment Stations, U.S. Department of Agriculture. CONTRIBUTIONS: Secured the establishment of the nation's first state agricultural station (1875). Obtained the passage of the Hatch Act (1887) providing federal funds for the maintenance of at least one agricultural experiment station in each state. Established administrative policies for the Office of Experiment Stations, which were continued through the next quarter century by his successor, the most important of which were insistence on high scientific standards for research and the application of science to agriculture. Conducted investigations that led to discovery that leguminous plants are able to assimilate atmospheric nitrogen (1885). In collaboration with Wesleyan physicist E. B. Rosa, perfected what came to be called the Atwater-Rosa calorimeter (1892-97); calorimetric studies demonstrated that the heat-energy output of the human body is exactly the same as the heat-energy potential of the foods ingested. Published tables showing the caloric value of various foods that are still widely used (1896); work was soon seen to have important health and public policy implications; absence of knowledge of vitamins and amino acid requirements led to recommendation that workingmen avoid "luxuries" such as green vegetables in favor of cheaper carbohydrates with high caloric value.

WRITINGS: "On the Acquisition of Atmospheric Nitrogen by Plants," *Am. Chem. J.* 6 (1885): 365-88; *A Digest of Metabolism Experiments in Which the Balance of Income and Outgo Was Determined* (1898); "Description of a New Respiration Calorimeter and Experiments on the Conservation of Energy in the Human Body," *U.S. Dept. of Agriculture, Office of Experiment Stations, Bull.* 63 (1899, with E. B. Rosa). Major works cited in *DAB*. REFERENCES: *BHM* (1976), 4; *DAB*, 1: 418-19; *DSB*, 1: 325-26; *NCAB*, 6: 262-63; *Who Was Who in Am.*, 1: 36.

S. Galishoff

AUER, JOHN (March 30, 1875, Rochester, N.Y.-April 30, 1948, St. Louis, Mo.). *Physician; Physiology; Pharmacology.* Son of Henry, brewer, and Luise (Hummel) Auer. Married Clara Meltzer, 1903; three children. EDUCATION: 1898, B.S., University of Michigan; Johns Hopkins University: 1902, M.D.; and 1903, resident house officer. CAREER: 1904-20, associated with Rockefeller Institute for Medical Research (later Rockefeller University) as assistant and close colleague of the physiologist Samuel J. Meltzer (q.v.); 1906-7, instructor in pharmacology, Harvard Medical School; 1917-18, medical reserve corps, U.S. Army; *post* 1920, pharmacological faculty, St. Louis University School of Medicine; *post* 1924, pharmacological staff, university group of hospitals in St. Louis; 1924-28, president, American Society of Pharmacology and Experimental Therapeutics. CONTRIBUTIONS: With Samuel J. Meltzer, demonstrated the anesthetic and relaxative effects of magnesium sulphate administered intravenously (was used in the treatment of tetanus, eclampsia, and other spasmodic conditions). Collaborated with Meltzer on devising a method of ventilating the lungs in surgery without breathing movements of the chest by blowing air into them through the trachea (intratracheal insufflation); by including an anesthetic vapor in the air stream, a patient could be kept under surgical anesthesia even after the chest was opened (1900-10); found worldwide use in thoracic surgery. Described hitherto unnoticed inclusions ("Auer bodies") in the large lymphocytes in acute leukemia (1906). With a junior colleague, Paul A. Lewis, discovered that sudden death from anaphylactic shock is caused by a spasm of the bronchial musculature; led Meltzer to propose the now accepted hypothesis that bronchial asthma results from anaphylactic sensitivity to foreign proteins. A founder of the American Society of Pharmacology and Experimental Therapeutics.

WRITINGS: "Physiological and Pharmacological Studies of Magnesium Salts," *Am. J. of Physiol.* 14 (1905): 366-88; 15 (1906): 387-405; 16 (1907): 233-51 (with Samuel J. Meltzer); "The Effects of Intraspinal Injection of Magnesium Salts upon Tetanus," *J. of Experimental Med.* 8 (1906): 692-706 (with Samuel J. Meltzer); "Continuous Respiration without Respiratory Movements," *ibid.*, 11 (1909): 622-25 (with Samuel J. Meltzer); "The Physiology of the Immediate Reaction of Anaphylaxsis in the Guinea Pig," *ibid.*, 12 (1910): 151-75 (with Paul A. Lewis). Scientific papers are in *Index Medicus*, 1904-48. REFERENCES: *DAB*, Supplement 4: 34; *NCAB*, 37: 302-3; *N.Y.Times*, May 2, 1948; *Who Was Who in Am.*, 2: 33.

S. Galishoff

AUGUSTA, ALEXANDER THOMAS (March 8, 1825, Norfolk, Va.-December 21, 1890, Washington D.C.). *Physician; General practice; Medical education.* EDUCATION: Sketchy information on his early education indicates studies performed under private tutors in Baltimore, Md., at the University of Pennsylvania, in Calif., and again in Philadelphia. 1856, M.B., Trinity Medical College, Toronto, Ontario, Canada. CAREER: 1856-61, practice, Toronto city hospitals and an industrial school, and perhaps private practice; 1861-63, perhaps practiced in West Indies, Baltimore, and Washington, D.C.; 1863-65, surgeon, U.S. Colored Troops, as chief medical officer at hospitals in Washington, D.C. (Freedmen's Hospital), and Savannah, Ga. (Lincoln Hospital); 1865-c.1867, assistant surgeon, Freedmen's Bureau, in charge of Lincoln Hospital, Savannah; c.1867-90, private practice, Washington, D.C.; 1868-77, anatomy demonstrator and then professor, Howard University Medical College; 1870-75, medical staff, Freedmen's Hospital, Washington, D.C. CONTRIBUTIONS: Only Negro on original faculty of Howard University Medical Department (1868). First Negro on any medical school faculty in United States. First Negro to hold medical commission in U.S. Army (1863). First Negro to be elevated to rank of lieutenant colonel (1865). First (with two others) black physician to be rejected for membership in Medical Society of District of Columbia (1869), which precipitated widespread discussion over racial exclusion of black physicians and founding of Medical-Chirurgical Society of D.C., the first black medical society in the United States (1884). Provided relief for many sick freedmen in Ga. as chief of Lincoln Hospital. REFERENCES: W. Montague Cobb, "Alexander Thomas Augusta," *JNMA* 4 (1952): 327-29; idem, *The First Negro Medical Society* (1939), 6-39; many papers and letters from Freedmen's Bureau duty and some from military service, National Archives, Washington, D.C.

T. Savitt

AVERY, OSWALD THEODORE (October 21, 1887, Halifax, Nova Scotia, Canada-February 20, 1955, Nashville, Tenn.). *Physician; Microbiology and immunology.* Son of Joseph Francis, Baptist clergyman, and Elizabeth (Crowdy) Avery. Never married. EDUCATION:1900, A.B., Colgate University; 1904, M.D.,

College of Physicians and Surgeons (Columbia); 1917, became U.S. citizen. CAREER: 1904-7, practiced medicine in N.Y.; 1907-13, bacteriology staff, Hoagland Laboratory (New York City); 1913-42, member, Rockefeller Institute for Medical Research. CONTRIBUTIONS: Made seminal discoveries in immunology and genetics in his investigations of pneumococcus infections.* Did early work on the classification of pneumococci into several distinct types. With Alphonse R. Dochez (q.v.) and others, demonstrated that the antigenic specificity of the pneumococcus resides in the polysaccharides of the bacterial capsule that envelops each pneumococcus (1917-23); led to the development of new diagnostic procedures; more important, showed that virulence and immunology could be measured biochemically apart from the organism as a whole in terms of some highly specialized cellular component; discovery constitutes one of the cornerstones of modern immunochemistry. With Walter F. Goebel, created an artificial antigen that called forth antibodies not only against itself but also against virulent pneumococci. With Colin M. MacLeod (q.v.) and Maclyn McCarty, made the epochal discovery that deoxyribonucleic acid (DNA) derived from one strain of pneumococcus produced inheritable changes when introduced into another strain (1944); indicated that DNA constitutes the chemical basis of heredity.

WRITINGS: "The Elaboration of Specific Soluble Substance by Pneumococcus During Growth," *J. of Experimental Med*. 26 (1917): 477-93, also in *Trans., Assoc. of Am. Physicians* 32 (1917): 281-98 (with A. Dochez); "Studies on the Chemical Nature of the Substance Inducing Transformation of Pneumococcal Types. . . ," *J. of Experimental Med*. 79 (1944): 137-58 (with C. M. MacLeod and M. McCarty). A bibliography is in *BMFRS* 2 (1956): 35-48 and *BMNAS* 32 (1958): 32-49. REFERENCES: *BHM* (1965-69), 18; (1970-74), 14; (1975), 4; (1977), 4; (1978), 4; *DAB*, Supplement 5: 25-26; *DSB*, 1: 342-43; *NCAB*, 44: 491-92; *Who Was Who in Am.*, 3: 37.

S. Galishoff

AWL, WILLIAM MACLAY (May 24, 1799, Harrisburg, Pa.-November 19, 1876, Columbus, Ohio). *Physician; Asylum superintendent*. Son of Samuel, lawyer and senator, and Mary (Maclay) Awl. Married Rebecca Loughey, 1830; five children. EDUCATION: Medical apprentice; 1819-20, attended lectures, medical department, University of Pennsylvania. CAREER: Began medical practice Harrisburg, Pa.; 1826, moved west to Lancaster, Ohio; practiced in several Ohio towns and finally settled in Columbus in 1833, where he took mental cases and saw the need for public facilities for the mentally disordered; elected to the state legislature, he and Marmaduke B. Wright, another physician-legislator, introduced a bill providing for the state care of the insane; 1838-50, superintendent of the then newly established Ohio State Asylum for the Insane (Columbus). CONTRIBUTIONS: Helped to establish the Ohio State Medical Society and played important role in founding of the Ohio Institution for the Blind. Gained professional acclaim for being the first surgeon in the West to tie the left carotid artery. One of the "original 13" founding fathers of the Association of Medical Superintendents of American Institutions for the Insane and served as president

(1848-51). An excellent administrator devoted to the concrete tasks and details of operating an asylum, practicing moral treatment, providing a humane institutional milieu approach that established a high quality of care in public mental institutions. Always stressed importance of the institution as the agency for curing the mentally ill.

WRITINGS: Asylum annual reports and some manuscripts on biblical subjects. REFERENCES: *DAB*, 1: 446; Kelly and Burrage (1928), 45; *NCAB*, 22: 133; *One Hundred Years of American Psychiatry* (1944), 53-54.

L. V. Bell

AYER, JAMES COOK (May 5, 1818, Ledyard, Conn.-July 3, 1878, Winchendon, Mass.). *Patent medicine entrepreneur*. Son of Frederick, miller, and Persis (Cook) Ayer. Married Josephine M. Southwick, 1850; three children. EDUCATION: 1838-41, read medicine under Dr. Samuel L. Dana and Dr. John W. Graves, both of Lowell, Mass., while employed in a local apothecary shop; later claimed to have received M.D. from the University of Pennsylvania, a claim unsupported by university records. CAREER: April 1841, bought the Lowell apothecary shop for $2,500; manufactured proprietary medicines from his own formulas; introduced: 1841, Ayer's "Cherry Pectoral," a consumption remedy; 1848, Ayer's Sarsaparilla; 1850, Ayer's "Cathartic Pills"; 1854, Ayer's sugar-coated pills; and 1857, Ayer's "Ague Cure"; 1855, founded J. C. Ayer and Co. and in same year began to publish Ayer's *American Almanac*, an advertising device; 1850s, expanded into textile businesses and 1860s, into mining and timber enterprises; major stockholder for a time in the N.Y. *Tribune*; 1874, established railway line between Lowell and Boston after feuding with operator of existing line; 1874, unsuccessful Republican candidate for U.S. Congress in Groton Junction, Mass., renamed "Ayer" in his honor, March 6, 1871; 1874, donated a town hall to Ayer; was incapacitated by illness and periods of insanity during the last several years of his life. SIGNIFICANCE: Ayer and Co. (by the late 1860s) was among the leading patent medicine advertisers in the United States. Led in the use of advertising almanacs, spending $120,000 annually and printing as many as 16 million copies in up to 21 languages and dialects. Solicited and printed testimonials from a wide assortment of royalty and prominent political and theatrical figures, including at least two presidents, and claimed for the almanacs a circulation "second only to the Bible." The firm said it produced (1871) 630,000 doses of its preparations daily. Used profits to expand business enterprises while buying out competing manufacturers. Considered the wealthiest American patent medicine manufacturer when he died. The company remained in business well into this century, shifting gradually into cosmetics rather than medicines. Its founder retained in his lifetime a reputation for honest business practices undamaged by his patent medicine connections and apparently gave generously to a variety of causes.

WRITINGS: *Some of the Usages and Abuses in the Management of Our Manufacturing Corporations* (1863, 1971). REFERENCES: *DAB*, 1: 450-51; Henry W. Holcombe,

"J. C. Ayer and Company," in George B. Griffenhagen, comp., *Patent Medicine Tax Stamps* (1969), 8-19; *NCAB*, 26: 347; George P. Rowell, *Forty Years an Advertising Agent* (1906), 77; *Who Was Who in Am.*, Hist. Vol.: 101; James Harvey Young, *The Toadstool Millionaires* (1961), 138-41.

E. M. Shoemaker

B

BABCOCK, JAMES WOODS (August 11, 1856, Chester, S.C.-March 3, 1922, Richmond, Va.) *Psychiatrist.* Son of Sidney Eugene, physician, and Margaret (Woods) Babcock. Married Katherine Guion, 1892; three children. EDUCATION: 1874-78, Phillips Exeter Academy, Exeter, N.H.; Harvard University: 1882, A.B.; and 1886, M.D. CAREER: 1885, house officer, McLean Asylum for the Insane, and assistant physician after graduation until accepting superintendency of the South Carolina State Hospital; while at the hospital, drew attention to tuberculosis and pellagra conditions; brought about many changes there in mental health because of his influence in the General Assembly of which he was at one time member; 1914, established the Waverly Sanitorium for the Insane (Columbia, S.C.) and taught courses on mental disease at the South Carolina Medical College; 1909-12, president, South Carolina Medical College; later, secretary, Association for the Study of Pellagra; 1910-13, chairman, State Hospital Commission; 1898-1901, member, Columbia Board of Health; chairman: 1901-3, Columbia Sewerage Commission; and 1903-7, Columbia Water and Water Works Commission. CONTRIBUTIONS: Founder of the National Association for the Study of Pellagra. Established a nursing school at South Carolina Medical School. First physician in South to recognize and treat pellagra; known for his research of the disease and translation with Dr. C. H. Lavinder of Marie's *La Pellagra.*

WRITINGS: "The Colored Insane," *Alienist and Neurologist* (1895); "Prevalence of Pellagra," *J. of the S.C. Med. Assoc.* (1910); "State Hospital for the Insane," in Henry M. Hurd (q.v.), ed., *The Institutional Care of the Insane in the U.S. and Canada* 3 (1916-17); many other articles on black insanity, mental hospitals, tuberculosis, and pellagra. REFERENCES: *Charleston Med. J.*, 2nd series, 4 (1876); *DAB* 1: 458; William S. Hall, "Psychiatrist, Humanitarian, and Scholar, James Woods Babcock, M.D.," *J. of the S.C. Med. Assoc.* 66 (1970); Robert Somors, *The Southern States Since the War*

(1871); J. T. Walton, "The Comparative Mortality of the White and Colored Races in the South," *Charlotte Med. J.* (1897) 10; Joseph I. Waring, *History of Medicine in South Carolina, 1900-1970* (1971).

J. P. Dolan

BACHE, FRANKLIN (October 25, 1792, Philadelphia, Pa.-March 19, 1864, Philadelphia). *Physician; Educator; Chemistry; Materia medica.* Son of Benjamin Franklin, journalist, and Margaret (Markoe) Bache. Married Aglae Dabadie, 1818; six children. EDUCATION: Dr. Wylie's School, Philadelphia; University of Pennsylvania: 1810, A.B.; and 1814, M.D.; student of Dr. Benjamin Rush (q.v.). CAREER: 1813-16, surgeon's mate and surgeon, U.S. Army; *post* 1816, medical practitioner, Philadelphia; 1824-26, physician, Walnut Street Prison; 1829-36, physician, Eastern Penitentiary of Pennsylvania; 1826-32, lecturer in chemistry, Franklin Institute; 1831-41, professor of chemistry, Philadelphia College of Pharmacy; 1841-64, professor of chemistry, Jefferson Medical College; American Philosophical Society: 1843-52, vice-president; and 1853-55, president; 1855-64, vice-president, College of Physicians of Philadelphia. CONTRIBUTIONS: Contributor to the literature of chemistry. Experimented and wrote on acupuncture. With George B. Wood (q.v.), played a dominant role in the revision of the *Pharmacopoeia of the United States* (USP) from the first (Philadelphia) revision of 1831 through the fourth revision of 1863. Also with Wood, compiled the monumental, authoritative and widely circulated *Dispensatory of the United States* (USD).

WRITINGS: *A System of Chemistry for the Use of Students of Medicine* (1819); "Cases Illustrative of the Remedial Effects of Acupuncturation," *N. Amer. Med. & Surg. J.* 1 (1826): 311-21; *N. Amer. Med. & Surg. J.* (1826-31, co-editor); contributor of 15 monographs to I. Hays, *American Cyclopedia of Practical Medicine and Surgery* (1834-1836); *Dispensatory of the United States* (11 editions in Bache's lifetime, 1835-58, with G. B. Wood). REFERENCES: J. H. Cassedy, "Early Use of Acupuncture in the United States," *Bull., N.Y. Acad. of Med.* 50 (1974): 879-906; *DAB,* 1: 463-64; J. W. England, ed., *The First Century of the Philadelphia College of Pharmacy* (1922), 82-83, 399-400; *NCAB,* 5: 346; E. F. Smith, *Franklin Bache, Chemist* (1922); G. Sonnedecker, *Kremers and Urdang's History of Pharmacy,* 4th ed. (1976); *Trans., Med. Soc. State of Pa.,* 4th series, 1 (1965): 137-38; G. B. Wood, *Biographical Memoir of Franklin Bache* (1865).

D. Cowen

BAIRD, DAVID WILLIAM ECCLES (October 21, 1898, Baker, Oreg.-July 28, 1974, Portland, Oreg.). *Physician; Internal medicine; Medical educator.* Son of David, railroad conductor, and Mamie W. (Bernston) Baird. Married Mary Alexander, 1925; three children. EDUCATION: 1918-21, University of Oregon; 1926, M.D., University of Oregon Medical School; 1926-27, intern, Multnomah Hospital; 1927-28, resident, University of Oregon Medical School. CAREER: 1928-32, medical staff, Portland Clinic; at University of Oregon Medical School: 1929-36, faculty; 1937-42, associate dean; 1942-43, acting dean; and 1943-68, dean. CONTRIBUTIONS: During his deanship, the University of Oregon Medical

School grew from a faculty of 26 full-time members and 637 students to a faculty of 276 full-time members and 1,202 students. Under his administration, a teaching hospital (1956) and a medical research building (1962) were constructed. The Crippled Children's Division was created (1953) and the Portland Hearing and Speech Center (1962) and a women's residence (1965) were built. Research grants rose from an annual sum of less than $75,000 to more than $6 million during his administration. Value of the physical facilities rose from slightly more than $2 million to more than $47 million. Patient-care services more than doubled.

WRITINGS: "The Syndrome of Acute Coronary Occlusion as Produced by Thrombosis of the Auricle," *Northwest Med.* 27 (1928): 469-72 (with N. W. Jones); "Possible Ill Effects Following Intravenous Use of Ammonium Ortho-iodoxy-benzoate," *Am. J. of Med. Sci.* 179 (1930): 794-99 (with J. H. Fitzgibbon and A. S. Rosenfeld). REFERENCE: *Northwest Medicine* 67 (1967): 997-1002.

G. B. *Dodds*

BAKER, HENRY BROOKS (December 29, 1837, Brattleboro, Vt.-April 4, 1920, Ypsilanti, Mich.). *Physician; Vital statistics and public health.* Son of Ezra and Deborah Knowlton (Bigelow) Baker. Married Fannie H. Howard, 1867; at least one child. EDUCATION: Studied medicine with Dr. I. H. Bartholomew of Lansing, Mich.; 1861-62, University of Michigan medical department; 1866, M.D., Bellevue Hospital Medical College (N.Y.). CAREER: 1862-65, assistant surgeon, Twentieth Michigan Infantry; 1866-70, medical practice (with I. H. Bartholomew), Lansing, Mich.; 1870-73, first registrar of vital statistics for Mich.; 1873-1904, first secretary, Michigan State Board of Health; 1898-1905, lecturer on the administration of health laws, University of Michigan; 1890, president, American Public Health Association; vice-president: American Social Science Association, Michigan State Medical Society, and American Climatological Association; 1905-20, ran private health resort, Holland, Mich. CONTRIBUTIONS: "Father of public health work in Michigan," initiated campaigns leading to creation of the state health board and vital statistics registry. As first secretary of the health board, developed "Michigan Plan" for centralized collection of local disease reports; responsible for Mich. being the first state to make tuberculosis reportable (1893).

WRITINGS: *Annual Reports of the Michigan State Board of Health* (1873-1904), including "Typhoid Fever and Low Water in Wells" (1885); "The Michigan Plan for General Boards of Health," *Detroit Lancet* 5 (1882). Writings listed in *Representative Men of Michigan: American Biographical History of Eminent and Self-Made Men* (1878), district 6: 8; *Index-Catalog*, 2nd series, 2: 60. REFERENCES: C. B. Burr, *Medical History of Michigan* (1930), 1: 809; 2: 791; Thomas R. MacClure, *The State Board of Health and a Quarter Century of Public-Health Work in Michigan* (1897), 21, 43; *Michigan State Medical Society, Journal* 38 (1939): 663; *NCAB,* 12: 136; *Representative Men of Michigan,* district 6: 8.

M. *Pernick*

BAKER, S[ARA] JOSEPHINE (November 15, 1873, Poughkeepsie, N.Y.-February 22, 1945, New York, N.Y.). *Physician; Public health administrator;*

Pediatrics. Daughter of Orlando Daniel Mosher, attorney, and Jenny Harwood (Brown) Baker. EDUCATION: 1898, M.D., Woman's Medical College of the New York Infirmary for Women and Children; 1898-99, intern, New England Hospital for Women and Children (Boston, Mass.); 1917, D.P.H., Bellevue Medical College (New York University). CAREER: 1899-1914, practiced medicine, New York City; at New York City Health Department: 1901-6, medical inspector; 1907-8, assistant to commissioner of health; and 1908-23, director, bureau of child hygiene; 1914-17, founder, first president, and Executive Committee chairman, Babies Welfare Association (later Children's Welfare Federation of New York); in Association for Study and Prevention of Infant Mortality (American Child Health Association): 1909, co-founder; and 1917-18, president. CONTRIBUTIONS: Responsible for the creation of a Division (later Bureau) of Child Hygiene within the New York City Health Department, which she headed for 15 years (1908-23); was first government agency devoted exclusively to the medical problems of infancy and childhood. Placed the bureau's emphasis on preventive measures and health education; established "Baby Health Stations," which advised mothers on the care of their infants and distributed pure milk to the poor; instituted training courses and a licensing system for midwives; distributed pamphlets in several languages on baby care; organized Little Mothers' Leagues among schoolgirls of working mothers; measures helped reduce the city's infant mortality rate from 144 to 66 per 1,000 live births in 1923, the lowest rate of any major American or European city. Bureau's success caused other city and state governments to assume responsibility for child health protection and led to the establishment (1912) of the federal Children's Bureau, which she served for many years as a consultant.

WRITINGS: *Healthy Babies* (1923); *Healthy Children* (1923); *Healthy Mothers* (1923); *Child Hygiene* (1925); *Fighting for Life* (1939). REFERENCES: *DAB*, Supplement 3: 27-29; *NCAB*, 36: 91; *Notable Am. Women*, 1: 85-86; *Who Was Who in Am.*, 2: 39.

S. Galishoff

BALDWIN, ABEL SEYMOUR (March 18, 1811, Oswego County, N.Y.-December 8, 1898, Jacksonville, Fla.). *Physician; General practice.* Orphaned as an infant, adopted by uncle and aunt of Madison County, N.Y. Married Eliza Scott, 1838, one child; Mrs. Mary E. Dell, 1866, one child. EDUCATION: Cazenovia Seminary, Cazenovia, N.Y., and Chittenango Polytechnic Institute, Chittenango, N.Y. Geneva College (now Hobart), Geneva, N.Y.: 1834, B.A. and B.S.; 1838, A.M.; and 1838, M.D., medical department. CAREER: 1834-36, botanist for geological survey of state of Michigan; 1838-98, medical practitioner, Jacksonville, Fla., except for service, Confederacy, 1861-65; war service: medical officer in charge, General Confederate Hospital, Lake City, Fla., and later (February-April 1865) medical director, General Hospitals of Fla. and Quitman, Ga.; May 1865, resumed practice in Jacksonville, after recovering property confiscated by federal authority. CONTRIBUTIONS: Maintained a scientific interest in the climatology of Fla. as it related to public health. Most important were his professional concerns for the low quality of medical education and practice and the absence of standardized procedures for the licensing of physicians. Instrumental in the founding of the Duval County Medical Society (1853). Provided the leadership and major initiative for the establishment of the Florida Medical Association, launched in his Jacksonville office on January 14, 1874, with nine other physicians present. First president of the association, and at its second meeting (again in Jacksonville, February 1875), delivered the presidential address, "The Climatology of Florida." Best-known medical achievement, the development of a procedure for treating a bowel disorder, intussusception, by pumping large quantities of tepid water into the intestines, brought him national acclaim. Civic interests and contributions were numerous, relating mostly to the improvement of rail and steamship transportation for Jacksonville. Elected to the Fla. legislature for four terms: 1852, House; 1858, 1860, 1861, Senate.

WRITINGS: "The Climatology of Florida," *Proc., Fla. Med. Assoc.* (1875), 21-56. His personal medical records—A Medical Directory of Florida; Book of the Chief Surgeon, District of East Florida; and Case Book of the General Hospital, Lake City—are preserved in the Confederate Museum, Richmond, Va. REFERENCES: S. M. Day, "Medical Leadership," *J. Fla. Med. Assoc.* 52 (1865): 468-76; *Florida Times-Union and Citizen* (Jacksonville), December 9, 1898; Webster Merritt, *A Century of Medicine in Jacksonville and Duval County* (1949), 10-16; *NCAB*, 5:184; *Proc., Fla. Med. Assoc.* (1874-98).

E. A. Hammond

BALDWIN, WILLIAM OWEN (August 6, 1818, Montgomery County, Ala.- May 30, 1886, Montgomery, Ala.). *Physician*. Son of William and Cecelia (Fitzpatrick) Baldwin. Married Mary Jane Martin, 1843; seven children. EDUCATION: Academy in Montgomery County; studied medicine in the office of Dr. McLeod, Montgomery; 1837, M.D., Transylvania University. CAREER: 1837-86, practice in Montgomery; 1850, vice-president, Alabama State Medical Association, succeeding to the presidency on the death of the elected president; 1868, AMA president; 1872-86, elected member, Board of Trustees, Medical College of Alabama, Mobile, Ala.; 1882, member of the Montgomery County Board of Health. CONTRIBUTIONS: Helped to organize Alabama State Medical Association (1847) and Sydenham Medical Society of Montgomery (1850). Served on the committee to prepare a memo to the legislature on the need to construct a hospital for the insane in Alabama and to help Dorothea Dix (q.v.), in efforts in the same area (1850). Helped reorganize the Medical and Surgical Society of Montgomery County (1866). Elected president of the American Medical Association (1868); at the first meeting since the Civil War at which delegates from the South were present (1869), helped to reunify the profession.

WRITINGS: "Remarks on Mustard Poultices, Applied Extensively to the Surface," *Western J. of Med. and Surg.* 3 (1845): 11; "Observations on the Poisonous Properties of the Sulphate of Quinine," *Am. J. of Med. Sci.*, n.s., 14 (1847): 292-310; "Observations on Spotted Fever," *ibid.*, n.s., 52 (1866): 321-37; *Tribute to the Late James Marion Sims* (1884). REFERENCES: E. B. Carmichael, "William O. Baldwin," *Annals of Med.*

Hist., 3rd series, 4 (1942): 521-31; *J. of the Med. Assoc. of the State of Ala.* 5 (1936): 315, 319; *NCAB*, 12: 473; T. M. Owen, *History of Alabama* (1978).

S. Eichold

BANCROFT, FREDERICK JONES (May 25, 1834, Enfield, Conn.-January 16, 1903, San Diego, Calif.). *Surgeon.* Son of Caleb Jones and Chloe (Wolcott) Bancroft. Married Mary Caroline Jarvis, 1871; three children. EDUCATION: Westfield Academy (Mass.), Charlotteville Seminary (N.Y.); 1861, M.D., University of Buffalo. CAREER: 1862, surgeon, 76th Pennsylvania Infantry, Hilton Head, S.C.; 1863-65, post surgeon, Fortress Monroe, Va.; 1866, moved to Colo. and acted as surgeon for the Ben Holliday Overland Mail Express Company and the Wells Fargo stage lines; railway surgeon for every line serving Denver; 1881-87, chief surgeon, Denver & Rio Grande Railroad; 1872-76, president, Denver School Board; 1872-77, city physician of Denver; 1876-78, first president of the Colorado State Board of Health; 1881, president of the Colorado Medical Society. CONTRIBUTIONS: An organizer of the medical department, University of Denver (1881), where he served as professor of clinical surgery and fractures and dislocations (1881-94). Founder of the Colorado Historical and Natural History Society and first president (1879-97).

WRITINGS: His contributions to medical literature were sparse, on topics as disparate as *fragilitas ossium* and drainage in pulmonary consumption. Writings listed in *Medical Coloradoana* (1922). REFERENCES: Caroline Bancroft, "Pioneer doctor," *Colorado Mag.* 39 (Jul. 1962): 195-203; Kelly and Burrage (1920), 56; E. J. A. Rogers, "Dr. F. J. Bancroft," *Denver Med. Times* 23 (Jul. 1903): 24-30.

F. B. Rogers

BARBER, AMOS WALKER (April 26, 1861, Doylestown, Pa.-May 19, 1915, Rochester, N.Y.). *Physician; Surgeon.* Son of Alfred H., special service officer detective in the Civil War, and Asenath (Walker) Barber. Married Amelia Kent, 1892; two children. EDUCATION: Doylestown Academy; 1883, M.D., University of Pennsylvania. CAREER: 1883-85, resident physician, University of Pennsylvania Hospital, and staff physician, Children's Hospital and Pennsylvania Hospital; acting assistant surgeon, U.S. Military Hospital, Ft. Fetterman, Wyo.; 1886, resigned from the U.S. service to practice general medicine and surgery at Cheyenne, Wyo. CONTRIBUTIONS: Particularly noted for his reputation among settlers for treating rattlesnake bites with inoculations of potassium permanganate; also well known for treatment of gunshot wounds. Elected first secretary of state for Wyo. (September 11, 1890), serving from November 8, 1890, to January 7, 1895. When Governor F. E. Warren was elected to the U.S. Senate, Barber served as acting governor (November 14, 1890-January 2, 1893).

WRITINGS: Wrote about gunshot wounds and snakebites and stories about Western life for *Harpers Weekly*. REFERENCES: T. S. Chamblin, *Historical Encyclopedia of Wyoming* (1954), 143; *NCAB* 11: 482.; *N.Y Times*, May 20, 1915, p. 11; C. S. Peterson, *Men of Wyoming* (1915).

A. Palmieri

BARD, JOHN (February 1, 1716, Burlington County, N.J.-April 1, 1799, Hyde Park, N.Y.). *Physician*. Son of Pierre, merchant, and Dinah (Marmion) Bard. Married Suzanne Valleau; four children. EDUCATION: Early education with Mr. Annan of Philadelphia; at 18, apprenticed to Dr. John Kearsley (q.v.). CAREER: Practiced in Philadelphia until November 28, 1745, when Benjamin Franklin convinced him to go to N.Y., where an epidemic had taken the lives of physicians, creating a shortage; 1748, organized the Weekly Society of Gentlemen, one of the first American medical societies. CONTRIBUTIONS: Created an infirmary at the city's house of correction, which would later become Bellevue Hospital. Instrumental in getting the charter for King's (Columbia) College on October 31, 1754. Health officer for N.Y. (1755). First president of New York Medical Society (1787). Assisted his son Dr. Samuel Bard (q.v.) with the operation on George Washington (acute local inflammation of subcutaneous tissue), before Washington's inauguration as first president.

WRITINGS: *A Letter from the. . . . President of the Medical Society of the State of New York, to the Author of Thoughts on the Dispensary* (1791). Writings mentioned in *DAB*. REFERENCES: *DAB*, 1: 597-98; Kelly and Burrage (1920), 57-59; John Brett Langstaff, *Dr. Bard of Hyde Park* (1942); *NCAB*, 8: 209.

D. Rosner

BARD, SAMUEL (April 1, 1742, Philadelphia, Pa.-May 24, 1821, Hyde Park, N.Y.). *Physician; Medical education; Obstetrics*. Son of John (q.v.), physician, and Mary (Valleau) Bard. Married Mary Bard, cousin, 1770; four children. EDUCATION: King's College, N.Y.; 1760-62, studied in London; 1765, M.D., Edinburgh University. CAREER: 1765, began practice in N.Y. with his father; 1767, helped found school of medicine affiliated with King's College, served as professor of the theory and practice of physic; 1792-1804, united medical school with Columbia College; dean and trustee in addition to duties as professor of theory and practice of medicine; 1813-21, president, College of Physicians and Surgeons. CONTRIBUTIONS: Was prime mover in organizing N.Y.'s first medical school and the second in the American colonies, King's College, which later joined Columbia College as the College of Physicians and Surgeons. Respected physician. Operated on Gen. George Washington for large abscess of thigh. Wrote first systematic treatise of obstetrics in America, which had a wide influence. Dean and later president of College of Physicians and Surgeons. Helped establish New York Dispensary, New York Hospital, New York City Library, and Botanical Garden of New York. Wrote important work on sheep raising. President of Agricultural Society of New York.

WRITINGS: *An Enquiry into the Nature, Cause and Cure of the Angina Suffocativa, or Sore Throat Distemper* . . . (1771); *A Compendium on the Theory and Practice of Midwifery* . . . , 5 eds. (1807); "A Discourse on the Importance of Medical Education . . . ," *Am. Med. Philos. Register* 2 (1812): 369-82; *A Discourse on Medical Education* . . . (1819). REFERENCES: *DAB*, 1: 598-99; Henry W. Ducachet, "A Biographical Memoir of Samuel Bard, M.D., LL.D., Late President of the College of Physicians and Surgeons of the University of New York; with a Critique on His Writings," *Am. Med. Recorder* 4 (1821): 609-633; David C. Humphrey, "The King's College Medical School and the Professionalization of Medicine in Pre-Revolutionary New York," *Bull. Hist. Med.* 49 (1975): 206-34; Kelly and Burrage (1920), 59-60; John Brett Langstaff, *Doctor Bard of Hyde Park* (1942); John M'Vickar, *A Domestic Narrative of the Life of Samuel Bard* (1822); *NCAB*, 8: 209.

L. D. Longo

BARDEEN, CHARLES RUSSELL (February 8, 1871, Kalamazoo, Mich.-June 12, 1935, Madison, Wis.). *Physician; Anatomist; Educator.* Son of Charles William, educator and author, and Ellen Palmer (Dickerman) Bardeen. Married Althea Harmen, 1905, four children; Ruth Hames, 1920, one child. EDUCATION: 1893, B.A., Harvard; 1897, M.D., Johns Hopkins. CAREER: At Department of Anatomy, Johns Hopkins University Medical School: 1897-99, assistant; 1899-1901, associate; and 1901-4, associate professor; at University of Wisconsin Medical School: 1904-35, professor, Department of Anatomy; and 1907-35, dean. CONTRIBUTIONS: As professor of anatomy and first dean of the University of Wisconsin Medical School, shaped medical education in Wis. to a greater extent than any other individual. Teaching in Wis.'s two-year preclinical program for 18 years, helped build the foundation for a four-year medical school by promoting the development of clinical facilities (including general and children's hospitals and one of the nation's earliest comprehensive student health services) and by fighting a series of legislative battles for the survival and expansion of the program. With the advent of the four-year program, instituted a preceptor system that required students to apprentice themselves to distinguished Wis. physicians for one-quarter of their senior year, a system later adopted by other schools. Pioneered in the use of X-rays to determine heart size and to study and teach anatomy. His formulae relating heart size to growth rate, body build, and other characteristics were highly regarded. Editor, *Anatomical Record* (1906-8).

WRITINGS: "Anatomy in America," *Bull. of the Univ. of Wisconsin*, no. 115, Science Series, 3, no. 4 (1905): 85-208; "The Height-Weight Index of Build in Relation to Linear and Volumetric Proportions and Surface-Area of the Body during Post-Natal Development," *Carnegie Institution of Washington Contributions to Embryology* 9 (1920): 483-554. REFERENCES: *Anatomical Record* 65, no. 2 (May 1936): 3-5; Paul F. Clark, *The University of Wisconsin Medical School: A Chronicle, 1848-1948* (1967), 41-50; *Dict. of Wisconsin Biog.*, p. 26; *JAMA* 105 (1935): 63.

E. B. Keeney

BARKER, B[ENJAMIN] FORDYCE (May 2, 1818, Wilton, Maine-May 30, 1891, New York, N.Y.). *Physician; Obstetrician.* Son of John, physician, and

Phoebe (Abbott) Barker. Married Elizabeth Lee Dwight, 1843. EDUCATION: 1837, B.A., Bowdoin College; 1838-40, apprentice to Henry I. Bowditch (q.v.); studied in Edinburgh and Paris; 1841, M.D., Bowdoin Medical College. CAREER: Began practice, Norwich, Conn.; 1846, became professor of midwifery, Bowdoin Medical College; 1850, professor of midwifery and diseases of women, New York Medical College; 1852, obstetric physician, Bellevue Hospital; 1860, became professor of clinical midwifery and diseases of women, Bellevue Hospital Medical College; consulting physician: Bellevue Hospital, Nursery and Child's Hospital, St. Elizabeth's Hospital, Cancer Hospital, and Women's Hospital, all in New York City. CONTRIBUTIONS: Considered best-known obstetrician in America during his time. Claimed to have introduced the use of the hypodermic syringe into American medicine. Author of standard work on puerperal diseases (1874). First president, American Gynecological Society (1876).

WRITINGS: *The Puerperal Diseases* (1874); articles on childbearing cases related to the age of the mother, bloodletting in obstetric medicine, and reducing pain in labor. REFERENCES: W. C. Coe, *In Memoriam; B. F. Barker* (1891); *DAB*, 1: 601; Kelly and Burrage (1920), 60-62; P. F. Munde, *In Memoriam; B. F. Barker* (1891); obituaries, *Trans., Am. Gyn. Soc.* 16 (1891): 551-58; *Trans., N.Y. Acad. of Med.*, 2nd series, 8 (1892): 286-302.

D. Rosner

BARKER, JEREMIAH (March 31, 1752, Scituate, Mass.-October 4, 1835, Gorham, Maine). *Physician.* Son of Samuel and Patience (Howland) Barker. Married Abigail Gorham, 1775, four children; Susanna Garrett, 1790, one child; Eunice Riggs; Temperance (Garrett) Gorham, 1808. EDUCATION: Received a "thorough classical" education from Rev. Timothy Cutler, Congregational minister; studied medicine under Dr. Bela Lincoln of Cambridge, Mass. CAREER: 1771-72, practiced medicine, Gorham, Maine, but competition forced his removal to Barnstable, Mass., 1772-79; soon after the Battle of Bunker Hill, went to Boston to be inoculated for smallpox by Dr. Isaac Rand and remained as a student and assistant for several months; during the Revolution, served as an army surgeon, sometimes aboard ships, and with his preceptor Dr. Lincoln was on the ill-fated Bagaduce expedition; after the Revolution, settled briefly in Gorham, moved to Portland in 1792, and practiced there until 1818 when he returned to Gorham. CONTRIBUTIONS: Invented a sponge tent for emphysema. Developed a unique alkaline treatment for fevers. Emphasized the value of autopsies. Was a founder of the Maine Medical Society.

WRITINGS: Published accounts of amputations, fractures, tetanus, and epidemics, generally in Mitchell's *Repository*. A "Proposal for Publishing a History of Diseases in the District of Maine Commencing in 1772 and Continued to the Present Time Containing Also Some Account of Diseases in N.H., and Other Parts of New England with Biographical Sketches of Learned and Useful Physicians, Both in Europe and America, as well as Other Promoters of Medical Science . . . " was never published but is an invaluable source. Kept a number of case books and made notes of significant cases. REFERENCES: Howard Kelly, *Cyclopedia of Am. Med. Biog.* 1 (1912): 47-48; *DAB*, 1: 605-6; Maine

Historical Society, Collection #13, Jeremiah Barker Papers, 1771-1835; Maine Historical Society, Collection #513, Maine Physicians, compiled by James Spalding; Hugh Davis McLellan, *History of Gorham, Maine* (1903), 396-98; James Alfred Spalding, "After Consulting Hours: Jeremiah Barker, M.D., Gorham and Falmouth, Maine, 1752-1835," *Bull. Am. Acad. of Med.* 10, no. 3 (Jun.1909): 1-24; idem, *Maine Physicians of 1820* (1928), 31-33.

B. Lister

BARKER, LEWELLYS FRANKLIN (September 16, 1867, Norwich, Ontario, Canada-July 13, 1943, Baltimore, Md.). *Physician; Neurology.* Son of James Frederick and Sarah Jane (Taylor) Barker. Married Lillian H. Halsey, 1903; five children. EDUCATION: 1881-84, attended Pickering College (Ontario); 1890, M.B., University of Toronto; 1890-91, intern, Toronto General Hospital; 1895, studied in Leipzig; and 1904, Munich and Berlin. CAREER: 1891-1900, 1905-21, medical staff, Johns Hopkins Hospital; at Johns Hopkins Medical School: 1894-99, anatomy faculty; 1899-1900, pathology faculty; and 1905-21, medicine faculty; 1899, Johns Hopkins medical commissioner to Philippine Islands; 1900-5, anatomy faculty, Rush Medical College (Chicago); 1901, member, U.S. commission to determine the existence of bubonic plague in San Francisco: *post* 1902, associate editor, *American Journal of Anatomy*; president: 1909-18, National Committee for Mental Hygiene; 1913, Association of American Physicians; and 1916, American Neurological Association. CONTRIBUTIONS: Reorganized the Department of Medicine at Johns Hopkins to emphasize research as well as teaching; established laboratories within the divisions of the department to investigate the medical problems encountered on the wards. Stressed the importance of research laboratories in clinical medicine both for studying fundamental disease processes and as an aid in diagnosis. Did important research on the anatomy, physiology, and pathology of the nervous system and the pathological-physiology of the heart. Helped eradicate bubonic plague in the Philippine Islands (1899) and San Francisco, Calif. (1901).

WRITINGS: *The Nervous System and Its Constituent Neurons* (1899); *Laboratory Manual of Human Anatomy* (1904, with Dean DeWitt Lewis and D. G. Revell); "The Laboratories of the Medical Clinic," *Bull., Johns Hopkins Hosp.* 18 (1907): 193; *The Clinical Diagnosis of Internal Diseases* (1916); *Time and the Physician* (1942). REFERENCES: Charles B. Austrian, "Lewellys Franklin Barker," *Bull., Johns Hopkins Hosp.* 73 (1943): 401-4; A. McGehee Harvey, "Creators of Clinical Medicine's Scientific Base . . . Franklin Barker . . . ," *Johns Hopkins Med. J.* 136, no. 4 (Apr. 1975): 168-77; Warfield T. Longcope, "Lewellys F. Barker," *Sci.* 98 (1943): 316-18; Miller, *BHM*, p. 7; *NCAB*, 32: 308-9; *N.Y. Times*, July 14, 1943; *Time and the Physician* (1942); *Who Was Who in Am.*, 2: 43.

S. Galishoff

BARLOW, WALTER JARVIS (January 22, 1868, Ossining, N.Y.-September 4, 1937, Sierra Madre, Calif.). *Physician; Internal medicine.* Son of William H., merchant, and Catharine S. (Lent) Barlow. Married Marion Brooks Patterson, 1898; three children. EDUCATION: 1892, M.D., College of Physicians and Surgeons, Columbia University; resident physician, Mt. Sinai Hospital, N.Y., for one year; postgraduate work, Sloane Memorial Hospital, N.Y. CAREER: Went to Calif. after developing pulmonary tuberculosis; 1897, began medical practice in Los Angeles, Calif.; 1908-14, professor of clinical medicine and dean of the faculty, Los Angeles Medical Department of the University of California; 1902, established and headed the Barlow Sanitorium; 1914, president, Los Angeles County Medical Association; 1912-13, chairman of the section on the practice of medicine, American Medical Association. CONTRIBUTIONS: Established the Barlow Sanitorium as a charitable institution for curable pulmonary tuberculosis patients of moderate means who were unable to finance the long period of inactivity necessary for recovery. Personally responsible for the acquisition of a generous endowment fund for this institution. Founded and donated the building for the Barlow Medical Library, which in 1934 was transferred to the Los Angeles County Medical Association, forming the nucleus of its library. Was the originator of the Barlow Trust, which supports the acquisition of materials of the Biomedical Library at the University of California, Los Angeles. REFERENCES: *California and Western Med.* 47, no. 4 (1937): 264-65; *NCAB*, 36: 250; obituaries, *Bull., Los Angeles County Med. Assoc.* 67, no. 18 (1937): 667; 67, no. 19 (1937): 733.

Y. V. O'Neill

BARNES, WILLIAM HARRY (April 4, 1887, Philadelphia, Pa.-January 15, 1945, Philadelphia). *Physician; Otolaryngology.* Son of George W. and Eliza (Webb) Barnes. Married Mattie E. Thomas, 1912; five children. EDUCATION: 1908, A.B., Central High School, Philadelphia; raised in impoverished circumstances in Philadelphia, worked throughout high school career and won a four-year scholarship to University of Pennsylvania Medical School in 1908, first black to earn this distinction; 1912, M.D., University of Pennsylvania; 1912-13, intern, Douglass and Mercy hospitals, Philadelphia; 1921, postgraduate courses, University of Pennsylvania, in Ear, Nose and Throat (ENT) and ENT operative surgery; 1924, 1926, postgraduate work in ENT and bronchoscopy in Paris and Bordeaux, France, Philadelphia, and New York City. CAREER: 1913-45, ENT staff, Douglass Hospital, Philadelphia; during career, also on ENT staffs, Mercy and Jefferson Medical School hospitals; 1931-45, lecturer in bronchoscopy, Howard University Medical School (commuted from Philadelphia); 1913-22, general medical practice, Philadelphia; 1922-45, ENT practice, Philadelphia. CONTRIBUTIONS: Served as 37th president of the NMA (1936). First black certified by an American specialty board (1927, American Board of Otolaryngology). Actively participated in NMA annual meetings, performing surgery and demonstrations or presenting papers. Founded, and served as executive secretary of, Society for the Promotion of Negro Specialists in Medicine. Three years as president of Philadelphia Academy of Medicine and Allied Sciences. Invented hypophyscope for visualizing pituitary gland. Developed a modification of the Myles lingual tonsillectomy. Devised new operative techniques for opening peritonsillar abscesses and for making incisions in myringotomy. Served black community of Philadelphia in numerous medical and nonmedical capacities. WRITINGS: About 25 articles on otolaryngology, published primarily in *JNMA*, 1913-39. "An Improved Hypophyscope," *Laryngos* 27 (1927): 379-80; "The Pituitary Gland (The Surgical Treatment of Disease of)," *JNMA* 19 (1927): 63-65. Writings listed in *JNMA* 47 (1955): 66, 69. REFERENCES: W. Montague Cobb, "William Harry Barnes, 1887-1945," *JNMA* 47 (1955): 64-66; "The President-Elect," *JNMA* 26 (1934): 176; *WWICA*, 6 (1941-43): 40; *WWAPS* 1 (1938): 55.

T. Savitt

BARRINGER, EMILY DUNNING (September 27, 1876, Scarsdale, N.Y.-April 8, 1961, New Milford, Conn.). *Gynecologist; Surgeon*. Daughter of Edwin J., broker, and Fanny Dunning. Married Benjamin Barringer, M.D., 1905; two children. EDUCATION: 1894-97, pioneering medical preparatory course, Cornell University; 1897-98, Medical College of the New York Infirmary (MCNYI); 1901, M.D., Cornell Medical School (which absorbed students of the MCNYI when the latter closed in 1898); 1902-4, house officer, Gouverneur Hospital, New York City (part of the municipal hospital system). CAREER: Practiced briefly with Mary Putnam Jacobi (q.v.); later, engaged in active private practice of gynecology, N.Y.; on staffs of the New York Infirmary and the Kingston Avenue Hospital; 1940, retired as director of gynecology, Kingston Avenue Hospital. CONTRIBUTIONS: Aided by a reform city administration, first woman to win a coveted residency position at Gouverneur, an emergency "feeder" hospital to Bellevue; thereby became the "first woman ambulance surgeon" in N.Y., rotating duty with her male colleagues; became the "Chief of Staff," that is, chief resident (1904). During later years of practice, studied the serologic diagnosis of gonorrhea and that disease's presentation in the female. Active in the National Prison Association, she urged better health care for female offenders. Served on the General Medical Advisory Board of the American Social Hygiene Association. Campaigned tirelessly for the commission of women physicians in the armed services. President of the New York Medical Women's Association and delegate to the AMA House of Delegates.

WRITINGS: "Problem of 'Clinical Gonorrhea' in the Female," *Am. J. of Obstet. & Gyn*. 25 (1933): 538; "Treatment of Gonorrhea in the Female," *JAMA* 103 (1934): 1825; "Complement Fixation Test: Diagnostic Aid in the Control of Gonorrhea," *N.Y. State J. of Med*. 38 (1938): 699; *Bowery to Bellevue: The Story of New York's First Woman Ambulance Surgeon* (1950). REFERENCES: *NCAB*, 50: 94; Iris Noble's *First Woman Ambulance Surgeon—Emily Barringer* (1962) adds little to Barringer's own autobiography.

S. J. Peitzman

BARRON, MOSES (March 8, 1893, Kovno, Russia-December 22, 1974, Minneapolis, Minn.). *Physician*. Son of Jacob, farmer and grocer, and Pauline Barron. Married Leah Fliegelman, 1913; four children. EDUCATION: University of Minnesota: 1910, B.S.; and 1911, M.D.; 1926, postgraduate work, University of Vienna. CAREER: At University of Minnesota: 1912-13, demonstrator in pathology and bacteriology; 1912-16, instructor in pathology and bacteriology; 1916-25, assistant professor; 1925-33, associate professor; and 1933-52, professor of medicine. CONTRIBUTIONS: Author of articles (1920) that provided the key for the discovery of insulin by Dr. Frederick Banting. Did scientific work on cancer of the lung and diseases of the pancreas, Hodgkin's Disease, hepatomegaly, and splenomegaly. Popularized the cause of the high incidence of bothriocephalus latus infestations in Jewish women (1921).

WRITINGS: "Relation of the Islets of Langerhans to Diabetes with Special Reference to Cases of Pancreatic Lithiasis" (1920); "Lead Poisoning with Special Reference to Poisoning from Cosmetics" (1921); "Carcinoma of the Lung" (1922). REFERENCES: *The Medical Way* 16 (Feb. 1954); *Minnesota Med.* 49 (1966): 689-90, 861-62.

R. Rosenthal

BARTHOLOW, ROBERTS (November 28, 1831, New Windsor, Md.-May 10, 1904, Philadelphia, Pa.). *Physician; Author*. Son of Jeremiah and Pleasants Bartholow. Was married and had children. EDUCATION: Calvert College (later New Windsor College): 1848, B.A.; and 1854, M.A.; 1852, M.D., medical department, University of Maryland. CAREER: 1852-55, practiced medicine, Baltimore, Md.; in medical corps, U.S. Army: 1855-60, service in the West during troubles with the Mormons and the Indians; and 1861-64, assigned to hospital service during the Civil War; 1864-79, practiced medicine, Cincinnati, Ohio; at Medical College of Ohio: 1864-67, medical chemistry faculty; 1867-74, materia medica faculty; and 1874-79, theory and practice of medicine faculty; *post* 1879, practiced medicine, Philadelphia; 1879-93, materia medica and therapeutics faculty, Jefferson Medical College; *post* 1879, medical staff, Philadelphia and Jefferson hospitals. CONTRIBUTIONS: Made one of the first studies of electrical stimulation of the human brain while treating a patient with a fatal malignant tumor of the scalp and skull (1874); work corroborated the results obtained by other researchers working with lower animals. Most important contributions were as an author and editor. Wrote *A Manual of Instruction for Enlisting and Discharging Soldiers* (1863), which was used by the army for many years; *Practical Treatise on Materia Medica and Therapeutics* (1876); and *Treatise on the Practice of Medicine* (1880), which went through 11 and 8 editions, respectively. Founded and edited the *Clinic*, the first weekly medical journal published in the West. Helped edit (beginning in 1882) *Medical News* (Philadelphia).

WRITINGS: "Experimental Investigations into the Functions of the Human Brain," *Am. J. of the Med. Sci.* 73 (Apr. 1874): 305-13; *Qualifications for the Medical Service* (1865); *Manual of Hypodermic Medication* (1868). REFERENCES: *DAB*, 2: 2-3; James W. Holland, "Memoir of Roberts Bartholow," *Trans., Coll. of Physicians of Phila.*, 3rd series, 26 (1904): 43-52; Kelly and Burrage (1928), 64; Miller, *BHM*, p. 8; *NCAB*, 22: 212-13; *Who Was Who in Am.*, 1: 63.

S. Galishoff

BARTLETT, ELISHA (October 6, 1804, Smithfield, R.I.-July 19, 1855, Smithfield). *Physician; Teacher; Author*. Son of Otis and Waite (Buffum) Bartlett. Married Elizabeth Slater, 1829; no children. EDUCATION: Studied medicine with George Willard of Uxbridge, Mass.; John Green and B. F. Heywood of Worcester, Mass.; and Levi Wheaton of Providence, R.I.; 1826, M.D., Brown University; 1826-27, studied in Europe. CAREER: 1827-c. 1847, practiced medicine, Lowell, Mass.; 1832-40, pathological anatomy and materia medica faculty, Berkshire Medical Institution; 1832-35, co-editor, *Medical Magazine* (Boston); 1841, 1846, theory and practice of medicine faculty, Transylvania University; spring and summer months, 1843-52, materia medica and obstetrics faculties, Vermont Medical College; on theory and practice of medicine faculty: 1844-46, University of Maryland; and 1849-50, University of Louisville; 1850-52, institutes and practice of medicine faculty, New York University; 1852-55, materia medica and medical jurisprudence faculty, College of Physicians and Surgeons (Columbia). CONTRIBUTIONS: In his treatise *The History, Diagnosis and Treatment of Typhoid and Typhus Fever. . .*(1842), gave a clear clinical description of typhoid fever, which, at the time, was often confused with typhus. Writings and teaching at many distinguished medical schools made him one of the country's best-known physicians. Most characteristic work was *An Essay on the Philosophy of Medical Science* (1844), in which he argued that the observation of facts was the sole path to medical enlightenment, and the only legitimate manipulations of facts were classification and generalization based on numerical analysis; ideas accorded with the teachings of the Paris school of medicine, of which he was an admirer. In most controversial work, *An Inquiry into the Degree of Certainty of Medicine, and into the Nature and Extent of Its Power Over Disease* (1848), urged that traditional practices be abandoned if they could not be supported by observation.

WRITINGS: *History, Diagnosis, and Treatment of Edematous Laryngitis* (1850); *A Discourse on the Times, Character, and Writings of Hippocrates* (1852). A bibliography is in Donald de F. Beuer, "Elisha Bartlett, A Distinguished Physician. . .," *Bull. Hist. Med.* 17 (1945): 85-92. REFERENCES: Erwin H. Ackerknecht, "Elisha Bartlett and the Philosophy of the Paris Clinical School," *Bull. Hist. Med.* 24 (1950): 43-60; *BHM* (1964-69), 23; *DAB*, 2: 3-5; Kelly and Burrage (1928), 65-66; Miller, *BHM*, p. 8; *NCAB*, 12: 70; R. F. Stone, *Biog. of Eminent Am. Physic. and Surg.* (1894), 29-30.

S. Galishoff

BARTLETT, JOSIAH (November 21, 1729, Amesbury, Mass.-May 17, 1795, Kingston, N.H.). *Physician.* Son of Stephen, shoemaker, and Hannah (Webster) Bartlett. Married Mary Bartlett, 1754; 12 children, including 3 physicians: Levi (1763-1828), Josiah (1768-1838), and Ezra (1770-1848). EDUCATION: 1745-50, apprenticed to Dr. Nehemiah Ordway, Amesbury, Mass.; at Dartmouth: 1790, A.M. (hon.); and 1792, M.D. (hon.). CAREER: 1750-95, practiced in Kingston, N.H.; 1791-93, founder and first president of New Hampshire Medical Society; much of his life was devoted to politics: 1765-67, selectman, justice of the peace; 1765-75, N.H. legislator; 1774-75, N.H. Provincial Congress delegate; 1774-84, member of the New Hampshire Committee of Safety; 1776-82, justice of

Inferior Court of Common Pleas, Rockingham County; 1782-90, justice of the N.H. superior court and 1790-94, its chief justice; and 1790-94, first chief executive of N.H.; 1788, declined election to the U.S. Senate; 1775-78,, delegate to the Continental Congress, one of the two physicians from his state to sign the Declaration of Independence. CONTRIBUTIONS: Although neither a leader nor an innovator in medical science, Bartlett's 45-year practice has been shown to provide an accurate reflection of that of the profession as a whole in colonial New England. REFERENCES: *BHM* (1975-79), 14; *DAB*, 2: 9-11; J. Worth Estes, "Therapeutic Practice in Colonial New England," in Philip Cash, Eric H. Christianson, and J. Worth Estes, eds., *Medicine in Colonial Massachusetts, 1620-1820* (1980), 289-383 (also see n.14 therein); Frank C. Mevers, ed., *The Papers of Josiah Bartlett* (1979).

J. W. Estes

BARTON, BENJAMIN SMITH (February 10, 1766, Lancaster, Pa.-December 19, 1815, Philadelphia, Pa.). *Physician; Botanist.* Son of Thomas, Episcopal clergyman, and Esther (Rittenhouse) Barton. Married Mary Pennington, 1792; two children. EDUCATION: Studied for two years at Edinburgh, Scotland; graduated from Göttingen, Germany. CAREER: At University of Pennsylvania: 1789-1813, professor of botany; and 1813-15, chair of practical medicine; 1804-9, editor, *Philadelphia Medical and Physical Journal.* CONTRIBUTIONS: Wrote first elementary botany text by an American. First professor of botany and natural history in the United States. As early as 1798, pointed to the need for a national pharmacopoeia and began to collect information that was published in 1804. President of the American Philosophical Society (1802).

WRITINGS: *Elements of Botany* (1803); *Collections for an Essay Towards a Materia Medica of the United States* (1804). REFERENCES: W. J. Bell, "Benjamin Smith Barton, M.D.," *J. Hist. Med.* 26 (1971): 197-203; *DAB*, 1, pt. 2: 17-18; *DSB*, 1 (1970): 484-86; *NCAB*, 8: 377; Francis W. Pennell, "Benjamin Smith Barton as Naturalist," *Proc., Amer. Philos. Soc.* 86 (1942): 108-22; F. Spencer, "Two Unpublished Essays on the Anthropology of North America by Benjamin Barton," *Isis* 68 (1977): 567-73.

J. Carvalho

BARTON, CLARA (December 25, 1821, North Oxford, Mass.-April 12, 1912, Glen Echo, Md.). *Nurse; Humanitarian.* Daughter of Capt. Stephen and Sarah (Stone) Barton, prosperous farmers. Never married. EDUCATION: Educated in local schools; 1850, student at the Liberal Institute, Clinton, N.Y. CAREER: 1840-49, taught school, Mass.; 1850-54, after studying in Clinton, N.Y., resumed teaching, Bordentown, N.J.; 1854-57, clerk, the U.S. Patent Office, Washington, D.C.; 1857-60, removed from her position due to Democratic political victory, returned to North Oxford: 1860-61, clerk, U.S. Patent office; 1861-62, supplied Union army with medical supplies, independently of the U.S. Sanitary Commission or Dorothea Dix's (q.v.) nursing corps; 1864, became head nurse, Benjamin Butler's Army of the James; 1865, headed office to search for missing soldiers; also directed the marking of graves at Andersonville prison, Ga.; 1866-

68, lectured on her wartime experiences; 1868-69, suffered a breakdown and on medical advice went to Europe where she learned of the International Red Cross (formed in 1862); 1870-71, served with the Red Cross, Franco-Prussian War; 1872-77, suffering a breakdown, remained in England, next went to Dansville, N.Y. to a water-cure sanitorium, and then to a house there; 1877-81, worked to develop an American organization of the Red Cross; 1881-1904, president, American Red Cross; 1904, resigned as president after a deep division within the Board of Directors of the American Red Cross; retired to Glen Echo, Md., where she lived, 1904-12. CONTRIBUTIONS: Known as "angel of the battlefield" for her work supplying and nursing the Union soldiers during the Civil War; was present at 16 battlefields during and after the fighting. Introduced the Red Cross to America, gained federal approval (1881-82); extended work of the Red Cross to natural disasters as well as wars, providing relief for the sufferers of the 1881 Mich. forest fires; 1882 Mississippi River floods; 1883 La. hurricane; 1886 Charleston, S.C., earthquake; 1887 Fla. yellow-fever epidemic; 1900 Galveston, Tex., hurricane and flood; and 1906 San Francisco, Calif., earthquake. Also distributed supplies to the men in the Spanish-American War, although over 75 at the time.

WRITINGS: *The Red Cross* (1898); *A Story of the Red Cross* (1904); *Story of My Childhood* (1907). Her 35 volumes of diaries are in the Library of Congress, along with her correspondence and records. REFERENCES: *BHM* (1964-69), 23; (1969-74), 18; *DAB* 2: 18-21; Foster Rhea Dulles, *The American Red Cross: A History* (1950); Miller, *BHM*, p. 8; *NAW*, 1: 103-8; *NCAB*, 15: 314; Ishbel Ross, *Angel of the Battlefield* (1956); Blanche Colton Williams, *Clara Barton* (1941).

M. Kaufman

BARTON, WILLIAM PAUL CRILLON (November 17, 1786, Philadelphia Pa.-March 27, 1856, Philadelphia). *Physician; Military medicine.* Son of Judge William and Elizabeth (Rhea) Barton. Married Esther Sergeant, 1814. EDUCATION: 1805, A.B., Princeton; studied medicine with Dr. Benjamin Smith Barton (q.v.), uncle; 1808, M.D., University of Pennsylvania. CAREER: 1809-14, surgeon, U.S. Navy; 1815, appointed professor of botany, University of Pennsylvania; professor of materia medica for three years, Jefferson Medical College; 1842-44, surgeon-general, U.S. Navy. CONTRIBUTIONS: Critical of military medicine during the War of 1812, became surgeon-general of the U.S. Navy (1842-44). Credited with providing the first modern medical view of sanitation and medical provision for sick naval personnel.

WRITINGS: *On the Chemical Properties and Exhilarating Effects of the Nitrous Oxide Gas* (1808); *A Treatise Containing a Plan for the Organization and Government of Marine Hospitals* (1814); *Vegetable Materia Medica of the United States* (1817-19); *Polemical Remonstrance Against the Project of Creating the New Office of Surgeon-General to the Navy* (1828). Writings listed in Kelly and Burrage (1920) and F. P. Henry, *Standard Hist. of Med. Profession in Phila.* (1897). REFERENCES: *Appleton's CAB; DAB*, 1: 25-26; Henry, *Standard Hist. of Med. Profession in Phila.*; Kelly and Burrage (1920); Miller, *BHM*, p. 8.

D. I. Lansing

BARUCH, SIMON (July 29, 1840, Schwersenz, Germany (now Poland)-June 3, 1921, New York, N.Y.). *Physician; General practitioner; Public health; Personal hygiene.* Son of Bernard and Teresa (Green) Baruch. Married Isabel Wolfe, 1867; four sons, including Bernard, a financier and public figure. ED-UCATION: Royal Gymnasium, Posen, Germany; 1859-60, apprentice to Drs. Workman and Deas, Camden, S.C.; 1862, M.D., Medical College of Virginia. CAREER: 1862-65, surgeon, Army of the Confederacy: 1865-81, general practice, Camden, S.C.; 1873, president, South Carolina Medical Association; 1880, acting chairman, South Carolina State Board of Health; 1881-1921, general and specialized practice, New York City, where his appointments included North-western Dispensary for Diseases of the Eye, Ear and Throat (1880-86); The New York Juvenile Asylum (1881-94); chief, medical staff (1884-92) and president, medical board, Montefiore Home for Chronic Invalids; and professor of hy-drotherapy, College of Physicians and Surgeons (N.Y.). CONTRIBUTIONS: An advocate of physiological remedies for chronic disease—particularly baths, diet, rest, and exercise, was also highly regarded as a general practitioner and diag-nostician. For example, made the first recorded accurate diagnosis of a case of perforated appendix that was successfully operated on. Best known for promoting public shower baths for the urban poor and the use of hydrotherapy in medical practice. The public bathhouses established in New York City (1891) and Chi-cago, Ill. (1894), the latter the first free public bath in the world, were direct results of his advocacy, as was the N.Y. State law of 1895 requiring cities with more than 50,000 population to offer free baths open 14 hours a day. A prolific speaker and writer and an active editor, contributed to medical journals and the popular press, and wrote books, several of which were translated into foreign languages. Public baths were named for him in Buffalo, N.Y., Chicago, New York City, and Philadelphia, as was a research laboratory at Saratoga Springs, N.Y., and a Center for Physical Medicine and Rehabilitation endowed by his son Bernard at the Medical College of Virginia.

WRITINGS: A bibliography of his writings is in Frances A. Hellebrandt, *Simon Baruch: Introduction to the Man and His Work* (1950). REFERENCES: "Simon Baruch, *British Med. J.* 2 (1940): 498; *DAB*, 2: 29-30; Kelly and Burrage (1928), 71: Thomas E. Keys and Frank H. Krusen, "Dr. Simon Baruch and His Fight for Free Public Baths," *Archives of Physical Med. and Rehab.* 26 (1945): 549-57, reprinted in 50 (1969): 41-46; Irving A. Watson, *Physicians and Surgeons of America* (1896), 534-35; Baruch wrote an in-tellectual history of his career, "Lessons of Half a Century in Medicine," reprinted from *The Old Dominion J. of Med. and Surg.* 11 (1910).

D. M. Fox

BATES, JAMES (September 24, 1789, Greene, Maine-February 25, 1882, Yarmouth, Maine). *Physician; Surgeon; Asylum superintendent.* Son of Solomon and Mary (Macomber) Bates. Married Mary Jones, 1815; five children. EDU-CATION: Public school education in Fayette, Maine; began the study of medicine with Dr. Charles Smith of Fayette, Maine, and Dr. Ariel Mann of Hallowell,

Maine; attended a course of lectures at Harvard Medical School. CAREER: 1813-15, U.S. Army, medical department, first as "surgeon's-mate" in Colonel McCobb's volunteer infantry regiment; 1814-15, on the Niagara frontier with Winfield Scott's forces; at the close of the war, was in charge of a general military hospital near Buffalo, N.Y., with 700 sick and wounded, and reportedly was the ranking medical officer at that time still in the service; 1815, entered into partnership with Ariel Mann, Hallowell; 1819-45, practiced medicine, Norridgewock, Maine; 1845-50, superintendent, state mental hospital, Augusta, Maine; when it burned in 1850, the governor commissioned him to investigate similar institutions in other states and report his findings for new construction at Augusta; 1851, practiced in Gardiner, Maine; 1851-58, served in Fairfield, Maine; finished out his medical career in North Yarmouth, Maine. CONTRIBUTIONS: An especially able surgeon, was called upon to operate and consult statewide. A founder of the Maine Medical Society. Frequent advocate, publically and privately, on temperance, public health, medical and agricultural topics. Possessed an extensive medical library—many works in Latin, Greek, and French—which he made available to all.

WRITINGS: "Local Blood-letting," *J. Med. Soc. Maine*, 1 (1834): 36-40. Presented a number of papers before the Maine Medical Society, including "On the Use of Artificial Leeches for Phlebotomy" and "Encephaloid Tumors." REFERENCES: *DAB*, 2: 51; Howard Kelly, *Cyclopedia of Am. Med. Biog.* 1: 59-60; Maine Historical Society Collections #513, Maine Physicians Compiled by James Spalding; *Maine Med. J.* 2, no. 6 (Jan. 1912): 594; *NCAB*; 21: 144; James Spalding, *Maine Physicians of 1820* (1928); *Trans. Maine Med. Assoc.* 7 (1882): 514-16.

B. Lister

BATTEY, ROBERT (November 26, 1828, Augusta, Ga.-November 8, 1895, Rome, Ga.). *Physician; Surgery.* Son of Cephas and Mary Agnes (Margruder) Battey. Married Martha B. Smith, 1849; 14 children. EDUCATION: Richmond Academy, Augusta, Ga.; Phillips Academy, Andover, Mass.; 1856, Philadelphia College of Pharmacy; apprentice to Dr. George M. Battey (brother), Rome, Ga., and Dr. Ellwood Wilson, Philadelphia, Pa.; 1857, M.D., Jefferson Medical College; 1859-60, studied in Paris. CAREER: 1857-95, surgeon, Rome, Ga.; except 1861-65, surgeon, Confederate Army (19th Regiment of Georgia Volunteers and Hampton's Brigade); 1872-75, professor of obstetrics, Atlanta Medical College; 1872-76, editor, *Atlanta Medical and Surgical Journal*. CONTRIBUTIONS: Developed "Battey's Operation"—bilateral oöphorectomy in premenstrual women for disturbances of menstruation accompanied by various nervous manifestations (severe headaches, pelvic pain, hystero-epileptic attacks, and so on). Contributed to the development of pelvic and abdominal surgery. Helped establish the functional relations between the gonads and menstruation, thus contributing to the emerging science of endocrinology. A founder of American Gynecological Society.

WRITINGS: "Normal Ovariotomy—Case," *Atlanta Med. & Surg. J.* 10 (1872-73):

321-29; "Normal Ovariotomy," *ibid.*, 11 (1873-74): 1-22; "Extirpation of the Functionally Active Ovaries for the Remedy of Otherwise Incurable Diseases," *Trans., Am. Gynec. Soc.* 1 (1876): 101-20; "A History of Battey's Operation," *Atlanta Med. & Surg. J.* 3 (1886-87): 657-75. REFERENCES: Joseph A. Eve, "A Sketch of the Life and Labors of Dr. Robert Battey, of Rome, Ga.," *Virginia Med. Monthly* 5 (1878): 1-9; *DAB*, 2: 55-56; Lawrence D. Longo, "The Rise and Fall of Battey's Operation: A Fashion in Surgery," *Bull. Hist. Med.* 53 (1979): 244-67; *NCAB*, 9: 349; Thaddeus A. Reamy, "Robert Battey, M.D., LL.D.," *Trans., Am. Gynec. Soc.* 21 (1896): 467-72.

L. D. Longo

BAYLESS, GEORGE WOOD (January 17, 1817, Washington, Mason County, Ky.-September 8, 1873, Rock Castle Springs, Rock Castle County, Ky.). *Physician; Surgeon; Educator.* Son of Benjamin, retail merchant, and Elizabeth (Wood) Bayless. Married Virginia Lafayette Browne, October 20, 1842; eight children. EDUCATION: Augusta College, Augusta, Bracken County, Ky.; 1836-37, studied medicine, office of Drs. Taliaferro and N. T. Marshall, Washington, Ky.; 1837-38, Louisville Medical Institute, Louisville, Ky.; 1838-39, University of Pennsylvania medical department, Philadelphia, Pa.; 1839, M.D., University of Pennsylvania Medical Department. CAREER: 1839-48, demonstrator in anatomy, Louisville Medical Institute and University of Louisville Medical Department, Louisville, Ky.; 1849-50, 1853-55, professor of anatomy, Medical College of Ohio, Cincinnati, Ohio: 1850-57, he and his family lived on a farm in western Mo., went to Cincinnati only to deliver lectures; 1857-61, professor of physiology and pathology, Kentucky School of Medicine, Louisville; at University of Louisville medical department: 1863-65, professor of physiology and pathological anatomy; 1865-66, professor of anatomy; 1864-66, dean; and 1866, professor of surgery; 1866, resigned in the fall. CONTRIBUTIONS: As demonstrator and prosector, taught anatomy with great skill and confidence. Was responsible as curator for the growth of the Pathological Museum at Louisville Medical Institute and University of Louisville medical department. One of the first faculty members in Louisville to use the microscope in his studies and private classes. An excellent and practical surgeon, was an early advocate of the use of anesthetics and not only used them in his surgical practice but conducted studies in their use on animals.

WRITINGS: Writings listed in *The Index Catalogue*. REFERENCES: E. Baker, "George W. Bayless" *J. of the Ky. Med. Assoc.* 57 (1959): 924-28; R. O. Cowling, "An Address on the Life and Professional Character of George Wood Bayless, M.D." *Am. Pract.* 8 (1873): 274; Charles Hentz diary in MSS. Collection, University of North Carolina, Chapel Hill, N.C.; O. Juettner, *Daniel Drake and His Followers* (1909).

E. H. Conner

BAYLEY, RICHARD (1745, Fairfield, Conn.-August 17, 1801, New York, N.Y.). *Physician; Surgeon.* Married "Dr. Charlton's sister." EDUCATION: 1766, apprentice to Dr. John Charlton, N.Y.; 1769-71, studied in London with Dr. William Hunter. CAREER: 1772-74, practice, N.Y.; 1775-76, studied in London;

1776-77, returned as surgeon to the British army in the American Revolutionary War; medical practice, New York City; 1792, joined medical faculty, Columbia College, in surgery and anatomy; 1795, health officer, New York City. CONTRIBUTIONS: Delivered anatomy lectures in New York City (1787), but in 1788 the "doctor's mob" destroyed his anatomy room. First doctor in America to amputate arm at the shoulder joint. Early supporter of the New York Dispensary. Wrote on the 1795 yellow-fever epidemic in N.Y. As city health officer, helped formulate early quarantine laws. Died of yellow fever.

WRITINGS: *A View of the Croup* (1781); *An Account of the Epidemic Fever Which Prevailed in the City of New York* . . . (1796). REFERENCES: *DAB*, 2: 74-75; Kelly and Burrage (1920), 76-77; John B. Langstaff, *Dr. Bard of Hyde Park* (1942); *Old New York* 1 (1890): 262-63; James Thacher, *American Medical Biographies* (1828).

D. Rosner

BAYNE-JONES, STANHOPE (November 6, 1888, New Orleans, La.-February 20, 1970, Washington, D.C.). *Bacteriologist; Medical educator and administrator.* Son of Stanhope, physician, and Minna Bayne; grandson of Joseph Jones (q.v.). Married Nannie Moore Smith, 1921; no children. EDUCATION: 1910, A.B., Yale University; Johns Hopkins: 1914, M.D.; 1914-15, intern; 1915-16, fellow in pathology; and 1917, M.A. CAREER: 1919-23, pathology and bacteriology faculties, Johns Hopkins Medical School; 1917-19, 1940-46, active duty, U.S. Army Medical Reserve Corps: 1923-32, bacteriology faculty, University of Rochester School of Medicine and Dentistry; 1923-32, director, Rochester Health Bureau Laboratories; at Yale Medical School: 1932-47, bacteriology faculty; and 1935-40, dean; 1941-46, administrator, Army Epidemiological Board; 1943-46, director, United States of America Typhus Commission; 1947-53, president, Joint Administration Board of New York Hospital-Cornell Medical Center; *post* 1947, advisor to U.S. Army Medical Corps, National Research Council, and U.S. Public Health Service; president: 1929, Society of American Bacteriologists; 1930, American Society of Immunologists; and 1940, American Association of Pathologists. CONTRIBUTIONS: Made significant discoveries in bacteriology early in his career but is best remembered for his administrative leadership and national medical activities. Co-authored the seventh and succeeding editions of *A Textbook of Bacteriology* by Hans Zinsser (qv.), one of the standard texts in its field (1934). Secured a new library at Yale Medical School that houses one of the nation's finest medical history collections (1941). Played a prominent role in the creation and work of the Army Epidemiological Board and served as its executive officer. Was a member of the U.S. Surgeon General's Commission on Smoking and Health, which linked smoking to cancer (1964). Oversaw the writing of the various histories of the army medical department during World War II and wrote a short monograph, *History of Preventive Medicine in the United States Army from Colonial Times* (1968).

WRITINGS: "The Titration of Diphtheria Toxin and Antitoxin by Ramon's Flocculation Method," *J. of Immunology* 9 (Nov. 1924): 481-504. REFERENCES: Morris C. Leikind,

"Stanhope Bayne-Jones . . . ,"*Bull., N.Y. Acad. of Med.* 48 (Apr. 1972): 584-95; John
R. Paul, "Stanhope Bayne-Jones . . . ," *Yale J. of Biol. and Med.* 45 (1972): 22-32;
Who Was Who in Am., 5: 45.

S. Galishoff

BAYNHAM, WILLIAM (December 7, 1749, Caroline County, Va.-December 8, 1814). *Physician; Surgeon; Anatomist.* Son of John Baynham, physician. EDUCATION: Five-year medical apprenticeship in Va. under Dr. Walker followed by several years study at St. Thomas's Hospital, London, England, where he gained considerable knowledge of anatomy. CAREER: 1772-75, employed by Charles Collignon, professor of anatomy, Cambridge University, England, to dissect and prepare specimens for lectures; 1776-81, employed by St. Thomas's Hospital, London, England, to instruct students in preparing anatomical specimens and to oversee the anatomical and dissecting rooms; 1781-85, after failing to win election by St. Thomas's governors to the professorship of anatomy, became a member of the "Company of Surgeons" and practiced surgery in London; 1785-1814, returned to Essex, Va., and successfully practiced medicine and surgery. CONTRIBUTIONS: Famous for outstanding ability as a surgeon and anatomist. Despite practice in rural Va., gained a national reputation as a surgeon and frequently traveled to other cities and states to practice surgery or give consultations. Did pioneering surgical work on laparotomies and is often credited with performing the first successful operation for extrauterine pregnancy (1785-1814). REFERENCES: "Biographical Sketch of William Baynham, Esq. Surgeon, Late of Essex County, Virginia," *Philadelphia J. of Med. and Physical Sci.* 4 (1822): 186-203; Wyndham Blanton, *Medicine in Virginia in the Eighteenth Century* (1931); *DAB*, 2: 80; Howard A. Kelly, *Cyclopedia of Am. Med. Bio.* 1 (1912); Benjamin Sheppard, "Dr. William Baynham of Virginia," *Virginia Med. Monthly* 81 (1954): 388.

P. Addis

BEACH, WOOSTER (1794, Trumbull, Conn.-January 28, 1868, New York, N.Y.). *Physician; Eclectic.* Son of Lewis Beach. Married Eliza de Grove, 1823; two children. EDUCATION: Studied medicine with Dr. Jacob Tidd, botanic physician of Hunterdon County, N.J.; 1825, College of Physicians and Surgeons, New York City, claimed an M.D. degree; 1832, elected to New York County Medical Society. CAREER: 1820s, practiced medicine, New York City; 1827, established U.S. Medical Infirmary; 1829, expanded the Infirmary into the New York Reformed Medical Academy; 1830, organized medical school, the Academy, Worthington, Ohio; 1832, in charge of the Cholera Hospital, New York City; 1833, published comprehensive text pointing out relationship between pathology and disease; 1836, established *Eclectic Medical Journal*; 1845, moved to Cincinnati, Ohio, to teach at Eclectic Medical Institute; 1849, a founder of National Eclectic Medical Association (president, 1855); 1852, moved to Boston, opened Reformed Medical College. CONTRIBUTIONS: Founder of a medical sect. Eclectics promised medical reforms along botanical lines as the heir of the better educated members of the Thomsonian sect. Opposed bloodletting and purging with mercurials and advocated medication derived from indigenous plants. Accepted the term *eclectic* for his theories, since he drew his ideas from a variety of sources. Edited *Journal* devoted to radical religious and political causes in the latter part of his life.

WRITINGS: *The American Practice of Medicine*, 3 vols. (1833); *Treatise Phthisis Pulmonales, with Remarks on Bronchitis* (1840); *The Family Physician; or the Reformed System of Medicine on Vegetable or Botanical Principles* (1842); *Improved System of Midwifery Adapted to the Reform Practice of Medicine—with Remarks on Physiological and Moral Elevation* (1851). REFERENCES: Miller, *BHM*, p. 9; *DAB*, 2: 85-86; *NCAB*, 23: 318-19; William Rothstein, *American Physicians in the 19th Century* (1972), 217-29.

                                                                              R. Edwards

BEARD, GEORGE MILLER (May 8, 1839, Montville, Conn.-January 23, 1883, New York, N.Y.). *Physician; Neurologist.* Son of Spencer and Lucy (Leonard) Beard. Married Elizabeth Alden, 1866. EDUCATION: 1854-58, Phillips Academy, Andover, Mass.; 1862, graduate, Yale University; 1866, M.D., College of Physicians and Surgeons, New York City. CAREER: 1868, lecturer on the diseases of the nerves, New York University; 1870-83, staff member, Demilt Dispensary, New York City. CONTRIBUTIONS: Published first works in the field of the medical use of electricity. One of the first American neurologists; first to formulate causes and treatment of seasickness. Pioneer in reforms for the care of the mentally ill. Made a specialty of the study of stimulants and narcotics. Developed the classic description of neurasthenia as a syndrome characterized as energy deficiency. Delegate to the International Medical Congress, London (1881).

WRITINGS: *Medical and Surgical Uses of Electricity* (1871); *Stimulants and Narcotics* (1871); *Nervous Exhaustion* (1880); *American Nervousness* (1881); *Sea Sickness* (1882). REFERENCES: G. M. Beard, *American Nervousness, Its Causes and Consequences* (1972), introduction by Charles E. Rosenberg; *DAB*, 1, pt. 2: 92-93; M. B. MacMillan, "Beard's Concept of Neurasthenia," *J. of the Hist. of Behavioral Sci.* 12 (1976): 376-90; *NCAB*, 8: 206; Charles E. Rosenberg, "The Place of George Miller Beard in 19th Century Psychology," *Bull. Hist. Med.* 36 (1962): 245-59; Barbara Sicherman, "The Uses of a Diagnosis," *J. Hist. Med.* 32 (1977): 33-54.

                                                                              J. Carvalho

BEARD, MARY (November 14, 1876, Dover, N.H.-December 4, 1946, New York, N.Y.). *Nurse; Public health.* Daughter of Ithamar Warren, Episcopal rector, and Marcy (Foster) Beard. Never married. EDUCATION: 1903, graduated from New York Hospital School of Nursing. CAREER: 1904-9, visiting nurse, Waterbury (Conn.) Visiting Nurse Association; 1910-12, worked in the Laboratory of Surgical Pathology, College of Physicians and Surgeons (Columbia); director: 1912-22, Boston Instructive District Nursing Association; and 1922-24, Boston Community Health Association; 1924-38, worked at Rockefeller

Foundation; 1938-44, director, American Red Cross Nursing Service; 1942-44, member, National Nursing Council and first chair, committee on nursing and health and medical committee, Office of Defense Health and Welfare Services. CONTRIBUTIONS: During early years in Boston, improved coordination of the work of voluntary health associations and government agencies, culminating in the establishment of the Community Health Association; organization fought for additional preventive health services, including government responsibility for the welfare of babies. Helped found (1912), and during World War I was president of, the National Organization for Public Health Nursing. With the Rockefeller Foundation, directed the spending of over $4 million on nursing projects. Part of money used to attract better educated women into nursing and to improve instruction by giving assistance to university schools of nursing and professional nursing associations. Other funds used to prepare American and foreign women for positions of leadership; travel grants and study programs arranged for approximately 428 nurses from 38 countries and 83 American nurses. Remainder of money used for studies of nursing care in Europe, Africa, and Asia, much of which she did herself, and to develop numerous foreign schools of nursing. Oversaw the recruitment, education, and distribution of nurses in the military and civilian services (1938-44) and put forth plan for fulfilling military needs without depriving the home front of adequate nursing or the nursing schools of qualified instructors.

WRITINGS: *The Nurse in Public Health* (1929). Other writings are mentioned in *DAB*. REFERENCES: *DAB*, Supplement 4 (1974): 64-66; *NCAB*, 35 (1940): 183-84; *Who Was Who in Am.*, 2: 52.

S. Galishoff

BEATTY, THEODORE BRUCE (June 2, 1863, Malden, Ill.-February 12, 1948, San Rafael, Calif.). *Public health administrator.* Son of Fulton H., farmer, and Mary J. (Sansom) Beatty. Married Adelaide Post, 1888; one child. EDUCATION: 1884, M.D., Rush Medical College; 1885, apprenticed to an uncle, Juanita, Ia.; 1886-87, assistant to Charles McBurney (q.v.), Roosevelt Hospital, N.Y.; 1894-95, postgraduate study, Berlin and Vienna. CAREER: 1891-1915, staff of St. Mark's Hospital, Salt Lake City; 1891, chairman, building committee, new St. Mark's Hospital; 1893-94, commissioner of health, Salt Lake City, Utah; 1898-1900, secretary, Utah State Board of Health; 1900-35, Utah State commissioner of health; 1932, president, State and Provincial Health Officers' Association; 1932, survey of child health in Europe for U.S. government. CONTRIBUTIONS: Created the special departments of the Utah State Department of Health. Enforced measures for sanitation and pure water throughout the state. Gained the passage of health education legislation (1907). Supervised a study (1919) of tularemia with U.S. Public Health Service assistance. Under provisions of the Sheppard-Towner Act, organized 194 local health units (1922) to examine preschool children. Supervised the only complete statewide goiter survey (1924-25) and introduced soon afterward the prophylactic use of iodized salt. Introduced

-the International Classification of the Causes of Death, qualifying Utah (1910) as the 23rd state admitted to the Registration Area.

WRITINGS: Annual reports, Utah State Board of Health, 1907-35; presidential address, *Proc., 47th Annual Meeting of the Conference of State and Provincial Health Authorities of North America* (1932). REFERENCES: Joseph R. Morrell, M.D., "The Beatty Period," in *Utah's Health and You. A History of Utah's Public Health* (1956), 77-166; Ralph T. Richards, M.D., *Of Medicine, Hospitals and Doctors* (1953), 44-50.

H. Bauman

BEAUMONT, WILLIAM (November 21, 1785, Lebanon, Conn.-April 25, 1853, St. Louis, Mo.). *Physician; Surgeon; Physiology.* Son of Samuel and Lucretia (Abel) Beaumont. Married Deborah Platt, 1821; three children. EDU-CATION: Lebanon, Conn. Common Schools; 1810-12, apprentice to Dr. Benjamin Chandler, St. Albans, Vt.; 1812, license, Third Medical Society of Vermont. CAREER: 1807-10, schoolteacher, Champlain, N.Y.; 1812-15, assistant surgeon, 6th Infantry Regiment, U.S. Army; 1816-20, private practice, Plattsburgh, N.Y.; 1820-39, surgeon, U.S. Army; 1839-53, private practice, St. Louis, Mo. CON-TRIBUTIONS: Most noted for his investigations of the physiology of digestion carried out on Alexis St. Martin, a French-Canadian hunter whom Beaumont treated for a shotgun wound (1822). When the wound healed, an external fistula allowed access to his stomach. Engaged in several series of experiments on St. Martin and published the results (1833).

WRITINGS: *Experiments and Observations on the Gastric Juice and the Physiology of Digestion* (1833). REFERENCES: *BHM* (1964-69), 25; (1970-75), 18-19; (1975-79), 15; *DSB*, 1: 542-45; Jesse S. Meyer, *Life and Letters of Dr. William Beaumont* (1912); Miller, *BHM*, pp. 9-10; *DAB*, 2: 104-10; R. L. Numbers, "William Beaumont and the Ethics of Human Experimentation," *J. Hist. Biol.* 12 (1979): 113-35; G. Rosen, *The Reception of William Beaumont's Discovery in Europe* (1942).

D. Sneddeker

BECK, CLAUDE SCHAEFFER (November 8, 1894, Shomokin, Pa.-Octo-ber 14, 1971, Euclid, Ohio). *Surgeon; Cardiovascular medicine.* Son of Simon and Martha (Schaeffer) Beck. Married Ellen Manning, 1933; three daughters. EDUCATION: 1916, A.B., Franklin and Marshall College; 1921, M.D., Johns Hopkins; 1922-23, interned, Johns Hopkins Hospital; 1922-23, assistant resident surgeon, New Haven Hospital; 1923-24, associate surgeon, Peter Bent Brigham Hospital. CAREER: 1923-24, Arthur Tracy Cabot fellow, surgical research, Har-vard; 1924-25, surgical staff, University and Lakeside hospitals, Cleveland, Ohio; Western Reserve University Medical School: 1925-28, instructor in sur-gery; 1928-33, assistant professor of surgery; 1933-40, associate professor of surgery; 1940-52, professor of neurosurgery; and 1952-65, professor of cardi-ovascular surgery (first such professorship in the United States); 1942-45, surgical consultant, Fifth Service Command, rank of colonel in the Medical Corps. CONTRIBUTIONS: Performed first mitral valve operation (1924). First successful removal of tumors of the heart (1942). First successful reversal of a fatal heart attack (1955). First successful defibrillation of the human heart (1947). Established the first teaching course in cardiac resuscitation. Helped organize the Resuscitators of America. Beck I Operation created a more even blood supply to the heart by the development of collateral circulation through intercoronary and extracoronary communications (1935); Beck II Operation arteriolized the venous system of the heart by vein graft between aorta and the coronary sinus as well as stimulating the growth of intercoronary communications.

WRITINGS: "The Surgical Treatment of Mitral Stenosis, Experimental and Clinical Studies," *Arch. Surg.* 9 (Nov. 1924): 689 (with E. C. Cutler [q.v.] and S. A. Levine); "The Development of a New Blood Supply to the Heart by Operation," *Annals of Surg.* 102 (1935): 801-13; "The Production of a Collateral Circulation to the Heart. I. An Experimental Study," *Am. Heart J.* 10 (1935): 849-73 (with Vladimir Leslie Tichy); "Resuscitation for Cardiac Standstill and Ventricular Fibrillation Occurring During Operation," *Am. J. Surg.* 54 (Oct. 1941); "Tumor of the Heart (Left Ventricular Wall) Successfully Removed by Operation," *Medico-Surgical Tributes to Harold Brunn* (1942); "Revascularization of the Brain Through Establishment of a Cervical Arteriovenous Fistula. Effects in Children with Mental Retardation and Convulsive Disorders," *J. Pediatrics* 35 (1949): 318-29 (with C. F. McKhann and W. D. Belnap). REFERENCES: Claude S. Beck, "Reminiscences of Cardiac Resuscitation," *Rev. of Surg.* 27 (Mar.-Apr. 1970); biography in *Postgraduate Med.* 1 (1947): 488; Robert M. Hosler, "Historical Notes on Cardiorespiratory Resuscitation," *Am. J. of Cardiology* (Mar. 1959): 416-19; *NCAB*, D: 305.

G. Jenkins

BECK, T[HEODRIC] ROMEYN (August 11, 1791, Schenectady, N.Y.-November 19, 1855, Utica, N.Y.). *Physician; Medical jurisprudence.* Son of Caleb, sailing master, and Catherine Theresa (Romeyn) Beck. Married Harriet Caldwell, 1814. EDUCATION: 1807, A.B., Union College; 1811, M.D., College of Physicians and Surgeons (New York City). CAREER: 1811-17, general practice, Albany, N.Y.; 1815-40, professor, College of Physicians and Surgeons, Fairfield, N.Y.; 1817-48, principal, Albany Academy; 1840-54, professor, Albany Medical College. CONTRIBUTIONS: Systematically and comprehensively reviewed the subject of medical jurisprudence and published a two-volume work (1823) that was regarded as the best publication of its kind in the English language. Twelve editions were eventually issued, and the work was translated into German and Swedish. Lectures and other publications helped to establish the importance of medical jurisprudence as a subject for serious study. President of the Medical Society of the State of New York for three consecutive years (1827-29). Also supported improvements in the care of the mentally ill; served as a member of the Board of Managers of the New York State Lunatic Asylum at Utica (1842-55) and edited the *American Journal of Insanity* (1850-54).

WRITINGS: *Elements of Medical Jurisprudence* (1823). REFERENCES: Chester R. Burns, "Theodric Romeyn Beck (1791-1855) and the Birth of Medical Jurisprudence in the United States," *The Bookman* (Moody Medical Library, University of Texas Medical

Branch), 2 (1975): 1-5; *DAB*, 1, pt. 2: 116-17; J. Lewi Donhauser, "The Life and Career of Dr. T. Romeyn Beck," *Union Worthies* 5 (1950): 5-8, 27-28; *NCAB*, 9: 350; Kelly and Burrage (1920), 87-88.

C. Burns

BECKER, HARRY FRANCIS (December 23, 1890, Knoxville, Ill.-July 25, 1969, Battle Creek, Mich.). *Physician; Health care administration; Pediatrics.* Son of Louis, general practitioner, and Addie (Rearick) Becker. Married Geta Tucker, 1918; three children. EDUCATION: 1917, B.S., Lombard College (Galesburg, Ill.); University of Illinois Medical School; 1919, M.D., University of Michigan Medical School; 1919, medical intern, University Hospital (Ann Arbor, Mich.); 1925, studied pediatrics, Tulane University Medical School. CAREER: 1919-24, general practice, South Haven, Mich.; 1924-25, medical director, Michigan Children's Hospital (Coldwater, Mich.); 1926-69, pediatric practice, Battle Creek, Mich.; 1942-45, colonel, Army Medical Corps; 1946-56, medical director, Michigan Hospital Service (Blue Cross). CONTRIBUTIONS: As medical director of Michigan Blue Cross, directed the nation's first statistical survey of hospital bed utilization, finding a correlation between hospitalization insurance coverage and "unnecessary" hospitalization (1954); pioneer of cost-control in Blue Cross. *Note*: Harry F. Becker should not be confused with Harry Becker (1909-75), long-time health-care activist with the United Automobile Workers in Detroit, Mich., and vice-president of national Blue Cross Association.
WRITINGS: "Controlling Use and Misuse of Hospital Care," *Hospitals* 28 (1954): 61-64. REFERENCES: George N. Fuller, ed., *Michigan: A Centennial History* 4 (1939): 430-31; *Michigan Med.* 68 (1969): 1098.

M. Pernick

BEDFORD, GUNNING (1806, Baltimore, Md.-September 5, 1870, New York, N.Y). *Physician; Obstetrician; Medical educator.* Married; at least two children. EDUCATION: 1825, B.A., Mt. St. Mary's College, Md.; 1829, apprentice to Dr. John D. Godman (q.v.); M.D., Rutgers College; 1829-33, study in Europe. CAREER: 1833, professor, Charleston Medical College, S.C. and then at Albany Medical College, N.Y.; 1836, went to New York City, developed an extensive and lucrative practice in obstetrics; 1840-62, professor of midwifery, University of New York; 1864, suffered a stroke, first of five similar attacks before his death. CONTRIBUTIONS: A well-known obstetrician, founded the first obstetrical clinic in America, at the University of New York medical department. A founder of the medical department of the University of New York (1840) and the New York Academy of Medicine (1848). It was estimated that over 10,000 poor patients per year were treated free of charge at his clinics.
WRITINGS: *The Anatomist's Manual or a Treatise on the Manner of Preparing All the Parts of the Anatomy, Followed by a Complete Description of These Parts* (1832); *A Practical Treatise on Midwifery* (1844); *Clinical Lectures on the Diseases of Women*

(1855); *The Principles and Practice of Obstetrics* (1861). REFERENCES: Kelly and Burrage (1920), 88; MS, New York Academy of Medicine, list of founders; *NCAB*, 9: 361; *N.Y. Times*, September 6, 1870.

D. Rosner

BEEBE, JAMES (May 19, 1881, Lewes, Del.-October 27, 1962, Lewes). *Physician; Surgeon.* Son of Richard, merchant, and Temperance (Magee) Beebe. Married Elsie Edna Kirkland, 1907; five children; Amelia Katherine Rifenbark, 1927; two children. EDUCATION: 1898, Goldey College; 1906, M.D., Jefferson Medical College, Philadelphia, Pa. Made frequent trips to recognized clinics, including the Mayo Clinic, to take short courses and attend lectures. CAREER: 1906-62, private practice; 1916, with brother, Dr. Richard C. Beebe, established Beebe Hospital; subsequently, this hospital served eastern and central Sussex County, Del. CONTRIBUTIONS: An outstanding diagnostician; president: Beebe Hospital (1935-62), Beebe Clinic (1935-62), Medical Society of Delaware (1917). President of Del. branch of American Cancer Society. During World Wars I and II, medical examiner for Sussex County Draft Board. Trustee and treasurer of Delaware State Hospital, the Hospital for the Mentally Retarded at Stockley, Del., and the Governor Bacon Health Center. REFERENCES: "James Beebe, Sr., M.D.," typed manuscript, Beebe Hospital, Lewes; Meridith I. Samuels, *Med. Soc. of Del., 150th Annual Session* (1939), 131-32; *Wilmington Morning News*, October 30, 1962.

W. H. Williams

BEECHER, CLARENCE HENRY (October 9, 1877, Granville, N.Y.-November 21, 1959, Burlington, Vt.). *Physician; Educator.* Son of David and Mary (Waring) Beecher. Married Florence Russell, 1904, two children; Reba Jones, 1931. EDUCATION: 1900, M.D., University of Vermont; 1910, graduate study in Vienna. CAREER: 1900-59, practice of internal medicine, Burlington, Vt.; at the University of Vermont: 1901-4, instructor of anatomy; and 1904-46, instructor, assistant professor, and professor of medicine; and 1941-45, dean; 1925-29, mayor, city of Burlington, Vt.; 1917, president, Vermont State Medical Society; 1953-54, president, Vermont Heart Association. CONTRIBUTIONS: Taught 52 classes of medical students at the University of Vermont, a total of 1,551 persons. At the time of his retirement, it was estimated that a majority of physicians practicing in Vt. had been personally trained by him. Served as dean of the medical college during the difficult war years when money and personnel were short and the future of the institution was being questioned.

WRITINGS: "The Management of Congestive Cardiac Failure," *New England J. of Med.* 209 (1933): 1226-28; "The Electrocardiographic Findings in 44 Cases of Trichinosis," *Am. Heart J.* 16 (1938): 219-24 (with E. L. Amidon). REFERENCES: Material in University of Vermont Archives.

L. J. Wallman

BEECHER, HENRY KNOWLES (February 4, 1904, Wichita, Kansas-July 25, 1976, Boston, Mass.). *Physician; Anesthesia; Educator; Ethics; History.* Son of, Harvard University: Mary Julia (Kerley) Beecher. Married ca. 1934; four children. EDUCATION: University of Kansas: A.B., 1926; Harvard University: M.A., 1927; M.D., 1932, 1932-34, intern, Mass. General Hospital; 1936, assistant resident in surgery, Mass. General Hospital; 1935, Moseley Traveling Fellow (Harvard) at lab of Professor August Krogh, Copenhagen. CAREER: 1936-69, anesthetist-in-chief, Mass. General Hospital; 1941-70, Henry I. Dorr Professor of Research in Anesthesiology, Harvard Medical School; 1943-76, U.S. Army, medical officer and consultant. CONTRIBUTIONS: As operator of the first laboratory devoted exclusively to anesthesia research, teacher of a generation of anesthesiologists, and author of the standard text, *Physiology of Anesthesia* (1938), stimulated the growth of that field. Established the danger of administering morphine to patients still in shock (early 1940s). Campaigned against unethical human research, exposing in print the most blatant examples (1966-76). Helped establish at Harvard a review committee to screen all research proposals for ethical breaches when human subjects were involved. Chaired the Harvard committee which established definition of brain death (1968). Devised methods widely used for the quantification of the effects of drugs on subjective responses, especially pain, drowsiness, sleep, nausea, anxiety (1959). Considered a founding father of scientific psychopharmacology. Wrote history of Harvard Medical School.

WRITINGS: Author of books and many articles, including *Experimentation in Man* (1959); *Measurements of Subjective Responses: Quantitative Effects of Drugs* (1959); "Ethics and Clinical Research," *New Eng. J. of Med.* (1966); *Research and the Individual: Human Studies* (1970); *Medicine at Harvard: The First Three Hundred Years* (1977) (with Mark D. Altschule). REFERENCES: *Anesthesiology*, 45 (1976), 377-78 (obituary); Beecher and Altschule, *Medicine at Harvard* (1977), 413-14; *New Eng. J. of Med.* 295 (1976): 730 (obituary); *N.Y. Times*, July 26, 1976, p. 26; *Who's Who in America*, 38 (1974-75), 1: 205.

                                                                                 T. L. Savitt

BEERS, CLIFFORD WHITTINGHAM (March 30, 1876, New Haven, Conn.-July 9, 1943, Providence, R.I.). *Founder of the mental hygiene movement.* Son of Robert Anthony, in the produce business, and Ida (Cooke) Beers. Married Clara Louise Jepson, 1912; no children. EDUCATION: 1897, Ph.B., Sheffield Scientific School, Yale University. CAREER: 1897, clerical worker, Tax Collector's Office, New Haven; 1899, similar post, New York City; 1899, on staff, Wall Street life insurance company; 1904-39, secretary, several mental hygiene societies he organized. CONTRIBUTIONS: While working in N.Y., suffered a mental breakdown and attempted suicide. From August 1900 to September 1903, spent most of his time in three Conn. mental hospitals. Indignities and violence that Beers and other patients endured in these institutions led him to formulate plans for their reform. After a brief return to the business world (1904), returned to the Hartford Retreat until January 1905, shortly after which he wrote *A Mind That Found Itself* (1908), an account of his illness and an exposition of his program to transform mental hospitals from essentially custodial into therapeutic institutions. With the collaboration of psychiatrist Adolf Meyer (q.v.), who coined the term *mental hygiene*, and Dr. William H. Welch (q.v.), of Johns Hopkins, established the movement with the founding of the Connecticut Society for Mental Hygiene (1908), the first such organization to be created in the world "to work for the conservation of mental health" and to raise standards of care for the mentally ill. Founded the National Committee for Mental Hygiene (February 1909); remained secretary and chief motivating force of the National Committee until 1939. Lack of an adequate and permanent source of support for the work of the National Committee caused Beers to found (May 24, 1928) the American Foundation for Mental Hygiene, of which he was secretary until 1939. Planned the First International Congress for Mental Hygiene (May 1930), resulting (1931) in the formation of the International Committee for Mental Hygiene, of which Beers served as general secretary until 1939.

WRITINGS: *A Mind That Found Itself*, which by 1966 had 38 printings, including 8 new editions with material added relative to the mental hygiene movement. REFERENCES: *DAB*; Norman Dain, *Clifford W. Beers* (1980); C. M. Hincks, "Clifford Whittingham Beers," *Mental Hygiene* 27 (Oct. 1943): 654-56; *NCAB*, 34: 140-41; Arthur H. Ruggles, "Clifford Beers and American Psychiatry," *Am. J. of Psychiatry* 100 (1944): 98-99; C.E.A. Winslow, "Clifford Whittingham Beers," *Mental Hygiene* 28 (Apr. 1944): 179-85; idem, "The Mental Hygiene Movement and Its Founder," in Wilber Cross, ed., *Twenty-Five Years After: Sidelights on the Mental Hygiene Movement and Its Founder* (1934); Eunice E. Winters, "Adolph Meyer and Clifford Beers, 1907-1910," *Bull. Hist. Med.* 43 (1969): 414-43.

J. Ifkovic

BEHLE, AUGUSTUS CALVIN (January 24, 1871, Moro, Ill.-July 26, 1951, Salt Lake City, Utah). *Surgeon.* Son of William H., Presbyterian minister, and physician after 1882, and Johanna (Busch) Behle. Married Daisy Harroun, 1905; three children. EDUCATION: 1890, licensed pharmacist, Blackfoot, Idaho; 1894, M.D., Rush Medical College; 1894-97, intern, St. Mark's Hospital, Salt Lake City; 1897-98, postgraduate study with William Welch (q.v.), William Osler (q.v.), William Halsted (q.v.), Howard Kelly (q.v.), and Joseph Bloodgood (q.v.), Johns Hopkins University; 1903-4, 1910-11, studied at the University of Vienna and the Allgemeines Krankenhaus in Vienna. CAREER: 1897-1931, staff, St. Mark's Hospital, Salt Lake City; in Utah State Medical Association: 1895, charter member; and 1922, president; 1920, elected Fellow, American College of Surgeons; 1906-7, lecturer, University of Utah Medical School. CONTRIBUTIONS: Introduced advanced surgical practices (1898) into St. Mark's Hospital, including the use of rubber gloves, aseptic surgery, sterilized catgut. Set up the first bacteriological laboratory at St. Mark's (1898). Helped acquire first X-ray equipment (1905). Led effort to gain accreditation for St. Mark's Hospital (1921).

WRITINGS: "Pyloric Obstruction," *Denver Med. Times* 23 (1903): 215-24; "The Surgery of the Thyroid Gland," *Utah Med. J.* 27 (1907): 146-52, 154-56; "The Pituitary Body and Its Importance to the Surgeon," *Northwest Med.* 11 (1912): 165-71; "Tuberculosis Peritonitis," *Northwest Med.* 13 (1914); "General Septic Peritonitis and Its Treat ment," *Northwest Med.*, 21 (1922): 361-65. REFERENCES: William H. Behle, *Biography of Augustus C. Behl, with an Account of St. Mark's Hospital, Salt Lake City* (1948); *NCAB* 51 (1969): 375-76; Ralph T. Richards, M.D., *Of Medicine, Hospitals and Doctors* (1953), 38-42.

H. Bauman

BÉKÉSY, GEORG VON   See VON BÉKÉSY, GEORG.

BELISLE, HENRI   (1675, Angers, France-September, 1740, Montreal, Quebec, Canada). *Surgeon; Military surgery.* Son of Anthony Lamarre, apothecary, and Marguerite (Levasseur) Belisle. Married Catherine Demosny, 1690, two children; Marie Francoise Perinne Dandonneau, 1705, no children; Jeanne Archambault, 1712, seven children. EDUCATION: Before 1690, supposed to have studied surgery in France. CAREER: Before 1690, arrived in Quebec; 1704-11, surgeon, Detroit, Mich.; 1712-40, surgeon, Montreal. CONTRIBUTIONS: First known medical practitioner in Detroit. Appears in the records as godfather to both French and Indian children. His stay in Detroit was marked by pay disputes with Antoin Cadillac. George Christian Anthon (1734-1815) is generally regarded as the first practitioner in British Detroit, 1760. REFERENCES: Fannie Anderson, *Doctors Under Three Flags* (1951), 15-16; C. B. Burr, *Medical History of Michigan* 1 (1930): 90; *Burton Historical Collections Leaflet* 8 (1929): 18; Kelly and Burrage (1928): 92.

M. Pernick

BELL, LUTHER VOSE   (December 20, 1806, Francestown, N.H.-February 11, 1862, Budd's Ferry, Md.). *Physician; Asylum superintendent.* Son of Samuel, member of N.H. legislature, chief justice of N.H., governor, and U.S. senator, and Mehitable (Dana) Bell. Married Frances Pinkerton, 1834. EDUCATION: 1823, A.B., Bowdoin College; 1826, M.D., Dartmouth College. CAREER: c. 1830, practiced medicine, Brunswick, Chester, and Derry, N.H.; 1835-36, served in state legislature; helped establish state asylum at Concord, N.H.; 1837-56, superintendent, McLean Asylum, Mass.; president: 1851-55, Association of Medical Superintendents of American Institutions for the Insane; and 1857-59, Massachusetts Medical Society; planner for Butler Hospital (Providence, R.I.) and Northampton State Asylum (Mass.); volunteer surgeon, Civil War; at the time of his death, division medical director, Army of the Potomac. CONTRIBUTIONS: Received the Boylston prize (1834) for a paper, "The Dietetic Regimen Best Fitted for the Inhabitants of New England." One of the most outstanding of the "original 13" founding fathers of the Association of Medical Superintendents of American Institutions for the Insane. A leading advocate of moral treatment, a legal expert of insanity, testifying in many important court cases, and a consultant on the planning of mental institutions. Gained professional stature for identifying "Bell's disease," often labeled "acute delirium" or "typhomania."

WRITINGS: Wrote on a range of topics including diet for laborers, heating and ventilation, crime and insanity, smallpox, and "Bell's disease." "On a Form of Disease Resembling Some Advanced Stages of Mania and Fever, but so Contradistinguished from any Ordinarily Observed or Described Combination of Symptoms, as to Render It Probable That It May Be an Overlooked and Hitherto Unrecorded Malady," *Am. J. of Insanity* 6 (1849-50): 97; His annual reports from McLean Asylum were highly informative on administrative subjects. REFERENCES: *DAB* 2 (1929): 160; Kelly and Burrage (1928), 90-91; *One Hundred Years of American Psychiatry* (1944), 54-56.

L. V. Bell

BELL, SIMEON BISHOP (May 13, 1820, Sussex County, N.J.-January 16, 1913, Rosedale, now Kansas City, Kans.). *Physician*. Son of Jabesh, farmer and builder of mills, and Gertrude (Nichols) Bell. Married Eleanor Taylor, 1846, ten children; Margaret Bellis, 1866, two children. EDUCATION: Unable to read or write at age 21, worked his way through school; 1853, M.D., Starling Medical College, Columbus, Ohio. CAREER: Began practice in Mansfield, Ohio, and then moved to Johnson County, Kans.; outspoken support of the Union brought him repeated grief, including a fractured skull, at the hands of Quantrill's men; after the war, accumulated considerable wealth through dealings in real estate. CONTRIBUTIONS: Offered land and money to the University of Kansas to establish a hospital and medical college (1874). Gift was accepted, but by 1903 nothing had happened, and Bell added land valued at $25,000. Three Kansas City proprietary medical schools merged (1905), and the legislature finally approved Bell's plan for the teaching hospital that became the clinical facility of the University of Kansas School of Medicine. Opposition to the new school continued, and it appeared (1913) that the center of Kans. medical education might be removed to Topeka. Wrote an impassioned plea to the legislature asking them to honor the commitment they assumed by accepting his previous gifts, and the legislature responded by appropriating money for a dispensary and laboratory. The Medical College of Topeka merged with the University of Kansas, and clinical instruction thereafter centered in the Kansas City area. REFERENCES: Robert H. Chesky, "Simeon B. Bell," *J. of the Kansas Med. Soc.* 67 (1966): 177-90, 199; Helen M. Sims, *Simeon Bishop Bell, M.D.* (1979).

R. Hudson

BENEDICT, FRANCIS GANO (October 3, 1870, Milwaukee, Wis.-May 14, 1957, Machiasport, Maine). *Physiological chemist*. Son of Washington Gano, businessman, and Harriet Emily (Barrett) Benedict. Married Cornelia Golay, 1897; one child. EDUCATION: Harvard University: 1893, A.B.; 1894, M.A.; University of Heidelberg, 1895, Ph. D. CAREER: 1892-94, chemistry faculty, Massachusetts College of Pharmacy; 1895-1907, physiological chemist, U.S. Department of Agriculture; 1896-1900, chemist, Storrs Agricultural Experiment Station; 1896-1907, chemistry faculty, Wesleyan University; 1907-37, director, Nutrition Laboratory of the Carnegie Institution of Washington. CONTRIBUTIONS: One of the world's leading authorities on animal calorimetry and respiration metabolism; equally renowned for the discoveries he made and the equipment and methods he devised. Most important invention was instrument to simultaneously and directly measure oxygen absorption, expired air, and heat (1910); led to development (1919) of basal metabolic rates of humans, which are still in use. Changed treatment of diabetics by demonstrating that their metabolic rate was higher than that of healthy persons (1912). Improved the Wilbur Atwater (q.v.)-Rosa respiration calorimeter by reducing its size and cost. Adopted the calorimeter to measure the heat production of animals ranging in size from elephants to mice (1907-38). Sought to reveal the laws governing heat production and heat loss in humans and animals; led to extensive comparisons of the metabolism of cold- and warm-blooded animals and the effects of age, race, sex, disease, and other factors. Concluded that except in emotional disturbances, basal rates were constant in humans, but that in some animal species, notably sheep and geese, there was lability of basal metabolism (1938). Accepted the idea (by 1910) that organisms do not generate heat in any simple, mechanical way, but largely ignored the work being done at this time on vitamins and the role of enzymes in cellular respiration.

WRITINGS: *Respiration Calorimeters for Studying the Respiratory Exchange and Energy Transformations of Man*, Carnegie Instit. of Wash., *Bull. No. 123* (1910, with T. M. Carpenter); *A Study of Metabolism in Severe Diabetes*, Carnegie Instit. of Wash., *Bull. No. 176* (1912, with E. P. Joslin); *Vital Energetics: A Study in Comparative Basal Metabolism*, Carnegie Instit. of Wash., *Bull. No. 503* (1938). For other writings, see *BMNAS*. REFERENCES: *BMNAS* 32 (1958): 66-98; *DSB*, 1: 609-11; Leonard A. Maynard, "Frances Gano Benedict—A Biographical Sketch," *J. of Nutrition* 98 (May 1969): 3-8; *Who Was Who In Am.*, 3: 66.

S. Galishoff

BENEDICT, STANLEY ROSSITER (March 17, 1884, Cincinnati, Ohio-December 21, 1936, Elmsford, N.Y.). *Chemist; Biological chemistry.* Son of Wayland Richardson, university professor, and Anne Elizabeth (Kendrick) Benedict. Married Ruth Fulton, 1913; no children. EDUCATION: 1906, B.A., University of Cincinnati; 1908, Ph.D., Yale University. CAREER: 1908-9, chemistry faculty, Syracuse University; 1909-10, associate in biological chemistry, Columbia University; at Cornell University Medical College: 1910-11, chemical pathology faculty; and 1911-36, chemistry faculty; 1919-20, president, American Society of Biological Chemists. CONTRIBUTIONS: With Otto Folin (q.v.), greatly improved analytical methods for investigating the chemistry of physiological processes; methods for analyzing uric acid, creatine and creatinine, total sulfur, sugar, and so on, developed by Folin, were improved shortly thereafter by Benedict; previous methods had required either special skills or impracticably large amounts of biological material; work made chemical analysis an important tool in the diagnosis and treatment of disease. Analyzed the principal nonprotein constituents of blood and urine in connection with the study of normal and abnormal metabolism. Developed Benedict's Solution, a reagent used to test for glucose in urine. Did important studies of quantitative blood chemistry and carbohydrate metabolism. Pioneered in disturbing the metabolic processes of tumors in an unsuccessful attempt to cause regression. Managing editor of *Journal of Biological Chemistry* (1920 until his death). WRITINGS: "The Estimation of Total Sulphur in Urine," *J. of Biological Chem.* 6 (1909): 363-71; "A Reagent for the Detection of Reducing Sugars," *ibid.*, 5 (1909): 485-87; "Studies in Creatine and Creatinine Metabolism. I. The Preparation of Creatine and Creatinine from Urine," *ibid.*, 18 (1914): 183-90; "The Determination of Uric Acid in Urine," *ibid.*, 51 (1922): 187-207. A bibliography is in *BMNAS*. REFERENCES: *BMNAS* 27 (1952): 155-71; *DAB*, Supplement 2: 35-36; Miller, *BHM*, p. 11; *Who Was Who in Am.*, 1: 82-83.

S. Galishoff

BENITES, JOSÉ MARIA (1790-1855). *Surgeon; Military surgery.* EDUCATION: Probably a Catalan; likely trained at one of the Catalonian schools for military or naval surgery. CAREER: 1803-6, surgeon-general of Alta Calif. CONTRIBUTIONS: September 1804, viceroy of Calif., Joseph de Iturrigaray, sent Benites a directive ordering the surgeon to investigate the causes and report on the high mortality rate among the soldiers, Indians, and colonists of Alta Calif.; detailed account, dated January 1, 1805, is first official report on health conditions in Alta Calif. written by trained practitioner.

WRITINGS: "Informe," *California Mission Document*, (January 1, 1805), 671. A bowdlerized version of Benites's report was translated and printed in Sherburne F. Cook, "California's First Medical Survey: Report of Surgeon-General José Benites," *California and Western Med.* 45 (1936): 352-54. "Certificate of Illness," *California Mission Document* (January 9, 1806), 716. REFERENCES: Cephas L. Bard, "Medicine and Surgery Among the First Californians," *Touring Topics* 22 (1930): 25-27; S. F. Cook, "The Monterrey Surgeons During the Spanish Period in California," *Bull. Hist. Med.* 5 (1937): 69-70; Zephyrin Engelhardt, *The Missions and Missionaries of California* (1930), 628-29; Henry Harris, *California's Medical Story* (1932), 28-29; G. D. Lyman, "The Scalpel Under Three Flags in California," *California Hist. Soc. Q.* 4 (1925): 6-7.

Y. V. O'Neill

BENJAMIN, DOWLING (January 23, 1849, Baltimore, Md.-November 20, 1930, Camden, N.J.). *Physician.* Son of Justus, railroader, and Anne (Dobson) Benjamin. Married Sarah Cooper White, 1879; five children. EDUCATION: Public schools, Baltimore; tutored privately; apprentice to Dr. J. H. Jamer (Port Deposit, Md.), Dr. J. M. Ridge (Camden), and Dr. D. Hayes Agnew (q.v.) (Philadelphia); 1877, M.D., University of Pennsylvania Medical School. CAREER: 1877-1920s, private practice, Camden; surgeon, obstetrician, gynecologist, Cooper Hospital, Camden; medical faculty: 1877, New Jersey Training School for Nurses; and 1890, Medico-Chirurgical College, Philadelphia; president: New Jersey Sanitary Association; and New Jersey State Board of Health; died of cancer of the bladder. CONTRIBUTIONS: Pioneer advocate (1877) of bacteriological pathology. M.D. thesis, "Infection and Antiseptic Practices," endorsed by his professors as "the first clear, logical and convincing presentation of the germ theory by an American medical writer." Performed (1888) the first successful hysterectomy in N.J. Instrumental in persuading the N.J. legislature to establish (1890) a State Board of Medical Examiners. WRITINGS: Writings listed in William M. Brown, ed., *Biographical, Genealogical and Descriptive History of the State of New Jersey* (1900), 447. REFERENCES: *Biographical Review: Camden and Burlington Counties*, 19 (1897): 319-23; Brown, *Biographical Genealogical and Descriptive History of the State of New Jersey*, pp. 444-48; Francis Bazley Lee, "Genealogical and Memorial History of the State of New Jersey," *JAMA* 95 (1930): 1852; "Resolution of Camden County Medical Society on the Death of Dr. Dowling Benjamin," *J. of the Med. Soc. of N.J.* 28 (1931): 84; John R. Stevenson, *History of Medicine and Medical Men of Camden County* (1886), 140, 199, 202, 222, 260.

W. Barlow

BENTLEY, EDWIN (July 3, 1824, New London County, Conn.-February 5, 1917, Little Rock, Ark.). *Physician; Educator*. Son of William and Hannah (Phillips) Bentley. Married Marguerite Williams, 1872; one son. EDUCATION: 1849, M.D., medical department, University of the City of New York; 1878, postgraduate terms, Bellevue Hospital Medical College and College of Physicians and Surgeons, Columbia University. CAREER: 1849-61, private practice, Norwich, Conn.; 1861-88, U.S. Army Medical Corps; 1879-84, 1888-1916, medical department, Arkansas Industrial University (University of Arkansas after 1899); 1904-7, dean, medical department, University of Arkansas. CONTRIBUTIONS: Helped organize the medical department of the College of the Pacific (1869) and became a charter faculty member. Urged the establishment of the medical department of Arkansas Industrial University (1879) and became a charter faculty member. Established the first free clinic in Little Rock (1879). Worked to restore harmony to a divided regular profession in Arkansas (beginning in 1878). Contributed occasionally to the fledgling *Journal of the Arkansas Medical Society*. Was honored as president of the Pulaski Medical Society (Little Rock) and the Arkansas State Medical Society (1888). REFERENCES: W. David Baird, *Medical Education in Arkansas* (1979), 27; *Goodspeed Biographical and Historical Memoirs of Central Arkansas* (1978), 462-63; *NCAB*, 6: 374; *Who Was Who in Am.*, 4 (1970): 78.

D. Konold

BERTNER, ERNST WILLIAM (August 18, 1889, Colorado City, Tex.-July 28, 1950, Houston, Tex.). *Gynecologist; Medical administration*. Son of Gustave, German immigrant, and Anna (Miller) Bertner. Married Julia Williams, 1922; no children. EDUCATION: 1903-6, New Mexico Military Institute, Roswell, N.M.; 1911, M.D., University of Texas Medical Branch, Galveston, Tex.; 1911-13, intern, St. Vincent's Hospital, Willard Parker Hospital, and the Manhattan Maternity Hospital; 1921-22, postgraduate study in surgery, gynecology, and urology, Johns Hopkins. CAREER: 1913-17, practice, Houston; 1917-19, medical corps, World War I: with the British army and the American Expeditionary

Force, wounded and discharged as a major; 1919-21, practice, Houston; 1922 (after postgraduate work in Baltimore, Md.), practice, Houston; 1943-50, professor of gynecology, Baylor University College of Medicine; president: 1933, Harris County Medical Society; and 1938-39, Texas Medical Society; 1935, chief of staff, Hermann Hospital; 1942-46, acting director, M. D. Anderson Hospital for Cancer Research; 1945-50, president, Board of Trustees, Texas Medical Center. CONTRIBUTIONS: Prime organizer and administrator of the Texas Medical Center, M.D. Anderson Hospital, and Baylor University College of Medicine in Houston. Personal physician to Jesse Jones, business magnate and philanthropist. With a score of outstanding men, worked together to put Houston's Texas Medical Center in position for take-off to prominence.

WRITINGS: Papers are at the Houston Academy of Medicine-Texas Medical Center Library; completed a paper after his year at Hopkins, "Adenocystomata of the Ovary," *Texas State J. of Med.* 18 (1922): 355-60; "The Future of the Medical Center," *ibid.*, 41 (1946): 625-28. REFERENCES: *The First Twenty Years of the University of Texas M.D. Anderson Hospital and Tumor Institute* (1964); N. Don Macon, *A Story of the Texas Medical Center* (1973); Walter H. Moursund, *History of the Baylor University College of Medicine* (1956); William D. Seybold, "E. W. Bertner: Cancer Fighter (address to the Texas Surg. Soc., October 4, 1971, unpublished ms. by Seybold and source materials of Dr. Lee Clark, Houston); *Texas State J. of Med.* 46 (1950) : 728-29.

J. Morris

BEVAN, ARTHUR DEAN (August 9, 1861, Chicago, Ill.-June 10, 1943, Lake Forest, Ill.). *Surgeon; Reformer of medical education.* Son of Thomas and Sarah (Ramsey) Bevan. Married Anna L. Barber, 1896; no children. EDUCATION: 1878-79, Sheffield Scientific School (Yale); 1883, M.D., Rush Medical College. CAREER: 1883-87, U.S. Marine Hospital Service; 1886-87, professor of anatomy, Oregon State University, Portland, Ore.; 1887-1934, professor of anatomy and surgery, Rush Medical College; 1892-1943, Presbyterian Hospital surgical staff (chief, 1894-1934). CONTRIBUTIONS: Helped reform American medical education. Chairman, AMA Committee on Medical Education (1902-4) and Council on Medical Education (1904-16, 1920-28). Worked closely with the Carnegie Foundation on developments leading to the Flexner Report on American medical education (1910). As a surgeon, developed several procedures, and his name was long associated with an operation for hydrocele of the testis. Developed the "hockey stick" incision for gallbladder operation and (1923) performed first operation in which ethylene oxygen was used as an anesthetic. President, AMA (1918-19). A founder and member, first board of directors, American College of Surgeons. President, American Surgical Association (1932).

WRITINGS: Compiled two textbooks, including an American edition of Lexer's *General Surgery.* REFERENCES: *DAB,* Supplement 3: 67; *NCAB,* D: 90; and 31: 282; *Who Was Who in Am.*, 2: 61.

J. Carvalho

BIDDLE, ANDREW PORTER (February 25, 1862, Detroit, Mich.-August 2, 1944, Detroit). *Surgeon; Dermatology.* Son of William Shepherd, lawyer and gentleman, and Susan Dayton (Ogden) Biddle. Married Grace Wilkins, 1892; one child. EDUCATION: Briefly attended U.S. Naval Academy; 1886, M.D., Detroit College of Medicine; 1885-87, intern and resident physician, Harper Hospital, Detroit; 1890, studied dermatology in Leipzig. CAREER: 1887, practice with Detroit police surgeon James Burgess Book; 1892, lecturer in dermatology, Detroit College of Medicine; 1898, major surgeon, 31st Michigan Volunteer Infantry and U.S. Typhoid Fever Commission; 1902-18, professor of dermatology, Wayne University College of Medicine; 1902-6, founding editor, Michigan State Medical Society, *Journal*; 1913-19, member, Michigan State Board of Health; 1916-18, president, Michigan State Medical Society; 1917-25, member, and 1918-19, president, Detroit Board of Education; president: 1925-26, American Dermatological Association; and 1931, 1943, Detroit Library Commission; consulting dermatologist to St. Mary's, Woman's, and Detroit Receiving Hospitals and Protestant Children's Home. CONTRIBUTIONS: With Leartus Connor (q.v.), led the reorganization and revival of the Michigan State Medical Society and founded the society's journal (1902). An early promoter of postgraduate medical education.

WRITINGS: "Supervision of Specialism," *Michigan State Med. Soc., J.* 32 (1933): 456-57; "Medicine: Influence of Social Forces," *ibid.*, 34 (1935): 645-49. REFERENCES: *Annals of Internal Med.* 21 (1944): 931-32; *Arch. of Dermatology and Syphilis* 50 (1944): 333; C. B. Burr, *Medical History of Michigan* (1930), 1: 646; 2: 427-28; C. M. Burton, *City of Detroit* 4 (1922): 740-44; *JAMA* 125 (1944): 1156; Paul Leake, *History of Detroit* 3 (1912): 1041-44; A. N. Marquis, *Book of Detroiters* (1914), 59; *Michigan State Med. Soc., J.* 43 (1944): 782, 830; *Who Was Who in Am. J.*, 2: 61.

M. Pernick

BIERRING, WALTER LAWRENCE (July 15, 1868, Davenport, Ia.-June 24, 1961, Des Moines, Ia.). *Physician; Bacteriology; Education; Public health.* Son of Jeppe and Catherine Elizabeth (Jessen) Bierring. Married Sadie Byrnes, 1896; two children. EDUCATION: 1892, M.D., State University of Iowa; 1892-93, postgraduate studies in bacteriology with Ernst at Heidelberg; 1893, Vienna; 1894-95, with Pasteur, Metchnikoff, Borrell, and Roux, Pasteur Institute, Paris; 1896, 1901, six-month courses of study, London, Paris, Berlin, Prague, and Vienna. CAREER: At State University of Iowa College of Medicine: 1892-1903, professor and head, Department of Pathology and Bacteriology; 1903-10, professor and head, Department of the Practice of Medicine; 1910-13, professor and head, Department of Medicine, Drake University, Des Moines; 1913-33, private practice in internal medicine, Des Moines; 1915-35, founding member, National Board of Medical Examiners; 1915-60, secretary-editor, Federation of State Medical Boards of the U.S.; 1918, member, National Commission on Medical Education; 1925-32, AAMC-AMA Commission on Medical Education; 1933-53, Iowa State commissioner of health; organizing member: 1936, American Board of Internal Medicine (1936-39, first chairman, holder of Certificate No. 1); and 1947, American Board of Preventive Medicine (1947-56, first chairman, holder of Certificate No. 1); 1953-60, director, Division of Gerontology, Heart and Chronic Diseases, Iowa State Department of Health. CONTRIBUTIONS: Sometimes called the "Dean of the Iowa Medical Profession," was the first professor of bacteriology at Iowa, and instituted the first formal graduate course in the medical school (1895, "Pasteur Course in Practical Bacteriology"). Prepared and distributed the first diphtheria antitoxin west of the Mississippi (1895). Through his efforts, the State Hygienic Laboratory was established (1903, Iowa City, Ia.). As an organizer of the National Board of Medical Examiners and as secretary-editor of the Federation of State Medical Boards for 48 years, directly influenced raising the standards of licensure examinations and thus of clinical practice. Helped establish both the American Board of Internal Medicine and the American Board of Preventive Medicine and was also influential in establishing aviation medicine as a specialty. During his 20-year tenure as Iowa State health commissioner, important public health legislation was implemented (especially in regard to venereal disease and to sewage disposal). Will always be thought of as personifying the development of public health work in Iowa.

WRITINGS: A prolific writer. "Modern Treatment of Diphtheria with Demonstration of Preparing Antitoxin," *Trans., Iowa Med. Soc.* (1895), 54-61 (and *J. Iowa Med. Soc.* 15 [1925]: 171); "The Role of Pathology and Physiology in Preventive Medicine," *JAMA* 55 (Aug. 13, 1910): 554; "Early Regulation of the Practice of Medicine in America," *Federation Bull.* 10 (1924): 295; "Undulant Fever: Clinical Characteristics Based on a Study of 150 Cases in Iowa," *JAMA* 93 (Sept. 21, 1929): 897; "The Function of the State in Relation to Specialized Practice," *Federation Bull.* 19 (1933): 215. Many of his works are included in "A Selected Bierring Bibliography," *J. Iowa State Med. Soc.* 47 (1957): 475. REFERENCES: William B. Bean, "Walter L. Bierring: An Appreciation," *Geriatrics* 16 (Jul. 1961): 355; Walter L. Bierring, *A History of the Department of Internal Medicine, State University of Iowa College of Medicine, 1870-1958* (1958); Morris Fishbein, *A History of the American Medical Association, 1847-1947* (1947); Daniel J. Glomset, "Recollections of Walter Lawrence Bierring, M. D.," *J. Iowa State Med. Soc.* 47 (1957): 478; Philip G. Kiel, "Walter Lawrence Bierring and the Specialty of Aviation Medicine," *J. Iowa State Med. Soc.* 47 (1957): 485; Miller, *BHM*, p. 12; *One Hundred Years of Iowa Medicine, 1850-1950* (1950); Joseph B. Priestley, "Iowa's Osler," *J. Iowa State Med. Soc.* 47 (1957): 471; *WWAPS*; University of Iowa Archives, Iowa City, Ia.; *Who's Important in Medicine* (1945); *Who's Who in Am. Med.* (1925).

R. E. Rakel

BIGELOW, HENRY JACOB (March 11, 1818, Boston, Mass.-October 30, 1890, Newton, Mass.). *Medical educator; Surgeon; Orthopedics; Urology.* Son of Jacob (q.v.), physician, and Mary (Scollay) Bigelow. Married Susan Sturgis, 1847; one child. EDUCATION: Boston Latin; 1837, A.B., Harvard; 1837-39, studied medicine with his father; 1837-38, Dartmouth Medical School; 1840-44, medical study in London and Paris; 1841, M.D., Harvard Medical School (during visit home). CAREER: 1844, opened with Dr. Henry Bryant a "Charitable Institution for Outdoor Patients" and ran into strong criticism for advertising the fact; 1845-58, faculty, Tremont Street Medical School; at Harvard Medical

School: 1849-82, medicine faculty; and 1882-90, emeritus; 1846-86, medical staff, Massachusetts General Hospital. CONTRIBUTIONS: Although only an observer at the epic public ether demonstration by W. T. G. Morton (q.v.) and John C. Warren (q.v.) at the Massachusetts General (October 16, 1846), may have played an important role in bringing it about and certainly played a major role in publicizing its success. May have collaborated with Morton in experimenting with ether in a number of private operations before the public demonstration (see statement by Morton's son in *JAMA* 56 [1911]: 1677). Following this, reported the successful result to the American Academy of Arts and Sciences (November 3) and the Boston Society for Medical Improvement (November 9) and published the first printed account in the *Boston Medical and Surgical Journal* (November 18). A major innovator in orthopedic surgery. Won the Boylston Prize (1844) for his *Manual of Orthopedic Surgery*, the first comprehensive treatment of the subject in America and a superb summary of the French orthopedic surgery of the day. Performed the first known excision of the hip joint in the United States (1852). Described the structure and function of the accessory Y (iliofemoral) ligament of capsular ligament of the hip joint (1861), which clarified the pathology of dislocation of the hip, and published (1869) *Mechanism of Dislocation and Fracture of the Hip with Reduction of Dislocation by the Flexion Method*, an outstanding summary of his eight years' research in this area. In urological surgery, improved the lithotrite used for crushing bladder stones and developed a large caliber evacuation tube to remove effectively the debris. Also an early expert in microscopy. Was also a bitter opponent of the admission of blacks and women to Harvard Medical School, of the modernizing reforms of President Eliot, and of venesection. Slow to comprehend and accept Listerism.

WRITINGS: *Manual of Orthopedic Surgery* (1845); "Insensibility During Surgical Operations, Produced by Inhalation," *Boston Med. and Surg. J.* 35 (1846): 309-17, 379; "Resection of the Head of the Femur," *Am. J. of Med. Sci.*, n.s., 24 (1852): 90; *Mechanism of Dislocation and Fracture of the Hip with Reduction of Dislocation by the Flexion Method* (1869); *Lithotrity by a Single Operation* (1878); *Surgical Anesthesia, Addresses and Other Papers* (1894). REFERENCES: [William Sturgis Bigelow], *A Memoir of Henry Jacob Bigelow* (1900); *DAB* 1, pt. 2: 256-57; O. W. Holmes, "Memoir of Henry Jacob Bigelow," *Proceedings of the Am. Acad. of Arts and Sci.* 26 (1890-91): 339-50; G. H. Jackson, Jr., "Henry Jacob Bigelow, Orthopedic Surgeon," *Arch. of Surg.* 46 (1943): 666-72; Kelly and Burrage (1920), 98-100; *NCAB*, 7: 37.

P. Cash

BIGELOW, JACOB (February 27, 1786, Sudbury, Mass.-January 10, 1879, Boston, Mass.). *Physician; Medical educator; Pharmacologist; Botanist.* Son of Jacob, a Congregational minister, and Elizabeth (Flagg) Bigelow. Married Mary Scollay, 1817; five children, including Henry J. (q.v.). EDUCATION: 1806, A.B., Harvard University; studied medicine with Dr. John Gorham of Boston and the Harvard Medical School; 1810, M.D., University of Pennsylvania Medical School. CAREER: Following graduation from medical school, began an as sociation with Dr. James Jackson (q.v.) in Boston; won Boylston Prize for four successive years; 1815-55, faculty, Harvard Medical School; 1816-27, first Rumford professor, Harvard University; 1838-58, faculty, Tremont Street Medical School; 1842-47, president, Massachusetts Medical Society; 1846-54, Harvard overseer; 1847-63, president, American Academy of Arts and Sciences. CONTRIBUTIONS: A leading early botanist and pharmacologist, lectured on botany at Harvard, compiled the pioneering *Flora Bostonienses* (1814; enlarged, 1824) and *American Medical Botany* (3 vols., 1817-20). A major contributor to the first *United States Pharmacopoeia* (1820) and author of *Treatise on Materia Medica* (1822). Responding to the work of Pierre Louis and the Paris School, became the leading American champion of the doctrine that nature cures most diseases and opponent of the excessive use of drugs and bleeding ("heroic therapy"). His paper "Self-limited Diseases" was of primary importance in advancing these concepts in America. A prodigious and multitalented worker, originated the concept and design of the famous Mount Auburn Cemetery (1831), a new style, rural, garden-type burial ground intended to avoid unhealthful urban interments. A founder of the *New England Journal of Medicine and Surgery* (1812), the Tremont Street Medical School (1838), and M.I.T. (1861). Coined the term *technology*. A social conservative, firmly opposed the admission of blacks and women to the Harvard Medical School.

WRITINGS: *Elements of Technology* (1829); *A Discourse on Self-limited Diseases, Delivered Before the Massachusetts Medical Society at Their Annual Meeting, May 27, 1835* (1835); *Nature in Disease and Other Writings* (1854); *Brief Expositions of Rational Medicine* (1858); *Modern Inquiries* (1867). REFERENCES: *BHM* (1964-69), 33; (1970-74), 23; (1980), 7; *DAB*, 1, pt. 2: 257-58; G. E. Ellis, *Memoir of Jacob Bigelow, M.D., LL.D.* (1880); O. W. Holmes, "Jacob Bigelow," *Proc. of the Am. Acad. of Arts and Sci.* 14 (1878-79): 332-42; Kelly and Burrage (1920), 100-101; *NCAB*, 4: 526; *Vital Records of Sudbury, Massachusetts, to the Year 1850* (1903), p. 18.

P. Cash

BIGGS, HERMANN MICHAEL (September 29, 1859, Trumansburg, N.Y.-June 28, 1923, New York, N.Y.). *Physician; Pathologist; Microbiology.* Son of Joseph H. and Melissa (Pratt) Biggs. Married Frances M. Richardson, 1898; two children. EDUCATION: 1882, B.A., Cornell University; 1883, M.D., Bellevue Hospital Medical College; intern, Bellevue Hospital; postgraduate study at Berlin and Greifswald, Germany. CAREER: 1886, appointed to house staff, Bellevue, as pathologist; first director, Carnegie Laboratory of the Bellevue Hospital Medical College; taught bacteriology, Bellevue Hospital Medical College, after graduation; 1901-14, general medical officer, New York Department of Health, while continuing as professor of therapeutics and medicine, Bellevue Hospital Medical College; 1914, accepted position as state health commissioner. CONTRIBUTIONS: Director of the first American laboratory devoted to microbiology and responsible for using bacteriological methods in sanitary surveillance of infectious diseases. Introduced diphtheria antitoxin into America and directed production of first serum (1895). Directed and formulated work for the prevention of tuberculosis and established tuberculosis clinics and dispensaries run by the New York City Department of Health. As state health commissioner (after 1914), responsible for much of N. Y.'s legislation on public sanitation.

WRITINGS: *The Health of the City of New York* (1895); *Report of Bacterial Investigations and Diagnosis of Diphtheria* (1895); *Preventive Medicine in the City of New York* (1897); *The Administrative Control of Tuberculosis* (1904); *Tuberculosis Campaign: Its Influence on the Methods of Public Health Work Generally* (1913). REFERENCES: *BHM* (1975-79), 18; *DAB*, 2: 262-63; John Duffy, *History of Public Health in New York City (1866-1966)* (1974); Miller, *BHM*, p. 12; *N.Y. Times*, June 30, 1923; C. E. A. Winslow, *Life of Hermann Biggs* (1929).

D. Rosner

BILDERBACK, JOSEPH BROWN (November 2, 1869, Philadelphia, Pa.-September 19, 1969, Portland, Oreg.). *Physician; Pediatrician; Medical educator*. Son of William, ship captain, and Margaret (Palmer) Bilderback. Married Carolyn Leete, 1911, two children; Gwendolyn Johnston, 1933, three children. EDUCATION: 1905, M.D., University of Oregon Medical School; 1906-7, intern, Good Samaritan Hospital, Portland, Oreg.; postgraduate study, New York, Vienna, Berlin, and London. CAREER: 1907-69, practice, Portland, Oreg.; 1911-12, clinical attendent, Portland Free Dispensary; 1918-50, medical faculty, University of Oregon Medical School. CONTRIBUTIONS: First pediatrician to practice privately in Portland, Oreg., and the first person in the city to organize a private clinic for children. Pediatrics remained his specialty throughout his lifetime. Founder of the pediatrics department at the University of Oregon Medical School. Assisted in establishing the American Academy of Pediatrics and also the Pacific Northwest Pediatric Society and was president of both organizations. A moving spirit in the provision of a children's hospital for Portland. Helped persuade Mrs. E. W. Morse and Edward Doernbecher to give $200,000 (1924) to establish the Doernbecher Memorial Hospital for Children as a part of the University of Oregon Medical School and served a term as chief of staff of the hospital. A consulting physician and enthusiastic supporter of the Waverly Baby Home in Portland (now the Waverly Children's Home), an institution designed to care for and adopt legally homeless children. One of the first to recognize acrodynia as a clinical entity and author of a classic description of the disease.

WRITINGS: "Acrodynia," in Waldo Nelson, ed., *Mitchell-Nelson Textbook of Pediatrics*, 5th. ed. (1950), 417-21. REFERENCES: S. Gorham Babson, comp., *A History of Pediatrics in the North Pacific* (1970); Waldo E. Nelson, "A Century of Pediatrics," *J. of Pediatrics* 75 (1969): 739-41.

G. Dodds

BILLINGS, FRANK (April 2, 1854, Highland, Wis.-September 20, 1932, Chicago, Ill.). *Physician; Medical educator*. Son of Henry Mortimer and Ann (Bray) Billings. Married Dane Ford Brawley, 1887; one child. EDUCATION: State Normal School, Platteville, Wis.; 1881, M.D., Northwestern University; 1881-

82, intern, Cook County Hospital, Chicago; 1885-86, postgraduate studies in Europe; 1890, M.S., Northwestern University. CAREER: Schoolteacher, Wis.; 1881, began practice, Chicago; at Northwestern University: 1882-86, demonstrator of anatomy; 1886-91, professor of physical diagnosis; and 1891-98, professor of medicine; 1898-1924, faculty, Rush Medical College; at University of Chicago: 1898-1924, professor of medicine; 1900-24, dean of the faculty; and 1905-24, professor of medicine; 1918-19, during World War I, served as medical advisor to the marshall-general and chief of the division of reconstruction, surgeon-general's office. CONTRIBUTIONS: As dean of Rush Medical College, developed an efficient teaching unit, coordinating laboratory, preclinical, and clinical teaching. After affiliation with the University of Chicago, built Senn Hall to house clinical and laboratory facilities. Able to obtain funds from philanthropists to rebuild and equip Presbyterian Hospital, to organize the John McCormick Memorial Institute (1902), to construct the Anna W. Durand Contagious Hospital (1911) and (1909) the Sprague Institute, which supported the Children's Hospital. President, AMA (1902); Chairman, Illinois Board of Charities (1906-12).

WRITINGS: *General Medicine* (1901); *Modern Clinical Medicine* (1906); *Forcheimer's Therapeusis of Internal Diseases*, 5 vols. (1914, editor). REFERENCES: *BHM* (1975-79), 19; J. A. Capps, "Dr. Frank Billings," *Q. Bull., Northwestern Univ. Med. School* 30 (1956): 376-86; *DAB*, Supplement 1: 80-81; E. F. Hirsch, *Frank Billings* (1966).

J. Carvalho

BILLINGS, JOHN SHAW (April 12, 1838, Switzerland County, Ind.-March 11, 1913, New York, N.Y.). *Hospital administrator; Librarian*. Son of James, farmer, and Abby (Shaw) Billings. Married Katharine Mary Stevens, 1862; six children. EDUCATION: 1857, A.B., Miami University (Ohio); 1860, M.D., Medical College of Ohio. CAREER: 1860-61, anatomy faculty, Medical College of Ohio; in U.S. Army: 1862-64, in-hospital service as surgeon and medical statistician; 1865-83, in charge of library of surgeon-general's office; and 1884-95, curator of medical museum and library; 1879, president, American Public Health Association; 1878, vice-chairman, National Board of Health; at University of Pennsylvania: 1891, hygiene faculty; and 1893-96, director, University Hospital; 1896-1913, director, New York Public Library; 1905-13, chairman, Board of Trustees, Carnegie Institution. CONTRIBUTIONS: Increased the size of the surgeon-general's library from 600 volumes (1865) to 50,000 (1873), making it the nation's most important medical library. With Robert Fletcher, began publication (1880) of the monumental *Index Catalogue* of the library, which had run to 16 volumes when Billings retired in 1895. With Fletcher, started publication (1879) of the *Index Medicus*, a monthly guide to current medical literature; two works gave physicians a set of incomparable tools for doing research in the medical literature, both past and present. Drafted plans for the organization and construction of the Johns Hopkins University Hospital (1873); recommended the adoption of the pavilion plan of hospital construction, which was soon widely used throughout the country. Authored several reports on hospital administration and the training of hospital personnel that are regarded as classics. Served as medical adviser to the trustees of the Hopkins estate in which capacity he played a key role in determining the organization, philosophy, and faculty of the Johns Hopkins Medical School. Supervised the compilation of vital statistics for the U.S. censuses of 1880 and 1890.

WRITINGS: *A Report on Barracks and Hospitals* . . . (1870); "Hospital Construction and Organization," in *Hospital Plans* . . . *Johns Hopkins Hospital* (1875), 3-46; *Medical Education* (1878); *National Medical Dictionary* (1889); *On Vital and Medical Statistics* (1889). A bibliography is in Fielding H. Garrison, *John Shaw Billings: A Memoir* (1915). REFERENCES: *BHM* (1964-69), 33; (1970-74), 24; (1975), 5; (1976), 5; (1977), 6; *DAB*, 2: 266-69; A. McGehee Harvey, "John Shaw Billings: Forgotten Hero of American Medicine," *Perspectives in Biol. and Med.*, 21 (Autumn 1977): 35-57; Miller, *BHM*, p. 12; *NCAB*, 4: 78; *Who Was Who In Am.*, Hist. Vol.: 95.

S. Galishoff

BINGHAM, ARTHUR WALTER (May 19, 1872, Milwaukee, Wis.-May 18, 1943, Orange, N.J.). *Physician; Obstetrician.* Son of Webster Adams, businessman, and Fanny (Bird) Bingham. Married Mary Condit Dodd, 1900; three children. EDUCATION: Public schools, Milwaukee and West De Pere, Wis.; 1893, B.S., Cornell University; 1896, M.D., College of Physicians and Surgeons of Columbia University; 1896-97, intern, New York General Hospital; 1898, intern, Infant Asylum and Sloan Maternity Hospital. CAREER: 1899-1942, medical staff, Orange Memorial Hospital; consulting obstetrician, Dover (N.J.) General Hospital and Presbyterian Hospital, Newark, N.J.; chief advisory obstetrician, New Jersey State Department of Health. CONTRIBUTIONS: Organized and directed (1914-37) the obstetrics department of the Orange Memorial Hospital and was responsible for the hospital's outstanding reputation in maternity cases. Founder (1921) and chairman of the Maternity Center of the Oranges. Organizer (1923) and president of the Essex County Medical Commission for Maternal Welfare. Established (1930) and chaired the Maternal Welfare Committee of the Medical Society of New Jersey. Through his efforts and in cooperation with the Bureau of Child Hygiene of the New Jersey State Department of Health, maternal deaths per thousand births reduced from 5.9 percent (1931) to 1.8 percent (1941).

WRITINGS: "The Prevention of Obstetric Complications by Diet and Exercise," *Am. J. Obst. and Gynecol.* 23 (1932): 38-44; "The Treatment of Repeated Still-Births and Miscarriages," *J. of the Med. Soc. of N. J.* 30 (1933): 444-45. Wrote series (more than 50 items) for *ibid.* entitled "A Lesson from a Death Certificate" dealing with maternal care. REFERENCES: Samuel Cosgrove, "In Appreciation: Arthur W. Bingham—1872-1943," *J. of the Med. Soc. of N.J.* 40 (1943): 6; "Dr. Arthur W. Bingham Receives the Edward J. Ill Award," *ibid.*, 40 (1943): 109-11; Walter B. Mount, "Arthur Walter Bingham, B.S., M.D., F.A.C.S., 1872-1943: Maternal Welfare Article Number Eighty-Four," *ibid.*, 40 (1943): 424-25; Hammell P. Shipps, "Advances in Maternal Welfare, 1903-1953," *ibid.*, 50 (1953): 391-93; *NCAB*, 33: 98; *Newark News*, May 19, 1943;

W. Barlow

BISHOP, GEORGE HOLMAN (June 27, 1889, Durand, Wis.-October 11, 1973, St. Louis, Mo.). *Neurophysiologist.* Son of George Stephen and Harriet Amanda (Holman) Bishop. Married Ethel Ronzoni, 1919. EDUCATION: 1912, A.B., University of Michigan; 1919, Ph.D., University of Wisconsin. CAREER: 1919-20, instructor, zoology, Northwestern University; 1920-21, assistant professor, histology, University of Tennessee Medical School; at Washington University School of Medicine: 1921-30, assistant and associate professor of physiology; 1930-32, professor, applied physiology in ophthalmology; 1932-47, professor of biophysics and laboratory neurophysiology; 1954-73, professor emeritus, neurophysiology, and lecturer in neurophysiology, Department of Neurology and Psychiatry. CONTRIBUTIONS: With Herbert Gasser (q.v.) and Joseph Erlanger (q.v.), Washington University School of Medicine, made fundamental contributions to the understanding of nerve impulse activity in unmyelinated fibers. With Peter Heinbecker and James O'Leary (q.v.), continued research on nerve fibers (1930s); turned from experiments on sensation to the visual system. Active as a scientist until shortly before his death; turned to electron microscopy and fiber-size distribution counts of subcortical white matter in his later years. Publications stretched over 54 years (1917-71). Several of his research contributions are among the classics of electrophysiology.

WRITINGS: "The Action Potential Waves Transmitted Between the Sciatic Nerve and Its Spinal Roots," *Am. J. of Physiol.* 78 (1926): 574-91 (with Erlanger and Gasser); "Experimental Analysis of the Simple Action Potential Wave in Nerve by the Cathode Ray Oscillograph," *ibid.*, 78 (1926): 537-73 (with Erlanger and Gasser); "The Function of the Non-myelinated Fibers of the Dorsal Roots," *ibid.*, 106 (1933): 647-69 (with Heinbecker and O'Leary); "Analysis of Function of Nerve to Muscle," *ibid.*, 110 (1935): 636-58 (with O'Leary and Heinbecker); "Radiation Path from Geniculate to Optic Corex in Cat," *J. Neurophysiol.* 15 (1952): 201-20 (with M. H. Clare). REFERENCES: Bishop's own autobiographical essay, "Life Among the Axons," *Annual Review of Physiology* 27 (1965): 1-18, is of great interest. See also James O'Leary's obituary of Bishop: "George Holman Bishop," *J. Neurophysiol.* 37, no. 2 (1974): 382-83.
M. Hunt

BLACK, GREENE VARDIMAN (August 3, 1836, Scott County, Ill.-August 31, 1915, Chicago, Ill.). *Dentist; Educator.* Son of William and Mary S. (Vaughn) Black. Married Jane L. Coughennower, 1860; Elizabeth Akers Davenport, 1865, two children. EDUCATION: 1854-56, studied medicine with his brother Dr. Thomas G. Black; 1856-57, studied dentistry with Dr. J. C. Speer, Mt. Sterling, Ill.; 1877, D.D.S., Missouri Dental College, St. Louis; 1884, M.D., Chicago Medical College. CAREER: 1857, began dental practice, Winchester, Ill.; 1862-63, served in Illinois Infantry in Civil War; was injured and discharged; 1864, practice of dentistry in Jacksonville, Ill.; 1870-80, lectured on pathology, histology, and operative dentistry, Missouri Dental College; 1883-89, professor of dental pathology, Chicago College of Dental Surgery; 1890-91, professor of dental pathology and bacteriology, University of Iowa; 1891-1915, professor of operative dentistry, pathology, and bacteriology and dean (1897-1915), Northwestern University Dental School. CONTRIBUTIONS: Developed methods of making alloys for amalgam (fillings) that were more stable than previous methods. Described pathological histology of mottled enamel caused by fluorosis. Formulated doctrine of extension of cavity to prevent further decay. Invented several dental instruments. First president of the Illinois Board of Dental Examiners. President, American Dental Association (1901).

WRITINGS: *Formation of Poisons by Micro-Organisms* (1884); *A Study of the Histological Characters of the Periosteum and Peridental Membrane* (1887); *Anatomy of the Human Teeth* (1891); *Operative Dentistry*, 2 vols. (1908); *Diseases and Treatment of the Investing Tissues of the Teeth and the Dental Pulp* (1915). REFERENCES: *BHM* (1964-69), 34; (1970-74), 24; (1980), 7; B. M. Black and C. E. Black, *From Pioneer to Scientist* (1940); C. E. Black, "The Blacks in Dentistry," *Ill. Dent. J.* 9 (1940): 318-24, 345; *DAB*, 2: 308-10; R. W. Edwards, "G. V. Black," *J. Amer. Coll. of Dentistry* 32 (1965): 336-38; Kelly and Burrage (1920), 104; Miller, *BHM*, p. 13; H. B. Robinson, "America's Pioneer Dental Educator," *J. Am. Dental Assoc.* 84 (May 1972): 940-43.

J. Carvalho

BLACK, JOHN JANVIER (November 6, 1837, Delaware City, Del.-September 27, 1909, New Castle, Del.). *Physician; Psychiatry.* Son of Charles H., physician, and Anne (Janvier) Black. Married Jane Sarah Groome, 1872; two children. EDUCATION: 1858, A.B., Princeton; 1859, U.S. Marine Hospital, San Francisco, Calif.; 1862, M.D., University of Pennsylvania; 1865-67, studied in Europe. CAREER: 1862-64, assistant surgeon, U.S. Army; 1867-1909, private practice, New Castle, Del. CONTRIBUTIONS: Leader in Del. in the fight against tuberculosis; first director of Hope Farm, the forerunner of the Brandywine Sanatorium. Led fight for better mental health in Del.; campaigned for the merger of county asylums into one institution; a founder and first president of the Board of Trustees, Delaware State Hospital.

WRITINGS: *Forty Years in the Medical Profession* (1900); *Consumptives in Delaware* (1902); *Eating to Live, with Some Advice to the Gouty, the Rheumatic and the Diabetic* (1906). REFERENCES: Kelly and Burrage (1928); Meridith I. Samuels, *Med. Soc. of Del., 150th Annual Session* (1939), 64, 65; *Who Was Who in Am.*, 1: 101; *Wilmington Morning News*, September 28, 1909.

W. H. Williams

BLACKFAN, KENNETH DANIEL (September 9, 1883, Cambridge, N.Y.-November 29, 1941, Louisville, Ky.). *Physician; Pediatrics.* Son of Harry Smith, physician, and Estella (Chase) Blackfan. Married Lulie Henry (Anderson) Bridges, 1920; no children. EDUCATION: 1905, M.D., Albany Medical College. CAREER: 1905-6, pathology and bacteriology faculty, Albany Medical College, pathology staff, Albany Hospital; 1906-9, practiced medicine, Cambridge; 1910-11, pediatrics staff, Philadelphia Polyclinic Hospital; pediatrics faculty: 1911-12, Washington University; 1912-20, Johns Hopkins Medical School; 1920-23, University of Cincinnati College of Medicine; 1923-41, Harvard Medical School; and physician-in-chief, Boston Children's Hospital; 1938, president, American Pediatric Society. CONTRIBUTIONS: Was one of the world's foremost authorities on diseases of childhood. Advanced the treatment of infant diarrhea and introduced (1918) the treatment of dehydration by intraperitoneal injection of salt solutions. Improved the diagnosis and treatment of meningococcus meningitis in children. With Walter E. Dandy (q.v.), made a definitive study of hydrocephalus. Made important hematological studies and described a blood disorder in which only the red cells fail to regenerate ("hypoplastic anemia"). Made Harvard Medical School and Boston Children's Hospital a preeminent center for research and training in pediatrics.

WRITINGS: "Internal Hydrocephalus," *Am. J. of Diseases of Children* 14 (1917): 424-43 (with Walter E. Dandy); "Some Observations upon Bacteria in Children," *Trans., Assoc. of Am. Physicians* 32 (1917): 16-31 (with M. D. Batchelor); "The Intraperitoneal Injection of Saline Solution," *ibid.*, 15 (1918): 19-28 (with Kenneth F. Maxcy [q.v.]); "The Early Recognition of Hydrocephalus in Meningitis," *ibid.*, 18 (1919): 525-36. REFERENCES: *BHM* (1970-74), 25; *DAB*, Supplement 3: 74-75; Miller, *BHM*, p. 13; *NCAB*, 32: 162-63; *N.Y. Times*, November 30, 1941; *Who Was Who in Am.*, 1: 102.

S. Galishoff

BLACKWELL, ELIZABETH (February 3, 1821, Counterslip, England-May 31, 1910, Hastings, England). *Physician; Medical educator; Reformer*. Daughter of Samuel, sugar refiner, reformer, and dissenting lay preacher, and Hannah (Lane) Blackwell. Never married. EDUCATION: Private tutors; 1845-47, read medicine with Samuel Dickson, Joseph Warrington, and William Elder; 1848, Blockley Hospital; 1849, M.D., Geneva Medical College; 1849-50, studied abroad in Birmingham and London, England, and La Maternité in Paris, France; 1850, studied with Sir James Paget at St. Bartholomew's Hospital, London. CAREER: 1851-57, private practice, New York City; 1857, founded New York Infirmary for Women and Children; 1859, first woman to have her name entered on the Medical Register of the United Kingdom; 1861-65, selected and trained nurses for the U.S. Sanitary Commission and chaired registration committee, Women's Central Association of Relief; 1868, founded Woman's Medical College of the New York Infirmary; and 1868-69, professor of hygiene; 1871, after returning to England (in 1869), founded National Health Society; 1875, professor of gynecology, New Hospital and London School of Medicine for Women; *post* 1875, devoted time to her writing and hygienic reform activities. CONTRIBUTIONS: First woman to graduate with a medical degree in the United States (1849). Indefatigable pioneer advocate of women's medical education (1857-1910). Founder of two exemplary and innovative institutions for the training of women in medicine (New York Infirmary, 1857; Woman's Medical College, 1868).

Outspoken proponent of social hygiene, sanitation, and preventive medicine (1868-1910). Opponent of vaccination, animal experimentation, and bacteriology (1871-1910). Important role model for generations of women physicians who followed her into the medical profession.

WRITINGS: *Pioneer Work in Opening the Medical Profession to Women* (1895); *Essays in Medical Sociology*, 2 vols. (1902). Writings listed in *Pioneer Work*, app. REFERENCES: *BHM* (1964-69), 34; (1970-74), 25; (1975-79), 19; (1980), 7; *DAB*, 1, pt. 2: 320-21; Elinor Rice Hays, *Those Extraordinary Blackwells* (1967); Kelly and Burrage (1920); Miller, *BHM*, p. 13; *NCAB*, 9: 127; Ishbel Ross, *Child of Destiny* (1944); Nancy Sahli, "Elizabeth Blackwell, M.D.: A Biography" (Ph.D. thesis, University of Pennsylvania, 1974); Elizabeth H. Thomson, "Elizabeth Blackwell," *Notable Am. Women* 1 (1971): 161-65.

R. M. Morantz

BLACKWELL, EMILY (October 8, 1826, Bristol, England-September 7, 1910, York Cliffs, Maine). *Physician; Surgeon; Medical educator*. Daughter of Samuel, sugar refiner, reformer, and dissenting lay preacher, and Hannah (Lane) Blackwell. Never married. EDUCATION: Private tutors; 1848, read medicine with Dr. John Davis, Cincinnati, Ohio; 1852, walked wards at Bellevue Hospital; 1852-53, Rush Medical College; 1854, M.D., Western Reserve; 1854-55, studied with Sir James Y. Simpson in Edinburgh, Scotland; 1855-56, clinics in London, Paris, Berlin, and Franz von Winckel's in Dresden, Germany. CAREER: 1856-1900, surgeon and administrator, New York Infirmary for Women and Children; 1869-99, dean and professor of obstetrics and diseases of women, Woman's Medical College of the New York Infirmary. CONTRIBUTIONS: Among the first pioneer women physicians to gain advanced training in surgery (1855-56). Chief administrator of the New York Infirmary, one of the finest institutions run by women physicians for the care of women and children in the country (1869-99). Made important contributions to the upgrading of medical education, including the introduction (1876) of a full three-year graded curriculum earlier than most other medical schools (1856-1910). Provided inspiration and support of a concrete nature to generations of women combating discrimination and prejudice in order to study medicine.

WRITINGS: *Address on the Medical Education of Women* (1864). REFERENCES: Elinor Rice Hays, *Those Extraordinary Blackwells* (1967); Miller, *BHM*, p. 13; *NCAB*, 9: 124; Elizabeth H. Thomson, "Emily Blackwell," *Notable Am. Women* 1 (1971): 165-67.

R. M. Morantz

BLAIR, VILRAY PAPIN (June 15, 1871, St. Louis, Mo.-November 24, 1955, St. Louis). *Plastic surgeon*. Son of Edward H. and Mary C. (Papin) Blair. Married Kathryn Johnson, 1907; five children. EDUCATION: Christian Brothers' College: 1890, B.A.; and 1894, M.A.; 1893, M.D., St. Louis Medical College; licensed to practice in Missouri; 1893-95, internship, Mullanphy Hospital. CAREER: At Washington University School of Medicine: 1894-1941, faculty, anatomy and surgery; and 1941-55, professor emeritus; at Washington University

School of Dentistry: 1927-41, professor of oral surgery; and 1941-55, professor emeritus; June 1947, retired from active practice. CONTRIBUTIONS: A pioneer in the development of plastic surgery as a speciality, organized a plastic surgery unit for the U.S. Army during World War I. Played a key role in the formation of a National Board of Plastic Surgery (1938). In addition, research and clinical skills led to the improvement of surgical techniques for congenital and acquired facial defects. Published more than 200 papers in his field.

WRITINGS: *Surgery and Diseases of Mouth and Jaw* (1912); *Cancer of the Face and Mouth* (1941, with S. Moore and L. Byars); "The Use of Large Split-Skin Grafts of Intermediate Thickness," *Surg. Gyn. & Obst.* 49 (1929): 82-97 (with James B. Brown); "The Why and How of Harelip Correction," *Internat. J. Orthod.* 15 (1929): 1112-19; "The Role of the Plastic Surgeon in the Care of War Injuries," *Annals of Surg.* 113 (1941): 697-704. REFERENCES: BHM (1964-69), 34; *J. Mo. Med. Assoc.* 44 (1947): 574-84; Jerome P. Webster, M.D., "Vilray Papin Blair: In Memoriam," *Plastic and Reconstructive Surg.* 18 (1956): 2.

M. Hunt

BLAKE, FRANCIS GILMAN (February 22, 1877, Mansfield Valley, Pa.-February 1, 1952, Washington, D.C.). *Physician; Medical administrator; Microbiology.* Son of Francis Clark, mining engineer, and Winifred Pamelia (Ballard) Blake. Married Dorothy P. Dewey, 1916; three children. EDUCATION: 1908, A.B., Dartmouth College; 1913, M.D., Harvard Medical School; 1913-16, intern and resident, Peter Bent Brigham Hospital. CAREER: Medicine faculty: 1916-17, 1919-20, Rockefeller Institute for Medical Research; and 1917-18, University of Minnesota Medical School; 1918-19, medical reserve corps, U.S. Army; at Yale Medical School: 1921-52, medicine faculty; and 1940-47, dean; medical staff: 1921-51, New Haven Hospital (1946-51, Grace-New Haven Community Hospital); and 1921-51, New Haven Dispensary; 1925-52, member, National Research Council; on Board for the Investigation and Control of Influenza and other Epidemic Diseases in the Army (1946-49, Army Epidemiological Board; later, Armed Forces Epidemiological Board): 1941-46, president; and 1946-52, member. CONTRIBUTIONS: Gained national prominence for clinical investigations of epidemic diseases. With Russell Cecil, worked on the production of experimental bacterial pneumonia in monkeys and how to prevent it (1918-19); with J. D. Trask (q.v.), demonstrated the virus etiology of measles (1920-21); with Trask, proved the usefulness of antitoxin treatment for scarlet fever (early 1920s); at Yale, directed some of the first laboratory and clinical tests of sulfonamides and penicillin (1930s and early 1940s). As teacher, researcher, and administrator, helped to transform Yale Medical School from a mediocre institution into a first-rate medical center. Had outstanding career as a government and scientific advisor. Greatest achievement was his organization and direction of the Army Epidemiological Board, which was responsible for many new protective measures for both military and civilian populations.

WRITINGS: *Epidemic Respiratory Disease* (1921, with Eugene L. Opie [q.v.] et al.);

"Susceptibility of Monkeys to the Virus of Measles," *J. of Experimental Med.* 33 (1921): 385-412 (with J. D. Trask); "Observations on the Treatment of Scarlet Fever with Scarlatina Antistreptococci Serum," *Trans., Assoc. of Am. Physicians* 39 (1926): 141-54. Bibliography is in *BMNAS.* REFERENCES: *BMNAS* 28 (1954): 1-29; *Current Biog.* (1943): 53; *DAB,* Supplement 5: 63-64; Miller, *BHM,* p. 14; *Trans., Assoc. of Am. Physicians* 65 (1952): 9-13; *Who Was Who in Am.,* 3: 81.

S. Galishoff

BLAKE, JAMES (July 14, 1815, Gosport, England-November 18, 1893, Middletown, Calif.). *Physician.* Never married. EDUCATION: 1832, University College, London; 1838, studied in Paris with Francois Magendie; 1842, became fellow, Royal College of Surgeons. CAREER: 1840, began medical practice, London; 1847, came to United States and became professor of anatomy and surgery, St. Louis Medical School; 1850, settled in Sacramento, Calif., and began medical practice; 1862, medical practice, San Francisco; 1864, became professor of midwifery and diseases of women and children, Toland Medical School; president of the California Academy of Sciences; 1876, founded a tuberculosis sanitorium, Napa Valley, Calif.; 1880, moved to Middletown, where he continued his medical practice. CONTRIBUTIONS: Associated the physiological action of drugs with their gross structural properties. Insisted that the actual physical presence of a drug was necessary before it could exert an action. Recommended open-air rest treatment for tuberculosis.

WRITINGS: "Memoire sur les effets de Diverses Substances Saline," *Arch. Gen. Med.* 6 (1839): 289-300; "Observations and Experiments on the Mode in Which Various Poisonous Agents Act on the Animal Body, " *Edinburgh Surg. J.* 53 (1840): 35-49. Writings listed (partial) in C. Leake, "The Clinical Career of James Blake (1815-1893)," *Calif. and Western Med.* 47, no. 6 (1937): 405-7. REFERENCES: W. F. Bynum, "Chemical Structure and Pharmacological Action: A Chapter in the History of 19th Century Molecular Pharmacology," *Bull. Hist. Med.* 44, no. 6 (1970): 518-38; Henry Harris, *California's Medical Story* (1932), 342-47; Leake, "The Clinical Career of James Blake (1815-1893)," pp. 405-7.

Y. V. O'Neill

BLAKEMORE, ARTHUR HENDLEY (July 2, 1897, Senora, Va.-October 8, 1970, Larchmont, N.Y.). *Physician; Surgery.* Son of John Edward and Mary Virginia (Fallin) Blakemore. Married Catharine Rundlet, 1927; one child. EDUCATION: 1918, B.S., College of William and Mary; 1922, M.D., Johns Hopkins Medical School; 1922-26, surgical training: Johns Hopkins (Baltimore, Md., 1922-23), Henry Ford (Detroit, Mich., 1923-24), and Roosevelt (N.Y.C., 1924-26) hospitals. CAREER: 1926-27, U.S. marine surgeon, Cardova General Hospital, and territorial commissioner of health, Cardova, Alaska; *post* 1928, surgical staff, Columbia Presbyterian Medical Center (N.Y.); at College of Physicians and Surgeons (Columbia University): 1930-42, surgery faculty; and 1942-62, clinical surgery faculty; during World War II, director, National Research Council project in anastomosis of blood vessels for the wounded. CONTRIBUTIONS:

Pioneered in vascular surgery. With Jere W. Lord, developed the vitallium tube nonsuture blood vessel anastomosis technique for bridging arterial defects (1945). With Arthur B. Voorhees, Jr., introduced prosthetic materials for aortic grafting. Directed the development of the Sengstaken-Blakemore balloon tamponade for control of variceal hemorrhage in patients with portal hypertension (1954). Also developed the portocaval shunt operation for relief of portal hypertension.

WRITINGS: "A Nonsuture Method of Blood Vessel Anastomosis: Experimental and Clinical Study," *JAMA* 127 (Mar. 24, 1945): 685-91; (Mar. 31, 1945): 748-53 (with Jere W. Lord); "The Portocaval Shunt in the Surgical Treatment of Portal Hypertension," *Trans., Am. Surg. Assoc.* 66 (1948): 506-22; "The Use of Tubes Constructed from Vinyon "N" Cloth in Bridging Arterial Defects—Experimental and Clinical," *ibid.*, 72 (1954): 64-72 (with Arthur B. Voorhees, Jr.). REFERENCES: David V. Habif, "Arthur Hendley Blakemore, 1897-1970," *Trans., Am. Surg. Assoc.* 89 (1971): 61-62; Mark M. Ravitch, *A Century of Surgery*, 2 vols. (1981); *N.Y. Times*, October 10, 1970; *Who Was Who in Am.*, 5: 65.

S. *Galishoff*

BLALOCK, ALFRED (April 5, 1899, Culloden, Ga.-September 15, 1964, Baltimore, Md.). *Physician; Cardiac surgery*. Son of George Zadock, merchant, and Martha (Davis) Blalock. Married Mary Chambers O'Bryan, 1930, three children; Alice Seney Waters, 1959. EDUCATION: 1918, A.B., University of Georgia; 1922, M.D., Johns Hopkins Medical School; 1922-25, intern and resident, Johns Hopkins Hospital; 1925-26, resident surgeon, Vanderbilt University Hospital. CAREER: Surgery faculty: 1925-41, Vanderbilt Medical School; and 1941-64, Johns Hopkins Medical School; 1941-64, surgery staff, Johns Hopkins Hospital; 1957-62, visiting professor of surgery, various schools. CONTRIBUTIONS: Codeveloped the "blue-baby" operation (1944) and made fundamental discoveries about the physiology of shock. Demonstrated (late 1920s and early 1930s) that surgical shock resulted from the loss of blood and popularized the use of plasma or whole-blood transfusions to treat the condition. At Johns Hopkins, met Dr. Helen Taussig, head of the children's heart clinic, who theorized that the poor circulation of "blue babies" was due to a lack of oxygenated blood caused by a narrowness or the obstruction of passages from the heart to the pulmonary arteries. In experiments on dogs, demonstrated this to be the case and developed an operation to bypass the deformity by surgically joining the subclavian artery to the pulmonary artery; operation has since saved the lives of thousands of babies born with congenital cyanotic heart disease; marked the opening of the modern era of cardiac surgery. With E. A. Park, developed a bypass operation for coarctation of the aorta (1944). With C. R. Hanlon, developed a technique to overcome still another congenital defect, the transposition of the great blood vessels of the heart (1948).

WRITINGS: "Experimental Shock: The Cause of the Low Blood Pressure Produced by Muscle Injury," *Arch. of Surg.* 20 (1930): 959-96; "The Surgical Treatment of Malformations of the Heart in Which There Is Pulmonary Stenosis or Pulmonary Atresia," *JAMA* 128 (1945): 189-202 (with Helen B. Taussig); "Complete Transposition of the

Aorta and the Pulmonary Artery. . . ,'' *Annals of Surg.* 127 (Jan.-Jun. 1948): 385-97. A bibliography is in Mark M. Ravitch, ed., *Papers of Alfred Blalock* (1966). REFERENCES: *BHM* (1964-69), 35; (1970-74), 6; (1978), 6; *DAB*, Supp. 7: 59; *McGraw-Hill Modern Men of Sci.* (1966): 44-45; Ravitch, *Papers of Alfred Blalock*, pp. xv-lvii; Charles L. Van Doren and Robert McHenry, *Webster's Am. Biog.* (1974), 109; *Who Was Who in Am.*, 4: 92-93.

S. Galishoff

BLANEY, JAMES VAN ZANDT (May 1, 1820, New Castle, Del.-December 11, 1874, Chicago, Ill.). *Physician*; *Chemistry*. Son of Cornelius Dushane and Susan (Cannon) Blaney. Married Clarissa Butler, 1847; seven children. EDUCATION: 1838, B.A., Princeton University; 1841, M.A., Princeton University; 1842, M.D., University of Pennsylvania Medical School. CAREER: 1843-57, chemistry, pharmacy, and materia medica faculties, Rush Medical College; 1857-61, chemistry and natural philosophy faculties, Northwestern University; at Rush Medical College: 1861-71, toxicology faculty; and 1866-71, president. CONTRIBUTIONS: A founder of the Chicago Medical Society (1850) and Illinois State Medical Society (1850). Founding editor of the *Illinois Medical and Surgical Journal* (1844), first medical journal in the Midwest. Prime mover for the first general hospital in Chicago (1847). Played major roles in the early development of chloroform as an anesthetic and in urging the state to require registration of vital statistics. Testimony as chemist and physician had major effect in several legal cases. REFERENCES: Kelly and Burrage (1920), 112-13; J. Woodbridge, *Chicago Med. J.* 32 (1875): 3-8; also in *TAMA* 26 (1875): 456-60.

W. K. Beatty

BLANTON, WILLIAM P. (June 20, 1903, Buda, Tex.-April 4, 1960, Juneau, Alaska). *Physician*; *Surgeon*; *Urology*. Married Louise Nisbett, 1931; three children. EDUCATION: 1933, M.D., University of Colorado; 1934, interned, Swedish Hospital, Seattle, Wash. CAREER: 1934-60, U.S. jail physician, Alaska Juneau Mining physician, and physician for Standard Oil Company; 1934-36, private practice with Harry Carlos DeVighne, Juneau. CONTRIBUTIONS: Secretary, Alaska Medical Association, for 20 years and president (1954). Medical director, Alaska Cancer Society and Red Cross. Died suddenly during surgery (1960). St. Ann's Hospital (Juneau) medical library is dedicated to the memories of Drs. Blanton and John Harold Clements. REFERENCES: *Alaska Med.* 2, no. 2 (1960): 41; *Anchorage Times*, April 6, 1960.

A. R. C. Helms

BLANTON, WYNDHAM BOLLING (June 3, 1890, Richmond, Va.-January 6, 1960, Richmond). *Physician*; *Internist*; *Allergist*; *Medical historian*. Son of Charles Armistead, physician, and Elizabeth (Wallace) Blanton. Married Natalie Friend McFaden, 1918; four children. EDUCATION: 1910, B.A., Hampden-Sydney; 1912, M.A., University of Virginia; 1916, M.D., College of Physicians and Surgeons (Columbia University), N.Y.; postgraduate work, New York City,

Berlin, Edinburgh. CAREER: 1918-19, captain, U.S. Army Medical Corps, World War I; 1920-60, clinician, Richmond; 1930-50, faculty, Medical College of Virginia; 1932-42, editor, *Virginia Medical Monthly*; 1936-54, organized and directed the Immunology Clinic, Medical College of Virginia; consulting editor, *Journal of the History of Medicine*; associate editor, *Annals of Medical History*; president, Virginia Historical Society. CONTRIBUTIONS: Pioneering work as a medical historian and an expert in clinical medicine and allergies. Wrote the definitive three-volume *History of Medicine in Virginia*, a landmark in American medical history; wrote numerous other historical papers and organized the 1957 Medical Exhibit of the Jamestown 350th Anniversary Festival. Developed one of the largest allergy clinics associated with a medical school and contributed many important papers on clinical medicine and allergies.

WRITINGS: "Hay Fever with Comments on Post Season in Richmond," *Virginia Med. Monthly* 59 (1932): 140-44; "Incidence of Aspirin Hypersensitivity," *Am. J. of Med. Sci.* 200 (1940): 390-94 (with Emily Gardner); "Granulocytopenia Due Probably to Pyribenzamine," *JAMA* 134 (1947): 454-55 (with M. E. B. Owens, Jr.); "Death During Skin Testing," *Am. J. of Med. Sci.* 217 (1949): 169-73 (with Adney K. Sutphin); *Medicine in Virginia in the Seventeenth, Eighteenth and Nineteenth Centuries*, 3 vols. (1930, 1931, 1933). REFERENCE: Harry J. Warthen, Jr., "Dr. Wyndham Bolling Blanton, 1890-1960," *Bull. Hist. Med.* 38 (1964): 80-81. *Who Was Who in Am.*, 4: 93.

P. Addis

BLESH, ABRAHAM LINCOLN (January 6, 1866, Clinton, Pa.-February 20, 1934, Oklahoma City, Okla.). *Physician*; *Surgeon*. Son of Swiss immigrant parents, was influenced early in his life to become a physician by a kindly country doctor. EDUCATION: 1889, M.D., Northwestern University Medical School; 1902-3, postgraduate work in surgery, Johns Hopkins. CAREER: Worked his way to Europe as ship's doctor and then returned to practice in Kans.; 1893-1911, practice, Guthrie, Okla.; 1911-34, practice, Oklahoma City; 1912-34, associate professor of surgery, University of Oklahoma School of Medicine. CONTRIBUTIONS: A founding member and chief surgeon of Wesley Hospital, Oklahoma City. President of the Oklahoma Territory Medical Association (1903); helped to found the present state medical association. A founder of the American College of Surgeons (1912). Served as a major during World War I and as chief of surgery, Fort Sam Houston, Tex.

WRITINGS: "Therapeutics of Minute Doses," *Okla. Med. J.* 3 (1895): 423, 429; "Practical Suggestions in Alkaloidal Therapy," *ibid.*, 5 (1897): 712-15; "Multiple Ovarian Cystoma," *ibid.*, 7 (1898): 101-4; "Surgery of the Gall Bladder and Ducts," *Okla. Med.-News J.* 10 (1902): 207-16. REFERENCES: "A. L. Blesh" file, History of Medicine Collection, University of Oklahoma Health Sciences Center Library, Oklahoma City, Okla.; William F. Browne and R. Palmer Howard, "The Role of the Oklahoma County Medical Society in Territorial Medicine, 1904-1905," *Journal of the Oklahoma State Medical Association* 70 (1977): 92-98; Mark R. Everett, *Medical Education in Oklahoma: The University of Oklahoma School of Medicine and Medical Center 1900-1931* (1972);

R. Palmer Howard and Richard E. Martin, "The Contributions of B. F. Fortner, LeRoy Long, and Other Early Surgeons in Oklahoma," *Journal of the Oklahoma State Medical Association* 61 (1968): 541-49.

V. Allen

BLOODGOOD, JOSEPH COLT (November 1, 1867, Milwaukee, Wis.-October 22, 1935, Baltimore, Md.). *Physician*; *Surgery*. Son of Francis, lawyer, and Josephine (Colt) Bloodgood. Married Edith Holt, 1908; two children. ED-UCATION: 1888, B.S., University of Wisconsin; 1891, M.D., University of Pennsylvania; 1891-92, resident physician, Children's Hospital (Philadelphia); 1892, assistant resident surgeon, Johns Hopkins Hospital; 1892-93, attended European clinics and hospitals; 1893-97, resident surgeon, Johns Hopkins Hospital. CAREER: At Johns Hopkins University: 1895-1914, surgery faculty; 1914-35, clinical surgery faculty; and *post* 1897, hospital surgical staff; chief of surgery, St. Agnes Hospital (Baltimore); 1917, member, Army Medical Reserve Corps and medical advisory board, American Red Cross; member: 1930-35, advisory board, Radiological Research Institute; and 1931-35, editorial board, in charge of surgical pathology, *American Journal of Cancer*. CONTRIBUTIONS: Through his association with William S. Halsted (q.v.), at Johns Hopkins, extended the use of rubber gloves to include all members of the surgical team. Was best known for his work on cancer and surgical pathology. Demonstrated the importance of surgical pathology for the successful practice of surgery and made Johns Hopkins Hospital a leading center for its study. Was one of the world's foremost authorities on cancer. Proselytized physicians and the public on the importance of early detection and treatment and removing the so-called precancerous lesions, such as black moles and ulcers. Pioneered in the clinical study of cancer by bringing laboratory analysis into the operating room; began the use of microscopical examination of tissue sections from the patient before attempting the operation. Also instituted an extensive follow-up system on surgical patients, which, together with the laboratory studies he had made of them while in the hospital, increased greatly the knowledge of cancer. Demonstrated that many bone and breast tumors were not cancerous; pointed out the benign nature of the often histologically frightening lesions of chronic cystic mastitis and giant-cell tumors, thereby saving many persons from needless mutilation. Improved operative methods for the more complete removal of diseased tissue. Made fundamental contributions to the pathology of bone tumors and their diagnosis and treatment by X-ray and radium. Helped found the American Society for the Control of Cancer and the Association for the Study of Neoplastic Diseases.

WRITINGS: "Benign Bone Cysts, Otitis Fibrosa, Giant-Cell Sarcoma and Bone Aneurysm of the Long Pipe Bones. A Clinical and Pathological Study with the Conclusion that Conservative Treatment is Justifiable," *Trans., Am. Surg. Assoc.* 28 (1910): 116-86; "The Transplantation of the Rectus Muscle in Certain Cases of Inguinal Hernia in Which the Conjoined Tendon is Obliterated," *Bull., Johns Hopkins Hosp.* 19 (May 1918): 96-100; "The Pathology of Chronic Cystic Mastitis of the Female Breast; with Special Consideration of the Blue-Domed Cyst," *Arch. of Surg.* 3 (Nov. 1921): 445-

542. A bibliography, *Index to the Writings of Jos. Colt Bloodgood, M.D.* (n.d.), was prepared by Edith H. Bloodgood and V. H. Long. REFERENCES: *DAB*, Supplement 1: 90-91; *NCAB*, 26: 210-11; Mark M. Ravitch, *A Century of Surgery*, 2 vols. (1981); *Who Was Who in Am.*, 1: 109.

S. Galishoff

BLUMER, GEORGE (March 16, 1872, Darlington, Durham County, England-May 16, 1962, Balboa, Calif.). *Internist*; *Educator*. Son of John George, shipbuilder, and Julia Edith (Walford) Blumer. Married Anne Evans, 1906; Mabel Louise Bradley, 1909; five daughters. EDUCATION: 1891, M.D., Cooper Medical College, San Francisco, Calif.; 1891-92, intern, City and County Hospital, San Francisco; at Johns Hopkins Hospital: 1893, postgraduate work; 1893-94, surgical house officer; and 1894-95, medical house officer. CAREER: 1895-96, assistant in pathology, Johns Hopkins University; 1896-1903, director of the Bender Hygienic Laboratory, New York State Department of Health, Albany, N.Y.; 1896-1903, faculty, Albany Medical College; 1903-6, practiced medicine, San Francisco; 1903-4, associate professor of pathology, Stanford University Medical School; 1904-6, instructor in medicine, University of California; at Yale Medical School: 1906-10, professor of the theory and practice of medicine; 1910-20, dean; and 1920-39, clinical professor of medicine; until 1940, conducted a consultative practice in internal medicine, New Haven, Conn., and was at times either consulting or attending physician at various Connecticut hospitals; 1940-47, staff appointment, Huntington Memorial Hospital, Pasadena, Calif. CONTRIBUTIONS: While dean of the Yale Medical School, introduced several innovations that contributed to its recognized standing as a class A medical college. Entrance requirements were raised to three years of academic work, and (1912) a bachelor's degree became a requirement for admission. Persuaded the Yale Corporation to increase its support of the medical school from about $40,000 annually to well over $200,000. This permitted a reorganization of several departments and the establishment of a department of public health. Endowment fund was increased from $248,000 to $2,800,000 during Blumer's tenure. Due to his efforts, the Anthony N. Brady Memorial Foundation was established (1914), enabling the medical school to build the Brady Laboratory. Received the right of the medical school to nominate the entire staff of the New Haven Hospital and gained its complete teaching control. Noteworthy research resulted in the original isolation of the micro-organism, gonococcus, as a causative factor in ulcerative endocarditis (1896). Provided evidence that trichinosis was more prevalent in the United States than previously believed (1900) and gave a general critical review of infectious jaundice in the United States (1923). President of the Association of American Physicians (1942-43), Connecticut State Medical Society (1920-21), and New Haven County Medical Society.

WRITINGS: Author of 150 articles, among which are "Healed and Quiescent Pulmonary Tuberculosis: An Analysis of Five Hundred Cases, with Remarks on Pleural Tubercles," *Calif. State J. of Med.* (1904); "A Note on the Normal Peculiarities of the Heart Sound in the Region of the Sternum," *Arch. Int. Med.* (1914); and "The Digital Manifestations of Subacute Bacterial Endocarditis," *Am. Heart J.* (1926). He also edited and contributed to several works including *Blumer's Bedside Diagnosis.* REFERENCES: George Blumer, "Reminiscences of an Old-Time Doctor," *Yale J. of Biol. and Med.* 28 (1955-56): 1-28; *NCAB*, 49: 240-41.

J. W. Ifkovic

BOBBS, JOHN STOUGH (December 28, 1809, Green Village, Franklin County, Pa.-May 1, 1870, Indianapolis, Ind.). *Surgeon; Educator.* Son of Conrad and Elizabeth Bobbs. Married Catherine Cameron, 1840; no children. EDUCATION: Village school; 1827-30, apprentice to Dr. Martin Luther, Harrisburg, Pa.; 1836, M.D., Jefferson Medical College. CAREER: 1830-34, early practice, Middletown, Pa.; 1835, moved to Indianapolis; 1835-36, returned to Pa. to attend medical school; 1836-70, practice in Indianapolis; 1846-48, assistant commissioner in the erection of the state's first mental hospital; 1848, participated in the founding of the Indianapolis Medical Society and was its first secretary; 1849-52, founder, Indiana Central Medical College, and dean and professor of surgery; 1856-60, elected to the state senate; volunteer surgeon, Civil War, later serving as medical director, district of Indiana; 1868, president, Indiana State Medical Society; 1869, founder and president of the faculty, Indiana Medical College. CONTRIBUTIONS: Noted for performing the world's first cholecystotomy (1867). His patient Mary (Wiggins) Burnsworth survived and lived in good health (until 1913). A principal figure in Ind. medicine during its pioneer period. Instrumental in founding a local medical society and the Indiana State Medical Society and its publication *Transactions of the Indiana State Medical Society.* Instrumental in founding two medical colleges, the latter of which (Indiana Medical College) survived until the turn of the century and became incorporated into what is now Indiana University School of Medicine. His legacy provided for the Bobbs Medical Library and the Bobbs Free Dispensary, important adjuncts to the medical school.

WRITINGS: "Cases of Lithotomy of the Gall Bladder," *Trans., Indiana State Med. Soc.* (1868). Limited literary output consists of five additional clinical reports, a biographical memoir, and a presidential address, all in the same journal. REFERENCES: *J. of the Indiana State Med. Assoc.* 60 (1967): 541-48; Kelly and Burrage (1920), 115-16; *Trans., Indiana State Med. Soc.* (1871): 211-17; *ibid.* (1894): 212a-12p.

C. A. Bonsett

BODINE, JAMES MORRISON (October 2, 1831, Fairfield, Nelson County, Ky.-January 25, 1915, Louisville, Ky.). *Physician; Educator.* Son of Alfred, physician and merchant, and Fanny Maria (Ray) Bodine. Married Mary Elizabeth Crow, 1855, one child; Laura M. Williams, November 1903. EDUCATION: Grammar school, Fairfield, Ky.; St. Joseph's College, Bardstown, Ky.; Hanover College, Hanover, Ind.; 1852, began the study of medicine under H. M. Bullitt, Louisville; 1852-54, Kentucky School of Medicine, Louisville; M.D., 1854. CAREER: 1854-55, practiced in Austin, Tex.; 1856-57, practiced in Louisville;

1857-62, practiced in Leavenworth, Kans.; 1862-63, practiced in Fairfield; 1864-1915, practiced in Louisville; at Kentucky School of Medicine: 1856-57, demonstrator in anatomy; and 1864-66, professor of anatomy; at University of Louisville medical department: 1866-1907, professor of anatomy; 1867-1907, dean; and 1907-15, president of the faculty. CONTRIBUTIONS: One of a group of physician-teachers who organized (1876) the Association of American Medical Colleges (AAMC). President of AAMC (1881); president of the Southern Medical College Association (1892); and president of the reorganized AAMC (1896). Major contribution to medicine was as dean and president of the faculty, for his wisdom and understanding guided the successful merger of the medical department of Kentucky University with the University of Louisville medical department (1907) and the merger of the Louisville College of Medicine, Kentucky School of Medicine, and Hospital College of Medicine with the University of Louisville (1908).

WRITINGS: Prepared very little for the press except for several addresses. REFERENCES: "Professor James Morrison Bodine, M.D.," in *History of the Ohio Falls Cities and Their Counties* 1 (1882): 447-48; H. A. Cottell, "The Life and Character of the Late Professor James Morrison Bodine, M.D., LLD.," *Louisville Monthly J. of Med. & Surg.* 22 (1915): 33-36; Kelly and Burrage (1920), 116-17.

E. H. Conner

BOND, THOMAS (May 2, 1713, Herring Creek, Md.-March 26, 1784, Philadelphia, Pa.). *Physician; Surgeon.* Son of Richard, Quaker tobacco farmer, and Elizabeth (Chew) Bond. Married Susannah Roberts, 1735, two children; Sarah Weymouth, 1742, six children. EDUCATION: ?-1732, probably apprenticed to his half-brother Dr. Samuel Chew; 1738-39, studied in London hospitals and the Hôtel-Dieu, Paris. CAREER: c.1732-84, general practitioner, Philadelphia; 1752-84, physician, Pennsylvania Hospital; 1752-84, clinical lecturer, Pennsylvania Hospital; 1766-76, faculty, College of Philadelphia (later University of Pennsylvania); 1769-79, physician, Philadelphia Almshouse (later Philadelphia General Hospital). CONTRIBUTIONS: Founder (with B. Franklin) of Pennsylvania Hospital, first in the country exclusively for care of the sick (1751), and member, Board of Managers (1751-52). Founding member and trustee, Philadelphia Academy (1749-84), which became College of Philadelphia in 1753 and University of Pennsylvania in 1779. Port physician, with Lloyd Zachary, 1741. A founding member, American Philosophical Society (1743), and vice-president, 1769-84. Member, Common Council, city of Philadelphia (1745-76). President, Philadelphia Humane Society, first in America, 1780-84. Concerned about better treatment for the insane, advocating cold or warm baths as soothing remedies. Donated meteorological apparatus to the hospital for study of effect of weather on illness. Contributed lecture fees to found a medical library. Advocated autopsies for teaching purposes. Promoted interest in public health, imposing, as port physician, strict quarantine on ships arriving with contagious disease on board. Worked with Franklin on better lighting for city streets and improvement in sewage disposal.

WRITINGS: *Anniversary Oration, Delivered May 21st, Before the American Philosophical Society, Held in Philadelphia, for the Promotion of Useful Knowledge; for the Year 1782*. The *Rank and Dignity of Man in the Scale of Being* (1782); *Défense de l'Inoculation, et Relation des Progrès qu'elle a Faits à Philadelphie en 1758* (1784). Writings listed in E. H. Thomson, *J. Med. Ed.* 33 (1958): 622-23. REFERENCES: C. Bridenbaugh and J. Bridenbaugh, *Rebels and Gentlemen: Philadelphia in the Age of Franklin* (1942); G. W. Corner, *Two Centuries of Medicine. A History of the School of Medicine, University of Pennsylvania* (1965); *DAB*, 2: 433-34; Miller, *BHM*, p. 14; T. G. Morton and F. Woodbury, *History of the Pennsylvania Hospital, 1751-1895* (1897); J. A. Scott, "A Sketch of the Life of Thomas Bond, Clinician and Surgeon," *U. of Pa. Med. Bull.* 18 (1905-6): 306-18; E. H. Thomson, "Thomas Bond, 1713-84: First Professor of Clinical Medicine in the American Colonies," *J. Med. Ed.* 33 (1958): 614-24; W. H. Williams, *America's First Hospital: The Pennsylvania Hospital, 1751-1841* (1976).

E. H. Thomson

BOSWELL, HENRY (March 26, 1884, Hinton, Ala.-December 16, 1957, Sanatorium, Miss.). *Physician; Diseases of the chest*. Son of John Wesley and Georgiana (Neal) Boswell. Married Iola Saunders, 1910; five children. EDUCATION: Rock Springs (Ala.) High School; 1908, M.D., University of Nashville (Tenn.); postgraduate study, Nashville General Hospital. CAREER: 1908-9, house surgeon, Providence Hospital, Mobile, Ala.; 1909-10, general practice of medicine, Laurel, Miss.; 1910, developed tuberculosis and was treated in El Paso (Tex.) Sanatorium; 1910-16, field director, Mississippi State Board of Health; 1916-17, health officer, Prentiss County, Miss.; 1917-57, director of the bureau of tuberculosis and superintendent of the Mississippi State Tuberculosis Sanatorium. CONTRIBUTIONS: Nationally recognized authority on tuberculosis; instrumental in providing improved care for patients with tuberculosis in Miss. President: Mississippi State Medical Association (1922-23); American Sanatorium Association (1929); and National Tuberculosis Association (1930). Also president of the Mississippi State Hospital Association, Mississippi State Tuberculosis Association, Southern Tuberculosis Association, and American Trudeau Society. REFERENCE: *J. Miss. Med. Assoc.* 1 (1960): 317-19.

M. S. Legan

BOSWORTH, FRANCKE HUNTINGTON (January 25, 1843, Marietta, Ohio-October 17, 1925, N.Y., N.Y.). *Laryngologist*. Son of Daniel P., merchant, and Deborah (Wells) Bosworth. Married Mary Hildreth Putnam, 1871; two surviving children. EDUCATION: 1858-60, attended Marietta College; 1860-62, Civil War service; 1862, Yale College, A.B.; 1863-65, Civil War service; 1868, M.D., Bellevue Hospital Medical College, interned at Bellevue. CAREER: 1871, appointed to medical faculty at Bellevue Hospital Medical College, became professor in 1881, and continued in that position after Bellevue merged with New York University (1898) until retirement. CONTRIBUTIONS: Pioneering laryngologist, credited with having developed the science of rhinology as a well-defined field of medical specialization. Contributed to the understanding of the physiology and pathology of the sinuses and nasal obstruction. Developed a nasal saw to remove septal spurs and other obstructions. A founder of the New York Laryngological Society (1873), first in the world devoted to that specialty.

WRITINGS: *Handbook upon Diseases of the Throat for the Use of Students* (1879); *Manual of the Diseases of the Throat and Nose* (1881); *A Treatise on Diseases of the Nose and Throat*, 2 vols. (1889, 1892); *Diseases of the Nose and Throat* (1896). REFERENCES: *DAB*, 1, pt. 2: 466-67; Kelly and Burrage (1928), 125-26; *Laryngoscope*, 35 (1925): 950-60.

M. Kaufman

BOUSFIELD, MIDIAN OTHELLO (August 22, 1885, Tipton, Mo.-February 16, 1948, Chicago, Ill.). *Physician.* Son of Willard Haymen, barber, and Cornelia Catherine (Gilbert) Bousfield. Married Maudelle Tanner Brown, 1914; one child. EDUCATION: 1907, A.B., University of Kansas; 1909, M.D., Northwestern University; 1909-10, Freedmen's Hospital, Washington, D.C. CAREER: 1910, 1912-14, private practice, Kansas City, Mo.; 1911, prospecting in Brazil; 1912, railroad employee (barber, porter, etc.); 1910, 1912-14, visiting physician, Kansas City General Hospital; 1914-48, private practice, Chicago; 1914-16, school health officer and school tuberculosis physician, Chicago; 1919-48, officer and medical director, Liberty Life Insurance Co., Chicago; 1934-42, director, Negro Health Program, Julius Rosenwald Fund, Chicago; 1942-45, U.S. Army Medical Corps, Station Hospital, Fort Huachuca, Ariz.; 1946-48, technical director, Provident Medical Associates, Chicago. CONTRIBUTIONS: Through Rosenwald Fund, aided many blacks in obtaining advanced training in medicine, hospital work, and public health. Served the cause of black health before federal committees and public health agencies at all levels. Very influential in establishing Infantile Paralysis Unit at Tuskegee Institute and at Provident Hospital in Chicago. Helped finance and provide opportunities for medical education of many Chicago blacks through the Provident Medical Associates. President of NMA (1933-34). Organized, staffed, and directed the Station Hospital at Fort Hauchuca, Ariz. (first black Army Medical Center). Served Liberty Life Insurance Company (1919-25) as incorporator, board member, medical examiner, and vice-president and (1925-29) as president and medical examiner. First vice-president and medical director (1929-48), Supreme Liberty Life Insurance Company, Liberty's successor. Involved in black Chicago activities such as YMCA and Urban League. One of first four black physicians appointed to staff of Kansas City's (Old) General Hospital (1910). As secretary of the Railway Men's Association, a pioneer Negro labor organization (1915-20), increased membership from 250 to 10,000.

WRITINGS: "Reaching the Negro Community," *Am. J. of Public Health* 24 (1934): 209-15; "Internships, Residencies and Post-Graduate Training," *JNMA* 32 (1940): 24-30; "Economics of a Tuberculosis Case Finding Campaign," *Med. Care* 1 (1941): 148-

56; "An Account of Physicians of Color in the United States," *Bull. Hist. Med.* 17 (1945): 61-84; "A Control Program in a Metropolitan Area for Tuberculosis Among Negroes," *JNMA* 38 (1946): 45. REFERENCES: Edwin R. Embree and Julia Waxman, *Investment in People* (1949), 117-118; Peter Marshall Murray, "Midian O. Bousfield, M.D., 1885-1948," *JNMA* 40 (1948): 120; *Who Was Who in America*, 2: 72; *WWICA*, 6: 67.

T. Savitt

BOWDITCH, HENRY INGERSOLL (August 9, 1808, Salem, Mass.-January 14, 1892, Boston, Mass.). *Physician; Diseases of the chest.* Son of Nathaniel, mathematician, and Mary (Ingersoll) Bowditch. Married Olivia Yardley, 1838; four children. EDUCATION: At Harvard University: 1828, graduated; and 1832, M.D.; 1831-32, house officer, Massachusetts General Hospital; 1832-34, studied medicine in Paris with Pierre Louis. CAREER: *Post* 1834, practiced medicine, Boston; 1838-92, staff member, Massachusetts General Hospital; 1859-67, clinical medicine faculty, Harvard Medical School; 1869-79, original member, Massachusetts Board of Health. CONTRIBUTIONS: Pioneered the operation for removal of pleural effusions (paracentesis thoracis) with trocar and suction pump (1851). Operation had first been suggested by Morrill Wyman (q.v.), who devised the suction pump, but was most successfully employed by Bowditch, who won for it the support of the medical profession. Published *The Young Stethoscopist; or the Student's Aid to Auscultation* (1846), which for 50 years instructed medical students in the art of auscultation and percussion of the chest. Translated several of Louis's works, including two monographs, *Fever* (typhoid) and *Phthisis*. An active investigator of tuberculosis; believed it occurred in places where there was damp soil and advocated open-air treatment. Following the death of his son who was left unattended for 24 hours on a Civil War battlefield, wrote *A Brief Plea for an Ambulance System for the Army of the United States* . . . (1863), which led to the establishment of a much improved ambulance corps. Greatly stimulated the public health movement in Mass. and in the nation. In his influential book *Public Hygiene in America* (1877), called attention to the nation's backwardness in matters of preventive medicine and vital statistics.

WRITINGS: "On Pleuritic Effusions and the Necessity of Paracentesis for Their Removal," *Am. J. of Med. Sci.* 23 (Apr. 1852): 320-50; *Consumption in New England; or Locality One of Its Chief Causes* (1862). Scientific works are found in *Index Catalogue*, 1st, 2nd, and 3rd series. REFERENCES: *BHM* (1964-69), 40-41; *DAB*, 2: 492-94; Kelly and Burrage (1928), 127-31; Miller, *BHM*, p. 14; *NCAB*, 8: 214; *Who Was Who in Am.*, Hist. Vol.: 134.

S. Galishoff

BOWDITCH, HENRY PICKERING (April 4, 1840, Boston, Mass.-March 13, 1911, Boston). *Physiologist; Educator.* Son of Jonathan Ingersoll, merchant, and Lucy Orne (Nichols) Pickering. Married Selma Knauth, 1871; survived by seven children. EDUCATION: At Harvard University: 1861, B.A.; 1866, M.A.; and 1868, M.D.; 1868-71, studied in France and Germany with Carl Ludwig.

CAREER: 1861-64, officer, First Massachusetts Cavalry; 1864-65, officer, Fifth Massachusetts Cavalry (black); at Harvard University: 1871-1906, physiology faculty; and 1883-93, dean, medical school; 1888, 1891-95, president, American Physiological Society; 1886, 1900, vice-president, American Academy of Arts and Sciences; active in Boston civic affairs. CONTRIBUTIONS: Demonstrated the *Treppe*, or steplike increase of heart-muscle contraction in response to successive uniform stimuli (1871) and, in same experiment, established the "all-or-nothing" principle of cardiac muscle contraction: that independently of the strength of the stimulus, it will contract either to the maximum or not at all. Established the first physiological laboratory in the United States (1871). Attracted to it many of the nation's leading scientific investigators, with whom he collaborated on several important studies. With Charles S. Minot (q.v.), showed that chloroform had a more pronounced effect than ether in depressing vasomotor reflexes (1874). Work of laboratory extended well beyond physiology to include experimental pharmacology, psychology, experimental pathology, bacteriology, and experimental surgery. Showed that nerve fiber cannot be exhausted by stimulation (1885). In making this proof, produced a functional nerve-block with curare, which led subsequently to the introduction of conduction anaesthesia in surgery. Made important anthropometric examinations of the rate of growth of schoolchildren (1875-91); showed that a loss of weight in growing children was a warning of impending illness. Extended the course of instruction at Harvard Medical School to four years and oversaw a large building program. Successfully opposed the attempts of antivivisectionists to limit the work of medical researchers. Helped organize the American Physiological Society (1887). An American editor for the English *Journal of Physiology* (*post* 1877), a founder of the *American Journal of Physiology* (1898), and a member of its first editorial board.

WRITINGS: "Über die Eigenthümlichkeiten der Reizbarkeit, welche die Muskelfasern des Herzens zeigen," *Berichte über Verhandlungen der Königlichen Sächsischen Gesellschaft der Wissenschaften zu Leipzig, Math.-phys. Klasse* 23 (1871): 652-89; "The Growth of Children," *8th Annual Report of the State Board of Health of Massachusetts, 1877*, pp. 275-325; "Note on the Nature of Nerve Force," *J. of Physiol.* 6 (1885): 133-35; "The Medical School of the Future," *Phila. Med. J.* 5 (May 5, 1900): 1011-18. A bibliography is in *BMNAS*. REFERENCES: *BHM* (1970-74), 28; *BMNAS* 17 (1922): 183-96; *DAB*, 2: 494-96; *DSB*, 2: 365-68; Kelly and Burrage (1928), 131-33; *Who Was Who in Am.*, 1: 121.

S. Galishoff

BOWLING, WILLIAM KING (June 5, 1808, Westmoreland County, Va.-August 6, 1885, Monteagle, Tenn.). *Physician; Medical educator; Editor; Writer.* Son of James B. Bowling, physician. Married Mrs. Melissa (Saunders) Cheatham, 1837; one child. EDUCATION: private tutors, a public library of 500 volumes, which he had read before the age of 14; medical preceptor, Lyman Martin, Owen County, Ky.; c. 1829-30, attended 1st course of lectures, Medical College of Ohio; 1836, M.D., medical department, Cincinnati College, where he was a pupil of Daniel Drake. CAREER: c. 1830-35, practiced medicine, northern Ky. (probably Owen County); 1836-50, practiced near Adairville, Logan County, Ky., where he set up a medical school in a cave and filled all the professorships himself; 1850-85, practice, Nashville, Tenn.; at University of Nashville: 1851-73, professor of theory and practice of medicine, and 1877-79, professor of malarial diseases and medical ethics; 1879-85, professor of theory and practice of medicine, University of Tennessee, Nashville; 1851-75, founder and editor, *Nashville Journal of Medicine and Surgery*; 1874-75, president, American Medical Association. CONTRIBUTIONS: Active participant in the founding of the medical department, University of Nashville, and held a professorship in that institution for 28 years. Taught more than 3,000 medical students (1851-61), delivering lectures that were both learned and practical. J. B. Lindsley said of Dr. Bowling, "Gifted with a creative fancy, a poetic imagination, and a delivery combining the graces of the orator with the arts of the actor, he kept large classes in rapt attention. He was the Rush, the Chapman, and the Drake of the South all in one." Contributions as a medical writer and editor were numerous and influential. Throughout his career, was a consistent advocate of universal public education for all races. As early as the 1850s, advocated the educating of women in medicine.

WRITINGS: A prolific writer, but no list of his published works has been compiled. REFERENCES: Morris Fishbein, *History of the American Medical Association* (1947), 625-26; Kelly and Burrage (1920), 132-33; J. B. Lindsley, "Biographical Sketch of W. K. Bowling, M.D., LL.D.," *Southern Pract.* 4 (1882): 1-6; *NCAB*, 12: 225.

S. R. Bruesch

BOYD, ROBERT FULTON (July 8, 1858, Giles County, Tenn.-July 20, 1912, Nashville, Tenn.). *Physician; Dentist; Educator.* Son of Robert and Mariah Boyd (both slaves). Never married. EDUCATION: Educated in Pulaski, Tenn., public schools and in Nashville night school; 1882, M.D. (honors), Meharry Medical College; 1886, A.B., Central Tennessee College, Nashville; at Meharry Medical College: 1887, D.D.S.; and P.H.C. (certificate of Pharmacy); 1890, 1892, postgraduate course in surgery, Ann Arbor, Mich.; postgraduate courses in diseases of women and children, Postgraduate Medical School and Hospital, Chicago, Ill. CAREER: 1875-80, public schoolteacher, night schoolteacher, public school principal, College Grove and Pulaski, Tenn.; 1882, medical practitioner and high school principal, New Albany, Miss.; 1887-1912, dental and medical practice, Nashville; 1882-1912, teacher of numerous subjects and professor and chairman of several departments, Meharry Medical College; 1900, became superintendent and surgeon-in-chief, Mercy Hospital, Nashville. CONTRIBUTIONS: A founder and first president of the NMA (1895-98); first full-time black physician with M.D. to practice in Nashville; respected teacher of a number of black medical students in the early days of black medical education. President of People's Savings Bank and Trust Co., Nashville (first black trust company in

United States). Founded Boyd Infirmary in Nashville (1893), which served for many years as teaching hospital for Meharry. Acknowledged leader (1890s) of the black medical profession in United States. REFERENCES: "Dr. Robert Fulton Boyd," in James T. Haley, ed., *Afro-American Encyclopedia* (1895): 59-62; W. Montague Cobb, "Robert Fulton Boyd," *JNMA* 45 (1953): 233-34; Leslie Falk and James Summerville, "History of Meharry Medical College," ms., pp. 63-66 (at Meharry Archives); John A. Kenney, *The Negro in Medicine* (1912), 25-26; obituary, *JNMA* 4 (1912): 282.

T. Savitt

BOYLSTON, ZABDIEL (March 9, 1679, Muddy River, then part of Boston, now Brookline, Mass.-March 1, 1766, Brookline). *Physician; Inoculist*. Son of Thomas, prosperous farmer and earliest physician of Muddy River, and Mary (Gardner) Boylston. Married Jerusha Minot, 1705; eight children. EDUCATION: Studied medicine with his father and Dr. John Cutler, Boston. CAREER: c. 1700-1740s, practitioner, Boston; 1721, invited by Sir Hans Sloan to go to England to tell of his smallpox inoculation accomplishments; 1724-26, spent two years there and lectured to both the Royal Society, which made him a member, and the Royal College of Physicians; lived in England, went into semiretirement on his estate in Brookline where he bred horses. CONTRIBUTIONS: Pioneer lithotomist, smallpox inoculator. At the urging of the Rev. Cotton Mather (q.v.) and with the support of most of the town's ministers and many of the colony's well-to-do, but with strong opposition from much of the general public, the Boston selectmen, and most of the city's doctors, led by William Douglass (q.v.), the town's best educated and most distinguished physician, conducted the first large-scale (247) inoculation in the Western world during the Boston epidemic of 1721. His work has been hailed by Richard H. Shryock (q.v.) as "the chief American contribution to medicine before the mid-nineteenth century." During his visit to London, Boylston published *An Historical Account of the Small Pox Inoculated in New England*, and subsequently printed in Boston. This was a classic clinical and statistical study based on careful records, clearly tabulated and the results logically set forth.

WRITINGS: *An Historical Account of the Small Pox Inoculated in New England* (1726; rep. 1730). REFERENCES: J. B. Blake, "The Inoculation Controversy in Boston, 1721-1722," *New Eng. Q*. 25 (1952): 489-506; *DAB*, 1, pt. 2: 535-36; G. M. Mager, "Zabdiel Boylston: Medical Pioneer of Colonial Boston" (Ph.D. diss., University of Illinois, 1975); *NCAB*, 7: 27; J. M. Toner, "History of Inoculation in Massachusetts," Massachusetts Med. Soc., *Publications* 2 (1867): 153-90: O. E. Winslow, *A Destroying Angel: The Conquest of Smallpox in Colonial Boston* (1974).

P. Cash

BOZEMAN, NATHAN (March 26, 1825, Greenville, Ala.-December 16, 1905, New York, N.Y.). *Physician; Gynecology*. Son of Nathan and Harriet (Knotts) Bozeman. Married Fannie Lamar, 1852, three children; a cousin of the first wife, no children. EDUCATION: Early education was limited; 1845, studied in office of Dr. James A. Kelly, Coosa County, Ala.; 1846-48, studied medicine, University of Louisville, Ky., M.D., 1848; after graduation, was private assistant to Dr. Samuel Gross (q.v.); demonstrator of anatomy at the University of Louisville under Dr. Thomas G. Robinson; assistant in the Louisville Marine Hospital. CAREER: 1849, practiced medicine, Montgomery, and then specialized in diseases of women; for a brief period, had a partnership with Dr. J. Marion Sims (q.v.); July 1858, visited Europe, performed vesico-vaginal fistula operations in London, Edinburgh, Glasgow, and Paris; 1858, after returning from Europe, opened a private hospital in New Orleans for the treatment of women; 1861, appointed attending surgeon to the Charity Hospital; during the Civil War, was surgeon in the Confederate Army and served on the medical board for the examination of surgeons; 1866, practiced in N.Y.; 1874-76, demonstrated the practicability of his theories in Europe by successful operations in Germany and France; 1877, returned to N.Y. to practice medicine; 1878-89, appointed to the attending staff, New York Women's Hospital; 1889, opened a private sanitarium. CONTRIBUTIONS: Soon after graduation (1848), administered chloroform in an operation of ovariotomy, performed by Professor Henry Miller (q.v.) of Louisville; said to have been the first successful one of its kind performed under anesthesia in the United States. Beginning with his brief partnership with Dr. J. Marion Sims, became noted for his successful operations for vesico-vaginal fistula. Performed the first operation in which a button-suture was used; was able to effect cures without endangering the organs involved (1855). Advocated a system of preparatory treatment in performing an ovariotomy; performed two successful operations (May 1878).

WRITINGS: "Urethro-vaginal and Vesico-vaginal Fistules; Remarks upon Their Peculiarities and Complications; Their Classification and Treatment; Modifications of the Button-suture; Report of Cases Successfully Treated," *North Amer. Med.-Chir. Rev.* (1857); "Removal of a Cyst of the Pancreas Weighing Twenty and One-half Pounds," *Med. Record* 21 (1882): 46-47; "The Gradual Preparatory Treatment of the Complications of Urinary and Fecal Fistula," *Trans. Internat. Med. Cong., Washington* 2 (1887): 514-58; "Chronic Pyelitis: Successfully Treated by Kolpo-uretero Cystotomy," *Am. J. of Med. Sci.* 95 (1888): 255-65, 368-76. REFERENCES: E. B. Carmichael, "N. Bozeman," *Ala. J. Med. Sci.* 6 (1969): 233-36; *DAB*, 1, pt. 2 : 538-39; Fielding Garrison, *Introduction to the History of Medicine* (1929); T. M. Owen, *History of Alabama*, 4 vols. (1978).

S. Eichold

BRACKETT, CYRUS FOGG (June 25, 1833, Parsonsfield, Maine-January 29, 1915, Princeton, N.J.). *Physician; Physicist; Sanitarian.* Son of John, farmer and carpenter, and Jemime (Lord) Brackett. Married Alice A. Briggs, 1864; no children. EDUCATION: Parsonsfield Seminary; 1859, A.B., Bowdoin College; 1863, M.D., Medical School of Maine; 1864, advanced study, Harvard Medical School. CAREER: 1860, principal, Limerick (Maine) Academy; faculty: 1861-62, New Hampton (N.H.) School; 1863-73, Bowdoin College; and 1873-1908, Princeton University; after retirement, pursued scientific experiments until the last week before his death. CONTRIBUTIONS: Founded (1889) and directed (until

1908) Princeton University's School of Electrical Engineering, first in the United States. Collaborated in testing and patent litigation involving Thomas A. Edison's incandescent lamp (1879), the electric storage battery, and the "Edison Effect" (1880); helped establish (1883, 1884) first practical system of electrical units. As chairman, New Jersey State Board of Health (1888-1908), played a significant role in the establishment of the first State Laboratory of Bacteriology and Hygiene at Princeton (1896), the institution of training in sanitary sciences for health personnel at Rutgers University (1897), and the certification of professional health officers and sanitary inspectors (1903).

WRITINGS: *Elementary Textbook of Physics* (1884, with William A. Anthony); *Electricity in Daily Life* (1890, editor). REFERENCES: "Cyrus Fogg Brackett—An Appreciation," *Princeton University Alumni Weekly* 15 (1915): 407-8; Kenneth H. Condit, *Cyrus Fogg Brackett (1833-1915) of Princeton: Pioneer in Electrical Engineering Education* (1952); Donald Drew Egbert, "Cyrus Fogg Brackett, 1833-1915," in *Princeton Portraits* (1947), 120-22; David C. English, "Cyrus F. Brackett, M.D., LL.D.," *J. of the Med. Soc. of N.J.* 12 (1915): 83; H. McClenahan, *Cyrus Fogg Brackett, 1833-1915: A Centenary Tribute to One of Princeton's Greatest and Most Beloved Teachers* (1934); Charles Penrose, *Brackett of Maine—A Fragment of the 1850s* (1948), 1-36; *N.Y. Times*, January 30, 1915; Fred B. Rogers, "Cyrus Fogg Brackett (1833-1915): Physicist and Physician," in *Help-Bringers: Versatile Physicians of New Jersey* (1960), 108-17.

W. Barlow

BRACKETT, JOSHUA (May 5, 1733, Greenland, N.H.-July 17, 1802, Portsmouth, N.H.). *Physician.* Son of Capt. John, lawyer, and Elizabeth (Pickering) Brackett. Married Hannah Whipple, 1761; no children. EDUCATION: 1752, A.B., Harvard College; pupil of Dr. Clement Jackson, Portsmouth, N.H.; 1792, M.D. (hon.), Harvard. CAREER: c. 1759 to his death, practiced in Portsmouth, N.H.; in New Hampshire Medical Society: 1791, charter member and first vice-president, and 1793-99, president. CONTRIBUTIONS: A local opinion leader among the profession, was widely known for his obstetrical skills, as recognized by his honorary degree from Harvard and by his election to honorary fellowship in the Massachusetts Medical Society (1783). Name often appears among the correspondents, and in the correspondence, of contemporary New England physicians. Gift of books to the New Hampshire Medical Society was designed to be the nucleus of a statewide information resource. Will endowed the Mass. professorship of natural history at Harvard. Like many of his colleagues, was active in local politics, as a member of the Revolutionary period Committee of Safety and as a judge of the Admiralty Court (1761-84). REFERENCES: Kelly and Burrage (1928); *Sibley's Harvard Graduates* 13 (1965): 197-201.

J. W. Estes

BRADFORD, CLAUDIUS B. (October 3, 1855, Savannah, Mo.-July 24, 1921, Oklahoma City, Okla.). *Physician.* Son of J. H. Bradford, physician. EDUCATION: Graduated from Council Grove (Kans.) High School; began study of medicine with his father and then attended Kansas City Medical College, M.D.,

1882. CAREER: Practice, Council Grove; May 3, 1889, moved to the newly settled Okla. Territory. CONTRIBUTIONS: Leader in promotion of professional medical societies in the new Okla. Territory. First meetings of the Oklahoma Medical Society were held in his office. Charter member, secretary, and president of the society. Became charter member of the Territorial Medical Association and president (1899-1900). Served for 7 years on the U.S. Board of Pension Examiners and was member of the Oklahoma City School Board for 14 years. A strong advocate of public education.

WRITINGS: "Fever—What Is It? How Shall We Treat It?" *Okla. Med. J.* 9 (1901): 33-39; "What Do We Know of Typhoid Fever?" *K. C. Med. Lancet* 12, no. 4 (Apr. 1891): 129-31; "Unavoidable and Accidental Hemorrhage Complicating Pregnancy and Labor," *Okla. Med. News J.* 15 (1907): 264-71. REFERENCES: "C. B. Bradford" file, History of Medicine Collection, University of Oklahoma Health Sciences Center Library, Oklahoma City, Okla.; William F. Browne and R. Palmer Howard, "The Role of the Oklahoma County Medical Society in Territorial Medicine, 1904-1905, *Journal of the Oklahoma State Medical Association,* 70 (Mar. 1977): 92-98; R. Palmer Howard and Rose C. Gideon, "The Beginning of Medical Organization in Oklahoma, 1889-1893," *Journal of the Oklahoma State Medical Association* 67 (Nov. 1974): 45-54.

V. Allen

BRADFORD, EDWARD HICKLING (June 9, 1848, Roxbury, Mass.-May 7, 1926, Boston, Mass.). *Orthopedic surgeon.* Son of Charles Frederic, merchant, and Eliza E. (Hickling) Bradford. Married Edith Fiske, 1900; four children. EDUCATION: Attended Roxbury Latin School; 1869, A.B., Harvard College; 1872, M.A., Harvard Medical School; 1873, M.D., Harvard Medical School; 1872-73, surgical house pupil at Massachusetts General Hospital; 1873-75, postgraduate study in Berlin, London, Paris, and Vienna. CAREER: 1875, general practice in Boston; 1876, medical staff at Boston Dispensary; 1878-1909, surgeon, and later chief of the orthopedic staff at Boston Children's Hospital; 1880-94, visiting staff at Boston City Hospital; 1880-1912, medical faculty of Harvard University, serving as its first professor of orthopedic surgery; 1912, retired from teaching and became dean of Harvard Medical School, serving until 1918. Blind late in life, learned to read Braille and was led by an assistant to meetings of organizations in which he held office. CONTRIBUTIONS: A founder of the American Orthopedic Association (1887), and president in 1889; helped to raise standards of the new specialty. Founded the Boston Industrial School for Crippled and Deformed Children (1893), the first of its kind in America. Convinced state authorities to establish the Massachusetts Hospital School for Crippled Children, at Canton (1904) and served as chairman of the board until his death. Developed the "Bradford Frame" to straighten physical deformities.

WRITINGS: *Treatise on Orthopedic Surgery* (1890 and four more editions, with Robert W. Lovett). REFERENCES: *DAB,* 1 pt. 2: 555-56; Kelly and Burrage (1928), 138-39;

obituaries in *Boston Med. and Surg. J.* (July 1926) and *J. of Bone and Joint Surg.* (July 1926).

M. Kaufman

BRAINARD, DANIEL (May 15, 1812, Oneida County, N.Y.-October 9, 1866, Chicago, Ill.). *Surgeon; Educator.* Son of Jeptha, Jr., well-to-do farmer, and Catherine (Comstock) Brainard. Married Evelyn Sleight, 1845; four children. EDUCATION: 1834, M.D., Jefferson Medical College; 1839-41, studied in Paris. CAREER: 1836-39, 1843-66, practiced surgery and taught in Chicago; 1842-43, anatomy and surgery faculties, St. Louis University; at Rush Medical College: 1843-66, anatomy and surgery faculties; and 1843-66, president. CONTRIBU-TIONS: Founder of Rush Medical College (1837, chartered; 1843, classes begun), Chicago Medical Society (1850), Illinois State Medical Society (1850), and first general hospital in Chicago (1847). Performed earliest recorded necropsy in Chicago (1844). Pioneered in treatment of ununited fractures (1854). Major contributor to surgical anesthesia and plastic surgery.

WRITINGS: "On the Inhalation of Etherial Vapor for the Prevention of Pain During Surgical Operations," *Ill. Ind. Med. and Surg. J.* 1 (1847): 544-49; "Essay on a New Method of Treating Ununited Fractures and Certain Deformities of the Osseous System," *TAMA* 7 (1854): 557-600. REFERENCES: *Chicago Med. J.* 23 (1866): 529-38; *DAB*, 1, pt 2: 589-90; E. Fletcher Ingals, "The Life and Work of Dr. Daniel Brainard," *Bull. Alumni Assoc. Rush Med. Coll.* 8 (Jul. 1912): 1-13; *NCAB*, 20: 309.

W. K. Beatty

BRANCHE, GEORGE CLAYTON (January 10, 1896, Louisburg, N.C.-September 10, 1956, Tuskegee, Ala.). *Neuropsychiatrist.* Son of Joel, minister, and Hannah (Shaw) Branche. Married Lillian V. Davidson, 1924; three children. EDUCATION: 1917, A.B., Lincoln University (Pa.); 1923, M.D., Boston University; 1923, intern, Boston Psychopathic Hospital; 1927, postgraduate course in neuropsychiatry, Veterans Administration Hospital, New York City. CAREER: 1917-19, master sergeant, U.S. Army; 1923-44, 1946-56, staff, Veteran's Hospital, Tuskegee, Ala. (1927-44, chief, neuropsychiatric service; 1946-56, director of professional services); 1944-46, lieutenant colonel, U.S. Army Medical Corps. CONTRIBUTIONS: New treatment for neurosyphilis in blacks (1936), introduction of quartan malarial parasites which replaced injection of patients with tertian malarial parasites. Thought blacks had become immune to the tertian plasmodium owing to its endemic nature in the South.

WRITINGS: "Syphilis of Brain and Cord," *JNMA* 21 (1929): 52-57; "Tryparsamide Therapy of Neurosyphilis in Negroes," *U.S. Vet. Bur. Med. Bull.* 7 (1931): 476-80; also in *JNMA* 23 (1931): 120-23; "Therapeutic Quartan Malaria in Treatment of Neurosyphilis Among Negroes," *J. Nervous and Mental Disorders* 83 (1936): 177-88. REFERENCES:

Obituary, *JNMA* 50 (1958) : 139-40; *WWAPS* 1 (1938): 130.

T. Savitt

BRANDRETH, BENJAMIN (January 9, 1807, Leeds, England-February 19, 1880, Sing Sing, N.Y.). *Proprietary medicine manufacturer; Eclectic physician.* Married Harriet Smallpage, 1829; Virginia Graham, 1840; 17 children. EDUCATION: Learned medicine from paternal grandfather; attended Eclectic Medical College, New York City. CAREER: 1835, went to N.Y. and began to market a formula said to be that of his grandfather as Dr. Benjamin Brandreth's Vegetable Universal Pills, which contained strong botanical cathartics and sarsaparilla; 1837, moved manufacturing to Sing Sing (later renamed Ossining); 1848, purchased Allcock's Porous Plasters; at his death, was making 2 million boxes of pills and 5 million plasters annually with worldwide distribution; president of Sing Sing; 1850, 1858, twice elected to state senate. SIGNIFICANCE: Unostentatious in personal life, was a lavish, flamboyant advertiser, using penny and rural press and wide-circulation magazines like *Harper's Weekly*. A congressional committee (1849) deemed Brandreth the largest proprietary advertiser in nation. Courted controversy to bring attention to his pills, as with New York Academy of Medicine, publisher James Gordon Bennett, and alleged counterfeiters of his pills. Advertising based on theory that corruption of the blood, largely through indigestion, caused all illness and that purgation was a universal panacea. Heirs continued business.

WRITINGS: Compiled promotional book *The Doctrine of Purgation, Curiosities from Ancient and Modern Literature, from Hippocrates and Other Medical Writers, Covering a Period of Over Two Thousand Years, Proving Purgation Is the Cornerstone of All Curatives* (1867 and two subsequent editions). REFERENCES: *Democratic Register* (Sing Sing), February 25, 1880; *Harper's Weekly*, February 19, 1859; Henry W. Holcombe, *Patent Medicine Tax Stamps* (1979), 47-56; *N.Y. Herald* and *Sun*, 1837; *N.Y. Times* and *Tribune*, February 20, 1880; John T. Scharf, *History of Westchester County* (1886), 358-61; James H. Young, *The Toadstool Millionaires* (1961), 75-89.

J. H. Young

BRIGGS, WILLIAM THOMPSON (December 4, 1828, Bowling Green, Ky.-June 12, 1894, Nashville, Tenn.). *Surgeon.* Son of John McPherson, physician and surgeon, and Harriet (Morehead) Briggs. Married Annie E. Stubbins, 1850; four children. EDUCATION: Literary education at Bowling Green, Ky.; served a medical preceptorship under his father; 1849, M.D., Transylvania University, Lexington, Ky. CAREER: 1849-51, practiced medicine with his father, Bowling Green, Ky.; 1852, became a surgeon, Nashville; 1852-68, held various chairs, medical department, University of Nashville; 1868-94, professor of surgery, University of Nashville and Vanderbilt University. CONTRIBUTIONS: As a surgeon, performed several unusual and difficult operations: removed the entire upper jaw following a gunshot injury and extirpated the lower jaw for a gunshot wound (1863); ligated the common and internal carotid artery for traumatic aneurysm (1871); did a hip-joint amputation for elephantiasis arabicum (1875). Also devised a new operative procedure for lithotomy and reported performing 254 operations for vesical calculus with six deaths. Made several important contributions to organized medicine: a founder of the American Surgical Association and its president (1885); chairman of the section on surgery of the International Medical Congress (1887); 43rd president of the American Medical Association (1890-91).

WRITINGS: Listed in Irving A. Watson, *Physicians and Surgeons of Am.* (1896), 43-44. REFERENCES: *JAMA* 22 (1894): 966-67; Kelly and Burrage (1920), 143-44; W. S. Speer, *Sketches of Prominent Tennesseans* (1888), 105-8; *Trans., Med. Soc. of Tenn.* (1895), 31-45.

S. R. Bruesch

BRIGHAM, AMARIAH (December 26, 1798, New Marlboro, Mass.-September 8, 1849, Utica, N.Y.). *Physician; Asylum superintendent.* Son of John and Phoebe (Clark) Brigham. Married Susan C. Root, 1833; five children. EDUCATION: 1812, medical apprentice to his uncle Dr. Origin Brigham, Schoharie, N.Y., and later with Dr. Edmund C. Peet, New Marlboro, Mass., and Dr. Ovid Plumb, Canaan, Conn.; 1828-29, visited hospitals and attended lectures throughout Europe; took courses at the School of Medicine, Sorbonne, Paris. CAREER: Practice: 1819-21, Enfield, Mass.; 1821-28, 1829-31; Greenfield, Mass.; 1828-29, European educational and cultural tour; 1831-37, 1838-40, practiced in Hartford, Conn., where he was profoundly influenced by Dr. Eli Todd (q.v.), superintendent of the Hartford Retreat; 1837-38, lectureship in anatomy, College of Physicians and Surgeons, N.Y.; 1838, assistant editor, *American Journal of Medical Sciences*; superintendent: 1840-42, Hartford Retreat; and 1842-48, New York State Lunatic Asylum, Utica; 1844, founder and the first editor, *American Journal of Insanity.* CONTRIBUTIONS: One of the "original 13" founding fathers of the Association of Medical Superintendents of American Institutions for the Insane and its vice-president (1848). Made the New York State Lunatic Asylum into a model institution where patients received medical and moral treatment in a warm familial atmosphere. Within this therapeutic milieu, they were expected to work, attend classes and lectures, and participate in recreational activities. Worked to inform the public about mental illness. One of the major objectives of his *American Journal of Insanity* was to disseminate knowledge about insanity and its treatment. Believed broad public understanding of mental health issues would facilitate the institutional care of the mentally ill.

WRITINGS: *Remarks on the Influence of Mental Cultivation upon Health* (1832); *Observations on the Influence of Religion upon Health and Physical Welfare of Mankind* (1835); *An Inquiry Concerning the Diseases and Functions of the Brain, Spinal Cord and Nerves* (1840). Complete writings listed in *Am. J. of Psychiatry* (1956). REFERENCES: Eric Carlson, "Amariah Brigham: I. Life and Works," *Am. J. of Psychiatry* 112 (1956): 831-36; idem, "Amariah Brigham: II. Psychiatric Thought and Practice," *ibid.*, 113 (1957): 911-16; *DAB*, 3: 42-43; Kelly and Burrage (1928), 145-46; *NCAB*, 10: 270.

L. V. Bell

BRILL, ABRAHAM ARDEN (October 12, 1874, Kanczuga, Austria-March 2, 1948, New York, N.Y.). *Physician; Psychoanalysis.* Son of Philip, noncommissioned army officer, and Esther (Seitelbach) Brill. Immigrated to the United States, 1889; naturalized, 1899. Married Kitty Rose Owen, 1908; two children. EDUCATION: 1901, Ph.B., New York University; 1903, M.D., College of Physicians and Surgeons (Columbia); 1907-8, studied in Paris and Zurich and under Freud in Vienna. CAREER: 1903-7, medical staff, Central Islip (Long Island) State Hospital; *post* 1908, practiced psychiatry, New York City; 1912-13, chief of clinic in psychiatry, Columbia University; psychiatry faculty: New York Post Graduate Medical School; and New York University; psychoanalysis and psychosexual sciences faculty, Columbia University; 1934, first president, psychoanalytic section, American Psychiatric Association. CONTRIBUTIONS: Called the "father of American psychoanalysis." Proselytized the teachings of Freud among American physicians and the general public and opened the first psychoanalytic practice in America. Translated most of Freud's major works into English as well as some of those of Carl Jung. Authored several basic expositions of psychoanalysis including *Fundamental Conceptions of Psychoanalysis* (1921) and *Psychoanalysis: Its Theories and Practical Application* (1922). Founder and first chairman of the New York Psychoanalytic Society (1911). Through writings, editorial work, and personal persuasion, gained American acceptance of the use of psychoanalysis in the treatment of mental disorders.

WRITINGS: *Freud's Selected Papers on Hysteria* (1909, translator); *Jung's Psychology of Dementia Praecox* (1909, translator); English edition of *Bleuler's Text Book of Psychiatry* (1925, editor); *The Basic Writings of Sigmund Freud* (1938, editor). A bibliography is in *Psychoanalytical Q.* 17 (1948): 164-72. REFERENCES: *DAB*, Supplement 4: 107-9; Miller, *BHM*, p. 15; *NCAB*, E: 526; *N.Y. Times*, March 3, 1948; *Who Was Who in Am.*, 2: 79.

S. *Galishoff*

BRINKLEY, JOHN RICHARD (c. 1886, Beta, N.C.-May 7, 1942, San Antonio, Tex.). *Physician.* Middle name originally Romulus. Son of John Richard, country doctor, and Candace (Burnett) Brinkley. Orphaned at age ten. Another source says, at age five, sent to live with his uncle John Brinkley, country doctor, East La Port, N.C. Married Sally Wike, 1908, three children; Minnie T. Jones, 1922, one child. EDUCATION: 1908-11, courses in Bennett Medical College, Chicago, Ill.; May 7, 1915, diploma, Eclectic Medical University of Kansas City, Mo.; 1919, diploma, Kansas City College of Medicine and Surgery; July 1925, M.D., Royal University, Pavia, Italy (degree annulled in 1927). CAREER: 1913-16, practiced medicine in Ark. under the guise of "undergraduate license"; jailed for forged checks; 1918, settled in Milford, Kans.; opened a hospital for 16 patients; 1920, arrested for selling intoxicating liquors in violation of Kans. laws; 1920, moved to Chicago, run-in with police, traveled to Calif., and returned to Milford in 1923; 1930, Kansas Medical Board revoked his physician's license; shipped "special gland emulsion"; 1930, Federal Radio Commission stopped his radio station KFKB (Kansas First, Kansas Best) from broadcasting; 1930, 1932, 1934, ran for governor of Kans.; 1937, moved to Mexico; 1940s, antiwar advocate and friend of the German-American Bund; 1942, trial for his arrest was scheduled. SIGNIFICANCE: Began transplanting goat glands into men to rejuvenate them; called himself a "rejuvenation surgeon." Prepared special gland "emulsion" as a substitute for the operation; was administered with a rectal syringe. One of first users of radio advertisements to sell health products. Ran a mail order business as a Fountain of Youth. Was in constant trouble with the U.S. government after the Kansas Medical Society filed complaints. Rather than face a trial, settled in Mexico, where he beamed his radio reports into the United States. Excelled at reporting unsubstantiated claims and announcing his success over radio. Publicly supported by the town fathers of Milford and by a national following. REFERENCES: *BHM* (1975-79), 22; Gerald Carson, *The Roguish World of Doctor Brinkley* (1960); *DAB*, Supplement 3: 103-5; *JAMA*, 90 (1928): 134-37; Patrick M. McGrady, *The Youth Doctors* (1968); Miller, *BHM*, p. 15; *N.Y. Times*, May 27, 1942, p. 24.

R. Edwards

BRINTON, JOHN HILL (May 21, 1832, Philadelphia, Pa.-March 18, 1907, Philadelphia). *Surgeon*. Son of George and Mary M. Smith. Married Sarah Ward, 1866; three children. EDUCATION: University of Pennsylvania: 1850, B.A.; and 1853, A.M.; 1852, M.D., Jefferson Medical College; 1852-53, clinical training, Paris and Vienna. CAREER: 1853-61, general and surgical practice, Philadelphia; 1853-82, operative surgery faculty, Jefferson Medical College; 1861-65, brigade surgeon, (major) U.S. Volunteers; medical director at Battle of Donelson and in Nashville and Missouri campaigns; first curator of Army Medical Museum, founded in May 1862 (now Armed Forces Institute of Pathology); published first catalog of museum; inspector and director of patient evacuation after battles of Antietam, Fredericksburg, Gettysburg, and Chancellorsville; 1864-65, medical director of hospitals, Nashville, and the Army of the Cumberland; 1866-1906, surgical practice, Philadelphia, and surgeon, St. Joseph's Hospital; 1867-82, surgeon, Philadelphia Hospital, and Jefferson Hospital (1877); 1882-1906, followed Samuel D. Gross (q.v.) as professor of surgery at Jefferson; fellow, College of Physicians of Philadelphia; a founder, Pathological Society of Philadelphia and the Academy of Surgery. CONTRIBUTIONS: As first curator of the Army Medical Museum, founded by Surgeon-General William A. Hammond (q.v.), established a research and teaching institution that was the only federally supported biomedical research organization (1862-87). Established a collection of war-related pathology and laid the groundwork for what later also became a great public medical museum. Developed the plan and direction of the three-volume *Surgical History of the War of the Rebellion*, the first such military medical history ever written on that scale. Later years of active teaching and writing established him as a preeminent academic surgeon in this country.

WRITINGS: *Personal Memoirs of John H. Brinton* (1914). REFERENCES: *DAB*, 3: 51-

52; *Jeffersonian* 8 (1906-7); Kelly and Burrage (1920), 145-46; *Military Surgeon* 22 (1908); 221-22; *NCAB*, 37: 214; *N.Y. Med. J.* 85 (1907): 559.

R. J. T. Joy

BRÖDEL, MAX (June 8, 1870, Leipzig, Germany-October 26, 1941, Baltimore, Md.). *Medical illustrator; Anatomy.* Son of Louis, piano works manager, and Henrietta (Frenzel) Brödel. Married Ruth Marian Huntington, 1902; four children. EDUCATION: 1885-90, studied at the Leipzig Academy of Fine Arts. CAREER: 1885-90, freelance illustrator, Leipzig Anatomical Institute and Leipzig Physiological Institute; 1890-92, military service, German army; 1894, brought to Johns Hopkins by Franklin P. Mall (q.v.), where he illustrated the works of leading medical scientists and was an instructor (1907-10) and associate professor and director of the Department of Art as applied to medicine (1911-40). CONTRIBUTIONS: Founded the art of medical illustration in the United States and taught many of the leading illustrators of his time. Department of Art as applied to medicine was the first of its kind in the United States. Clear and informative drawings of operative procedures and pathological specimens for Howard Kelly's (q.v.) *Operative Gynecology* contributed to that work's revolutionary impact on that branch of medicine. These drawings plus those in Thomas Cullen's *Cancer of the Uterus* brought him recognition as the nation's foremost medical artist. Studied anatomy and physiology to improve his art. Dissection of the kidney and vascular injections led to discovery of an area of the kidneys relatively free of blood vessels, along which line the incision for the operation for stone could be made (Brödel's line). Also devised a suture for repairing a prolapsed kidney (Brödel's suture).

WRITINGS: Most famous works included the illustrations for Howard A. Kelly, *Operative Gynecology* (1898); Thomas S. Cullen, *Cancer of the Uterus* (1900); and some for *Atlas of Human Anatomy* (1935). REFERENCES: *BHM* (1964-69), 42; (1975), 5; (1975-79), 23; *DAB*, Supplement 3: 106-7; *DSB*, 2: 64-65; *Who Was Who in Am.*, 1: 142.

S. Galishoff

BRODIE, WILLIAM (c. July 28, 1823, Fawley Court, England-July 30, 1890, Detroit, Mich.). *Physician; Surgeon.* Son of a farm family. Married Jane Whitfield, 1851; three children. EDUCATION: Collegiate Institute, Brockport, N.Y.; 1847, studied medicine with William Wilson, Pontiac, Mich.; Berkshire Medical Institution (Pittsfield, Mass.) and Vermont Medical College (Woodstock, Vt.); 1850, M.D., College of Physicians and Surgeons (N.Y.); 1850-51, house surgeon, St. Mary's Hospital, Detroit. CAREER: 1850, surgical practice (with Zina Pitcher), Detroit; 1850-63, surgeon, St. Mary's Hospital, Detroit; 1852, a founder, and 1855, president, Detroit Medical Society; 1855-57, editor, *Peninsular Medical Journal*; 1857, secretary, and 1886, president, American Medical Association; 1861, surgeon, First Michigan Volunteers; 1866, president, Detroit Common Council, and long-term president, Detroit Board of Health; president:

1876, Michigan State Medical Society; and 1876-90 (except two years), Wayne County Medical Society; 1879-85, founding professor of clinical medicine, Michigan College of Medicine. CONTRIBUTIONS: Long the "motive power" of local professional societies in Detroit; leader of early AMA efforts to regulate medical school size and standards (1860); responsible for installing lateral drainage sewer system in Detroit. REFERENCES: C. B. Burr, *Medical History of Michigan* (1930) 1: 665, 722; 2: 58-60, 111; Martin Kaufman, *American Medical Education: The Formative Years* (1976), 106; Kelly and Burrage (1928), 149-50; Paul Leake, *History of Detroit* 3 (1912): 1077-81; *NCAB*, 12: 224; *Representative Men of Michigan: American Biographical History of Eminent and Self-Made Men* (1878), district 1: 13-14.

M. Pernick

BRONK, DETLEV WULF (August 13, 1897, New York, N.Y.-November 17, 1975, New York). *Physiologist; University president; Biophysics.* Son of Mitchell, Baptist minister, and Marie (Wulf) Bronk. Married Helen Alexander Ramsey, 1921; three children. EDUCATION: 1920, B.S., Swarthmore College; at University of Michigan: 1922, M.S.; and 1926, Ph.D.; 1928-29, National Research Council fellow, Cambridge, England. CAREER: 1918, executive secretary, Office of Food Administration, Philadelphia, Pa.; 1918-19, U.S. Naval Aviation Corps; at University of Michigan: 1921-24, physics faculty; and 1924-26, physiology faculty; 1927-29, physiology and biophysics faculty and dean of men, Swarthmore College; at University of Pennsylvania: 1929-49, biophysics faculty and director, Eldridge Reeves Johnson Foundation for Medical Physics; and 1936-40, 1942-49, head, Institute of Neurology; 1940-41, physiology faculty, Cornell Medical College; during World War II, served several federal offices in advisory capacities; 1946-50, chairman, National Research Council; 1949-53, president, Johns Hopkins University; 1950-62, president, National Academy of Sciences; at Rockefeller Institute for Medical Research (in 1965, Rockefeller University): *post* 1946, member, Board of Scientific Directors; and 1953-68, president; member: 1948-58, National Advisory Committee for Aeronautics; 1950-70, Board of Trustees; and Committee on Scientific Policy, Sloan Kettering Institute. CONTRIBUTIONS: Studied the physical basis of the neuronal activity that is fundamental to the regulatory functions of the nervous system. Established the modern science of biophysics—the application of physics to the study of life systems. Investigated the molecular structure of nerve cells and measured the changes in nerve cells during the passage of stimuli to the brain. Studied the chemical excitation of nerves and nerve impulses and measured oxygen consumptions in nerve fibers. As coordinator of research in the Air Surgeon's Office of the U.S. Army Air Corps during World War II, directed important studies of the physiological aspects of aviation. Helped edit several journals including *Journal of Cellular and Comparative Physiology* (1939-53), *Proceedings of the Society of Experimental Biology and Medicine* (1935-41), and the *American Journal of Physiology* (1938-43). After World War II, was an outstanding college administrator and "statesman of science" who played a leading role in the organization of scientific research in the United States. As president of the Rockefeller Institute for Medical Research, oversaw its transition from a distinguished medical facility to one of the best graduate universities in the world. WRITINGS: "Afferent Impulses in the Carotid Sinus Nerve," *J. of Cellular and Comparative Physiol.* 1 (1932): 113 (with G. Stella); "Oxygen Supply and Oxygen Consumption in the Nervous System," *Trans., Am. Neurological Assoc.* 70 (1944): 141-44; "Physical Structure and Biological Action of Nerve Cells, with Some Reference to Problems of Human Flight," *Am. Scientist* 34 (1946): 55-76; "Prolonged Facilitation of Synaptic Excitation in Sympathetic Ganglia," *J. of Neurophysiology* 10 (1947): 139-54; "The Role of Scientists in the Furtherance of Science," *Science* 119 (1954): 223-27. A bibliography is in *BMNAS*. REFERENCES: *BHM* (1964-69), 43; (1975-79), 23; *BMNAS* 50 (1979): 3-87; *Current Biog.* (1949), 76-78; *McGraw-Hill Modern Men of Sci.* 2 (1966): 56-57; *N.Y. Times*, November 18, 1975.

S. Galishoff

BROOMALL, ANNA ELIZABETH (March 4, 1847, Upper Chichester Township, Delaware County, Pa.-April 4, 1931, Chester, Pa.). *Obstetrician; Medical educator.* Daughter of John Martin, lawyer, farmer, and congressman, and Elizabeth (Booth) Broomall. Never married. EDUCATION: 1866, Bristol Boarding School; 1871, M.D., Woman's Medical College of Pennsylvania; 1871-75, studied obstetrics in Vienna with Carl and Gustav Braun and in Paris. CAREER: 1875-83, chief resident physician, Woman's Hospital, Philadelphia; 1875-1903, instructor and then (1880) professor of obstetrics, Woman's Medical College of Pennsylvania; 1888, established one of first obstetrical out-patient practice clinics, connected with Woman's Medical College; 1883, gynecologist to Friends' Asylum for the Insane, Frankford, Philadelphia, Pa.; 1892, among first women to be admitted to Philadelphia Obstetrical Society. CONTRIBUTIONS: Brought to women students most advanced European methods of obstetrical and gynecological care. Noted for extensive reading in French, German, and Italian medical literature. Among the first obstetricians to emphasize thorough prenatal care including pelvimetry; advocated episiotomy, Caesarian section, and symphysiotomy. Boasted of extremely low mortality rates at the Maternity Hospital of the Woman's Medical College and demonstrated the ability of women physicians to practice advanced and progressive obstetrics. Sincere and supportive teacher and friend to women medical students (1875-1903). First woman physician to publish in the *Transactions* of the Philadelphia Obstetrical Society (1878).

WRITINGS: "The Operation of Episiotomy as a Prevention of Perineal Ruptures During Labor," *Am. J. of Obstet. and Diseases of Women and Children* 11 (1878): 517-27; "Three Cases of Symphysiotomy, with One Death from Sepsis," *ibid.*, 28 (1893): 305-12. Writings listed in Clara Marshall, *The Woman's Medical College of Pennsylvania* (1897). REFERENCES: Gulielma Fell Alsop, *History of the Woman's Medical College* (1950); Marshall, *The Woman's Medical College of Pennsylvania*; *NCAB*, 24: 291; *Notable American Women* 1 (1971): 246-47.

R. M. Morantz

BROWN, CHARLOTTE AMANDA (BLAKE) (December 22, 1846, Philadelphia, Pa.-April 19, 1904, San Francisco, Calif.). *Physician.* Daughter of

Charles Morris, teacher and Presbyterian minister, and Charlotte A. (Farrington) Blake. Married Henry Adams Brown, bank clerk, 1867; three children. EDUCATION: 1861, Bangor (Maine) High School; 1866, B.A., Elmira College; 1874, M.D., Woman's Medical College of Pennsylvania. CAREER: 1875, founded Pacific Dispensary for Women and Children with Dr. Martha E. Bucknell in San Francisco; 1878-80, reorganized dispensary as a hospital and added one of the earliest nurses' training programs; 1885, incorporated hospital as San Francisco Hospital for Children and Training School for Nurses; 1876, accepted, along with four other women, to the California Medical Society; 1885-95, staff physician, Children's Hospital; 1895-1904, private practice. CONTRIBUTIONS: Member, committee on diseases of women and children, California Medical Society (1876). Outspoken advocate of medical innovation and public health measures, including the establishment of a "tumor registry" in San Francisco (1887), the use of incubators for premature babies (1893), the monitoring of adolescent health habits, milk sterilization, strict inspection and enforcement of public health regulations in new and old city buildings, improved training for nurses and doctors (1876-1904). Performed first ovariotomy by a woman on the Pacific Coast (1878). Strong, successful, and highly respected supporter of women in medicine.

WRITINGS: "The Health of Our Girls," *Calif. State Med. Soc. Trans.* 26 (1896): 193-202; "Practical Points in Obstetrics," *Occidental Med. Times* 14 (1900): 12-16. Writings listed in Clara Marshall, *The Woman's Medical College of Pennsylvania* (1897). REFERENCES: Adelaide Brown, "The History of the Development of Women in Medicine in California," *Calif. and Western Med.* (May 1925); *Notable American Women* 1 (1971): 251-53.

R. M. Morantz

BROWN, LAWRASON (September 29, 1871, Baltimore, Md.-December 26, 1937, Saranac Lake, N.Y.). *Physician; Tuberculosis.* Son of William Judson, commission merchant, and Mary Louise (Lawrason) Brown. Married Martha Lewis Harris, 1914; no children. EDUCATION: Johns Hopkins University: 1895, A.B.; and 1900, M.D. CAREER: At Adirondack Cottage Sanitarium (later Trudeau Sanitarium), Saranac Lake: 1900-1901, assistant resident physician; 1902-12, resident physician; 1912-14, visiting physician; 1916-29, chairman, medical board; and 1916-37, consulting physician; instructor, Trudeau School of Tuberculosis; president: 1919-23, American Sanitorium Association; 1920, American Clinical and Climatological Association; and 1922-23, National Tuberculosis Association. CONTRIBUTIONS: In capacity as medical director of the Trudeau Sanitarium, developed professional standards in the care of tuberculosis that were widely adopted throughout the United States; notable features included detailed clinical records and a follow-up system of postsanitarium medical observation. Helped found the National Tuberculosis Association and the closely related American Sanitorium Association. Pioneered in the roentgenographic

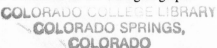

diagnosis of pulmonary and intestinal tuberculosis. Founded (1905) and edited (until 1910) *Journal of the Outdoor Life*, a magazine for tuberculosis patients.

WRITINGS: *Rules for Recovery from Pulmonary Tuberculosis* (1915); "A Study of the Occurrence of Hemoptysis, Pleurisy, Rales, Tubercle Bacilli and X-Ray Findings in 1,000 Consecutive Cases Admitted to the Trudeau Sanitarium" *Am. Review of Tuberculosis* (1926, with Homer L. Sampson); *The Lungs and the Early Stages of Tuberculosis* (1931); *The Story of Clinical Pulmonary Tuberculosis* (1941, posthumously). A bibliography is in S. Adolphus Knopf, *A History of the National Tuberculosis Association* (1922). REFERENCES: *DAB*, Supplement 2: 70-71; *NCAB*, 28: 130-31; *N.Y. Times*, December 27, 1937; *Who Was Who in Am.*, 1: 150.

S. Galishoff

BROWN, PERCY (November 24, 1875, Cambridge, Mass.-October 8, 1950, Egypt, Mass.). *Physician: Roentgenology*. Son of Isaac Henry and Mary Elizabeth (Kennedy) Brown. Married Bernice Mayhew, 1904; no children. EDUCATION: 1893-96, premedical study, Lawrence Scientific School; 1900, M.D., Harvard Medical School; 1901-3, intern, Boston Children's Hospital. CAREER: 1904-17, practiced medicine, Boston, Mass.; roentgenologist: 1903-6, 1910-22, Boston Infant's Hospital; 1903-10, Carney Hospital; 1905-11, St. Elizabeth's Hospital; and 1911-13, Long Island Hospital, Boston, Mass.; 1911, president, American Roentgen Ray Society; 1911-22, roentgenology faculty, Harvard Medical School; 1917-18, Medical Corps, U.S. Army, Harvard Unit, Base Hospital 5, France; after World War I, roentgenologist to several medical facilities, including St. Luke's Hospital, New York City (1924-29); Jackson Clinic, Madison, Wis.; and Grunow Clinic, Phoenix, Ariz.; 1934, retired from active practice because of lesions on his hands caused by radiation. CONTRIBUTIONS: Instrumental in the establishment of roentgenology as a separate medical specialty based on scientific principles. Used influence to establish professional standards and training for physicians practicing roentgenology (radiology). Designed several pieces of X-ray apparatus.

WRITINGS: *Science of Radiology for Fist* (1933); *American Martyrs to Science Through the Roentgen Rays* (1935). REFERENCES: *DAB*, Supplement 5: 111-12; George W. Holmes, "Percy Brown, 1870-1950," *Am. J. of Roentgenology* 65 (1951): 122-24; *Who Was Who in Am.*, 3: 112.

S. Galishoff

BROWN, SAMUEL (January 30, 1769, Augusta, now Rockbridge County, Va.-January 12, 1830, near Huntsville, Ala.). *Physician; Teacher*. Son of John, Presbyterian minister and schoolmaster, and Margaret (Preston) Brown. Married Catherine Percy, 1808; three children. EDUCATION: 1789, B.S., Dickinson College; c. 1790-92, studied medicine as private pupil of Alexander Humphreys, Staunton, Va.; and Benjamin Rush (q.v.), Philadelphia, Pa.; and at Edinburgh, Scotland; c. 1795, M.D., Aberdeen, Scotland. CAREER: 1795, practice, Bladensburg, Prince Georges County, Md.; 1795-1806, Lexington, Ky.; 1799, appointed professor of anatomy, surgery, and chemistry, Transylvania University medical department, Lexington; no regular classes or school building, but taught medical students; 1806-19, practiced medicine, New Orleans, La., and Natchez, Miss.; 1819-25, professor of theory and practice of medicine, Transylvania medical department. CONTRIBUTIONS: With Dr. Frederick Ridgely (q.v.), gave the first formal lectures in medicine at Lexington (1799). Authorized by Board of Trustees of Transylvania to spend $500 for the purchase of books for the first medical library (October 18, 1799). Introduced vaccination with the kine pox in Lexington in association with Dr. Ridgely (May 1801). A founder of the Kappa Lambda Society of Hippocrates at Transylvania medical department (1820).

WRITINGS: Five case reports were published in the *Med. Repository* 2, 4, and 5 (1806, 1808, 1809), and several short papers concerning sources and the manufacture of nitre appeared in *Trans., Am. Philos. Soc.* (1809) and *Am. J. of Sci. & Art* (1818). REFERENCES: *DAB*, 3: 152-53; [D. Drake], "Obituary of Professor Brown," *Western J. of Med. & Phys. Sci.* 3 (1830): 606-8; B. Hardin, "The Brown Family of Liberty Hall," *Filson Club Hist. Q.* 16 (1942): 75-87; Kelly and Burrage (1920), 154-55; *NCAB*, 4: 348; L. P. Yandell, "Dr. Samuel Brown as an Author," *Western J. of Med. & Surg.* 2 (1853): 175-82.

E. H. Conner

BROWN, SOLYMAN (November 17, 1790, Litchfield, Conn.-February 13, 1876, Dodge Center, Minn.). *Dentist.* Son of Nathaniel and Thankful (Woodruff) Brown. Married Elizabeth Butler, 1834; eight children. EDUCATION: Attended Morris Academy, Litchfield; Yale College: 1812, A.B.; 1817, M.A.; 1832-33, studied dentistry with Eleazar Parmly (q.v.), New York City. CAREER: 1813-18, Congregational minister in Conn. until he lost his license due to requirement that ministers needed two years of special study; 1820-32, taught in private schools in New York City while preaching in the New Jerusalem Church (Swedenborgian); 1834-37, practiced dentistry in N.Y. with Samuel Avery; 1837-44, practiced dentistry in N.Y. with Augustus Woodruff Brown, his brother; 1844, lived and worked in a Fourier phalanx at Leraysville, Pa.; 1846-50, practice of dentistry and preacher at Ithaca and Danby, N.Y.; 1850-62, dental practice of New York City, where he opened a dental supply depot and then was a partner in the New York Teeth Manufacturing Company; 1862-70, minister at Danby. CONTRIBUTIONS: Credited with elevating dentistry as a profession. With Eleazar Parmly, organized the Society of Surgeon Dentists of the City and State of New York, the world's first dental society. Edited the first dental journal, *American Journal of Dental Science* (1839-1842). An organizer of the first national dental society, the American Society of Dental Surgeons, which awarded him an honorary degree of Doctor of Dental Surgery. Author of the first treatise on orthodontia in America (1841). Publisher of the *Semi-Annual Dental Expositor* (1852-54).

WRITINGS: *Importance of Regulating the Teeth of Children* (1841); *Treatise on Mechanical Dentistry* (1843); numerous poems, including *Dentologia* (1833); and political writings, including *Union of Extremes: A Discourse on Liberty and Slavery* (1858).

REFERENCES: *DAB*, 2, pt. 1:155-56; C. R. E. Koch, *History of Dental Surgery* (1909), vol. 2, essay on Brown; J. A. Taylor, *Hist. of Dentistry* (1922).

M. Kaufman

BROWN, WILLIAM (1752, Haddingtonshire, Scotland-January 11, 1792, Alexandria, Va.). *Physician.* Son of Richard, minister, and Helen (Bailey) Brown. Married Catherine Scott; several children. EDUCATION: Early schooling in St. Mary's County, Md.; 1770, M.D., University of Edinburgh. CAREER: Returned to America; established practice in Alexandria; 1775, became surgeon, Woodford's Regiment; 1776, deputy to William Shippen (q.v.), director-general of medical services; 1778, replaced Benjamin Rush (q.v.) as physician-general of Middle Department; 1780, resigned to return to practice; voted special land bounty for services by General Assembly of Va. CONTRIBUTIONS: A competent practitioner, one of only 400 in colonies with an M.D., for Edinburgh thesis "De Viribis Atmosphaerae." Met critical need of army hospital physicians and surgeons during the Revolution for drug formulary and pharmacology text with his Lititz pharmacopeia, the first pharmacopeia published in the U.S.

WRITINGS: *Pharmacopoeia Simpliciorum et Efficaciorum in Usum Nosocomii Militaris* (1778). Writings listed in Robert B. Austin, *Early American Imprints*, no. 297 (1961). REFERENCES: *DAB*, 3: 157; Bessie W. Gahn, "Dr. William Brown," *J. of the Am. Pharmacy Assoc.* 16 (1927): 1090-91; "The Lititz Pharmacopeia," *The Badger Pharmacist* (1938): 22-25.

R. J. T. Joy

BROWN, WILLIAM EUSTIS (August 27, 1887, Jersey City, N.J.-January 5, 1968, Burlington, Vt.). *Physician; Administrator.* Son of John Lovell, businessman, and Susan (Ingersoll) Brown. Married Estelle Wolff, 1919; one child. EDUCATION: 1909, B.A., Lafayette; Harvard-MIT School of Public Health: 1915, C.P.H.; and 1916, M.P.H.; 1919, M.D., Harvard; 1919-21, surgical house officer, Peter Bent Brigham Hospital, Boston, Mass. CAREER: 1916, instructor and acting dean, Harvard School of Public Health; 1917, health officer, York, Maine; 1921-24, Franklin Hospital, Franklin, N.J.; 1925-45, associate professor and professor, preventive medicine, University of Cincinnati; 1945-52, professor, preventive medicine, and dean, University of Vermont; 1943-45, senior surgeon, U.S. Public Health Service. CONTRIBUTIONS: During the war years as a public health service officer (1943-45), was in charge of U.N. Relief and Rehabilitation Service for the Mid-East and Balkans. Following the German evacuation of Greece and during the Revolution, took over control of the civilian hospitals in Athens and Piraeus; was decorated by the Greek government. As dean at Vermont, revitalized the faculty that had been decimated during the war, reorganized the clinical facilities, gained the confidence of the medical community, and was largely responsible for developing the medical college into a national resource. REFERENCE: Paul K. French, "William E. Brown, Dean of the University of Vermont Medical College, An Oral History Interview," *Vermont Hist.* 41 (1973): 158-72.

L. J. Wallman

BROWN, WILLIAM WELLS (c. 1816, near Lexington, Ky.-November 6, 1884, Chelsea, Mass.). *Physician.* Said to be son of George Higgins (white) and Elizabeth (Lee?), slave of Dr. John Young (q.v.). Married Elizabeth Schooner, 1834 (d. 1850 or 1851), two children; Annie Elizabeth Gray, 1860, two children. EDUCATION: Self-educated. 1849-54, while in Europe, began reading books on medicine, especially those given him by Dr. John Bishop Estlin in England; during the Civil War, attended lectures on medicine and read medical books in Boston whenever possible; in late 1864 or early 1865, appended "M.D." to his name and took on patients in Boston area. CAREER: Born a slave; gained some education when hired out to Elijah P. Lovejoy, editor, *St. Louis Times*; 1834, escaped to Ohio, where he worked on Lake Erie steamer and began self-education; antislavery lecturer and writer: 1843-49, United States; and 1849-54, Europe; 1854-84, lectured, wrote, and practiced medicine (1865-84). CONTRIBUTIONS: Did not practice medicine much, owing to widespread activities: writing, lecturing, and generally advancing the black cause both before and after the Civil War. One of the early black healers in United States. Most famous as abolitionist and reformer.

WRITINGS: *Narrative of William W. Brown* (1847); *The Black Man and His Antecedents, His Genius, and His Achievements* (1863); *The Rising Son: or The Antecedents and the Advancement of the Colored Race* (1874). Writings listed in *DAB*, 2: 161; William Edward Farrison, *William Wells Brown, Author and Reformer* (1969), 459-60. REFERENCES: *DAB*, 2: 161; *Encyclopedia of Am. Biog.* (1934), 139-40; Farrison, *William Wells Brown*; William J. Simmons, *Men of Mark* (1887), 447-50; *Who Was Who in Am.*, Hist. Vol.: 80.

L. Falk and T. Savitt

BRUNK, ANDREW S. (1884, Elida, Ohio-February 3, 1952, San Antonio, Tex.). *Surgeon; Health insurance.* Son of Perry E. and Maria (Powell) Brunk. Married; one child. EDUCATION: 1909, M.D., Cleveland Homeopathic College. CAREER: 1911-24, surgeon, Southern Pacific Railroad, Colo.; 1924-39, practiced surgery, Detroit, Mich.; 1930-52, founder and director, Martin Place Hospital; 1939-48, founder, first president, and Executive Committee, Michigan Hospital Service (Blue Cross); 1940-52, founder and director, Michigan Medical Service (Blue Shield); 1943-50, founding president, Michigan Health Council; 1944-45, president, Michigan State Medical Society; 1945, founding president, Conference of State Medical Association Presidents. CONTRIBUTIONS: The key figure in organizing Blue Cross and Blue Shield plans in Mich. and a militant opponent of compulsory health insurance. Spearheaded the national organization of state medical association leaders to coordinate grass-roots medical opposition to government involvement in medicine.

WRITINGS: "Radio Broadcasting by the Medical Profession," *JAMA* 127 (1945): 283-84; "Aims and Purposes of the Conference of Presidents and Other Officers of State Medical Associations," Michigan State Med. Soc., *J.* 45 (1946): 479-80; "Prepaid Medical Care Plans," *Kentucky Med. J.* 44 (1946): 124-29. REFERENCES: *Detroit Free Press*, February 5, 1952, p. 21; *JAMA* 148 (1952): 950; *Michigan State Med. Soc., J.* 51 (1952): 374.

M. Pernick

BRYCE, PETER (March 5, 1834, Columbia, S.C.-August 14, 1892, Tuscaloosa, Ala.). *Physician; Psychiatry.* Son of Peter and Martha (Smith) Bryce. Married Marie Ellen Clarkson, 1860; no children. EDUCATION: Graduated from the Citadel in Charleston, S.C; 1859, M.D., New York University; postgraduate study, Europe, specializing in nervous diseases. CAREER: 1860, first superintendent of Alabama Hospital for the Treatment of the Insane in Tuscaloosa; Dorothea Dix (q.v.), national reform leader, urged Alabama authorities to appoint Bryce to this position; president: 1878, Alabama Medical Association; 1892, American Medico-Psychological Association; 1892, Commission of Lunacy, established by the Alabama legislature in reference to the custody and trial of the criminal insane; and National Association of Hospital Superintendents. CONTRIBUTIONS: Advocated the use of nonrestraint treatment for the mentally ill; due to this method, the Alabama Hospital for the Treatment of the Insane, later named Bryce Hospital, became a model institution known throughout the United States. Found employment for a large percentage of his patients in useful and congenial occupations.

WRITINGS: "The Mind and How to Preserve It," *Trans. Med. Assoc. Ala.*, 33 (1880): 243-91;"Moral and Criminal Responsibility" (Read before the National Conference of Charities and Corrections at its annual meeting in Buffalo, N.Y.); "The Non-restraint System" (Read before the Medico-Legal Society of New York). Published as "Mechanical Restraint and the Insane," *Medico-Legal J.* 8 (1890-91): 311-13, this paper formed the basis of a discussion among leading alienists and superintendents of hospitals for the insane in both England and America. Symposium was published in successive issues of the *Medico-Legal J.* (Dec. 1891-Jun. 1892), as well as in the British journals of that period. REFERENCES: Howard Holley, *History of Medicine in Alabama* (1982), 318-26; *J. Med. Assoc. of the State of Ala.* (Mar. 1936): 317; (Apr. 1936): 351; *Memorial Record of Ala.* (1976); T. M. Owen, *History of Alabama*, 4 vols. (1978).

S. Eichold

BUCKINGHAM, RICHARD GREEN (September 14, 1816, Troy, N.Y.-March 18, 1889, Los Angeles, Calif.). *Physician.* Son of Gideon and Maria (Jutau) Buckingham. Married Caroline DeForrest, 1839; three children. EDUCATION: Graduate of Rensselaer Institute; 1836, M.D., Berkshire Medical College. CAREER: 1837-41, practiced medicine, Ala.; moved: 1841-42, to St. Louis; 1842-63, to Lexington, Mo.; and 1863, to Denver, Colo.; first president: 1871, Denver Medical Society; and Colorado Territorial Medical Society; 1868-72, president,

Denver School Board; 1876, mayor, Denver. CONTRIBUTIONS: Member, Colorado Territorial Senate (1874), which at his urging passed a bill establishing Deaf Mute Institute in Colorado Springs, Colo.; was on its first Board of Trustees. A founder and first dean of the University of Denver medical department (1881-82) and taught forensic medicine there. Portrait in stained glass is in the rotunda of the Colorado State capitol building in Denver, one of 16 such portraits honoring the state's pioneers.

WRITINGS: Special interest in obstetrics is reflected in his few papers on that topic in the *Transactions* of the Colorado Medical Society (1871-83). REFERENCE: Judith Hannemann, "Richard Green Buckingham" (in three parts), *Denver Med. Bull.* 59 (Jan., Feb., and May 1969).

F. B. Rogers

BULL, WILLIAM (September 24, 1710, Charleston, S.C.-July 4, 1791, London, England). *Physician; Politician.* Son of William, lieutenant governor, and Mary (Quintyne) Bull. Married Hannah Beale, 1746; no children. EDUCATION: Charleston schools; 1734, M.D., Leyden, Netherlands. CAREER: In Charleston and S.C.: 1736, justice of the peace; 1736-49, House of Commons; 1740-42, 1744-49, Speaker of the House of Commons; 1740, captain in St. Augustine Expedition; 1740, assistant judge; 1749, Council; 1751, representative to Six Nations Day; 1751-59, brigadier of the Provisional forces; 1759, lieutenant governor; 1760-61, 1764-66, summer 1768, 1769-71, 1773-75, governor; 1760, president, Charleston Library Society. CONTRIBUTIONS: Although the first native-born American to receive the doctor of medicine, there is no evidence that he ever practiced medicine; however, is credited with being instrumental in the establishment of the College of Philadelphia. Promoted better regulation of "physic" and better protection against yellow fever and other diseases. Helped establish public schools and a college in S.C.

WRITINGS: *Letter to the Honorable Thomas Penn, Esq., Proprietary of Pennsylvania* (1740). REFERENCES: *DAB*, 3: 252-53; Gulielma Melton Daminer, *Dictionary of South Carolina Biography During the Period of Royal Government, 1719-1775* (M.A. thesis, University of South Carolina, 1926); J. H. Easterby, *Colonial Records of South Carolina* (1952); Charles Evans, ed., *Am. Biblio.* (1960); *J. of the Commons House of Assembly, 1742-1744* (1954); Eleanor W. Townsend, "William Bull, M.D., Lieutenant Governor of South Carolina under Royal Government," *Annals of Med. Hist.* (1935); Joseph Ioor Waring, *History of Medicine in South Carolina, 1670-1825* (1964).

J. P. Dolan

BURCH, FRANK EARL (March 27, 1876, Manomenie, Wis.-July 1, 1957, St. Paul, Minn.). *Ophthalmologist.* Son of Newell and Susan (Paris) Burch. Married Katharine Jackson, 1901; two children. EDUCATION: 1897, M.D., University of Minnesota; 1897-98, intern, St. Luke's Hospital; postgraduate work, Johns Hopkins and the London Royal Ophthalmic Hospital, as well as at Vienna University. CAREER: 1897, located in Minn.; 1898-1904, practiced at Glencoe, Minn., and then at St. Paul, where he specialized in ophthalmology until his retirement in 1946; at University of Minnesota: 1920-26, associate professor of ophthalmology; and 1926-43, professor and chief of the department. CONTRI-BUTIONS: An early investigator of retinal detachment and advanced ophthalmic surgery in this area. Work on cautery puncture operation (1929). Invented a special eyeglass frame for patients with miasthenia gravis. President: Minnesota Academy of Medicine (1927), Minnesota Academy of Ophthalmology (1919), and American Academy of Ophthalmology and Otolaryngology (1936). Founder, Minnesota Society for the Prevention of Blindness. REFERENCES: J. A. Myers, *Masters of Med.* (1968); *N.Y. Times,* July 3, 1957, p. 23; *Who Was Who in Am.,* 3: 122.

R. Rosenthal

BURGESS, ALEXANDER MANLIUS (May 4, 1885, St. Albans, Vt.-September 17, 1974, Providence, R.I.). *Physician; Internal medicine; Educator.* Son of Thomas M., Clergyman, and Mary T. (Sargent) Beck. Married Abby Bullock, 1910; four children. EDUCATION: St. Albans High School; 1906, A.B., Brown University; 1910, M.D., Harvard Medical School; 1910-11, Boston City Hospital; 1914, studied in Berlin, Germany. CAREER: 1910-11, assistant pathologist, Boston City Hospital; 1912-13, pathologist, Montreal General Hospital; 1913, assistant professor, pathology, McGill University; in Providence: 1914-49, private practice of internal medicine; 1925, chief of medicine, Miriam Hospital; 1945-48, Rhode Island Hospital; and 1926-40, Charles V. Chapin Hospital; at Brown University: 1924-44, assistant professor, biology, and chairman, Division of University Health; and 1944-50, professor, health and hygiene; 1949-55, area section chief in medicine, Veterans Administration; director of medical education: 1955-70, Miriam Hospital; 1955-58, Newport Hospital; and 1957-63, Pawtucket Memorial Hospital. CONTRIBUTIONS: Career was uniquely multifaceted, comprising clinical practice and consultation, original clinical investigation—particularly in oxygen therapy—and medical education. A founder and president of the Association of Hospital Directors of Medical Education and an examiner of the American Board of Internal Medicine (1946-51). Active in medical organizations, being elected second vice-president of the American College of Physicians (1953-54) and its awardee of the Alfred Stengel Prize for Distinguished Service (1958). Advocated innovation in medical economics, emphasizing public service by physicians and health insurance. First, on his own initiative, pre-World War II, and later as vice-chairman and chairman of the National Committee for Resettlement of Foreign Physicians (1949-64), aided in the rescue of colleagues from Hitler's regime and after the war from Displaced Person's camps.

WRITINGS: "Problems and Results in the Use of Insulin in Diabetics," *Rhode Island Med. J.* (1925); "Administration of Oxygen According to a New Principle," *ibid.* (1933); "Some Cytologic and Serologic Aspects of Infectious Mononucleosis," *Arch. Int. Med.* (1934) (with C. A. Stuart, H. A. Lawson, and H. E. Wellman); "Excessive Hypertension of Long Duration," *New England J. of Med.* (1948); "Resettlement of Refugee Physicians in the United States," *New England J. of Med.* (1952): 360. REFERENCE: *NCAB*, 58: 499.

I. A. Beck

BURROUGH, JAMES WILLIAM (December 11, 1800, Claverack, N.Y.-August 14, 1854, Santa Barbara, Calif.). *Physician*. Son of William Y. and Magdalena (Van Rensselaer) Burrough. Married Maria Isabel Lopez, 1825, two children; Leonarda Ayala, 1851, one son. CAREER: July 1, 1823, commandant of the Santa Barbara Presidio, Capt. José de la Guerra y Noriega, and Burrough signed a contract by which, and for the annual payment of 240 pesos, the physician would provide medical services for the soldiers and their families resident in Santa Barbara; unique document affords an early, and perhaps the earliest, instance of a group medical plan in Calif. REFERENCES: Hubert H. Bancroft, *History of California* 5 (1884-90): 632-33; Robert J. Moes, *The Elusive Dr. Burrough—Alta California's First Physician* (1980); Doyce B. Nunis, Jr., ed., *A Medical Journey in California by Dr. Pierre Garnier* (1967): 4-16.

Y. V. O'Neill

BURTON, DE WITT T. (November 15, 1892, Memphis, Tenn.-February 17, 1970, Detroit, Mich.). *Physician; Hospital administrator; Civic leader.* Orphaned early in life. Married Alice Boyd, 1922; three children. EDUCATION: Fisk University; 1920, M.D., Meharry Medical College; studied with James E. Davis, Grace Hospital, Detroit, at a time when few formal internships were open to blacks. CAREER: 1921-46, medical practice, Detroit; 1928-46, staff physician, Parkside and Grace Hospitals, Detroit; 1939-70, founder and administrator, Wayne Diagnostic, later Burton Mercy Hospital; 1959-68, Board of Governors, Wayne State University, Detroit; officer: NAACP, Urban League, United Negro College Fund, Boy Scouts of America, and Brandeis University Club; trustee, Meharry Medical College. CONTRIBUTIONS: Founded the leading black proprietary hospital in Detroit. Helped arrange the affiliation of Parkside (late 1920s), city's first black, nonprofit hospital, with Grace, a prestigious and large hospital. First black ever to hold statewide elective office in Mich. when elected to Wayne State University Board of Governors (1959). Sponsored the campaigns of most of Michigan's pioneer black public officials. REFERENCES: *Detroit Free Press*, February 18, 1970, p. 6B; Detroit Hist. Soc., *Bull.* 20, no. 3 (1963): 3; *JNMA* 55 (1963): 475-84; *JNMA* 61 (1969): 451; *JNMA* 63 (1971): 74; *Michigan Chronicle*, February 21, 1970, p. 1; February 28, 1970, p.8; *Michigan Med.* 69 (1970): 362.

M. Pernick

BUSEY, SAMUEL CLAGETT (July 23, 1828, Montgomery Co., Md.-February 12, 1901, Washington, D.C.). *Physician; Pediatrics.* Son of John, farmer, and Rachel (Clagett) Busey. Married Catherine Posey, 1849; no children. EDUCATION: 1841-45, Rockville Academy; 1845, studied medicine with Dr. Hezekiah Magruder; 1848, M.D., University of Pennsylvania. CAREER: 1848-95, private practice, District of Columbia; practice interrupted about ten years by illness; at Georgetown Medical School: 1853-58, professor of materia medica; 1875, professor of diseases of children; and 1876, professor of theory and practice of medicine. CONTRIBUTIONS: Founder of pediatric medicine in the District of Columbia. Helped to organize a dispensary in connection with the Columbia Hospital and took charge of its Department of Diseases of Infancy and Childhood (1869). Helped to establish the Children's Hospital (1870). Staff of the dispensary began the first postgraduate school of clinical medicine in the country (1872), and he taught the course on children's diseases. With Dr. Abraham Jacobi, founded the Section of Diseases of Children in the American Medical Association and was elected its first chairman (1881). A founder of the American Pediatric Society, American Dermatological Association, Washington Obstetrical and Gynecological Society, Garfield Memorial Hospital, American Gynecological Society, Association of American Physicians, Columbia Historical Society, and Washington Academy of Sciences. President of the Medical Association of the District of Columbia (1875), Medical Society of the District of Columbia (1877, 1894-99), Association of American Physicians (1890), and Washington Obstetrical and Gynecological Society. Vice-president of the American Gynecological Society and Washington Academy of Sciences. After retiring from practice (1895), devoted time to writing about his life and about the physicians and medical institutions of the District of Columbia.

WRITINGS: Wrote many articles on pediatrics, obstetrics, gynecology, public health, and other topics. A complete list of his publications (1869-94) is in his *Personal Reminiscences and Recollections of Forty-Six Years' Membership in the Medical Society of the District of Columbia and Residence in this City with Biographical Sketches of Many of the Deceased Members* (1895), 354-63. Additional works are listed in *Index Catalogue*, 2nd series, 2 (1897): 942, and 3rd series, 3 (1922): 622. Many of the more important articles are reprinted in *A Souvenir, with an Autobiographical Sketch of Early Life and Selected Miscellaneous Addresses and Communications* (1896). REFERENCES: Kelly and Burrage (1920), 177-78; G. M. Kober, ed., *Fiftieth Anniversary of the Graduation in Medicine of Samuel Clagett Busey, M.D., LL.D.* (1899); D. S. Lamb et al., *History of the Medical Society of the District of Columbia, 1817-1909* (1909), 240-42; *Nat. Med. Rev.* 2 (1893-94): 177; *Proc. Washington Acad. of Sci.* 5 (1903-4): 375-78; *Trans., Med. Soc. of District of Columbia* 6 (1901): 71-92.

R. Kondratas

BUSH, LEWIS POTTER (October 19, 1812, Wilmington, Del.-March 5, 1892, Wilmington). *Physician; Public health*. Son of David, shipper, and Martha (Potter) Bush. Married Maria Jones, 1839; five children. EDUCATION: 1831, A.M., Jefferson College; 1835, M.D., University of Pennsylvania; 1835-36, resident, Blockley (Philadelphia General) Hospital. CAREER: 1837-92, private practice, Wilmington. CONTRIBUTIONS: Leader of public health movement in Del. Led the effort to control typhoid fever in Del. and was one of the first American physicians to note the difference between typhoid and typhus. Active in the temperance movement; was particularly notable for willingness to treat charity patients. President of the American Academy of Medicine (1886) and Medical Society of Delaware (1860). A founder and president of Delaware Hospital (1891-92). REFERENCES: Kelly and Burrage (1928); *Morning News* (Wilmington), March 7, 1892; *NCAB*, 12: 398; Meridith I. Samuels, *Med. Soc. of Delaware, 150th Annual Session* (1939), 49, 50; J. Thomas Scharf, *History of Delaware* 1 (1888): 497, 498.

W. H. Williams

BUTLER, HENRY RUTHERFORD (April 11, 1862, Cumberland County, N.C.-December 17, 1931, Atlanta, Ga.). *Physician; General practice; Pediatrics.* Son of William T. and Caroline Butler. Married Selena Mae Sloan, 1893; one child. EDUCATION: Wilmington, N.C., public schools and special tutoring by Dr. E. E. Green; Lincoln University, Pa.: 1887, A.B.; and 1890, A.M.; 1890, M.D., Meharry Medical College; 1894, 1895, summer postgraduate courses in diseases of children and surgery, Harvard Medical School. CAREER: 1890-1931, practice of general medicine (*post* 1890) and pediatrics (*post* 1894), Atlanta, Ga.; staff of Fair Haven Infirmary, Atlanta, Ga. (served at times as superintendent and secretary-treasurer). CONTRIBUTIONS: A founder of NMA (1895), Atlanta Medical Association, and Association of Physicians, Pharmacists and Dentists of Georgia. He and Thomas H. Slater were first two black physicians to establish practices and remain in Atlanta (1890). Their drugstore was the first black-owned and operated in Atlanta (early 1890s). A founder of Fair Haven Infirmary, first hospital run by black physicians for blacks in Atlanta. Founder, dean, and principal teacher of Morris Brown College School of Nursing (associated with Fair Haven Hospital). Involved in black civic activities: helped establish YMCA, black Boy Scout Troop, and Interracial Commission in Atlanta.

WRITINGS: "The History of the Association of Physicians, Pharmacists and Dentists of Georgia," pamphlet (1910); published medical papers and regular column for *Atlanta Constitution* called "What Colored People are Doing" and for *Atlanta Independent* (black); *History of Masonry in Georgia among Colored Men* (1911); *Acute Gastro-Infection of Infants and Children* (1912). REFERENCES: W. Montague Cobb, "Henry Rutherford Butler, M.D., 1862-1931," *JNMA* 51 (1959): 406-8; John A. Kenney, *The Negro in Medicine* (1912), 25-26; *WWCR* 1 (1915): 54; *WWICA* 3 (1930-32): 74.

T. Savitt

BUXTON, LAUREN HAYNES (July 15, 1859, Londonderry, Vt.-October 11, 1924, Oklahoma City, Okla.). *Physician; Ear, nose, and throat.* Son of Stephen Andrew and Laura (Haynes) Buxton. Married Ella Gertrude Hooey, 1882; six children. EDUCATION: Londonderry Academy and Leland and Grey Seminary, Townshend, Vt.; taught school while studying medicine with Dr. Spafford, Windham and Cavendish, Vt.; 1882, studied law and served as principal of public schools, Bloomingdale, N.Y.; 1883, enrolled in medical department, University of New York; 1884, M.D., medical department, University of Vermont; 1907, postgraduate study, Vienna. CAREER: Practice: Plymouth

Union, Vt., Fulton, Ia.; 1888-99, Guthrie, Oklahoma Territory; and *post* 1899, Oklahoma City; professor of ophthalmology and president, Board of Directors, Epworth College of Medicine, Oklahoma City; first professor of ophthalmology, University of Oklahoma School of Medicine. CONTRIBUTIONS: Voluminous contributor to the secular, scientific, and religious press. 1898-1902, State Superintendent of Public Health; 1897-1901, President, Insane Commission of Okla.; Secretary, Medical Examiners Board.

WRITINGS: "Some Observations on Glaucoma," *K.C. Med. Index-Lancet* 31 (Jan. 1908): 12-18. REFERENCES: "Lauren H. Buxton" file, History of Medicine Collection, University of Oklahoma Health Sciences Center Library, Oklahoma City, Okla.; Bernice N. Crockett, *The Origin and Development of Public Health in Oklahoma 1830-1930* (1953); Mark R. Everett, *Medical Education in Oklahoma: The University of Oklahoma School of Medicine and Medical Center 1900-1931* (1972); *Who Was Who in Am.*, 1: 178.

V. Allen

BYFORD, WILLIAM HEATH (March 20, 1817, Eaton, Ohio-May 21, 1890, Chicago, Ill.). *Gynecologist.* Son of Henry T., mechanic, and Hannah Byford. Married Mary Anne Holland, 1840 (d.1864), five children; Lina W. Flershem, 1873, one child. EDUCATION: 1836-37, apprentice to Dr. Joseph Maddox, Vincennes, Ind.; 1845, M.D., Ohio Medical College, Cincinnati, Ohio. CAREER: 1838-50, practiced medicine, Ind.; 1850-56, anatomy, theory, and practice of medicine faculty, Evansville (Ind.) Medical College; obstetrics and diseases of women and children faculty: 1857-59, Rush Medical College; and 1859-79, medical department, Lind University (Chicago Medical College); 1879-90, gynecology faculty, Rush Medical College; 1870-90, obstetrics and gynecology faculty and president, Woman's Hospital Medical College. CONTRIBUTIONS: Founder of Woman's Hospital Medical College (1870). Developed use of ergot for expulsion of fibroid tumors of the uterus (1875). A founder of the medical department, Lind University (1859), later Northwestern University Medical School. Major role in founding Hospital for Women and Children, Chicago, Ill. (1865). A founder of the American Gynecological Society (1876). Wrote first textbook of gynecology in Chicago area (1864). Performed first ovariotomy in Chicago (1861).

WRITINGS: *A Treatise on the Chronic Inflammation and Displacements of the Unimpregnated Uterus* (1864; 2nd ed., 1871); *The Practice of Medicine and Surgery, Applied to the Diseases and Accidents Incident to Women* (1865; 4th ed., 1888); *A Treatise on the Theory and Practice of Obstetrics* (1870; 2nd ed., 1873). Writings listed in F. M. Sperry, comp., *A Group of Distinguished Physicians and Surgeons of Chicago* (1904), 14-15. REFERENCES: *Am. J. Obstet.* 23 (1890): 622-27; Leslie B. Arey, *Northwestern Univ. Med. School, 1859-1959: A Pioneer in Educational Reform* (1959), 333-38; *DAB*, 3: 379-80; Edward W. Jenks, *Trans., Am. Gyn. Soc.* 15 (1890): 401-6; Kelly and Burrage (1920), 182-83; *NCAB*, 2: 13; *Trans., Chicago Gyn. Soc.* 1 (1892-93): iii-vii; *Trans., Ill. State Med. Soc.* 41 (1891): 12-16.

W. K. Beatty

C

CABELL, JAMES LAWRENCE (August 26, 1813, Nelson County, Va.-August 13, 1889, Overton, Va.). *Physician; Teacher.* Son of George, physician, and Susanna (Wyatt) Cabell. Married Margaret Gibbons, 1839; no children. EDUCATION: 1833, M.A., University of Virginia; 1834, M.D., University of Maryland; continued studies, Baltimore Almshouse, several Philadelphia hospitals, and in Paris. CAREER: 1837-89, professor of anatomy, surgery, and physiology, University of Virginia; 1846-47, chairman of faculty; during the Civil War, chief surgeon, Confederate hospitals, Charlottesville, Va.; president: 1876, Medical Society of Virginia; 1879-84, National Board of Health; and 1879, American Public Health Association; chairman, National Sanitary Conference in Washington during the yellow-fever epidemic in Memphis, Tenn. CONTRIBUTIONS: Most important contributions were in the area of public health. Leader in the movement to introduce public health programs in Va. and in the country at large. Wrote extensively on hygiene and sanitation. Distinguished member of the medical faculty of the University of Virginia for many years.

WRITINGS: "Etiology of Enteric Fever," *TAMA* 28 (1877); "Address in State Medicine and Public Hygiene," *ibid.*, 29 (1878); "The National Board of Health and the International Sanitary Conference of Washington," *ibid.*, 32 (1881); *A Brief Historical Notice of the Origin and Progress of International Hygiene* (1882); "On Sanitary Conditions in Relation of the Treatment of Surgical Operations and Injuries," *Virginia Med. Monthly* 9 (1882-83); *Remarks Before the Committee on Public Health, 18 Cong., 1 Session, for the Protection of Public Health* (1884). REFERENCES: Wyndham Blanton, *Medicine in Virginia in the Nineteenth Century* (1933); Alexander Brown, *The Cabells and Their Kin* (1895); *DAB*, 3:386-87; Howard A. Kelly, *Cyclopedia of Am. Med. Biog.*, 1 (1912); obituary, *N.Y. Times*, August 15, 1889.

P. Addis

CABOT, HUGH (August 11, 1872, Beverly Farms, Mass.-August 14, 1945, Frenchman's Bay, Maine). *Surgeon; Medical educator.* Son of James Elliot and Elizabeth (Dwight) Cabot. Married Mary Anderson Boit, 1902, four children;

Elizabeth (Cole) Amory, 1938, no children. EDUCATION: Harvard University: 1894, A.B., and 1898, M.D.; internship at Massachusetts General Hospital. CAREER: 1900-1919, surgeon, New England Baptist Hospital; 1902-19, surgical staff, Massachusetts General Hospital; 1910-18, assistant professor of surgery, Harvard Medical School; 1918-19, served with Harvard unit, Royal Army Medical Corps, British Expeditionary Force, commanding General Hospital 22; at University of Michigan Medical School: 1919-30, professor of surgery and department head; and 1921-30, dean; 1930-39, professor of surgery, graduate school, University of Minnesota; 1930-39, consulting surgeon, Mayo Clinic; 1939-45, surgical practice, Boston, Mass. CONTRIBUTIONS: Supported prepayment and group practice. Advocate of hospital staff status for all physicians. Government witness in the 1938-43 AMA antitrust case. Headed the White Cross, a Boston health insurance group. President, American Association of Genito-Urinary Surgeons (1915).

WRITINGS: *Modern Urology*, 3 eds. (1918-36); *Surgical Nursing*, 4 eds. (1924-40); *The Doctor's Bill* (1935); *The Patient's Dilemma* (1940). REFERENCES: *DAB*, Supplement 3: 121-23; *NCAB*, 35: 547-48; *New England J. of Med.* 233 (1945): 706-7.

                                                                            J. Carvalho

CABOT, RICHARD CLARKE (May 21, 1868, Brookline, Mass.-May 8, 1939, Cambridge, Mass.). *Physician; Medical ethics; Medical education; Pathology.* Son of James Elliot and Elizabeth (Dwight) Cabot. Married Ella Lyman, 1894; no children. EDUCATION: 1892, M.D., Harvard Medical School. CAREER: 1899-1933, taught at Harvard Medical School; at Massachusetts General Hospital: 1898-1921, medical staff; and 1912-21, chief of staff; 1920-34, chair of social ethics, Harvard College. CONTRIBUTIONS: Initiated a medical social service unit at Massachusetts General Hospital (1905). Honesty was so forthright that the Massachusetts Medical Society considered (1916) his expulsion for "Publicly advertising the faults of general practitioners." Introduced a case method of teaching that drew together clinicians and pathologists (clinical-pathological conferences), and the cases studied were published in the *Boston Medical and Surgical Journal* and *New England Journal of Medicine* (since 1928). Devoted considerable attention to various forms of psychotherapy. Outlined the ethical obligations of the hospital physician. Analyzed 1,000 consecutive autopsies at the Massachusetts General Hospital and compared pathological findings and clinical judgments in each case; discovered that a large percentage of their judgments were incorrect and publicized the results of his findings.

WRITINGS: *Physical Diagnosis*, 10 eds. (1901-30); *Differential Diagnosis*, 2 vols: vol. 1 published in 4 eds. (1911-19); vol. 2 published in 3 eds. (1915-24); *Social Service and the Art of Healing*, 2 eds. (1909-28); *Case Histories in Medicine* (1906). REFERENCES: C. R. Burns, "Richard Clarke Cabot (1868-1939) and Reformation in American Medical Ethics," *Bull. Hist. Med.* 51 (1977): 353-68; *DAB*, Supplement 2: 83-85; J. Stoeckle, ed., *Richard Cabot on Practice, Training, and the Doctor-Patient Relationship* (1977);

Thomas F. Williams, "Cabot, Peabody, and the Care of the Patient," *Bull. Hist. Med.* 24 (1950): 462-81.

J. Carvalho

CADWALADER, THOMAS (1707 or 1708, Philadelphia, Pa.-November 14, 1779, Philadelphia). *Physician.* Son of John and Martha (Jones) Cadwalader. Married Hannah Lambert, 1738; six children. EDUCATION: Apprenticed as a teenager to his uncle, Dr. Evan Jones; at age 19 or 20, went to Europe for a year, where he studied medicine at the University of Rheims (France) and in England under William Cheselden. CAREER: Practiced medicine upon his return from Europe, probably in 1730, in Philadelphia and southern N.J.; 1751-79, consulting physician, Pennsylvania Hospital; 1768, vice-president, American Society for Promoting Useful Knowledge; active in civic and cultural affairs and in the early resistance to British rule. CONTRIBUTIONS: Described a common form of lead poisoning known as the "dry-gripes," later shown to have been caused by drinking punch made with Jamaica rum that had been distilled through lead pipes. Performed some of the earliest autopsies in the United States (1731, 1742). An early advocate of inoculation against smallpox. Helped found Pennsylvania Hospital (1751).

WRITINGS: *An Essay on the West-India Dry-Gripes . . . to Which Is Added an Extraordinary Case in Physick* [Osteomalacia] (1745). REFERENCES: *DAB*, 3: 400; John Spencer Felton, "Man, Medicine and Work in America: An Historical Series. IV. Thomas Cadwalader, M.D. Physician, Philadelphian and Philanthropist," *J. of Occupational Med.* 11 (Jul. 1969): 374-80; Kelly and Burrage (1928), 192-93; William Shainline Middleton, "Thomas Cadwalader and His Essay," *Annals of Med. Hist.*, 3rd series, 3 (1941): 101-13; Miller, *BHM*, p. 17; Stone, *Biog. of Eminent Am. Physicians and Surgeons* (1894), 71-72; *Who Was Who in Am.*, Hist. Vol.: 159.

S. Galishoff

CALDWELL, CHARLES (May 14, 1772, Orange County, now Caswell County, N.C.-July 9, 1853, Louisville, Ky.). *Physician; Educator.* Son of Lieut. Charles and Mrs. (Murray) Caldwell. Married Eliza Leaming, January 3, 1799, one son, divorced; Mrs. Mary (Warner) Barton, 1842. EDUCATION: 1791, began study of medicine under Dr. Harris (probably Thomas Harris), Salisbury, N.C.; 1792-94, medical department, University of Pennsylvania; summer 1793, private course in botany under Benjamin S. Barton (q.v.) and clinical study at Pennsylvania Hospital; 1796, M.D., medical department, University of Pennsylvania. CAREER: 1788-92, taught school, central N.C.; 1795-1819, practiced medicine, Philadelphia, Pa.; 1815-18, professor of geology and philosophy of natural history, "Physical Faculty," University of Pennsylvania; at Transylvania University medical department: 1819-37, institutes and clinical medicine faculty; 1819-21; dean; 1837-49; institutes of medicine and clinical practice and medical jurisprudence faculties, Louisville Medical Institute. (Dismissed from faculties at both Transylvania and Louisville). CONTRIBUTIONS: Introduced clinical instruction in medicine (1802) at the Blockley Alms House (Philadelphia General

Hospital). Gave one of the first courses in medical jurisprudence in the United States (1812). Appointed to Philadelphia Board of Health and modified maritime quarantine regulations by reducing the detention of vessels to a period sufficient to examine the passengers and cleanse the ships (1812). The example was followed in New York City, Boston, Mass., and Charleston, S.C. Received the Boylston Prize for his essay "Thoughts on Quarantine and other Sanitary Systems" (1834). Helped found medical department, Transylvania University (1819), and Louisville Medical Institute (1837). Went to Europe and purchased $20,000 worth of books and apparatus for the Louisville medical department and assembled a complete faculty (1837) after there had been several unsuccessful attempts by others (1833, 1836). Considered himself the man who introduced medicine to the West. Much embittered after dismissal in 1849, is said to have gone to Nashville, Tenn., to attempt to start another school, but no other information is available.

WRITINGS: Most of his medical papers appear in *Transylvania J. of Med. and the Associate Sci., Western J. of Med. & Surg., Transylvania Med. J.*, and in pamphlets. *Autobiography* with preface, notes, and appendix by Harriot W. Warner (1855). Writings listed in *Index Catalogue*, in the appendix of his *Autobiography*, and in E. F. Horine's *Biographical Sketch and Guide to the Writings of Charles Caldwell, M.D. (1772-1853)* (1960). REFERENCES: H. A. Cottell, "Doctor Charles Caldwell," *Ky. Med. J.* 15 (1917): 72-74; *DAB*, 2: 406; Kelly and Burrage (1920), 190; W. S. Middleton, "Charles Caldwell, A Biographical Sketch," *Annals of Med. Hist.* 3 (1921): 156-78; *NCAB*, 7: 276; L. P. Yandell [Sr.], "A Memoir of Dr. Charles Caldwell," *Western J. of Med. & Surg.*, 3rd series, 12 (1853): 101-16.

                                                                        E. H. Conner

CALDWELL, EUGENE WILSON (December 3, 1870, Savannah, Mo.— June 20, 1918, New York City). *Radiologist.* Son of W. W. and Camilla (Kellogg) Caldwell. Married Elizabeth Perkins, 1913. EDUCATION: 1872, B.S. in electrical engineering, University of Kansas; 1898-99, special student, College of Physicians and Surgeons, Columbia University; 1905, M.D., New York University and Bellevue Hospital Medical College. CAREER: 1893-95, worked for United States Lighthouse Establishment; 1895-97, worked for New York Telephone Company; director of the Edward N. Gibbs Memorial X-Ray Laboratory of Bellevue Medical College until 1908; physician and roentgenologist to the New York Orthopedic Hospital, the Neurological Institute, and to Presbyterian Hospital; served in the Medical Reserve Corps as a lieutenant and as a major in the U.S. Army Medical Corps (1918). CONTRIBUTIONS: A leading early radiologist. Invented many improvements on the Roentgen equipment, including an electrical interrupter, an induction coil, an X-ray generator, and various X-ray tubes. Researched the nasal accessory sinuses, using the X-ray machines. Death was caused by burns incurred during X-ray experiments.

WRITINGS: *The Practical Application of the Roentgen Rays in Therapeutics and Di-*

agnosis (1903, with William A. Posey). REFERENCES: *Am. J. of Roentgenology*, 5 (1918): 575; *DAB*, 2, pt. 2: 407-408; *JAMA*, June 29, 1918; Kelly and Burrage (1928), 193-194.

M. Kaufman

CALHOUN, ABNER WELLBORN (April 16, 1845, Newnan, Ga.-August 21, 1910, Atlanta, Ga.). *Physician; Ophthalmologist*. Son of Andrew B., physician, and Susan (Wellborn) Calhoun. Married Louise Phinizy, September 25, 1877; four children. EDUCATION: Private tutors; 1869, M.D., Jefferson Medical College; studied with his father; three years abroad studying eye, ear, and throat under Politzer in Vienna; additional work in Berlin and London. CAREER: 1873, returned to America; 1874, chair of diseases of eye, ear, and throat, Atlanta Medical College; 1889, president of faculty, new Atlanta College of Physicians and Surgeons, a position held until his death; several times president of the Medical Society of Georgia; 1904, chairman, AMA section on ophthalmology; at time of death, held the A. W. Calhoun Chair of Ophthalmology, Otology, and Laryngology; was clinical professor of ophthalmology, otology, and laryngology; and oculist and aurist to Grady, St. Joseph's, and Wesleyan Memorial Hospitals. CONTRIBUTIONS: One of the few ophthalmologists practicing in the Deep South; secured a far-flung reputation. Both his son and grandson, F. Phinizy Calhoun, Sr., and Jr., followed in his footsteps, and each became professor and chairman of the Department of Ophthalmology, Emory University School of Medicine, of which the Atlanta College of Physicians and Surgeons was a parent. In Calhoun's memory, the family established the A. W. Calhoun Medical Library at Emory.

WRITINGS: Published a number of articles, many of which are found in the *Atlanta Med. and Surg. J.* REFERENCES: F. Phinizy Calhoun, "The Founding and the Early History of the Atlanta Medical College, 1854-1875," *Georgia Hist. Q.* 9 (1925): 34-54; *Index-Catalogue*, 2nd series (1898): 87-88; Kelly and Burrage (1920): 191-92; *NCAB* 16 (1918): 303; *Who Was Who in Am.*, 1:183.

P. Spalding

CALLISTER, ALFRED CYRIL (September 24, 1894, Salt Lake City, Utah-February 9, 1961, Salt Lake City). *Plastic surgery; Medical education*. Son of Thomas A., printer and publisher, and Bertha (James) Callister. Married Vera Taft, 1916, five children; Lucie Christophersen, 1945, one child. EDUCATION: 1915, A.B., University of Utah; 1917, M.D., Harvard Medical School; at Boston City Hospital: 1917-18, surgical intern; and 1918-19, resident surgeon; 1922-40, numerous postgraduate courses. CAREER: 1920-21, county physician and surgeon, County Hospital, Salt Lake City; 1924-42, chief, Section of Plastic and Thoracic Surgery, Latter Day Saints Hospital; at University of Utah Medical School: 1921-42, lecturer, hygiene and preventive medicine; and 1942-45, dean; 1938, member, American Board of Plastic Surgery; 1941, president, Utah State Medical Association; 1924-50, member, Utah State Board of Health; 1942-45, procurement and assignment officer for Utah physicians. CONTRIBUTIONS: Assumed the leading role in transforming the two-year medical school at the University of Utah into a four-year school (1941-42). Served as first dean of the reorganized school (1942-45). Recruited the new faculty and integrated the preclinical with the clinical curriculum.

WRITINGS: "Hypoplasia of Mandible (Micrognathy) with Cleft Palate; Treatment in Early Infancy by Skeletal Traction," *Am. J. of Diseases of Children* 53 (Apr. 1937): 1057-59; "Congenital Defects of the Nose, Lip and Palate," *Rocky Mt. Med. J.* 35 (Sept. 1938): 698-701; "Hypertelorism with Facies Bovinia," *ibid.*, 40 (Jan. 1943): 36-40; "The Medical Profession's Ideals in Medical Service," *ibid.*, 38 (Jun. 1941): 106-13; "What Would Wagner Bill Do for American Medicine?" *ibid.*, 41 (Nov. 1944): 825-32; "Technique Designed to Prevent Lateral Creeping of Alar Cartilage in Repair of Hare-Lip," *Plastic & Reconstr. Surg.* 3 (Sept. 1948): 617-20; REFERENCES: *Who's Important in Med.* (1952), 177.

H. Bauman

CAMPBELL, ELIZABETH (February 3, 1862, Ripley, Ohio-June 7, 1945, Cincinnati, Ohio). *Physician; Social hygiene and maternal health.* Daughter of William Byington and Mary D. (Leavitt) Campbell. Never married. EDUCATION: 1892-94, studied at University of Michigan; 1895, M.D., Women's Medical College, Cincinnati; interned, Prison Hospital for Women, Framingham, Mass. CAREER: Maintained a large private practice, Cincinnati; 1902, first woman to serve on medical staff of Christ's Hospital. CONTRIBUTIONS: Founder of three welfare organizations: Visiting Nurse Association (1909), Cincinnati Social Hygiene Association (1917), and the Committee on Maternal Health (1932). Became prominent in national issues in public health. REFERENCES: *J. of Social Hygiene* 28 (1942): 151; *Med. Woman's J.* 52 (Jul. 1945): 55; Miller, *BHM*, p. 18; Cecil Striker, ed., *Medical Portraits* (1963); *Who Was Who in Am.*, 4:150.

G. Jenkins

CAMPBELL, HENRY FRASER (February 10, 1824, Savannah, Ga.-December 15, 1891, Augusta, Ga.). *Physician; Physiologist; Educator.* Son of James Colgan and Mary (Eve) Campbell. Married Sara Bosworth Sibley, 1844; one child. EDUCATION: Private; 1842, M.D., Medical College of Georgia. CAREER: Began practice, Augusta, at age of 18; at Medical College of Georgia: 1842-54, assistant demonstrator of anatomy; 1854-57, professor of surgical, comparative, and microscopic anatomy; and 1857-66, professor of anatomy; at New Orleans School of Medicine: 1866-67, professor of anatomy; and 1867-68, professor of surgery; at Medical College of Georgia: 1868-80, professor of operative surgery and gynecology; and 1881 until his death, professor of principles and practice of surgery and gynecology; during the Civil War, medical director, Ga. military hospitals, Richmond, Va.; member, Army Medical Examining Board of the Confederate States; 1849, with his physician-brother Robert, established in Augusta the Jackson Street Hospital for Negroes, where skilled health care was rendered to the blacks; in the American Gynecological Society: 1876, a founder; and 1881, vice-president; 1884, president, AMA; 1857-61, co-editor,

Southern Med. and Surg. J. CONTRIBUTIONS: Invented a number of specialized tools for use in gynecological operations and in lithotomy. Concentrated, as a physiologist, on the makeup and function of the nervous system and received an award from the AMA (1857) for his work on the excito-secretory function of the nervous system. This research led to international recognition when the distinguished Marshall Hall of England acknowledged his precedence over C. Bernard in this work.

WRITINGS: *Essays on the Secretory and the Excito-Secretory System of Nerves in Their Relations to Physiology and Pathology* (1857); *Report on the Nervous System in Febrile Diseases, and the Classification of Fevers by the Nervous System* (1858). Contributed the article on ligation of the arteries to the *Confederate Manual of Military Surgery* (1863) and published in the *Trans. of the Am. Surg. Assoc.* and *TAMA*, as well as in his own magazine. REFERENCES: William B. Atkinson, *Physicians and Surgeons of the U.S.* (1878), 402-3; *DAB*, 3 (1958): 453-54; William H. Goodrich, *The History of the Medical Department of the University of Georgia* (1928); Howard Kelly, *Cyclopedia of Am. Med. Biog.* 1 (1912): 159-60; Kelly and Burrage (1920): 193-94; *Memoirs of Georgia* 2 (1895): 180-85; Cecilia C. and Fred Mettler, "Henry Fraser Campbell," *Annals of Med. Hist.*, 3rd series, 1 (1939): 405-26; *National Union Catalogue, Pre-1956 Imprints* 92 (1970): 188-89; *NCAB* 12 (1904): 68; *Southern Med. and Surg. J.* (1850). *Index Catalogue* 1 (1873): 288, contains a partial listing of Campbell's writings, also 2nd series, 3 (1898): 102-3.

                                                                        P. Spalding

CAMPBELL, WILLIS COHOON (December 18, 1880, Jackson, Miss.-May 4, 1941, Chicago, Ill.). *Orthopedic surgeon.* Son of Charles C., clerk, and Lula (Cohoon) Campbell. Married Elizabeth Yerger, 1908; four children. EDUCATION: Literary education: Millsaps College, Hampden-Sydney College, Roanoke College, and University of Virginia; 1904, M.D., University of Virginia. CAREER: 1910-41, private practice of orthopedic surgery, Memphis, Tenn.; 1920-40, organized, built, and headed the Willis C. Campbell Clinic; developed this institution into one known internationally for the excellence of its diagnostic and therapeutic work in orthopedic surgery as well as its outstanding postdoctoral-level training program; 1911-41, organized and served as the first chairman, Department of Orthopedic Surgery, University of Tennessee, Memphis. CONTRIBUTIONS: Achieved international recognition for many contributions to orthopedic surgery, perhaps the most notable being improved methods of repairing damaged ligaments of the knee, use of sulfanilamide to prevent infections, surgical reconstruction of still joints, and bone grafting to promote healing of nonunited fractures. Organized the Crippled Children's Hospital in Memphis (1919) and was chief of staff until his death (1941). Organized the Hospital for Crippled Adults (1923). Also made major contributions as a leader in organized orthopedic surgery. President: Clinical Orthopedic Society (1928); and American Orthopedic Association (1931). Founder and first president of the American Academy of Orthopedic Surgeons (1933). President of American Board of Orthopedic Surgery (1937-40).

WRITINGS: Aside from numerous journal articles, is best known for three books, now regarded as classic works: *Orthopedics of Childhood* (1927), *Orthopedic Surgery* (1930), and *Operative Orthopedics* (1939). REFERENCES: *J. Bone & Joint Surg.*, 23 (1941): 716-17; *NCAB*, 31: 330.

S. R. Bruesch

CANNON, GEORGE EPPS (July 7, 1869, Fishdam [now Carlisle], S.C.-April 6, 1925, Jersey City, N.J.). *Physician*. Son of Barnett G., farmer, and Mary (Tucker) Cannon. Married Genevieve Wilkinson, 1901; two children. EDUCATION: Brainerd Institute (Chester, S.C.); 1893, A.B., Lincoln University (Pa.); 1900, M.D., New York Homeopathic Medical College. CAREER: 1893-96, worked to support his family, which had moved to Jersey City; 1900-25, medical practice, Jersey City. CONTRIBUTIONS: Leading black practitioner and among the most prominent citizens of Jersey City during early twentieth century. Served NMA as chairman of executive board for eight years. Became deeply involved in North Jersey medical affairs; Republican local, state, and national politics; and racial matters. Provided a haven for Dr. John A. Kenney (q.v.) (1923) when the Ku Klux Klan threatened Kenney's life over black staffing at Tuskegee (Ala.) Veterans' Hospital. Involved himself in many projects to better blacks in Jersey City and in nation. Had a national medical reputation. REFERENCES: Dennis Clark Dickerson, "George E. Cannon: Black Churchman, Physician, and Republican Politician," *J. of Presbyterian Hist.* 51 (1973): 411-32; *National Cyclopedia of the Colored Race* (1919), 210; obituary notice, *JNMA* 17 (1925): 76, 173.

T. Savitt

CANNON, IDA MAUD (June 29, 1877, Milwaukee, Wis.-July 8, 1960, Cambridge, Mass.). *Nurse; Social Worker*. Daughter of Colbert Hanchett, railroad traffic controller, and Wilma (Denio) Cannon, schoolteacher. Never married. EDUCATION: 1896-98, graduated Saint Paul City and County Hospital Training School for Nursing; 1900, took courses in sociology and psychology, University of Minnesota; 1907, graduated Boston School for Social Workers (Simmons College). CAREER: 1898-1900, organized hospital unit, State School for the Feeble-Minded, Faribault, Minn.; 1903-6, visiting nurse, Saint Paul Associated Charities; at Massachusetts General Hospital: 1906-7, volunteer social worker; 1907-8, social worker; 1908-14, head worker, social service; 1912, inaugurated special training program for hospital social workers; and 1914-45, chief of social service; 1918, a founder of American Association of Hospital Social Workers and president (1920-22); 1932-36, director, National Institute of Immigrant Welfare. CONTRIBUTIONS: A founder of medical social work in the United States. Chiefly responsible for the development of programs of the Massachusetts General Hospital social service department, which she joined one year after it was founded by Richard Clarke Cabot (q.v.). Spoke widely and wrote on medical social work education, practice, and organization; emphasized teamwork of physicians, nurses, and social workers in providing patient care. A leading advocate of the shift from the friendly visiting ideal to the concept of social work as a skilled professional service.

WRITINGS: *Social Work in Hospitals: A Contribution to Progressive Medicine* (1917); "Medicine as a Social Instrument: Medical Social Service," *New England J. of Med.* 244 (1951): 717-24; *On the Social Frontier of Medicine; Pioneering in Medical Social Service* (1952). REFERENCES: Harriet M. Bartless, "Ida M. Cannon: Pioneer in Medical Social Work," *Soc. Service Rev.* 49 (1975): 208-29; M. Antoinette Cannon, "Ida Cannon and Medical Social Work," *Bull Amer. Assoc. of Med. Soc. Workers* 19 (1946): 47-50; idem, *Social Frontier of Medicine; DAB*, Supplement 6: 97-98; Marian Cannon Schlesinger, *Snatched from Oblivion: A Cambridge Memoir* (1979), 49-64.

J. H. Warner

CANNON, WALTER BRADFORD (October 19, 1871, Prairie du Chien, Wis.-October 1, 1945, Franklin, N.H.). *Physiologist; Endocrinology; Neurology.* Son of Colbert Hanchett, railroad official, and Sarah Wilma (Denio) Cannon. Married Cornelia James, 1901; five children. EDUCATION: Harvard University: 1896, A.B.; 1897, M.A.; and 1900, M.D. CAREER: 1900-1942, physiology faculty, Harvard University; 1914-16, president, American Physiological Society. CONTRIBUTIONS: Introduced the use of radiopaque substances for X-ray examination of the soft organs of the alimentary canal (1897); facilitated the diagnosis and subsequent surgical treatment of diseases of the esophagus, stomach, and intestines. Used new X-ray method to investigate the physiology of digestion (1897-1911). Discovered several of the physiological mechanisms that trigger hunger and thirst which he summarized in *The Mechanical Factors of Digestion* (1911). Was struck by the cessation of digestive activities in animals that were frightened or otherwise disturbed; led to investigations of the physiology of emotions; found that adrenalin directly released from the adrenal medulla played a pivotal role in helping the body to deal with emergencies. Argued that the bodily changes mediated by the sympathetic nervous system were preparations for flight or fight (1911-15). Studied the functions and responses of the autonomic nervous system (1920s). From this research, developed the concept of homeostasis to explain the body's tendency to maintain physiological stability during periods of both stress and ordinary activity. Discovered an adrenalinlike hormone, which he named sympathin (1931). Made important investigations of the role of hormones in the transmission of nerve impulses in a period when this was thought to be a purely electrical phenomenon. During World War I, solved the problem of traumatic shock by showing that it was related to a decrease in blood circulation. Persuaded Harvard Medical School to adopt the case method system of teaching (c. 1900); idea was incorporated in several medical textbooks published shortly thereafter.

WRITINGS: *Bodily Changes in Pain, Hunger, Fear and Rage* (1915); *Traumatic Shock* (1923); *The Wisdom of the Body* (1932); *Autonomic Neuro-Effector Systems* (1937). REFERENCES: *BHM* (1964-69), 49; (1970-74), 34; (1975), 6; (1976), 7; C. M. Brooks et al., eds., *Life and Contributions of W. B. Cannon . . .* (1975); *DAB*, Supplement 3: 133-37; *DSB*, 15, Supplement 1: 71-77; Miller, *BHM*, p. 18; *NCAB*, D: 72-73; *N.Y.*

Times, October 2, 1945; M. C. Schlesinger, *Snatched from Oblivion* (1979); *Who Was Who in Am.*, 2: 101.

S. Galishoff

CARMALT, WILLIAM HENRY (August 3, 1836, Friendsville, Susquehanna County, Pa.-July 17, 1929, New Haven, Conn.). *Surgeon; Ophthalmologist.* Son of Caleb and Sarah (Price) Carmalt. Married Laura Woolsey Johnson, 1863; three children. EDUCATION: Friends' Boarding Schools, West Chester, Philadelphia, Pa.; Moorestown, N.J.; and Alexandria, Va.; 1854-55, Yale Scientific School; 1857, private medical school of Drs. Morrill Wyman (q.v.) and Jeffries Wyman (q.v.), Cambridge, Mass.; 1861, M.D., College of Physicians and Surgeons, New York City; 1861-62, intern, St. Luke's Hospital, New York City; 1870-74, studied with Samuel Stricker in Vienna and Waldeyeh in Breslau, Poland, and Strassburg and Paris, France. CAREER: 1862, began general practice, New York City; 1862-63, Civil War service as surgeon, Fortress Monroe, Va., and on the army transport *St. Marks*; 1863-70, clinical assistant, assistant surgeon, and surgeon, New York Eye Infirmary; 1866-70, ophthalmic surgeon to Charity Hospital, N.Y.; 1876, practice as an ophthalmologist, New Haven, Conn.; at Yale Medical School: 1876-79, lecturer in ophthalmology and otology; 1879-81, professor; 1881-1907, professor, principles and practice of surgery; and 1907-29, professor emeritus; at New Haven Hospital: 1879-1908, attending surgeon; and 1908-29, consulting surgeon. CONTRIBUTIONS: Greatly influenced the course of medical education at the Yale Medical School. Influence was directly exercised in the union of the Medical School and New Haven Hospital; the inauguration of the full-time professorial system; the location and erection of the building of the Wilbar Wirt Winchester Tuberculosis Hospital and the reorganization of the hospital (1919), which may have saved it from bankruptcy; and the improvement in the training of nurses. A pioneer in the field of surgery—such as operations under carbolic spray, asepsis, intestinal anastomosis, appendicitis, the treatment of peritonitis, the use of the Roentgen ray, and early interference in gallbladder disease—and from the beginning, published case reports on these and other subjects. One of the first to call attention to the epithelial origin of cancer and the connective tissue origin of sarcoma. Made improvements in various surgical instruments, including a modification of the Förster perimeter, cannular aural forceps, curved hemostat, and tongue forceps. A charter member of both the New York and American Ophthalmological Societies (both founded in 1864). President, Connecticut State Medical Society (1904) and American Surgical Association (1907). When the Congress of American Physicians and Surgeons was formed (1887), was elected its first secretary (office held until 1911). Elected chairman of the Executive Committee of the Congress (1907), which office he held until his death.

WRITINGS: A complete listing is in the *Yale J. Biol. & Med.* 2 (Dec. 1929): 111-12. REFERENCES: "William Henry Carmalt, 1836-1929," *Conn. State Med. J.* 20 (Jul. 1956): 544; Samuel C. Harvey, "Surgery of the Past in Connecticut," in Herbert Thoms, ed., *The Heritage of Connecticut Medicine* (1942), 172-87; John E. Lane, "William H. Carmalt," *Yale J. Biol. & Med.* 2 (Dec. 1929): 90-113; *NCAB*, 29: 122-23.

J. W. Ifkovic

CARPENTER, WALTER (January 12, 1808, Walpole, N.H.-November 9, 1892, Burlington, Vt.). *Physician.* Son of Sylvester, farmer, and Lydia (Bowker) Carpenter. Married Olivia Claire Blodgett, 1832, two children; Mrs. Anna Brown Troop, 1844, one child; Adelina Brown, 1872. EDUCATION: Chesterfield Academy, Allstead, N.H.; studied in office of his uncle, Dr. Davis Carpenter, Brockport, N.Y., and Dr. Amos Twitchell, Keene, N.H.; 1829, M.D., Dartmouth. CAREER: practiced medicine: 1829-30, Bethel, Vt.; 1830-58, Randolph, Vt.; and 1858-92, Burlington; 1854, helped S. W. Thayer reestablish the University of Vermont Medical College (which had ceased operations for 20 years) and became professor, materia medica and pharmacy; 1855, assumed financial responsibility for the college, which had ended the first term with a balance of $7.25; at University of Vermont Medical College: 1857-72, professor, theory and practice of medicine; and 1871-81, dean. CONTRIBUTIONS: Secured the donation for, supervised the construction of, and became physician-in-chief of the Mary Fletcher Hospital, the first teaching hospital of Vt. (1876-79). President, Vermont State Medical Society (1856). Assistant Surgeon, Second Vermont Volunteers (1861-64). REFERENCES: M. Kaufman, *Univ. of Vermont College of Med.* (1979), 53, 61, 66-67; Kelly and Burrage (1920), 197-98; obituary by Henry Holton, *Trans., Vermont State Med. Soc.* (1893): 224-30; William S. Rann, *History of Chittenden County* (1886): 807-11.

L. J. Wallman

CARREL, ALEXIS (June 28, 1873, Lyons, France-November 5, 1944, Paris, France). *Surgeon; Experimental biologist.* Son of Alexis, textile manufacturer, and Anne-Marie (Ricard) Carrel-Billiard. Married Anne de la Motte de Meyrie, 1913; no children. EDUCATION: University of Lyons: 1890, L.B.; and 1900, M.D.; 1896-1900, intern, Lyons Hospital; 1903-4, studied in Paris. CAREER: 1900-1902, prosector, University of Lyons; 1904, went to the United States; 1905-6, physiology faculty, University of Chicago; 1906-39, at Rockefeller Institute for Medical Research (later Rockefeller University); 1914-18, served in French Army; 1940, returned to France; 1941-44, founder and director, Foundation for the Study of Human Problems; at the time of his death, was under suspicion of being a collaborator for having accepted aid from the Vichy government in the establishment of his foundation. CONTRIBUTIONS: Developed technique for joining blood vessels end to end (1902). Used method to effect organ transplants in animals. For these ground-breaking advances, was awarded the 1912 Nobel Prize in medicine or physiology. Developed tissue culture techniques for cultivating the cells of warm-blooded animals; transplanted connective tissue cells from the heart of an embryo chick into an *in vitro* culture (1912), which he maintained for over 30 years; technique has been of great value in oncology and virology. During World War I, with the chemist Henry Dakin, developed an antiseptic solution for treating infected wounds that was credited with having prevented numerous amputations and deaths; was later superseded by antibiotic treatment. With the aviator Charles A. Lindbergh, developed a sterilizable glass pump for circulating a culture fluid through an excised organ, by means of which the organ could be kept alive for a short time (1930s).

WRITINGS: "Anastomosis and Transplantation of Blood Vessels," *Am. Med.* 10 (1904): 284; "The Ultimate Result of a Double Nephrectomy and the Replantation of One Kidney," *J. of Experimental Med.* 14 (1911): 124-25; "Artificial Activation of the Growth in Vitro of Connective Tissue," *ibid.*, 17 (1913): 14-19; *Man the Unknown* (1935); *The Culture of Organs* (1938, with C. A. Lindbergh). A bibliography is in Robert Soupault, *Alexis Carrel, 1873-1944* (1952). REFERENCES: *BHM* (1964-69), 50; (1970-74), 35; (1975-79), 26; (1980), 9; *DAB*, Supplement 3: 139-42; *DSB*, 3: 90-92; William S. Edwards, *Alexis Carrel, Visionary Surgeon* (1974); Theodore I. Malinin, *Surgery and Life* (1979); *NCAB*, 15: 301-3; *N.Y. Times*, November 6, 1944; *Who Was Who in Am.*, 2: 104.

S. Galishoff

CARROLL, JAMES (June 5, 1854, Woolwich, England-September 16, 1907, Washington, D.C.). *Microbiologist; Investigator of yellow fever.* Son of James and Harriet (Chiverton) Carroll. Married Jennie M. George Lucas, 1888; seven children. EDUCATION: Studied medicine: 1886-87, University of the City of New York; and 1889-91, University of Maryland, where he received an M.D. degree; 1891-93, attended postgraduate classes in bacteriology and pathology, Johns Hopkins University. CAREER: With U.S. Army: 1874-1907, infantry service; 1874-83, hospital steward; 1883-98, assigned to the Army Medical Museum as assistant to the curator, Maj. Walter Reed (q.v.); 1895-1902, member, Army Yellow Fever Commission; and 1900-1901, contracted yellow fever in Cuba, which left him with a permanent heart lesion that caused his death seven years later; 1895-1907, bacteriology and pathology faculty, Columbian (now George Washington) University; 1902-7, bacteriology and pathology faculty, Army Medical School. CONTRIBUTIONS: Working with Reed (1899), refuted Giuseppe Sanarelli's theory that *Bacillus icteroides* was the cause of yellow fever. Second in command of the Army Yellow Fever Commission, directed much of its actual work while Reed was occupied in Washington. Contracted yellow fever after allowing himself to be bitten by an infected *Aedes aegypti* mosquito; experiment helped prove Carlos Finlay's theory that yellow fever is transmitted by an insect vector. Demonstrated that the causative agent of yellow fever is ultramicroscopic; work was the first proof that a filterable virus was the cause of a human disease. During the Spanish-American War, aided the medical investigations of Major Edward O. Shakespeare (q.v.) by showing that the disease then prevailing in army camps was typhoid fever and not malaria.

WRITINGS: "The Specific Cause of Yellow Fever. A Reply to Dr. G. Sanarelli," *Med. News* 75 (1899): 321-29 (with Walter Reed); "The Etiology of Yellow Fever," *Phila. Med. J.* 6 (1900): 790-96 (with Walter Reed, Aristide Agramonte, and Jesse

William Lazear [q.v.]); "The Prevention of Yellow Fever," *Med. Record* 60 (1901): 641-53 (with Walter Reed). A bibliography is in John C. Hemmeter, *Master Minds in Medicine* (1927), 319-20. REFERENCES: *DAB*, 3: 525-26; *DSB*, 3: 94-95; Kelly and Burrage (1928), 201-2.

S. *Galishoff*

CARSON, SIMEON LEWIS (January 16, 1882, Marion, N.C.-September 8, 1954, Washington, D.C.). *Surgeon.* Son of Martin, farmer, later gardener at University of Michigan, and Harriet Carson. Married Carol H. Clark, 1905; two children. EDUCATION: 1903, M.D., University of Michigan. CAREER: 1903-8, U.S. government physician, Indian Reservation at Lower Brule, S.D.; 1908-18, assistant surgeon-in-chief, Freedmen's Hospital, Washington, D.C.; 1918 to shortly before his death, maintained private surgical practice, D.C.; 1919-38, operated Carson's Private Hospital for black patients (in segregated Washington); 1929-36, clinical professor of surgery, Howard University; 1938-54, part-time consultant and surgeon, Adams Hospital, Washington, D.C. CONTRIBUTIONS: Through his private proprietary hospital (1919-36), provided medical and surgical care to many blacks of Washington, D.C., who could not obtain good hospital care at segregated city hospitals. Known to students and patients as excellent bedside clinician and fine, reliable surgeon. Performed some surgery at all-white Garfield Hospital, Washington, D.C., where he had regular privileges (1910-54). Held many teaching clinics for black physicians throughout the country during his career.

WRITINGS: "Acute Indigestion," *JNMA* 7 (1915): 1-6. Writings listed in *JNMA* 46 (1954): 419. REFERENCES: W. Montague Cobb, "Simeon Lewis Carson, M.D., 1882-1954," *JNMA* 46 (1954): 414-19; *DAB*, Supp. 5:104-5; "Hospital Symposium: Carson's Private Hospital," *JNMA* 22 (1930): 148-51; John A. Kenney, *The Negro in Medicine* (1912), 29; *WWICA* 7 (1950): 90.

T. *Savitt*

CARTER, C. DANA (May 24, 1874, Washington, Ia.-March 20, 1945, Thermopolis, Wyo.). *Physician; Surgeon.* Son of John W., Methodist minister, and Allie (Perkins) Carter. Married Mary A. Curry, 1903; one son. EDUCATION: Apprentice to Drs. Libby and Brown of Tacoma, Wash.; 1895, M.D., Missouri Medical College; 1901, postgraduate work, Chicago Polyclinic; 1909, New York Polyclinic; 1913, New York School of Pathology and Surgery; intern, St. Louis County Hospital; studied in Vienna under Dr. Adolph Lorenz. CAREER: 1897, went to Big Horn Basin as the first physician in the region; 1911, built at Basin the first hospital on the western side of Wyo. between Rock Springs and Billings, Mont.; 1912, moved to Thermopolis; 1917, built hotel and sanitarium in Thermopolis (Hot Springs State Park); until January 1945, practiced medicine. CONTRIBUTIONS: Performed the first caesarian in Wyo. at Basin (1900). Served on the Wyoming State Board of Health (1919-23) and as health officer of Hot Springs County (1919-23, 1942-45).

WRITINGS: Pamphlet on injuries of bones of skull read before C. B. & Q. (Chicago,

Burlington, and Quincy) Medical Society (1909). REFERENCES: *History of Wyoming* (1918), 92; *Men of Wyoming* (1915), 50.

A. Palmieri

CARTER, HENRY ROSE (August 25, 1852, Clifton plantation, Caroline County, Va.-September 14, 1925, Washington, D.C.). *Sanitarian; Epidemiologist.* Son of Henry Rose, planter, and Emma Caroline (Coleman) Carter. Married Laura Eugenia Hook, 1880; three children. EDUCATION: University of Virginia: 1873, C.E. and 1874-75, postgraduate work in mathematics and applied chemistry; 1879, M.D., University of Maryland School of Medicine. CAREER: 1879, practiced medicine, Baltimore, Md., in partnership with Dr. Frank West; 1879-1919, with Marine Hospital Service (now, U.S. Public Health Service): 1888, assigned to Gulf Quarantine Station at Ship Island; 1893, 1897-98, national government's representative to southern states afflicted with yellow fever; 1899-1900, organized Cuban quarantine service; 1904-8, inaugurated quarantine service and became director of hospitals in Panama; 1913-19, directed malaria eradication program in the South; 1915-25, member, Yellow Fever Council, International Health Board, Rockefeller Foundation; active in campaigns in Central and South America. CONTRIBUTIONS: Scientific investigations and field work helped eradicate yellow fever and malaria in the United States and parts of Latin America. Determined that the incubation period of yellow fever lasts from three to six days (1898). Discovered that there is also an extrinsic incubation of the disease; work led Walter Reed (q.v.) to reconsider Carlos Finlay's theory that yellow fever was transmitted by a mosquito. Father of modern quarantine (late 1880s, 1890s); established the efficiency of sulphur fumigation and began the disinfection of vessels at ports of departure or en route; of greatest importance, replaced arbitrary local and state regulations with a uniform federal code; reforms freed commerce from cumbersome restrictions and expensive delays while improving the nation's safeguards against yellow fever. Directed the first systematic campaign against malaria in the South.

WRITINGS: "A Note on the Interval Between Infecting and Secondary Cases of Yellow Fever from the Records of Yellow Fever at Orwood and Taylor, Mississippi, in 1898," *New Orleans Med. & Surg. J.* 52 (1900): 617-36; *Yellow Fever, an Epidemiological and Historical Study of its Place of Origin* (1931, published posthumously). Scientific writings are briefly described in Kelly and Burrage (1928) and John C. Hemmeter, *Master Minds in Medicine* (1927), 343-44. REFERENCES: *BHM* (1964-69), 51; *DAB*, 3: 535-36; T. H. D. Griffitts, "Henry Rose Carter: The Scientist and the Man," *Southern Med. J.* 32 (1939): 841-48; Kelly and Burrage (1928), 203-4; Miller, *BHM*, p. 18; *NCAB*, 25: 346-47.

S. Galishoff

CARTER, WILLIAM SPENCER (April 11, 1869, Warren County, N.J.-May 12, 1944, Auburndale, Mass.). *Physician; Physiology.* Son of William and Ann (Stewart) Carter. Married Lillian V. McCleavy, 1894; two daughters. EDUCA-

TION: 1887, Easton High School, Pa.; 1890, M.D., University of Pennsylvania. CAREER: 1891-97, faculty in pathology and physiology, University of Pennsylvania; at University of Texas Medical Branch, Galveston, Tex.: 1897-1938, faculty; and 1903-22, 1935-38, dean; in Association of American Medical Colleges: 1917-18, president; and 1919-20, chairman, Committee on Education and Pedagogy; with Rockefeller Foundation: 1922-23, University of Philippines; and 1922-24, survey of medical education in the Far East; 1925-34, associate director, Peking Union Medical College. CONTRIBUTIONS: Original investigations, surveys, and reports in physiology, public health, pedagogy, medical education, administration. Won Boylston Prize for work on uremia (with W. E. Hughes); Alvarenza Prize, College of Physicians (1903).

WRITINGS: More than 30 published articles. *Notes on Pathology and Bacteriology* (1895, with D. Riseman); *Physician as Sanitarian* (1900); *Laboratory Exercises in Physiology* (1908); *Safe and Convenient Anesthetic* (1913); "A Decade of Progress in the Medical Department," *The Alcade* (1914); "Dean Carter in the Far East," *The Alcade* (1923); "The First Five Years of the Peking Union Medical College," *China Med. J.* 40 (1926): 726-43. REFERENCES: *JAMA* 125 (Jun. 3, 1944): 374; Moody Medical Library Archives, Galveston, Tex.; reports, correspondence and diary (1924-34) in the Rockefeller Archive Center, N. Tarrytown, N.Y.; *Texas State J. of Med.* 40 (Sept. 1944): 310-11; *The University of Texas Medical Branch at Galveston* (1967), 79-80.

J. Morris

CARTWRIGHT, SAMUEL ADOLPHUS (November 30, 1793, Fairfax County, Va.-May, 1863, Miss.) *Physician.* Son of John S. Cartwright (minister). Married Mary Wrenn, 1825; at least one child. EDUCATION: Before 1812, apprentice to Dr. John Brewer, Fairfax Co., Va.; 1812, apprentice to Benjamin Rush (q.v.); c. 1812-13, attended University of Pennsylvania Medical School. CAREER: Medical practice in Huntsville, Ala. (c. 1813-22), Natchez, Miss. (1822-48), and New Orleans, La. (1848-62); 1862-63, Confederate army physician focusing on sanitary improvement of soldiers' camps around Vicksburg and Port Hudson, Miss. CONTRIBUTIONS: As a proponent of idea that blacks were medically different from whites, wrote numerous articles and presented many talks which earned him national notoriety. Used medical ideas to justify enslaving blacks. Strongly advocated study of Southern medicine since it was different from the rest of the nation in diseases and treatments needed. Gained respect and admiration among planters around Natchez for his successful and untiring efforts during 1832 cholera epidemic.

WRITINGS: Many articles, including "Report on the Diseases and Physical Peculiarities of the Negro Race," *New Orleans Medical and Surgical Journal* (1851-1852); "Philosophy of the Negro Constitution," *ibid.*, (1852); "The Caucasians and the Africans," *DeBow's Review* (1858). Partial list of writings in *Transactions of the AMA* 24 (1873): 348. REFERENCES: *Appleton's Cyclopedia of Am. Biog.*, 1: 545; J.D. Guillory, "The Pro-Slavery Arguments of Dr. Samuel A. Cartwright," *Louisiana History*, 9 (1968), 209-27; Mary L. Marshall, "Samuel A. Cartwright and States' Rights Medicine," *New*

Orleans Med. and Surg. J. 93 (1940): 74-78; *Transactions of the AMA*, 24 (1873): 345-48.

T.L. Savitt

CARY, EDWARD HENRY (February 28, 1872, Union Springs, Ala.-December 11, 1953, Dallas, Tex.). *Surgeon; Eye, Ear, Nose & Throat.* Son of Joseph Milton and Lucy Janette (Powell) Cary. Married Georgia Fonda Schneider, April 19, 1911; four children. EDUCATION: 1898, M.D., Bellevue Hospital Medical College; 1898-1901, intern, chief of Eye Clinic, Bellevue Dispensary; and taught ophthalmology, New York Polyclinic. CAREER: 1901-3, professor and dean, Dallas Medical College; at Baylor University College of Medicine: 1903-22, dean; 1921-29, chairman, Department of Surgery; and 1929-43, dean emeritus; 1917-18, president, Texas Medical Association; 1925-29, AMA trustee; 1932-33, president, AMA; 1939, organizer and president, Southwestern Medical Foundation; 1941-43, attempted transfer of control of Baylor University College of Medicine from parent University board in Waco to the Southwestern Medical Foundation and Dallas interests, to assure funding and survival with nonsectarian focus; 1943, instead, medical school moved to Houston; 1942-46, National Physicians Committee for the Extension of Medical Service; 1943, founder, Southwestern Medical College of the Southwestern Medical Foundation; 1943-49, complex negotiations for state support while the college operated independently. CONTRIBUTIONS: Dynamic physician, medical educator, administrator. Skillfully orchestrated the fortunes of three successive medical schools in Dallas, finally achieving a viable medical center through state funding as the University of Texas Southwestern Medical School at Dallas (1949).

WRITINGS: Listed in card file, "Writings of Dallas Physicians" and archive material, University of Texas Southwestern Medical School Library, Dallas; bibliography in Booth Mooney, *More Than Armies: The Story of Edward H. Cary* (1948), 271-72. REFERENCES: John S. Chapman, *Southwestern Medical School* (1976); Samuel W. Geiser, *Medical Education in Dallas, 1900-1910* (1952); *JAMA* 154 (Jan. 2, 1954): 75; Walter H. Moursund, *History of Baylor College of Medicine, 1900 to 1953* (1956); Catherine Schulze, "What Happened During 1943-48," Archives, University of Texas Southwestern Medical School Library, Dallas; *Texas State J. of Med.* 50 (1954): 60-61.

J. Morris

CAVERLY, CHARLES SOLOMON (September 3, 1856, Troy, N.H.-October 16, 1918, Rutland, Vt.). *Physician; Epidemiologist.* Son of Abiel Moore, physcian, and Sarah (Goddard) Caverly. Married Mabel Alice Tuttle, 1885; one son. EDUCATION: Kimball Union Academy, Meriden, N.H.; 1878, B.A., Dartmouth; 1881, M.D., University of Vermont; 1881-82, postgraduate study, College of Physicians and Surgeons, N.Y. CAREER: 1883-1918, medical practice and health officer, Rutland; on Vermont State Board of Health: 1890, member; and 1891-1918, president; at University of Vermont: 1903-10, professor of hygiene; and 1911-19, professor of hygiene and preventive medicine. CONTRIBUTIONS: Helped to establish the Vermont State Laboratory (1898). Identified an outbreak of paralytic disease of children in Vt. as poliomyelitis (1895); was the largest epidemic reported anywhere at that time and the first one to be studied by a public health official. First to recognize cases of nonparalytic polio. Following the larger epidemic of 1910, secured a generous grant from the Proctor family to set up a research laboratory and clinics for treatment, the latter serving as model for Handicapped Children's Clinics. Known for his work on the diagnosis, treatment, and prevention of tuberculosis; efforts led to the establishment of the Vermont Tuberculosis Sanitarium (1907) and the ''Preventorium'' (1918, named for him) to which children of infected parents were sent.

WRITINGS: Many of Caverly's papers were reprinted in *Infantile Paralysis in Vermont, 1894-1922—A Memorial to Charles S. Caverly* (1924). The book contains an obituary and papers by other workers in the field. REFERENCES: Kelly and Burrage (1920), 202; John R. Paul, *A History of Poliomyelitis* (1971), 79-86.

L. J. Wallman

CHAILLÉ, STANFORD EMERSON (July 9, 1830, Natchez, Miss.-May 27, 1911, New Orleans, La.). *Anatomist; Educator; Editor; Medical reformer*. Son of William Hamilton, planter, and Mary Eunice Priscilla (Stanford) Chaillé. Married Laura E. Mountfort, 1857 (d. 1858), one child; Mary Louise Napier, 1863. EDUCATION: Phillips Academy, Andover, Mass.; 1851, A.B., Harvard University; 1853, M.D., University of Louisiana; 1854, A.M., Harvard University; 1860-61, 1866-67, postgraduate medical study in Europe. CAREER: 1854, resident physician, U.S. Marine Hospital, New Orleans; 1854-60, resident physician, Circus Street Hospital; 1857-61, proprietor and co-editor, *New Orleans Medical and Surgical Journal*; 1858-61, demonstrator of anatomy, medical department, University of Louisiana; 1861-65, served in Confederate forces respectively as private, medical inspector, and surgeon; 1865-66, demonstrator of anatomy, medical department, University of Louisiana; 1866, proprietor and editor, *New Orleans Medical and Surgical Journal*; at Tulane University: 1867-1908, professor of physiology, pathological anatomy, and hygiene; and 1886-1908, dean of medical faculty; 1879, chairman, Havana Yellow Fever Commission; 1880-82, supervising inspector, National Board of Health. CONTRIBUTIONS: Outstanding medical professor, administrator, journalist, and public health leader. A major force in improving medical education and constantly stressed the need for laboratory and clinical teaching. Under his leadership, Tulane Medical School became one of the three best medical schools in the South. An advocate of the use of statistics in medical and public health research, and his papers and speeches on ''State Medicine'' or public health profoundly influenced state and national developments.

WRITINGS: A frequent contributor to the *New Orleans Med. and Surg. J.*, writing 18 articles alone (1854-76) on diverse topics such as clinical medicine, vital statistics, medical jurisprudence, physiology, medical education, and the opium habit. In addition, contributed articles to the *Transactions* of the American Public Health Association, American Public Health Association *Reports, Reports* of the National Board of Health (1879), *Sanitarian, JAMA*, and other journals. ''The Yellow Fever, Sanitary Condition, and Vital Statistics of New Orleans During Its Military Occupation, the Four Years 1862-65,'' *New Orleans Med. and Surg. J.* 23 (1870): 563-98, ''Origin and Progress of Medical Juris-

prudence, 1776-1876. A Centennial Address," *Trans. of the Internat. Med. Cong., 1876,*
pp. 167-204; "History of the Laws Regulating the Practice of Medicine, etc. in Louisiana,
1808 to 1878," *New Orleans Med. and Surg. J.,* n.s., 5 (1878): 909-26; "State Medicine
and State Medical Societies," *TAMA* 30 (1879): 299-355. REFERENCES: Stanford Emerson Chaillé, *Collected Reprints, 1855-1908,* Rudolph Matas Med. Library, Tulane University, New Orleans, La.; George Denegre, "Dr. Stanford E. Chaillé," *New Orleans
Med. and Surg. J.* 65 (1912): 49-57; John Duffy, *The Rudolph Matas History of Medicine
in Louisiana* 2 (1962); Albert E. Fossier, "History of Medical Education in New Orleans
from Its Birth to the Civil War," *Annals of Med. Hist.* 4 (1934): 320-52, 427-47; Miller,
BHM, p. 19; F. W. Parham, "Address for the Louisiana State Medical Society, in
Memorial of Stanford Chaillé" (1912), 42-49; Kenneth Ray Whitehead, "A Biography
of Stanford Emerson Chaillé, 1830-1876" (M.A. thesis, Louisiana State University,
1961).

J. Duffy

CHANDLER, CHARLES FREDERICK (December 6, 1836, Lancaster,
Mass.-August 25, 1925, New York, N.Y.). *Industrial chemist; Public health.*
Son of Charles, merchant, and Sarah (Whitney) Chandler. Married Anna Maria
Craig, 1862, one child; Augusta P. Berard, 1905. EDUCATION: Lawrence Scientific School, Harvard University; 1855-56, studied at the universities of Göttingen and Berlin; 1856, A.M., Ph.D., University of Göttingen. CAREER: 1857-
64, chemistry faculty, Union College; at Columbia School of Mines: 1864, co-
founder; 1864-1911, analytical and applied chemistry faculty; 1864-97, dean;
1866-1904, chemistry faculty and president, New York College of Pharmacy
(later, a department of Columbia University); at New York Metropolitan Board
of Health (*post* 1870, New York City Board of Health): 1867-73, chemist; and
1873-83, president; at Columbia University: 1872-96, chemistry and medical
jurisprudence faculty; 1877-1910, chemistry faculty; and 1897, dean of science
faculty. CONTRIBUTIONS: During years with Metropolitan Board of Health, initiated and directed a wide variety of reforms, including regulation of noxious
trades, installation of plumbing and house drainage, prevention of milk adulteration, and abatement of the gas nuisance; opposition of corrupt politicians
and powerful commercial interests caused some reforms to be short-lived. Established flash-point tests for kerosene that helped prevent lamp explosions (1870).
Invented the modern flush toilet, which he gave to the public unpatented. Organized a summer corps of visiting physicians (1879) to care for the children of
the poor in their homes, which, it was estimated, saved the lives of 5,000 children
annually. Created a permanent vaccination squad that reduced deaths from smallpox. Made studies of the water supply of several N.Y. cities and was an expert
in the field. Lifted the New York College of Pharmacy into the first rank of
pharmacy colleges.

WRITINGS: *Report on the Quality of the Kerosene Oil Sold in the Metropolitan District*
(1870). A bibliography is in *BMNAS.* REFERENCES: *Appleton's CAB,* 1: 571-72; *BMNAS*

14 (1932): 127-81; *DAB*, 3: 611-13; Miller, *BHM*, p. 19; Charles L. Van Doren and Robert McHenry, *Webster's Am. Biog.*(1974), 189; *Who Was Who in Am.*, 1: 210.

S. Galishoff

CHANNING, WALTER (April 15, 1786, Newport, R.I.-July 27, 1876, Brookline, Mass.). *Physician; Obstetrics.* Son of William, attorney, and Lucy (Ellery) Channing. Married Barbara Higginson Perkins, 1815; Elizabeth Wainwright, 1831; four children. EDUCATION: 1808, A.B., Harvard College; 1809, M.D., University of Pennsylvania; 1812, M.D., Harvard Medical School; 1812, studied obstetrics, Edinburgh University and London hospitals. CAREER: At Harvard Medical School: 1812-15, lecturer on obstetrics; 1815-54, first professor of obstetrics and medical jurisprudence; and 1819-47, dean; in Massachusetts Medical Society: 1822-25, librarian; and 1828-40, treasurer; 1828-c. 1848, visiting staff, Massachusetts General Hospital; c. 1832, one of first attending physicians, Boston Lying-In Hospital. CONTRIBUTIONS: Soon after first demonstration of ether anesthesia at the Massachusetts General Hospital (1846), studied and became the chief American proselytizer of etherization in childbirth. A founder of the *New England Journal of Medicine and Surgery* (1812), *Boston Medical and Surgical Journal* (1828); and Boston Lying-In Hospital (1832). First to describe pregnancy anemia (1842). Social reformer concerned with temperance, peace, pure water, and prevention of pauperism.

WRITINGS: *Remarks on the Employment of Females as Practitioners in Midwifery, by a Physician* (1820); *Lecture on the Moral Uses of the Study of Natural History* (1836); *Annual Address Delivered Before the Massachusetts Temperance Society* (1836); *An Address on the Prevention of Pauperism* (1843); *Cases of Inhalation of Ether in Labor* (1847); *A Treatise on Etherization in Childbirth* (1848); *Bedcase: Its History and Treatment* (1860). REFERENCES: *BHM* (1970-74), 37; Kelly and Burrage, (1920), 205-6; Walter Channing, *A Physician's Vacation* (1856); *DAB*, 2, pt. 2: 3-4; Gordon W. Jones, "An American Gift to the World," *Virginia Med. Monthly* 99 (1972): 326-27; "The Late Dr. Channing," *Bost. Med. and Surg. J.* 95 (1876): 237-38; Miller, *BHM*, 19; *NCAB*, 13: 431; Herbert Thoms, "Channing and Simpson in Edinburgh," *Yale J. of Bio. & Med.* 30 (1958): 374-81.

J. H. Warner

CHAPIN, CHARLES VALUE (January 17, 1856, Providence, R.I.-January 31, 1941, Providence). *Physician; Public health.* Son of Joshua Bicknell, physician and photographer, and Jane Catherine Louise (Value) Chapin, painter. Married Anna Augusta Balch, 1886; one child. EDUCATION: 1872, graduated from English and Classical High School for Boys, Providence; 1876, A.B., Brown University; 1876-77, apprentice to George D. Wilcox and Joshua B. Chapin; 1877-78, College of Physicians and Surgeons of New York; 1879, M.D., Bellevue Hospital Medical College; 1879-80, intern, Bellevue Hospital. CAREER: 1880-83, private practice, Providence; 1880-83, attending physician, Providence Dispensary; 1882-83, lecturer on anatomy and physiology, Rhode Island Hospital Training School for Nurses; 1882-86, pathologist and librarian, Rhode Island

Hospital; at Brown University: 1882-95, professor of physiology; and 1891-95, director of physical culture; in Providence: 1884-1932, superintendent of health; and 1888-1932, city registrar; 1913-22, lecturer, Harvard-MIT School for Health Officers; 1922-32, lecturer, Harvard School of Public Health. CONTRIBUTIONS: Leader of the American movement to bring the findings of bacteriology into public health work. Discredited outmoded general sanitary theories and procedures by use of specific measures directed against specific diseases. Organized the first municipal bacteriological laboratory (1888). Made exhaustive field studies of the common infectious diseases of temperate climates. Organized the Providence City Hospital (1910), the first American infectious disease hospital operated on the principle of aseptic nursing. With his volume *The Sources and Modes of Infection* (1910), provided the definitive text of the "New Public Health." Stimulated the elevation of American vital and sanitary statistics in completeness and accuracy. Helped rejuvenate the specialty of epidemiology in this country. Conducted the first evaluation of state public health work (1913-16) and established a realistic scale of priorities for both state and municipal health work.

WRITINGS: *Municipal Sanitation in the United States* (1901); *The Sources and Modes of Infection* (1910); *Report on State Public Health Work* (1916); *How to Avoid Infection* (1917); *Papers of Charles V. Chapin, M.D.* (1934, ed. Clarence L. Scamman). REFERENCES: James H. Cassedy, *Charles V. Chapin and the Public Health Movement* (1962; also diss., 1959); *Encyclopedia of Am. Biog.* (1974), 188-89; Miller, *BHM*, p. 19; *NCAB*, 39:99; *DAB*, Supplement 3 (1973): 157-59; Irving A. Watson, ed., *Physicians and Surgeons of Am.* (1896), 141.

J. H. Cassedy

CHAPMAN, NATHANIEL (May 28, 1780, Fairfax County, Va.-July 1, 1853, Philadelphia, Pa.). *Physician; Medical educator.* Son of George and Amelia (Macrea) Chapman. Married Rebecca Biddle, 1804. EDUCATION: Alexandria (Va.) Academy; studied medicine with Dr. Benjamin Rush (q.v.), Dr. John Weems, and Dr. Elisha Cullen Dick; 1801, M.D., University of Pennsylvania; 1801-4, study in Edinburgh and London. CAREER: 1804, medical practice, Philadelphia; 1810-50, faculty, University of Pennsylvania school of medicine (midwifery, materia medica, theory and practice of medicine); 1820, became editor, *Philadelphia Journal of Medical and Physical Sciences* (still in existence as the *American Journal of Medical Sciences*); 1817, founded the Medical Institute of Philadelphia. CONTRIBUTIONS: The leading medical man in Philadelphia after the passing of Benjamin Rush. Founded the Medical Institute of Philadelphia, first postgraduate medical school in America. First president of the American Medical Association (1848).

WRITINGS: *Elements of Therapeutics and Materia Medica* (1817); *Lectures on the More Important Diseases of the Thoracic and Abdominal Viscera* (1844); *Lectures on the More Important Eruptive Fevers* (1844); *A Compendium of Lectures on the Theory and Practice of Medicine* (1846). Writings listed in Kelly and Burrage (1920), 208. REFERENCES: *Appleton's Cyclopedia of Biog.* (1888); *BHM* (1964-69), 54; *DAB*, 2, pt.

2: 19-21; F. P. Henry, *Standard Hist. of Med. Profession in Philadelphia* (1897); Kelly and Burrage (1920); Miller, *BHM*, p. 19; *NCAB*, 3: 294.

D. I. Lansing

CHASE, WILL HENRY (January 19, 1874, Warsaw, N. Y.-October 1, 1964, Seattle, Washington). *Physician and Surgeon.* Son of Leander and Almeda (Mallison) Chase. Married Ellen Fraisure, 1920; one child. EDUCATION: Attended Mills Training School for Male Nurses and Eclectic Medical Training School at Bellevue Hospital, New York City. Also pursued special studies in natural history. Licensed to practice under the "grandfather laws" of the Territory of Alaska. CAREER: 1897, entered Alaska; 1900-1907, practice in Dawson, Yukon Territory, and in Fairbanks; 1908, staff of hospital in Cordova; 1912-26, U.S. Indian Medical Service; 1909-17, Alaska Commissioner of Health. CONTRIBU-TIONS: 1897, reported to have performed the first appendectomy (at Sheeps Camp) in Skagway. 1906, performed first post mortem in Valdez. Treated patients by dogsled, 1900-1907. Helped establish first Alaska Medical Association, *circa* 1906. 1908, helped set up first hospital in Cordova in an abandoned cannery building. 1919, when he was filling in for the Kennicott Copper Mine surgeon, he crawled over a collapsed railroad bridge to treat survivors of a mine accident. During career, delivered more than 3000 infants. Was aspiring naturalist and provided expert assistance to United States Biological Service. Medical member, Cordova Selective Service Board, World War II. Served as Mayor of Cordova for 24 terms.

WRITINGS: Several books of anecdotal history; a scientific treatise on *Alaska's Mammoth Brown Bears.* REFERENCES: *Anchorage Times,* October 8, 1964, p. 3; *Cordova Times,* October 2, 1964, pp. 1, 6.

A. R. C. Helms

CHEATHAM, ANDERSON WILLIAM (April 6, 1880, Nashville, Tenn.-May 4, 1936, St. Louis, Mo.). *Physician; General medicine; Surgery.* EDU-CATION: A.B., Fisk University; 1909, M.D., Northwestern University; 1909-10, intern, Provident Hospital, Chicago, Ill. CAREER: 1910-36, private practice, general medicine and surgery, St. Louis; chief, Department of Obstetrics and Gynecology, People's Hospital, St. Louis; associate director of obstetrics and gynecology, Homer G. Phillips Hospital, St. Louis. CONTRIBUTIONS: Active in breaking racial barriers in medically segregated St. Louis in early twentieth century. Helped found People's Hospital, St. Louis branch of Urban League, and YMCA branch. Involved in making arrangements for black physicians at St. Mary's Infirmary. Organized, among local black physicians, first medical study club, which became involved in medical-social programs and dissemination of medical information to the public. Encouraged and trained young black physicians during era of segregation and open racism. Mound City Medical Forum named annual lecture for him (1945). REFERENCES: W. Montague Cobb, "Anderson William Cheatham, 1880-1936," *JNMA* 50 (1958): 400-401.

T. Savitt

CHEEVER, DAVID WILLIAMS (November 30, 1831, Portsmouth, N.H.-December 27, 1915, Boston, Mass.). *Physician; Surgery.* Son of Charles Augustus, physician, and Adeline (Haven) Cheever. Married Anna C. Nichols, 1860; six children. EDUCATION: Harvard University: A.B., 1852; M.D., 1858. CAREER: 1858-60, practiced medicine in Boston; Harvard University: anatomy faculty, 1861-66; surgery faculty, 1866-93; member, Board of Overseers, 1896-1908; 1864-95, surgeon, Boston City Hospital; 1864-*c*.-1907, first president, medical staff, Boston City Hospital; editor of the *Boston Medical and Surgical Journal*; president: Massachusetts Medical Society (1888-90); American Surgical Association (1889); Boston Medical Library (1896-1906). CONTRIBUTIONS: Originated or revived several operations including displacement of the upper jaw for nasopharyngeal tumors, removal of tumors of the tonsil by external incision, pharyngotomy, esophagotomy to remove foreign bodies in the esophagus, and the radical cure for hernia. One of the first in New England to do Caesarean sections and ovariotomies. Aided Charles W. Eliot (q.v.) in his reform of medical education at Harvard University. The dominant medical figure at Boston City Hospital, fought a long and ultimately unsuccessful battle against municipal politicians to maintain the institution's aristocratic traditions.

WRITINGS: Editor, *Medical and Surgical Reports of* [Boston] *City Hospital* (5 vols.). Won the Boylston Prize Essay in 1860 and was the author of several monographs, essays, case reports, and hospital reports. REFERENCES: Kelly and Burrage (1928), 217-19; F.B. Lund, "David Williams Cheever," *New Eng. J. Med.*, 220 (1939): 321-26; *NCAB*, 13: 515; Morris J. Vogel, *The Invention of the Modern Hospital: Boston, 1870-1930* (1980), passim; *Who Was Who in Am.*, 1: 214.

S. Galishoff

CHESNEY, ALAN MASON (January 17, 1888, Baltimore, Md.—September 22, 1964, Baltimore). *Physician; Immunologist; Historian.* Son of Jesse Mason and Annie (Atkinson) Chesney. Married Cora Chambers, 1917; three children. EDUCATION: 1905, Baltimore City College; Johns Hopkins: 1908, A.B.; and 1912, M.D.; 1913, intern and assistant resident in medicine, Johns Hopkins Hospital; 1914-17, worked under Rufus Cole (q.v.) and O.T. Avery (q.v.), Rockefeller Institute; 1921, worked with Wade Brown and Louise Pearce (q.v.), Rockefeller Institute, in preparation for his appointment to the new Syphilis Division at Johns Hopkins' Department of Medicine. CAREER: 1912, began practice, Baltimore; 1917-19, served in France and Germany in the Army Medical Corps, where he advanced from first lieutenant to major; 1919-21, head of Infectious Disease Division, Department of Medicine, Washington University at St. Louis; 1921, appointed associate professor of medicine in charge of the Syphilis Division at Johns Hopkins, where he remained until his death; 1923-

47, editor, *Medicine*; at School of Medicine: 1927-29, assistant dean; and 1929-53, dean; president: 1937-38, American Association of Medical Colleges; and 1952-53, Medical and Chirurgical Faculty of Maryland; 1953, became dean emeritus, School of Medicine; 1959-61, president, Johns Hopkins Medical and Surgical Association. CONTRIBUTIONS: By public referendum (1950), won his long battle with Baltimore's antivivisectionists and founded the Maryland Society for Medical Research. Proved that immunity to syphilis continued even after the agent causing the original infection was destroyed by a specific treatment; showed that patients with early syphilis harbored *Treponema pallidum* in their blood, spinal, and joint fluid; exhibited that, in both early and latent syphilis, almost all organs of rabbits were susceptible to infection by the disease; made further contributions through his later studies of penicillin's biological and therapeutic role in treating syphilis. Had observed (by 1928) that many of his experimental rabbits had developed goiter; eventually helped show that goiter, rather than being caused strictly by iodine deficiency, could be caused by specific goitrogens first found in cabbage; in a paper co-authored with Bruce Webster ("Studies in the Etiology of Simple Goiter," *Am. J. of Pathology* 6, no. 3 [May 1930]), helped show that iodine could prevent goiter.

WRITINGS: "The Use of Phenol Red and Brom-cresol Purple as Indicators in the Bacteriological Examination of Stools," *J. of Experimental Med.* 35 (Feb. 1922): 181; *Immunity in Syphilis* (1927); *The Flowering of an Idea: A Play Presenting the Origin and Early Development of the Johns Hopkins Hospital* (1939); *The Johns Hopkins Hospital and The Johns Hopkins University School of Medicine,* 3 vols. (1943, 1958, 1963). REFERENCES: A. McGehee Harvey, *Adventures in Medical Research* (1976): 317-20; "Scientists in the News," *Science* 118 (Aug. 14, 1953): 3059; Thomas B. Turner, *Heritage of Excellence: The Johns Hopkins Medical Institutions, 1914-1947* (1974), esp. 501-5; *Who Was Who in Am.,* 4: 169.

C. Donegan

CHISOLM, JULIAN JOHN (April 16, 1830, Charleston, S.C.-November 2, 1903, Petersburg, Va.). *Physician; Surgeon; Oculist.* Son of Robert Trail and Harriett Emily (Schutt) Chisolm. Married cousin Mary Edings Chisolm, 1852, two children; after her death, M. Elizabeth Steele, 1888, one child. EDUCATION: 1850, M.D., Medical College of South Carolina; 1850-51, studied in Paris and London. CAREER: 1857, he and Dr. D. J. C. Cain opened and conducted a hospital for slaves; 1858, professor of surgery, Medical College of South Carolina; 1859, observed medical treatment of wounded soldiers in Italy; 1860, assumed professorship in Charleston; 1861, received first commission bestowed on a medical officer of the Confederacy; 1862, elected vice-president of the South Carolina Medical Association; later served as chief surgeon in a Richmond, Va., hospital; directed a pharmaceutical plant in Columbia, S.C.; served in the Wayside Hospital in Columbia and as a surgeon-purveyor in Newberry, S.C.; at Medical College of South Carolina: after the war, resumed practice and chair of surgery; and 1865, dean of faculty; 1866, spent year in Europe; 1869, assumed chair of eye and ear surgery created for him at University of Maryland, later that year, dean; 1871, visited Europe to study eye and ear surgery; 1877, chief surgeon, Presbyterian Eye and Ear and Throat Hospital, Baltimore, Md.; 1887, chairman, Ophthalmological Section, Ninth International Medical Congress. CONTRIBUTIONS: Devised a chloroform inhaler that was first used during war. One of first to experiment with cocaine as anesthesia (1884). Cleansed the eye before and after operating (1887). Began sterilizing the instruments in boiling water (1891). Instrumental in establishment of the Baltimore Eye and Ear Institute (1870). Instrumental in establishment of the Presbyterian Eye and Ear and Throat Hospital in Baltimore (1877).

WRITINGS: *A Manual of Military Surgery for the Use of Surgeons in the Confederate States Army* (1861); "Treatment of Wild Hairs More Especially by Electrolysis," *Maryland Med. J.* (1880); "Cataract Extraction with Iridectomy in an Infant Six Months Old," *Arch. Ophthal.* (1882); "An Obscure Case in Nerve Pathology Accompanying Optic Neuritis," *ibid.* Wrote over one hundred papers. Writings listed in *Va. Med. Monthly* (Jan. 1879). REFERENCES: *DAB* 4:76-77; James Wood Davidson, *The Living Writers of the South* (1869); J.W. Jervey, "John Julian Chisolm [sic] and Hospital Expense," *Recorder of the Columbia (S.C.) Med. Soc.* (1964); Kelly and Burrage (1920), 217.

J. P. Dolan

CHITTENDEN, RUSSELL HENRY (February 18, 1856, New Haven, Conn.-December 26, 1943, New Haven). *University professor and director; Physiological chemistry.* Son of Horace Horatio, factory superintendent, and Emily Eliza (Doane) Chittenden. Married Gertrude Louise Baldwin, 1877; three children. EDUCATION: Sheffield Scientific School (Yale University): 1875, Ph.B.; and 1880, Ph.D.; 1878-79, studied at University of Heidelberg under Wilhelm Kühne. CAREER: At Sheffield Scientific School: 1874-1922, physiological chemistry faculty; and 1898-1922, director; 1898-1903, physiological chemistry faculty, Columbia University; 1908-15, member, referee board of consulting scientific experts to U.S. secretary of agriculture; 1918, U.S. representative on Inter-Allied Scientific Food Commission at London, Paris, and Rome. CONTRIBUTIONS: Considered to be the father of American biochemistry; established the study of physiological chemistry through his research, influence as a teacher, and promotion of professional publications and societies. Scientific work falls broadly into three categories: (1) enzyme studies; with Kühne, investigated the enzymatic splitting of proteins (1895); also studied the enzymatic digestion of starch; (2) toxicology studies; examined the effects of heavy metals, drugs, and alcohol on the body (1903-5, 1908-15); (3) nutrition, especially man's minimum daily protein requirement; concluded that a diet providing 50 grams of protein and 2,600 calories was sufficient to maintain good health (1904-7); isolated glycogen, the body's principal carbohydrate reserve, and demonstrated the occurrence of free glycine in nature (1875). Taught the first American laboratory course in physiological chemistry and opened it to medical students. Developed the Sheffield Scientific School into a prestigious institution. Taught some of the most eminent biochemists of his time and trained generations of college and university instructors. Helped organize the American Physiological Society (1887) and the American Society of Biological Chemists (1906) and served as president of each. Member of the editorial board of several journals, including *American Journal of Physiology, Journal of Experimental Medicine,* and *Journal of Biological Chemistry.* Wrote extensively on the history of physiological chemistry (1922-44).

WRITINGS: *Physiological Economy in Nutrition* . . . (1907); *The Development of Physiological Chemistry in the United States* (1930). A bibliography is in *BMNAS.* REFERENCES: *BHM* (1964-69), 55; *BMNAS* 24 (1947): 59-104; *DAB,* Supplement 3: 162-64; *DSB,* 3: 256-58; Miller, *BHM,* p. 20; *Who Was Who in Am.,* 2: 114.

S. Galishoff

CHURCH, BENJAMIN (August 24, 1734, Newport, R.I.-1778, lost at sea). *Physician; Surgeon.* Son of Benjamin Church, merchant. Married Hannah Hill, 1758; several children. EDUCATION: Boston Latin School; 1754, A.B., Harvard College; apprenticed in medicine, Dr. Joseph Pynchon, Boston, Mass.; 1757-59, clinical training, London hospitals. CAREER: 1757, ship surgeon; practice in Boston as surgeon and physician and expert on smallpox inoculation; active in Whig politics; widely known as a poet and orator; published verse and satire in newspapers; 1774, delegate, Mass. Provincial Congress; member Committee of Safety of Mass. and Boston Committee of Correspondence; active in planning for defense of Bunker Hill; 1775, delegate, Continental Congress; July 1775, appointed by the Continental Congress as director-general and chief physician of the Hospital of the Army; same month, mistress was intercepted trying to smuggle an encoded letter to General Gage in Boston; code was broken, and she confessed; October 4, 1775, Church was court-martialed for engaging in treasonous correspondence with the enemy; November 11, was tried and expelled from the Mass. General Court (legislature). By order of the Continental Congress, was jailed that month in Norwich, Conn.; May 1776, was paroled due to ill health; 1778, permitted to leave for the West Indies; lost at sea when his ship disappeared. CONTRIBUTIONS: Established examining boards for surgeons for the army (the first "licensure") and as director-general, tried to establish rational systems for medical supply and patient care. Lacked the diplomatic and executive skills to deal with the separately appointed regimental surgeons whose political power fostered a series of bitter quarrels over hospital policy and medical supply. Medical work was overshadowed by his political roles.

WRITINGS: *The Choice: A Poem* (1757); *The Times: A Poem* (1763); *An Oration...to Commemorate the Bloody Tragedy of the Fifth of March, 1770* (1773). REFERENCES: *BHM* (1975-79), 28; Philip Cash, *Medical Men at the Siege of Boston* (1973); *DAB,* 2, pt 2:100-101; Louis C. Duncan, "Medical Men in the American Revolution," *U.S. Army Med. Bull.* (1931); Kelly and Burrage (1920), 221; *NCAB,* 7: 167; William F. Norwood, "The Enigma of Dr. Benjamin Church," *Med. Arts and Sciences* 10 (1956): 71-93; James M. Phalen, "Chiefs of the Medical Department, U.S. Army," *U.S. Army Med.*

Bull. (Apr. 1940); James E. Pilcher, *The Surgeon Generals of the Army of the United States* (1905); *Sibley's Harvard Graduates* 13: 380-98.

R. J. T. Joy

CHURCHILL, EDWARD DELOS (December 25, 1895, Chenoa, Ill.-August 28, 1972, Strafford, Vt.). *Physician; Surgery; Medical education.* Son of Ebenezer Delos, farmer and businessman, and Maria Atkins (Farnsworth) Churchill. Married Mary Lowell Barton, 1927; four children. EDUCATION: Northwestern University: 1916, B.S.; and 1917, A.M.; 1920, M.D., Harvard Medical School; 1920-24, intern and resident, Massachusetts General Hospital; 1926-27, studied in Europe as a Moseley fellow. CAREER: 1922-62, surgery faculty, Harvard Medical School; 1924-72, surgical staff, Massachusetts General Hospital; 1928-30, associate surgeon and director, Surgical Research Laboratory, Boston City Hospital; 1943-46, chief surgical consultant, North African and Mediterranean theaters of operation; chairman: 1946-48, medical advisory committee to secretary of war; and 1946-49, committee on surgery, National Research Council; 1948-49, 1953-55, vice-chairman, Task Force of the Federal Medical Services of the Commission on Organization of the Executive Branch of the Government; 1948-51, member, Armed Forces Medical Advisory Committee to secretary of defense; 1953-72, senior civilian consultant in thoracic surgery to Surgeon General; 1954-55, consultant to Surgeon General; 1958, on a Rockefeller Foundation grant, visited medical centers in India, where he helped establish a residency program at Lucknow University's King George Medical College; 1959-60, surgery faculty, American University, Beirut, Lebanon; member, editorial board, *Annals of Surgery*; president: 1946-47, American Surgical Association; 1948-49, American Association for Thoracic Surgery; and 1949-50, Society of Clinical Surgery. CONTRIBUTIONS: Advanced the frontiers of thoracic and cardiac surgery through new operative procedures, laboratory research, and teaching. Pioneered in surgical treatment of tuberculosis and lung cancer. Performed the first successful operation in the United States to relieve constrictive pericarditis. Established the role of parathyroidectomy in the treatment of hyperparathyroidism. Introduced a new procedure for primary resection by lobectomy (1939), which, after World War II, in conjunction with the use of antibiotics, superceded collapse therapy in the treatment of pulmonary tuberculosis. As chief surgical consultant in the North African and Italian campaigns, developed new techniques for the care of the wounded on the battlefield. Developed an outstanding Department of Surgery at the Massachusetts General Hospital and taught a generation of young physicians who later became leading surgeons.

WRITINGS: *To Work in the Vineyard of Surgery: The Reminiscences of J. Collins Warren (1842-1927)* (1958, editor); "The Operative Treatment of Hyperparathyroidism," *Trans., Am. Surg. Assoc.* 52 (1934): 255-59; "Pericardial Resection in Chronic Constrictive Pericarditis," *ibid.*, 54 (1936): 43-54; "The Surgical Management of the Wounded in the Mediterranean Theater at the Time of the Fall of Rome," *ibid.*, 62 (1944): 268-83; *Surgeon to Soldiers* (1972). REFERENCES: *Current Biog.* (1963), 68-70;

NCAB, 57: 643-44; N.Y. Times, September 4, 1972; Mark M. Ravitch, A Century of Surgery, 2 vols. (1981); Who Was Who in Am., 5: 131.

S. Galishoff

CLAPP, ASAHEL (October 5, 1792, Hubbardstown, Mass.-December 17, 1862, New Albany, Floyd County, Ind.). Physician; Botanist; Geologist. Son of Reuben, farmer, and Hepzibah (Gates) Clapp. Married Elizabeth Scribner; two children. EDUCATION: Early schooling near Montgomery, Vt.; c. 1810-12, medical apprenticeship served under Benjamin Chandler (1772-1818) of St. Albans, Vt. CAREER: Before 1810, taught school, Shelton, Vt.; 1813-14, practiced in or near St. Albans or Plattsburg, N.Y.; 1817, moved to New Albany; 1817-62, practiced in New Albany; president: 1820-21, Medical Society, State of Indiana; and 1850-51, reorganized Indiana State Medical Society; 1834, founder, New Albany Lyceum, which existed for over a decade; held no academic appointments and had never enrolled in a medical school, although he made it a practice to attend the introductory lectures of medical schools whenever possible in Louisville, Ky., Cincinnati, Ohio, and Philadelphia, Pa. CONTRIBUTIONS: An excellent practical botanist, largely self-taught through personal visits, correspondence, and the exchange of botanical specimens with other botanists throughout the United States. Chairman, American Medical Association Committee on Indigenous Medical Botany and Materia Medica (1850-51).

WRITINGS: Report of Committee on Indigenous Medical Botany and Materia Medica, TAMA 5 (1852): 689-906. REFERENCES: G. W. H. Kemper, A Medical History of the State of Indiana (1911), 48, 251-52; MSS. Journal, April 6, 1819-December 11, 1862 (missing March 30, 1824-March 21, 1831), photostatic copy in Indiana State Library, Indianapolis, Ind.; obituary, New Albany Daily Ledger, December 17, 1862, p. 2, col. 1.

E. H. Conner

CLARK, SAM LILLARD (October 5, 1898, Nashville, Tenn.-July 1, 1960, Nashville). Physician; Neuroscientist; Medical educator. Son of Martin and Margaret Ransom (Lillard) Clark. Married Nettie Lee Petrie, 1922; four children. EDUCATION: 1922, B.S., Vanderbilt; 1926, Ph.D. (Anatomy), Washington University; 1930, M.D., Vanderbilt. CAREER: 1926-27, assistant professor of anatomy, Washington University; 1927-30, assistant professor of anatomy, Northwestern University; at Vanderbilt University: 1930-31, assistant professor of anatomy; 1931-37, associate professor of anatomy; 1937-60, professor and head of anatomy; 1945-50, associate dean of College of Medicine; and 1958, acting dean; at American Journal of Anatomy: 1940-57, associate editor; and 1957-59, manager-editor. CONTRIBUTIONS: Pioneered the techniques of studying the function of the nervous system unencumbered by anesthetic agents in the early 1930s and used this technology most effectively in his studies on the function of the cerebellum. Interest in the cerebral cortex became the basis for obtaining the first EEG machine in the South (1939); for many years, read the

EEGs for Vanderbilt Hospital. A superb teacher, dedicated to stimulating the habit of inquiry in the young medical student and providing him with awareness of when he resorts to hypothesis.

WRITINGS: Numerous scientific articles mainly on the structure and function of the brain. Best known for his three revisions of Stephen W. Ranson's textbook *The Anatomy of the Nervous System* (1947, 1953, 1959). REFERENCES: *Anatomical Record* 140 (1961): 225-29.

S. R. Bruesch

CLARKE, EDWARD HAMMOND (February 2, 1820, Norton, Mass.-November 30, 1877, Boston, Mass.). *Physician; Materia Medica; Otology.* Son of Pitt, Congregational minister, and Mary Jane (Stimson) Clarke, poet. Married Sarah Loud, 1852; two children. EDUCATION: 1841, A.B., Harvard College; 1846, M.D., University of Pennsylvania Medical School. CAREER: 1855-72, professor of materia medica, Harvard Medical School; 1872-77, member, Board of Overseers, Harvard University. CONTRIBUTIONS: In controversial book, *Sex in Education* (1873), claimed that the health of adolescent women could be seriously endangered by the rigors of academic work and thus argued against co-education and the admission of women to medical school (especially Harvard Medical School). Numerous critics, including Julia Ward Howe, Mary Putnam Jacobi (q.v.), and Eliza Bisbee Duffee, responded with studies refuting his views on feminine weakness and questioning the authenticity of his clinical evidence. Joined in the revival of the Boston Society for Medical Observation (1846). Founder, Boylston Medical School of Boston, an avowed rival of Harvard (1850).

WRITINGS: *Observations on the Nature and Treatment of Polypus of the Ear* (1867); *The Physiological and Therapeutical Action of the Bromide of Potassium and Bromide of Ammonium* (1872; 1874, with Robert Amory); *The Building of the Brain* (1874); *A Century of American Medicine, 1776-1876* (1876); *Visions: A Study of False Sight (Pseudopia)* (1878, posthumously). REFERENCES: "The Death of Dr. Clarke," *Boston Med. and Surg. J.* 97 (1877): 657-59; Oliver Wendell Holmes, "Introduction and Memorial Sketch," in Edward H. Clarke, *Visions* (1878), vi-xxii; *NCAB*, 8: 213; Mary Roth Walsh, *"Doctors Wanted: No Women Need Apply"* (1977), 106-46.

M. H. Warner

CLEMENT, KENNETH WITCHER (February 24, 1920, Vashti, Pittsylvania County, Va.-November 29, 1974, Cleveland, Ohio). *Physician; Surgeon.* Son of Harry Leonard and Inez (Mae) Clement. Married Ruth Doss, 1942; three children. EDUCATION: 1942, A.B., Oberlin College; 1945, M.D., Howard University; 1945-46, intern, Harlem Hospital, N.Y.; 1946-51, resident in surgery, Cleveland City (now Metropolitan General) Hospital. CAREER: 1951-53, U.S. Air Force, deputy commanding officer and chief of professional services, Lockbourne Air Force Base Hospital, Columbus, Ohio; 1953-74, private surgical practice, Cleveland; 1953-74, surgical faculty (1953-58, demonstrator; 1959-64, clinical instructor; 1964-68, senior clinical instructor; 1968-74, clinical assistant professor), Case-Western Reserve University. CONTRIBUTIONS: In addition to maintaining a surgical practice among the black citizens of Cleveland, also served on government agency boards and panels, for example, National Advisory Council on Social Security (1963), Governor Rockefeller's "Blue Ribbon Panel" on New York City's hospital problems (1967), the first Federal Hospital Insurance Benefits Advisory Council (1964-68), and on several nonmedical boards, for example, National Selective Service Appeals Board (1965-69), consultant to Office of Economic Opportunity (1967-68). President, NMA (1963-64), and active member of local medical societies and medical charitable groups. Deeply involved in black support organizations such as NAACP and Urban League, both locally and nationally, including health committees. Involved in religious, business, and political activities.

WRITINGS: Wrote some 37 articles in professional journals, popular magazines, and newspapers primarily on surgery and black health concerns, for example, "Carcinoma of Cervical Stump: Its Incidence and Prophylaxis," *Ohio State Med. J.* 47 (1951): 733-35; "Cecostomy and Colostomy in Acute Colon Obstructions: Experiences in Eighty-Nine Cases," *JAMA* 28 (1953): 896-902; "Statement of Objection to AMA Proposed Hill-Burton Amendment in the New Harris-Hill Bill," *JNMA* 56 (1964): 287; "AMA Versus Medicare," *The Crisis* (Apr. 1965): 214-19; "The New Separatism, Will It Work?" *St. Louis-Globe Democrat*, April 18, 1968. Writings listed in *JNMA* 67 (1975): 255. REFERENCES: W. Montague Cobb, "Kenneth Witcher Clement," *JNMA* 67 (1975): 252-55; obituary (brief), *JAMA* 231 (1975): 1097; *Who's Who in Am.*, 38 (1974-75): 582.

T. Savitt

CLENDENING, LOGAN (May 25, 1884, Kansas City, Mo.-January 31, 1945, Kansas City). *Physician; Popular medical writer.* Son of Edwin McKaig, businessman, and Lide (Logan) Clendening. Married Dorothy Hixon, 1914; no children. EDUCATION: Undergraduate collegiate work, University of Michigan; 1907, M.D., University of Kansas, followed by medical study in England and Scotland. CAREER: Gradually moved from private and academic medicine to popular medical writings; 1912 until death in 1945, excepting two years as a major in the Medical Corps (1917-19), was on the faculty of the University of Kansas School of Medicine. CONTRIBUTIONS: *Modern Methods of Treatment* (1924) was read by Henry Mencken who persuaded Alfred Knopf that Clendening was the man to author a popular work on human physiology. Result was *The Human Body* (1927), an instantaneous success, selling more than half a million copies. This led to a daily column on health advice, which at the time of his death appeared in 383 daily newspapers with a combined circulation of 25 million. Early in life, became interested in the history of medicine. Elected vice-president, American Association of the History of Medicine (1942), and became president on the death of Dr. Jabez Elliott. With the aid of his wife, amassed a collection of rare medical books that, on his death, he bequeathed to the University of Kansas and that led to the formation of a Department of the History of Medicine of which he became the first professor (1940).

WRITINGS: *The Care and Feeding of Adults* (1928); *The Romance of Medicine* (1933); *A Handbook to Pickwick Papers* (1936); *Health Chats* (1936); *Workbook of Elementary Diagnosis* (1938); *The Balanced Diet* (1942); *Source Book of Medical History* (1942); *Methods of Diagnosis* (1947, with E. H. Hashinger). REFERENCES: *BHM* (1964-69), 56; "A Clendening Sampler," *J. Kans. Med. Soc.* 70 (1969): 151-55; Robert P. Hudson, "Logan Clendening: The Anatomy of A Teacher," *ibid.*, 69 (1968): 154-56, 160; Ralph Major, *Logan Clendening* (1958); Miller, *BHM*, p. 21; *NCAB*, 34: 434.

R. Hudson

CLEVELAND, EMELINE (HORTON) (September 22, 1829, Ashford, Conn.-December 8, 1878, Philadelphia, Pa.). *Surgeon; Medical educator.* Daughter of Chauncey, farmer, and Amanda (Chaffee) Horton. Married Rev. Giles Butler Cleveland, Presbyterian licentiate, 1854; one son. EDUCATION: Private tutors; 1853, B.A., Oberlin College; 1855, M.D., Woman's Medical College of Pennsylvania; 1861, diploma, School of Obstetrics, Maternité, Paris. CAREER: 1855, private practice, Oneida, N.Y.; 1856-61, professor of anatomy and histology, Woman's Medical College of Pennsylvania; 1862-69, chief resident,Woman's Hospital of Philadelphia; at Woman's Medical College of Pennsylvania: 1862-78, professor of obstetrics and diseases of women and children; and 1872-74, dean; 1878, gynecologist, Department for the Insane, Pennsylvania Hospital. CONTRIBUTIONS: Sought postgraduate training abroad specifically to bring increased professional skills and knowledge of hospital management to chief residency of the newly chartered Woman's Hospital of Philadelphia (1860-62). Inaugurated one of earliest programs for nurse's aide training at Woman's Hospital (1862-69). Performed among first major surgical operations by a woman physician (1862-75). One of first professional woman ovariotomists in America. Warm and supportive teacher, especially significant as a role model because of her successful attempt to combine marriage, family, and career before her life was cut short by tuberculosis.

WRITINGS: "Successful Ovariotomy at the Woman's Hospital of Philadelphia," *Clinic* (Cincinnati) 9 (1875); 100-102; "A Complicated Case of Vesico-Vaginal Fistula," Obstetrical Society of Philadelphia, *Transactions* (1877). Writings listed in Clara Marshall, *The Woman's Medical College of Pennsylvania* (1897). REFERENCES: Gulielma Fell Alsop, *History of the Woman's Medical College* (1950); Mary Putnam Jacobi, "Woman in Medicine," in Annie Nathan Meyer, ed., *Woman's Work in America* (1891); Kelly and Burrage (1920), 229; Clara Marshall, *The Woman's Medical College of Pennsylvania* (1897); *Notable Am. Women* 1 (1971): 349-50.

R. M. Morantz

CLINTON, FRED SEVERS (April 15, 1874, near Okmulgee, Creek Nation-April 25, 1955, Tulsa, Okla.). *Physician; Surgeon.* Son of Charles, rancher, and Louise (Atkins) Clinton, a member of the Creek Nation. Married Jane Heard, 1897 (d. 1945), no children; Beulah Jane Elliott, 1946, no children. EDUCATION: Presbyterian Mission, Muskogee, Indian Territory; St. Francis Institute, Osage, Kans.; and Drury College, Springfield, Mo.; 1897, M.D., Kansas City Medical College. CAREER: Practice: 1895, 1896 (summers), in Red Fork, near Tulsa;

1897-early 1930s, Tulsa. CONTRIBUTIONS: Built Tulsa's first permanent hospital and nursing school (1905). Pioneered in the oil industry, drilling first well in Tulsa County (1901). President, Indian Territory Medical Association (1902-3). Participated in combination of Territorial and Oklahoma branch medical societies into a single association (1906). Organized and built Oklahoma Hospital (Tulsa, 1915), which pioneered in fire protection for patients and nurses. Organized Oklahoma Hospital Association at Muskogee (1919) and elected president every year until 1926, when he was elected honorary life president (1927). Chief surgeon of every transportation company operating in Tulsa. Advocated and promoted rewriting provisions of the Oklahoma State Workman's Compensation Law, greatly increasing its effectiveness.

WRITINGS: "University of Oklahoma Medical School Crisis Averted," *Chronicles of Oklahoma* 24 (1947): 352-57. REFERENCES: "Fred S. Clinton" file, History of Medicine Collection, University of Oklahoma Health Sciences Center Library, Oklahoma City, Okla.; Mark R. Everett, *Medical Education in Oklahoma: The University of Oklahoma School of Medicine and Medical Center 1900-1931* (1972); R. Palmer Howard, and Richard E. Martin, "The Contributions of B. F. Fortner, Leroy Long, and Other Early Surgeons in Oklahoma," *Journal of the Oklahoma State Medical Association* (Nov. 1968): 541-49; *NCAB*, 41: 601; L. M. Witham, "Fred Severs Clinton, M.D., F.A.C.S.," *Chronicles of Oklahoma* 33 (1955): 467-71.

V. Allen

COAKLEY, CORNELIUS GODFREY (August 14, 1862, Brooklyn, N.Y.-November 22, 1934, New York, N.Y.). *Physician; Laryngology.* Son of George Washington, university professor, and Isabella Hoe (Godfrey) Coakley. Married Annette Perry, 1890; Mary Louise Perry, 1924; no children. EDUCATION: College of the City of New York: 1884, A.B.; and 1887, A.M.; 1887, M.D., New York University Medical School; 1887-88, intern, Bellevue Hospital. CAREER: *Post* 1888, practiced medicine, New York City; 1888-89, director, histology department, Loomis Laboratory; at New York University Medical School: 1889-90, anatomy faculty; and 1889-96, histology faculty; 1898-1914, laryngology faculty, University and Bellevue Hospital Medical College; *post* 1914, laryngology and otology faculty, College of Physicians and Surgeons (Columbia); consulting surgeon, ear, nose and throat service, Bellevue Hospital; attending otolaryngologist, Presbyterian Hospital; consulting surgeon, several New York metropolitan area hospitals; president: 1918, American Laryngological Association; and 1933, New York Laryngological Society. CONTRIBUTIONS: Best known for his excision of the larynx in cases of cancer. Published *A Manual of Diseases of the Nose and Throat* (1899), which went through numerous editions and was widely used as a textbook in medical colleges.

WRITINGS: "Observations on Pneumococcus Infection of the Nasal Accessory Sinuses," *Trans., Am. Laryngological Assoc.* 40 (1918): 307. Also published in *Annals of Otology, Rhinology, and Laryngology* 27 (1918): 1127; *Boston Med. and Surg. J.* 179 (1918): 647; *Laryngoscope* 28 (1918): 915; "External Surgery of the Nasal Accessory Sinuses," *Surg. Gyn. & Obst.* 30 (1920): 309; "Tumors of Larynx," *Surgical Clinics of North Am.* 13 (1933): 295. A bibliography is in *Trans., Am. Laryngological Assoc.* (1935). REFERENCES: *DAB*, Supplement 1: 181-82; *NCAB*, 26: 87; *Who Was Who in Am.*, 1: 233.

S. Galishoff

COCA, ARTHUR FERNANDEZ (March 20, 1875, Philadelphia, Pa.-December 12, 1959, Ridgewood, N.J.). *Physician; Allergy; Immunology.* Son of Joseph Fernandez and Augustine (Ware) Coca. Married Marietta A. Clews, 1905, two children; Ella Foster Grove, 1930. EDUCATION: Haverford College: 1896, A.B.; and 1899, A.M.; 1900, M.D., University of Pennsylvania; 1905-9, studied at University of Heidelberg. CAREER: 1900-3, demonstrator, University of Pennsylvania; 1907-9, chemical assistant, Cancer Institute, University of Heidelberg; 1909-10, bacteriologist, Bureau of Science, Manila, Philippine Islands; at Cornell University Medical School: 1910-19, pathology and bacteriology faculty; and 1919-32, immunology faculty; 1928-40, medical director, Blood Transfusion Betterment Association; 1931-35, clinical medicine faculty, New York Postgraduate Medical School, Columbia University; 1931-49, medical director, Lederle Laboratories, Inc. CONTRIBUTIONS: Helped establish allergy as a medical discipline. Prepared allergenic extracts and offered classifications of hypersensitivity. Wrote several books on food, dust, and pollen allergies. Founded *Journal of Immunology* (1916) and served as its editor-in-chief for more than 30 years. Made important studies of blood transfusion, including a compatibility test for direct matching of blood samples.

WRITINGS: "The Examination of the Blood Preliminary to the Operation of Blood Transfusion," *J. of Immunology* 3 (Jan. 1918): 93-100; *Essentials of Immunology for Medical Students* (1925); "Studies in Specific Hypersensitiveness. III. A Study of the Atopic Reagins," *J. of Immunology*, 10 (1925): 471-81 (with Ella Foster Grove); *Asthma and Hay Fever in Theory and Practice* (1931, with Matthew Walzer and A. A. Thommen); *Familial Nonreaginic Food Allergy* (1943). REFERENCES: Merrill W. Chase, "Irreverent Recollections from Cooke and Coca, 1928-1978," *J. of Allergy and Clinical Immunology* 64, no. 5 (Nov. 1964): 306-20; "In Memoriam, Arthur F. Coca, Founder of the *Journal of Immunology*," *J. of Immunology* 85 (1960): 330-31; *N.Y. Times*, December 13, 1959; *Who Was Who in Am.*, 6: 84.

S. Galishoff

COCHRAN, JEROME (December 4, 1831, Moscow, Tenn.-August 17, 1896, Montgomery, Ala.). *Physician; Public health.* Son of Augustine Owen and Frances (Bailey) Cochran. Married Sarah Jane Collins, 1856; three children. EDUCATION: Had few early educational advantages; however, being eager to learn, used every book; at age 19, began to teach; 1857, graduated from the Botanical Medical School of Memphis, Tenn., M.D.; 1861, graduated from the medical department, University of Tennessee, and while attending college, was private student of Professor W. K. Bowling (q.v.); studied mental diseases in the insane hospital, Tuscaloosa, Ala., during the Civil War. CAREER: 1857, practiced medicine, Miss.; 1860, resident physician, State Hospital of Tennessee;

later became contract physician in Confederate Hospital, Okalona, Miss.; 1862, promoted to full rank of surgeon; later in the year, was designated president of a conscript board in Tuscaloosa; 1865, practiced medicine in Mobile, Ala.; 1868-73, professor, chemistry, Medical College of Alabama; 1871, 1872, 1874, Mobile health officer; 1873-77, appointed to the chair of public hygiene and medical jurisprudence, Medical College of Alabama; 1873-96 chairman, Board of Censors of the Alabama Medical Association; 1877-96, chairman, Board of Medical Examiners; 1878, physician, Quarantine Station, Fort Morgan; resigned in September to accept position on National Yellow Fever Committee; 1879-96, first state health officer for Ala. CONTRIBUTIONS: Through a series of papers on public hygiene entitled "The Origin and Prevention of the Endemic and Epidemic Diseases of Mobile," a city health ordinance creating a health officer and a Board of Health, elected by the Mobile Medical Society, was established (1871). Established a Board of Censors of the Alabama Medical Association (1873). Through his efforts, a State Board of Medical Examiners began regulating the practice of medicine in Ala. (1877). Gave form to the laws that established the state health department in Ala. (1879).

WRITINGS: Wrote a large number of pamphlets and articles on diseases and their control, among them: "Yellow Fever, in Relation to Its Causes"; "Sanitary Administration"; "Theory and Practice of Quarantine"; "The Act Establishing Boards of Health in Alabama"; "The Alcohol Question"; "Leading Indication for Treatment of Yellow Fever"; "The White Blood Corpuscle in Health and Disease." REFERENCES: *J. Med. Assoc., Alabama* (1936); *Memorial Record of Ala.* (1976); Kelly and Burrage (1920), 232-33; Miller, *BHM*, p. 21; *NCAB*, 5: 225; T. M. Owen, *History of Alabama*, 4 vols. (1978).

S. Eichold

COCHRAN, JOHN (September 1, 1730, Chester County, Pa.-April 7, 1807, Palatine, N.Y.). *Physician.* Son of James, farmer, and Isabella Cochran. Married Mrs. Gertrude Schuyler, 1760; five children. EDUCATION: Studied medicine under Dr. Robert Thompson of Lancaster, Pa. CAREER: 1754-61, surgeon's mate, British hospital department; 1761-63, practiced medicine, Albany, N.Y.; 1763-76, practiced medicine, New Brunswick, N.J.; 1776-77, volunteered medical services in the American army commanded by George Washington; 1777-81, physician and surgeon-general to the Army of the Middle Department; 1781-83, director-general of the Military Hospitals of the United States; 1783-90, practiced medicine, New York City; 1786-89, receiver of continental taxes, state of N.Y.; 1790-95, commissioner of loans of the United States, state of N.Y. CONTRIBUTIONS: The last American medical director of the Revolutionary War, placed the army medical department on a relatively efficient basis and ended the unseemly squabbling that had occurred under his predecessors, William Shippen, Jr. (q.v.), and John Morgan (q.v.). Gave up a successful inoculation practice to serve in the Revolutionary War. Attracted Washington's attention with his knowledge of military medicine, acquired during the French and Indian War, and his diligence in treating smallpox patients and wounded soldiers. Was the physician Washington most relied on during the N.J. campaign. Aided Shippen in producing a plan for reorganizing the medical department (1777). Received large stores of medical supplies from France, which together with the decline in casualties after the battle of Yorktown (1781) resulted in a significant improvement in the medical care of American soldiers. A founder (1766) and third president (1768-70) of the New Jersey Medical Society. REFERENCES: *DAB*, 4: 251-52; Kelly and Burrage (1928), 240; Miller, *BHM*, p. 21; Morris Harrold Saffron, *Surgeon to Washington, Dr. John Cochran (1730-1807)* (1977).

S. Galishoff

CODMAN, ERNEST AMORY (December 30, 1869, Boston, Mass.-November 23, 1940, Ponkapog, Mass.). *Orthopedic surgeon; Crusader for hospital standards.* Son of William Coombs, international trade, then Boston real estate and insurance, and Elizabeth (Hurd) Codman. Married Katharine Putnam Bowditch, 1899; no children. EDUCATION: A.B., 1891, Harvard College; M.D., 1895, (cum laude) Harvard Med. School; 1894-95, surgical intern, Mass. General Hospital. CAREER: 1895-1940, general surgeon, Boston, Mass.; 1895-1914, faculty member, Harvard Medical School; 1899-1914, 1929-40, surgeon, Mass. General Hospital. CONTRIBUTIONS: Became the first American expert on diseases and injuries of the shoulder (1900-30s), first to do original work on and to describe subdeltoid bursitis. Developed "end-result plan" of tracking hospital patients long enough to determine effectiveness of treatments so that competence of hospital physicians, surgeons, and staff could be evaluated (1900-10). As chair of Committee on Hospital Standardization of Clinical Congress of Surgeons of North America initiated and crusaded for improvement and standardization of hospital treatment nationally (1910). Lost staff privileges at Mass. General Hospital (1914) in dispute over evaluating competence of surgeons there, but seniority system was dropped. Established at Harvard first bone tumor registry in U.S., setting precedent for national exchange of information on bone tumor cases (1920). Co-founded American College of Surgeons (1913).

WRITINGS: "The Use of the X-Ray and Radium in Surgery," in W.W. Keen, *Surgery* (1909); *A Study in Hospital Efficiency, As Demonstrated by the Case* (1915); *The Shoulder* (1934); numerous articles on surgery and hospitals. REFERENCES: Henry K. Beecher and Mark D. Altschule, *Medicine at Harvard* (1977), 322-24; F.D. Moore, "Surgical Biology and Applied Sociology; Cannon and Codman 50 Years Later," *Harvard Medical Alumni Bulletin* 49 (1975): 12-21; *NCAB*, 30: 66-67; *Who Was Who in Am.*, 1: 237.

T. L. Savitt

COFFEY, ROBERT CALVIN (October 20, 1869, Caldwell County, N.C.-November 9, 1933, Portland, Oreg.). *Surgeon; Medical educator.* Son of Patterson Vance, farmer, and Nancy (Estes) Coffey. Married Clarissa Coffey, 1893; three children. EDUCATION: 1892, M.D., Kentucky Medical School; 1896, intern, Louisville City Hospital. CAREER: Practice: 1892-95, 1896-97, Moscow, Idaho;

and 1897-1900, Colfax, Wash.; 1900-1910, operated North Pacific Sanitarium; 1911-14, medical staff, St. Vincent's Hospital, Portland; 1915-33, operated Portland Surgical Hospital; 1920-33, medical faculty, University of Oregon Medical School. CONTRIBUTIONS: Founded, with Andrew C. Smith (q.v.), the first specialized hospital (the North Pacific Sanitorium) in the Pacific Northwest (except for insane asylums). First medical doctor in the region to maintain an experimental surgical laboratory, where he repeated operative procedures on dogs. Perfected an application of the quarantine drain in abdominal surgery. Perfected the technique of transplanting the ureters into the large intestine. Contributed the hammock operation for ptosis and a method for treatment of the displaced uterus. One of the early advocates of the two-stage operation for carcinoma of the rectum. As a member of the Oregon State Medical Examining Board, fought for higher standards. Founded Portland Surgical Hospital in Portland, now Physicians and Surgeons Hospital. A founder and fellow, American College of Surgeons.

WRITINGS: *Gastro-enteroptosis* (1923); "The Relative Merits of Three Types of Technic for Submucous Implantation of the Ureters into the Large Intestine," *Western J. of Surg., Obstet. and Gyn.* 41 (1933): 311-17; "Application of Quarantine Drain in Abdominal Surgery," *Am. J. of Surg.* 24 (1934): 417-46. REFERENCES: O. Larsell, *The Doctor in Oregon* (1947); [Fred M. Lockley], *History of the Columbia River Valley* 2 (1928): 588-89; *NCAB*, 25: 380.

G. B. Dodds

COFFIN, NATHANIEL, JR. (May 3, 1744, Portland, Maine-October 18, 1826, Portland). *Physician; Surgeon.* Son of Nathaniel, doctor, and Patience (Hale) Coffin. Married Eleanor Foster, 1770; 11 children. EDUCATION: Studied medicine with his father, who frequently invited ships' surgeons just out from England to his home to learn of medical progress—many had recently graduated from the famous London hospitals; 1764-66, sent to England, where he worked in London medical institutions under luminaries such as John Hunter. CAREER: 1766, returned to Portland to assume his father's extensive practice, the elder Coffin having died in January. CONTRIBUTIONS: Active in the Revolution, one of the commissioners sent to plead with Captain Mowatt not to bombard Portland—this being an unsuccessful effort, he fled to the countryside with other exiles and cared for their needs. As the war progressed, cared for the sick and wounded brought into Portland on men-of-war and privateers. After the war, served as hospital surgeon for marine patients in the Portland area and established for a brief period a private hospital on Bramhall's Hill, Portland, and with Dr. John Merrill, tried to establish some system of marine hospital service. As a member of the Massachusetts Medical Society, petitioned for power to set up a district society in Maine (1804). First president of the Maine Medical Society. Performed many trephining operations as well as amputations of the feet from frostbite and of the extremities from injuries and gangrene. Often called upon to treat wounds caused by gunshot or Indian weaponry. Regarded by Jeremiah

Barker (q.v.), himself a noted surgeon, "as the most skillful surgeon east of the Massachusetts Bay Colony"—especially in "tapping for dropsies" and in fractures. REFERENCES: Howard Kelly, *Cyclopedia of Am. Med. Biog.* 1 (1912): 191-92; Maine Historical Society Coll. #1606, Spalding Papers, "Old Doctors of Portland"; James Spalding, *Maine Physicians of 1820* (1928).

B. Lister

COFFMAN, VICTOR H. (September 10, 1839, Zanesville, Ohio-August 4, 1908, Omaha, Neb.). *Physician; Surgeon.* Son of William, farmer, and Mary (Gates) Coffman. Married Rose Devoto, September 10, 1879; four children. EDUCATION: 1858, Iowa Wesleyan College; 1858-59, preceptorship, C. W. Davis, M.D., Indianola, Ia.; 1859-62, Chicago Medical College; 1866, M.D., Jefferson Medical College; 1866-67, postgraduate study, College of Physicians and Surgeons, N.Y. CAREER: 1862, commissioned assistant surgeon, U.S. Army; 1863, surgeon of the regiment, later chief medical officer, 13th Army Corps; 1865, commissioned brevet-lieutenant colonel; at Omaha Medical College: 1880, organizer; 1882-87, professor of theory and practice of medicine; and 1882-84, president, Board of Trustees; at Nebraska State Medical Society: 1872, organizer and secretary; and 1884, president; 1871, president, Omaha Medical Society, and author of its "Fee Bill." CONTRIBUTIONS: With only two years formal medical training, was commissioned assistant surgeon and gained the rank of lieutenant-colonel by distinguished service in many Civil War campaigns. Practiced medicine and surgery in Omaha (1867-1908). First in Neb. to use plaster of paris dressing for curvature of the spine and to perform an ovariotomy. First in America to remove a tumor of the thyroid gland. An early advocate of a state board of health. City health commissioner, Omaha (1900-1902). Member of both Fire and Police Commission. Noted for his outstanding health care of the poor.

WRITINGS: "Ovariotomy," *Proc., Nebraska State Med. Soc.* 5 (1873): 9-10; "Report of a Case of Ovariotomy," *ibid.*, 14 (1882): 146-49; "Injections of Carbolic Acid in Treatment of Hydrocele Ganglia of the Wrist, Housemaid's Knee, and Tuberculosis of Cervical Glands," *Western Med. Rev.* 1 (Jul. 15, 1896): 53-55. REFERENCES: J. S. Morton, *History of Nebraska* 2 (1907): 609-11; Alfred Sorenson, *The Story of Omaha* (1923), 397-98; A. T. Tyler and E. F. Auerbach, *History of Medicine in Nebraska* (1977, enlarged by B. M. Hetzner), 63-66, 325-330.

B. M. Hetzner

COGSWELL, MASON FITCH (September 28, 1761, Canterbury, Conn.-December 10, 1830, Hartford, Conn.). *Physician; Surgeon.* Son of the Rev. Dr. James and Mrs. (Fitch) Cogswell. Married Mary Austin Ledyard, 1800; four children. EDUCATION: 1780, A.B., Yale College, valedictorian; studied medicine under his brother James in Stamford, Conn. and New York City and later pursued studies in anatomy by dissection in Hartford. CAREER: 1789-1830, practiced medicine and surgery, Hartford. CONTRIBUTIONS: Among the first in the United

States to operate upon the eye for cataracts. For the first time in this country, ligated the carotid artery (November 1803), although it had been done two years previously in London. Played an important part in the founding of the American Asylum for the Deaf in Hartford (beginning in 1812). Interest in the matter grew from his solicitude for his deaf and dumb daughter Alice. With Mr. Silbert, an attorney from Hebron with five deaf children, ascertained the number of deafmutes in Conn. and then unsuccessfully attempted to obtain funds from the state legislature. A few years later, he and six other persons collected sufficient money to enable Dr. Thomas Gallaudet (q.v.) to journey to Europe to acquire the necessary knowledge to start a school for the deaf (1817). Alice Cogswell was the first pupil registered. Also a founder of the Connecticut Retreat for the Insane in Hartford. When the Medical Institute of Yale College was established (1812), was invited to fill the chair of surgery but withdrew when Dr. Nathan Smith (q.v.) was available. Active in the founding of the State Medical Society and its secretary, vice-president, and then president (1812-22). First presiding officer of the Hopkins Medical Society, which preceded the Hartford Medical Society.

WRITINGS: A description of the removal of a tumor from the parotid gland of a woman in 1803 in the *New Eng. J. of Med. & Surg.* 13 (1824): 356. Cogswell's manuscripts are in the Yale University Library, New Haven, Conn. and the Connecticut Historical Society, Hartford. REFERENCES: *Appleton's Cyclopedia of Am. Biog.* 1: 679-80; Franklin B. Dexter, *Yale Biographies and Annals* 4 (1885): 141-43; Samuel C. Harvey, "Surgery of the Past in Connecticut," in Herbert Thoms, ed., *The History of Connecticut Medicine* (1942), 112-87; Kelly and Burrage (1920), 237; Edward R. Lampson, "Mason Fitch Cogswell," *Yale J. Bio. & Med.* 3, no. 1 (Oct. 1930): 3-9; *NCAB*, 8: 207.

J. W. Ifkovic

COGSWELL, WILLIAM F. (December 5, 1868, Fort Williams, Nova Scotia, Canada-May 26, 1956, Helena, Mont.). *Physician; Public health.* EDUCATION: 1894, M.D., Dalhousie University, Halifax, Nova Scotia, Canada. CAREER: 1896, migrated to Mont.; miners' physician, Sand Coulee and Stockett, Mont.; Western Federation of Miners recruited him for coal fields in Aldridge and Horr in Park County, Mont.; 1908, county health officer; 1912, secretary, Montana State Board of Health; chief state health officer for 33 years; chairman, State Board of Entomology; 1910, president, Montana Medical Association; helped found Aldridge hospital; created divisions of industrial hygiene, communicable disease, rural health nursing, vital statistics, sanitary engineers, food and drug, hygienic laboratory, and tuberculosis control. CONTRIBUTIONS: Most important public health officer in Mont. State history. Recruited and trained cadre of public health specialists. Established (1931-32) Rocky Mountain Laboratory (National Institutes of Health, Division of Allergy and Infectious Disease) in Hamilton, Mont., and school for water works officials. Placed Indian Reservation health boards under jurisdiction of State Board of Health. Responsible for prevention of arsenical sprays in pear and apple orchards and registration of new water wells. President: Western Branch American Public Health Association; State and

Provincial Health Officers of North America; and Association of State and Territorial Health Officers. Pioneered in county health boards.
WRITINGS: Numerous reports, recommendations, and pieces of legislation. REFERENCES: *Billings Gazette*, May 28, 1956; L. W. Brewer, ed., *First Hundred Years: History of the Montana Medical Association* (1978); *Great Falls Tribune*, May 28, 1956; Esther G. Price, *Fighting Spotted Fever in the Rockies* (1948).

P. Mullen

COHN, ALFRED EINSTEIN (April 16, 1879, New York City-July 20, 1957, New Milford, Conn.). *Physician; Cardiovascular diseases.* Son of Abraham, tobacco merchant, and Maimie (Einstein) Cohn. Married Ruth Walker Price, 1911; no children. EDUCATION: 1900, A.B., Columbia College; 1904, M.D., Columbia University; 1904-7, internship at Mount Sinai Hospital, New York; 1907-9, postgraduate study in Freiburg and London where he studied under Wilhelm Trendelenberg, Ludwig Aschoff, James Mackenzie, and Thomas Lewis. CAREER: 1909-11, staff at Mount Sinai Hospital, New York City; 1911-44, staff of the Rockefeller Institute for Medical Research. CONTRIBUTIONS: Helped set up an electrocardiograph at University College, London after Willem Einthoven introduced the string galvanometer and made electrocardiography possible. (August 1909) brought the first electrocardiograph to the western hemisphere using it at Mount Sinai (1909-11) and at the Rockefeller Institute after 1911. An early specialist in diseases of the cardiovascular system. An early member of the Association for Prevention of Heart Disease which later became the New York Heart Association and was a model for the American Heart Association. Tried to help refugees during World War II, and participated in the American Committee for Emigre Scholars, Writers and Artists.

WRITINGS: *Medicine, Science and Art* (1931); *Minerva's Progress* (1946); *No Retreat from Reason* (1948); *The Burden of Diseases in the United States* (1950) with Claire Lingg. REFERENCES: G. E. Burch and N. P. DePasquale, *A History of Electrocardiography* (1964); G. W. Corner, *History of the Rockefeller Institute* (1964); *DAB*, Supplement 6:117-18.

M. Kaufman

COHN, EDWIN JOSEPH (December 17, 1892, New York, N.Y.-October 1, 1953, Boston, Mass.). *Biochemist; Blood fractionation; Protein chemistry.* Son of Abraham, tobacco merchant, and Maimie (Einstein) Cohn. Married Marianne Brettauer, 1917, two children; Rebekah Higginson, 1948. EDUCATION: University of Chicago: 1914, B.S.; and 1917, Ph.D.; 1915-17, graduate student, Harvard University; 1919-20, studied chemistry, Copenhagen and Cambridge. CAREER: At Harvard University: 1920-53, biochemistry faculty; 1936-49, chairman, division of medical sciences; 1949-53, director, laboratory of physical chemistry related to medicine and public health. CONTRIBUTIONS: Discovered several medically important blood fractions and was a leader in the study of the physical chemistry of proteins. Investigated the solubility of proteins in various media, their sizes and shapes, and their molecular electric charges under various conditions (1920s). Sought to isolate and purify the active factor in liver that George R. Minot (q.v.) had shown to be effective in the treatment of pernicious anemia; failed in this effort but did prepare a concentrated liver extract of great clinical value. Investigated the amino acids, peptides, and other molecules that make up proteins. During World War II, planned and directed a major program for fractioning of human blood plasma; led to the development of purified serum albumin for treatment of shock, gamma globulin for passive immunization against measles and hepatitis, fibrinogen and fibrin for neurosurgery, and many other protein fractions of blood plasma.

WRITINGS: *Proteins, Amino Acids and Peptides as Ions and Dipolar Ions, American Chemical Society Monograph No. 90* (1943, with J. T. Edsall); "Chemical, Clinical, and Immunological Studies on the Products of Human Plasma Fractionation," *J. Clin. Invest.* 23 (1944): 417-606 (with others). A bibliography is in *BMNAS* 35 (1961): 47-84. REFERENCES: *BHM* (1970-74), 40; *DAB*, Supplement 5: 121-23; *DSB*, 3: 335-36; *N.Y. Times*, October 3, 1953; *Who Was Who in Am.*, 3: 170.

S. Galishoff

COIT, HENRY LEBER (March 16, 1854, Peapack, N.J.-March 12, 1917, Newark, N.J.). *Physician; Originator of certified milk.* Son of John Summerfield, Methodist minister, and Ellen (Neafie) Coit. Married Emma Gwinnell, 1886; five children. EDUCATION: 1876, graduated from New York College of Pharmacy; 1883, M.D., College of Physicians and Surgeons (Columbia). CAREER: 1876-82, chemist, Tarrant and Company (N.Y.); 1883-1916, practiced medicine, Newark, specializing in pediatrics; 1896-1913, founder and medical director, (Newark) Babies' Hospital; 1907, founder and first president, National Association of Medical Milk Commissions; vice-president, International Society of Milk Dispensaries (Brussels). CONTRIBUTIONS: Has been called "the father of clean milk." Proposed the formation of a nongovernmental medical milk commission (1890) composed of physicians who would supervise and certify the dairy production of a high-grade milk for women unable to breast feed. Gave successful demonstration of plan (1893) on a farm near Fairfield, N.J., and in that year established the Essex County Medical Milk Commission. Movement soon spread to other states and nations. Responsible for many innovations in dairying, including immediate cooling and bottling of milk and the medical supervision of herds and employees. Established physical, chemical, and bacteriological standards of milk purity and wholesomeness. Aroused interest in milk reform and in the whole question of infant and child welfare. Work was later largely taken over by government and certified milk superseded by pasteurized milk. Founded (Newark) Babies' Hospital (1896), the second institution of its kind in the United States. A founder of the New Jersey Pediatrics Society.

WRITINGS: *The Feeding of Infants* (1890); *The Care of the Baby* (1894); *Certified Milk* (1912). REFERENCES: *BHM* (1970-74), 40; *DAB*, 4: 277-78; Stuart Galishoff,

Safeguarding the Public Health, Newark, 1895-1918 (1975), 81, 84-86, 93-95, 102, 109-10; Miller, *BHM*, p. 21; *NCAB*, 22: 102-3.

S. *Galishoff*

COLDEN, CADWALLADER (February 7, 1688, Enniscorthy, County Wexford, Ireland-September 28, 1776, Flushing, Long Island, N.Y.). *Physician; Naturalist; Author; Public official.* Son of Rev. and Mrs. Alexander Colden. Married Alice Christie, 1715; three children. EDUCATION: 1705, A.B. (A.M. in some sources), Edinburgh, Scotland, where he was educated for the Presbyterian ministry; 1705-8 (1710 in some sources), studied anatomy and chemistry in London. CAREER: 1708-15, practice of medicine and importer of commodities from the West Indies to Philadelphia; 1715-16, medical and scientific activities in England and Scotland; 1716-18, medical practice and commerce in Philadelphia; 1718-76, medical practice, (which he eventually abandoned), scientific correspondence, philosophical and medical authorship, and official duties in New York City. Public duties included membership on the Governor's Council and the offices of surveyor general, master in chancery, and lieutenant governor (1761-76). CONTRIBUTIONS: More important as a public figure—a government official, author, organizer, promoter, disseminator of scientific knowledge—than as a physician, historical reputation is controversial. One of the leading "early American naturalists" who introduced the Linnaean system into America. A significant figure in the history of American medicine because of his contributions to the organization of scientific and medical knowledge, his successful agitation for the first law to regulate the practice of medicine in the colonies, and the wealth of primary source material assembled in his papers.

WRITINGS: The best bibliography of Colden's publications is Saul Jarcho, "Biographical and Bibliographical Notes on Cadwallader Colden," *Bull. Hist. Med.* 32 (1958): 322-34, which supplements *The Letters and Papers of Cadwallader Colden*, 11 vols. (1917-35). REFERENCES: John Duffy, *A History of Public Health in New York City, 1625-1866* (1968); Claude E. Heaton, "Medicine in New York During the Early Colonial Period, 1664-1775," *Bull. Hist. Med.* 17 (1945): 9-37; Alfred H. Hoermann, "Cadwallader Colden and the Mind Body Problem," *ibid.*, 50 (1976): 392-404; Jarcho, "Biographical and Bibliographical Notes"; idem, "Cadwallader Colden as a Student of Infectious Disease," *Bull. Hist. Med.* 29 (1955): 99-115; idem, "The Correspondence of Cadwallader Colden and Hugh Braham on Infectious Disease, 1716-19," *ibid.*, 30 (1956): 195-212; idem, "The Therapeutic Use of Resin and Tar Water by Bishop George Berkeley and Cadwallader Colden," *N.Y. State J. of Med.* 55 (1955): 834-40; Kelly and Burrage (1928), 246; Alice Maplesden Keys, *Cadwallader Colden: A Representative Eighteenth Century Official* (1906); *DAB* 4 (1958): 286-87; Byron Stookey, *A History of Colonial Medical Education in the Province of New York . . .* (1962).

D. M. *Fox*

COLE, FERN MORTON (January 18, 1876, Durand, Ill.-April 2, 1950, Caldwell, Idaho). *Physician.* Son of Edward VanSickle, hotel keeper, and Flora Maria (Crowley) Cole. Married Leila Jane Smylie, 1898; no children. EDUCA-

TION: 1894-96, Grinnell College; 1897, M.D., Northwestern University. CAREER: 1897-1907, practice, Battle Creek, Ia.; 1907-50, practice, Caldwell; World War I, served in the U.S. Army Medical Corps. CONTRIBUTIONS: Founder, Caldwell Sanitarium, later the Caldwell Memorial Hospital (1919). President, Idaho State Medical Association (1940). Active in civic organizations: founder and first president, Caldwell Kiwanis Club; and president, Caldwell Chamber of Commerce. REFERENCES: *Daily Statesman*, (Boise), April 3, 1950; M. D. Beal and M. Wells, *History of Idaho* 3 (1959): 93.

A. A. Hart

COLE, RICHARD BEVERLY (August 12, 1829, Manchester, Va.-January 15, 1901, San Francisco, Calif.). *Physician; Obstetrics and gynecology.* Son of John, mine owner, and Pamelia (Wooldrich) Cole. Married Eugenie Irene Bonaffon, 1848; three children. EDUCATION: Apprentice to Dr. Benjamin Dudley (q.v.), Lexington, Ky. Enrolled at Transylvania University, transferred to Jefferson Medical College, M.D., 1849. CAREER: 1849-52, practiced medicine, Philadelphia; 1852, went to San Francisco and established medical practice; 1859-64, professor of obstetrics and diseases of women and children and of physiology, medical department, University of the Pacific, also dean of the faculty; later dean and president of the faculty, Toland Medical College; and professor of obstetrics and clinical diseases of women, medical department, University of California; editor, *San Francisco Medical Press* and *San Francisco Western Lancet*; 1895-96, president, American Medical Association; 1901, coroner, city of San Francisco. CONTRIBUTIONS: Deeply involved in the medical and political affairs of San Francisco. Involvement with the Toland Medical College helped lead to its transfer to the University of California. Helped face the smallpox crisis (1868) as the medical man on the Hospital Committee and took an active part in dealing with public health matters in the city.

WRITINGS: "Alum in the Treatment of Uterine Hemorrhage," *San Francisco Med. Press* 1 (1860) 15-19; Writings listed in F. T. Gardner, "King Cole of California," *Annals of Med. Hist.* 3rd series, 2, no. 3 (1940): 245-58; 2, no. 4 (1940): 319-47; 2, no. 5 (1940): 432-42. REFERENCES: Gardner, "King Cole of California"; Henry Harris, *California's Medical Story* (1932), 355-60; Kelly and Burrage (1920), 239; *NCAB*, 7: 288.

Y. V. O'Neill

COLE, RUFUS (April 30, 1872, Rowsburg, Ohio-April 21, 1966, Washington, D.C.). *Physician; Microbiology.* Son of Ivory S., physician, and Ruth (Smith) Cole. Married Annie Hegeler, 1908; three children. EDUCATION: 1896, B.S., University of Michigan; 1900, M.D., Johns Hopkins Medical School. CAREER: 1899-1907, medical staff, Johns Hopkins Hospital; 1901-7, medicine faculty, Johns Hopkins Medical School; 1908-37, director, Hospital of the Rockefeller Institute (N.Y.); 1937, president, Association of American Physicians. CONTRIBUTIONS: Fought to bring research to the bedside and to establish clinical investigation as a science. Trained numerous clinical investigators who carried the gospel of laboratory research to medical institutions throughout the nation. Pioneered in the use of blood cultures for medical diagnosis. Made a lifelong study of pneumococcal pneumonia, which contributed to the discovery of fundamental concepts of immunochemistry and heredity. With Alphonse Dochez (q.v.) and Oswald T. Avery (q.v.), developed a method for the typing of pneumococci and produced a serum treatment for lobar pneumonia that saved many lives before it was superseded by the discovery of antibiotics.

WRITINGS: "Note on the Production of an Agglutinating Serum for Blood Platelets," *Bull., Johns Hopkins Hosp.* 18 (Jun.-Jul. 1907): 261-62; *Acute Lobar Pneumonia; Prevention and Serum Treatment. Monographs of the Rockefeller Institute for Medical Research, No. 7* (1917, with Oswald T. Avery, H. T. Chickering, and Alphonse Dochez). REFERENCES: A. McGehee Harvey, "Creators of Clinical Medicine's Scientific Base: Franklin Paine Mall, Lewellys Franklin Barker, and Rufus Cole," *Johns Hopkins Med. J.* 136 (1975): 168-77; *N.Y. Times,* April 22, 1966; *Who Was Who in Am.,* 5: 143.

S. Galishoff

COLEY, WILLIAM BRADLEY (January 12, 1862, Westport, Conn.-April 16, 1936, New York, N.Y.). *Physician; Surgery.* Son of Horace Bradley and Clarine Bradley (Wakeman) Coley. Married Alice Lancaster, 1891; three children. EDUCATION: 1884, B.A., Yale University; 1888, M.D., Harvard University; 1888-90, intern, New York Hospital. CAREER: *Post* 1888, practiced medicine, New York City; 1890-1931, surgical staff, Hospital for Ruptured and Crippled; 1908-32, surgeon, New York Central Railroad; at Memorial Hospital: surgical staff, more than forty years; *post* 1902, member, Board of Managers; and 1909-36, chairman, research fund; at Cornell University Medical College: 1909-15, clinical surgery faculty; and 1915, clinical cancer research faculty; 1918-36, surgical staff, Mary McClellan Hospital (Cambridge, N.Y.); consulting surgeon, Fifth Avenue (N.Y.) and Sharon (Conn.) hospitals. CONTRIBUTIONS: An authority on cancer, malignant tumors, and abdominal surgery. One of the first in America to adopt the Bassini method of operating for the radical cure of hernia (1890); had outstanding success with it and pioneered in extending operative treatment of hernia to children. Best known for the development of "Coley's toxin," a preparation consisting of the killed cultures of erysipelas streptococcus combined with the toxines of bacillus prodigiosus, which he used in the treatment of certain types of malignant tumors, especially sarcoma; advocated its use only for inoperable sarcoma or as a prophylactic measure after surgery for bone sarcoma and not for malignant tumors in general; is considered to be the beginning of adjuvant immunotherapy for cancer. Was instrumental in the development of Memorial Hospital and (1902) persuaded one of his patients, Mrs. C. P. Huntington, to endow it with the nation's first fund for cancer research.

WRITINGS: "The Treatment of Malignant Tumors by Repeated Inoculations of Erysipelas with a Report of Ten Original Cases," *Am. J. of the Med. Sci.* 105 (May 1893): 487-511; "Radical Cure of Inguinal and Femoral Hernia with a Report of Eight Hundred and Forty-Five Cases," *Trans., Am. Surg. Assoc.* 19 (1901): 338-55. REFERENCES: Carl

G. Burdick, "William Bradley Coley," *Trans., Am. Surg. Assoc.* 54 (1936): 415-18; *N.Y. Times*, April 17, 1936; Mark M. Ravitch, *A Century of Surgery*, 2 vols. (1981); *Who Was Who in Am.*, 1: 243.

S. Galishoff

COLLER, FREDERICK AMASA (October 2, 1887, Brookings, S.Dak.-November 5, 1964, Ann Arbor, Mich.). *Physician; Surgery.* Son of Granville James, physician, and Helen Rosalie (Underwood) Coller. Married Jessie E. Bernsen, 1917; two children. EDUCATION: South Dakota State College: 1906, B.S.; and 1908, M.S.; 1912, M.D., Harvard University; 1912-15, intern and resident, Massachusetts General Hospital. CAREER: 1915, surgical staff, American Ambulance Hospital, Neuilly-sur-Seine, France; officer, Harvard Unit, Royal Army Medical Corps, British Expeditionary Force, northern France; 1915-16, surgical staff, American Woman's War Hospital, Paighton, Devonshire, England; 1916-17, practiced surgery, Los Angeles, Calif.; 1917-18, officer, Medical Corps, U.S. Army, assigned to the 316th Sanitary Train, 91st Division, and later to units in England and France; 1920-57, surgery faculty, University of Michigan; and surgical staff, University Hospital; *post* 1932, surgical staff, St. Joseph's Mercy Hospital; during World War II, member, Surgical Committee, National Research Council, and surgical consultant to Surgeon General of the U.S. Army; 1957, consultant for special projects involving a study of medical practices in hospitals of the U.S. Armed Forces; lecturer or visiting professor, at 16 medical institutions in the United States and Canada; president: 1943-44, American Surgical Association; and 1949-50, American College of Surgeons. CONTRIBUTIONS: Internationally known as a surgeon, medical investigator, and teacher. With Eugene B. Potter, conducted extensive studies (1930s) of water and electrolyte metabolism in surgical patients. Demonstrated that the insensible loss of the sick surgical patient averaged two liters per day. Showed that abnormal water and electrolyte losses could lead to severe shock from acute dehydration or hypopotassemia and developed a course of therapy aimed at replacement of urinary losses of sodium, potassium, and water. An authority on surgery of the thyroid gland and gastrointestinal surgery, particularly as related to neoplasms of the colon. Adopted and developed new methods of transverse abdominal incisions and wound closure that reduced postoperative complications.

WRITINGS: "The Water Requirements of Surgical Patients," *Trans., Am. Surg. Assoc.* 51 (1933): 467-76 (with Walter G. Maddock); "The Development of the Techniques of Thyroidectomy," *Surg. Gyn. & Obst.* 64 (1937): 405 (with A. K. Boyden); "The Role of the Transverse Abdominal Incision and Early Ambulation in the Reduction of Post-Operative Complications," *Arch. of Surg.* 50 (1949): 1267 (with J. B. Thompson and K. F. Maclean); "Diverticulosis and Diverticulitis of the Colon," *Abdominal Surgery* (1961, with Marion S. DeWeese). A bibliography is in the Frederick A. Coller Commemorative Issue of *Annals of Surg.* 154 (Dec. 1951). REFERENCES: Marion S. DeWeese, "The Frederick A. Coller Surgical Society: Past, Present, and Future," *Univ. of Mich. Med. Center J.* 36 (Jan.-Mar. 1970): 1-7; *NCAB*, 51: 458; *N.Y. Times*, November 6,

1964; *Who Was Who in Am.*, 4: 190; Philip D. Wilson, "Frederick Amasa Coller, 1887-1964," *Trans., Am. Surg. Assoc.* 3 (1965): 481-87.

S. Galishoff

COLLISTER, GEORGE (October 16, 1856, Willoughby, Ohio-October 18, 1935, Boise, Idaho). *Physician.* Son of Thomas, stonemason, and Fannie (Young) Collister. Married M. E. Marden, 1898; one adopted daughter. EDUCATION: 1876, Ohio State University; 1877-79, Herron Medical College of Cleveland (later called the Homeopathic Medical College), M.D., 1879. CAREER: 1881, established medical practice, Boise, which continued for 54 years. CONTRIBUTIONS: A founder, St. Alphonsus Hospital (1894), and president, Idaho State Medical Association (1903). Served two terms on the Boise City Council and was city and county physician. Physician, Idaho State Penitentiary, for over 30 years. Considered an outstanding surgeon and diagnostician. REFERENCES: *Daily Statesman* (Boise), October 19, 1935; H. T. French, *History of Idaho* (1914), 827; J. H. Hawley, *History of Idaho* (1920), 135.

A. A. Hart

COLWELL, NATHAN PORTER (May 25, 1870, Osceola, Ia.-January 6, 1936, Wilmette, Ill.). *Physician; Medical education.* Son of Fernando N. and Mary Ellen (Shields) Colwell. Married Agnes Louise Peterson, 1903; two children. EDUCATION: 1900, M.D., Rush Medical College. CAREER: 1900-31, practiced medicine, Chicago, Ill.; 1900-1906, associate instructor, Rush Medical College; 1905-31, secretary, Council on Medical Education, American Medical Association; 1913-30, collaborator, U.S. Bureau of Education; *post* 1915, managing editor, monthly bulletin of Federation of State Medical Boards; 1918, contract surgeon, assigned to Office of Surgeon General, U.S. Army. CONTRIBUTIONS: As the first secretary of the American Medical Association Council on Medical Education, played a leading role in the reform of American medical education. Helped direct the council's investigation of some 160 medical schools (1906-7). Schools were graded in ten categories, including performance of graduates before state boards of licensure, preliminary education requirements, and laboratory and clinical facilities; on the basis of their scores, they were classified into three groups: Class A (acceptable), Class B (doubtful), and Class C (unacceptable). Results were not published but were distributed to the colleges studied resulting in a widespread movement to improve medical education. Investigation also provided the framework for the landmark study of the Carnegie Foundation for the Advancement of Teaching about American medical education (the "Flexner Report") begun (1908) by Abraham Flexner (q.v.) with the help of Colwell. Was instrumental in organizing the Federation of State Medical Boards of the United States. Played an important part in the campaign to reduce injuries and deaths associated with Fourth of July accidents.

WRITINGS: "The Need, Methods and Value of Medical College Inspection," *JAMA* 53 (Aug. 14, 1909): 512-15; "Progress in Medical Education," in *U.S. Commissioner of Education Report, 1913*, 1: 31-56; "Medical Education," *U.S. Commissioner of Education Report, 1915*, 1: 185-220. REFERENCES: Morris Fishbein, *History of the American Medical Association, 1847 to 1947* (1947), 891-99; *JAMA* 106 (Jan.-Jun. 1936): 231; *Who Was Who in Am.*, 1: 247.

S. Galishoff

CONNOR, LEARTUS (January 29, 1843, Coldenham, N.Y.-April 16, 1911, Detroit, Mich.). *Educator; Editor.* Son of Hezekiah, stone mason and farmer, and Caroline (Corwin) Connor. Married Anna A. Dame, 1870; two children. EDUCATION: Wallkill Academy (Middletown, N.Y.); at Williams College: B.A., 1865; and M.A., 1868; studied medicine with George L. Dayton; 1867-68, University of Michigan medical department; 1870, M.D., College of Physicians and Surgeons (N.Y.). CAREER: 1870, practiced surgery, Searsville, N.Y.; at Detroit Medical College: 1871-72, lecturer in chemistry; 1872-79, professor of physiology and clinical medicine; and 1878-81, professor of ophthalmology and otology; 1871-95, editor, *American Lancet*; 1876-83, secretary, American Medical College Association; 1877, 1888, president, Detroit Academy of Medicine; 1882-83, vice-president, American Medical Association; president: 1883-84, American Medical Editors' Association; 1888-89, American Academy of Medicine; and 1902-3, Michigan State Medical Society; attending surgeon, St. Mary's, Woman's, Children's hospitals. CONTRIBUTIONS: Rewrote the constitution and led the reorganization of the Michigan State Medical Society (1902); with Andrew Biddle, established the society's journal. Led and almost succeeded in national effort to get medical colleges to adopt a three-year curriculum (1876-83); opposed all cooperation with homeopaths. Both sons became physicians; Guy Leartus Connor (1894-1943) was a long-term secretary of the State Board of Medical Registration, overseeing medical licensing policy.

WRITINGS: "Glaucoma Caused by Mental Worry," *Detroit Lancet* 5 (1881): 3; "Tobacco Amblyopia," *JAMA* 14 (1890): 217-25; "Amblyopia from Suppression, Congenital Imperfection, or Disuse: Which or All?" *ibid.*, 30 (1898): 203-7. Many contributions to Kelly and Burrage (1928). Writings listed in *Index Catalogue*, 2nd series, 3: 851-52. REFERENCES: C. B. Burr, *Medical History of Michigan* 1 (1930): 523-25; 2: 404, 434; *Compendium of History and Biography of the City of Detroit and Wayne County* (1909), 453-56; *Detroit Free Press*, April 17, 1911, p. 1; Martin Kaufman, *American Medical Education; The Formative Years* (1976), 135-39; Kelly and Burrage (1928), 253-54; A. N. Marquis, *Book of Detroiters* (1914), 120-21; *Michigan State Med. Soc. J.* 10 (1911): 241; *NCAB*, 12: 456; *Who Was Who in Am.*, 1: 252.

M. Pernick

COOKE, JOHN ESTEN (March 2, 1783, Boston, Mass.-October 19, 1853, near Louisville, Ky.). *Physician; Theorist.* Son of Stephen, a prominent Va. physician, and Catherine (Esten) Cooke, daughter of one of the leading families of Bermuda. Married. EDUCATION: Medical apprenticeship in his father's office; 1805, M.D., University of Pennsylvania. CAREER: 1805-20, practice, Warrenton, Va.; 1821-26, practice, Winchester, Va.; 1827-36, succeeded Daniel Drake (q.v.), in the chair of theory and practice of medicine, Transylvania University Medical School, Lexington, Ky.; 1837-44, professor of the theory and practice of medicine at Louisville Medical Institute, of which he was a co-founder; 1844, forced to retire because of widespread opposition to his medical theories. CONTRIBUTIONS: Best known for support of the theory of the universal origin of disease. Thought "all autumnal fevers were but varieties of one disease, and typhus, typhoid and yellow fever, plague, cholera and dysentery were modifications of the same"; theorized that fever was a necessary stage in the process of getting well. Championed the use of therapeutics to remove congestion around large internal veins. As a leading exponent of "heroic medicine," favored using large doses of calomel, other purgatives, and bleeding. Helped found the *Transylvania Journal of Medicine and the Associate Sciences* in the hope of establishing an independent American medical literature (1827).

WRITINGS: *Account of the Inflammatory Bilious Fever Which Prevailed in the Summer and Fall of 1804 in the County of Loudon, Virginia* (1805); "Essays on the Autumnal and Winter Epidemics," *Transylvania J. of Med.* (1828); *Treatise on Pathology and Therapeutics*, 2 vols. (1828). REFERENCES: *BHM* (1975-79), 30; Wyndham Blanton, *Medicine in Virginia in the Nineteenth Century* (1933); Jas. Craik, "Memoir," *Southern Literary Messenger* 24 (1857): 286-93; *DAB* 4: 384-85; Howard A. Kelly, *Cyclopedia of Am. Med. Biog.* (1912); Lunsford Yandell, "The Life and Writings of John Esten Cooke," *Am. Practitioner* 12 (1875): 1-27; *Who Was Who in Am., History Vol.*: 120.

P. Addis

COOKE, ROBERT ANDERSON (August 17, 1880, Holmdel, N.J.-May 7, 1960, New York, N.Y.). *Physician; Allergies.* Son of Henry Gansevoort, physician, and Maria (Cowdrey) Cooke. Married Florence Rogers, 1916, one child; A. Louise Hegan, 1929; Marie McNally Salman, 1950. EDUCATION: Rutgers University: 1900, A.B.; 1904, A.M.; and 1925, D.Sc.; 1904, M.D., College of Physicians and Surgeons (Columbia); 1905-7, intern, Presbyterian Hospital (N.Y.); 1910-14, research fellow, Cornell University Medical College. CAREER: *Post* 1907, practiced medicine, N.Y.; at Cornell University Medical College: 1920-32, immunology faculty; and 1932-40, clinical medicine faculty; *post* 1932, director, allergy department, Roosevelt Hospital (N.Y.); 1944-47, civilian consultant, U.S. Surgeon General; attending physician: 1907-10, New York City; 1910-14, Bellevue; 1914-21, Postgraduate Medical School hospitals. CONTRIBUTIONS: Made pioneering studies of the nature and treatment of allergies. Promoted the use of intradermal skin tests to determine hypersensitivity and treated symptoms by neutralization of allergic reactions. Developed the first treatment for desensitization for hay fever and demonstrated the development of a blocking antibody after desensitization. Stressed the importance of standardizing doses for desensitization and introduced the protein nitrogen unit for that purpose. His book *Allergy in Theory and Practice* (1947) was long a standard reference. Founded and directed the first clinic devoted to allergy at New York Hospital (1919); was world renowned when it was moved to Roosevelt Hospital (1932), where it was renamed the Institute of Allergy (1950). Established the field of allergy as a medical specialty. Founded and was first president (1923), American Society for the Study of Allergy and Allied Conditions (later the American Academy of Allergy). Founded and was chairman (1938), Association of Allergy Clinics of Greater New York.

WRITINGS: "The Treatment of Hay Fever by Active Immunization," *Laryngoscope* 25 (1915): 108-12. Many of Cooke's articles are cited in his *Allergy in Theory and Practice* (1947). REFERENCES: Merrill W. Chase, "Irreverent Recollections from Cooke and Coca, 1928-1978," *J. of Allergy and Clinical Immunology* 64, no. 5 (Nov. 1979): 306-20; *DAB*, Supplement 6: 123-24; Miller, *BHM*, p. 22; *N.Y. Times*, May 8, 1960; *Who Was Who in Am.*, 4: 199-200.

S. Galishoff

COOLEY, THOMAS BENTON (June 23, 1871, Ann Arbor, Mich.-October 13, 1945, Bangor, Maine). *Physician; Pediatrics.* Son of Thomas McIntyre, distinguished law professor and judge, and Mary Elizabeth (Horton) Cooley. Married Abigail Hubbard, 1903; two children. EDUCATION: At University of Michigan: 1891, A.B.; and 1895, M.D.; 1895-97, intern, Boston City Hospital; 1901, studied in Germany; 1902, resident in contagious diseases, Boston City Hospital. CAREER: University of Michigan: 1897, instructor of hygiene and physiological chemistry; 1903-5, assistant professor of hygiene; 1905-41, practice of pediatrics, Detroit, Mich.; 1918-19, American Red Cross, France; 1921, chief of staff, Children's Hospital (Detroit); 1934-35, founder and president, American Academy of Pediatrics; 1936, professor of pediatrics, Wayne University College of Medicine; 1940-41, president, American Pediatric Society. CONTRIBUTIONS: Published the first description of "Cooley's Anemia" or thalassemia and hinted at its genetic etiology. Pioneer in the formal organization of pediatrics.

WRITINGS: "A Series of Cases of Splenomegaly in Children, with Anemia and Peculiar Bone Changes," *Trans., Am. Pediat. Soc.* 37 (1925): 29 (with P. Lee); "Anemia in Children," *Am. J. of Diseases of Children* 34 (1927): 347-63 (with E. Witwer and P. Lee). REFERENCES: Thomas E. Cone, Jr., *History of American Pediatrics* (1979), 208-9; *DAB*, Supplement 3: 189-90; *NCAB*, 33: 93-94; *Who Was Who in Am.*, 2: 127.

M. Pernick

COOPER, ELIAS SAMUEL (November 25, 1820, near Somerville, Ohio-October 13, 1862, San Francisco, Calif.). *Surgeon.* Son of Jacob and Elizabeth (Walls) Cooper, Quaker farmers. Never married. EDUCATION: Studied medicine with his brother Dr. Esaias Cooper, Galesburg, Ill.; c. 1838, studied medicine in Cincinnati, Ohio; 1841, M.D., St. Louis University. CAREER: c. 1841-44, practice, Danville, Ill.; 1844-54, practice, Peoria, Ill., where he established a surgical reputation extending into other states; 1853, president, Knox County (Ill.) Medical Society; 1854, visited various European clinics; 1855, in San Francisco, established a busy surgical practice as well as Dr. Cooper's Eye, Ear and Feet Clinic, which was later known as the Pacific Clinical Infirmary. CONTRIBUTIONS: Helped found the short-lived California State Medical Society (1856).

Successfully organized the medical department, University of the Pacific (1858), the first medical college on the Pacific Coast. Afterwards reorganized as the Medical College of the Pacific, later known as the Cooper Medical College. Served this institution as president of the medical faculty and professor of surgery (1858-death). Began publishing the *San Francisco Medical Press* (1860), a quarterly journal of medicine and surgery, continuing as its editor until his death when he was succeeded by his nephew Dr. Levi Cooper Lane (q.v.) and Dr. Henry Gibbons (q.v.). The medical school he founded (1858) was continued by Lane and ultimately became the medical department of Stanford University.

WRITINGS: Some of his many articles appeared in: *Calif. State J. of Med.* (1856); *Trans., Med. Soc. of the State of Calif.* (1858). REFERENCES: *DAB*, 2 pt. 2: 397; Henry Harris, *California's Medical Story* (1932), 366-69; Kelly and Burrage (1920); *NCAB*, 22: 128; *San Francisco Med. Press* (Oct. 1862).

Y. V. O'Neill

COPELAND, ROYAL SAMUEL (November 7, 1868, near Dexter, Mich.-June 17, 1938, Washington, D.C.). *Physician; Ophthalmology; Public health*. Son of Roscoe Pulaski, farmer, and Frances Jane (Holmes) Copeland. Married Frances Spalding, 1908; two children. EDUCATION: Michigan State Normal College, Ypsilanti, Mich.; 1889, M.D., University of Michigan; 1889-90, intern, University of Michigan hospital (homeopathic); 1890, postgraduate study, Europe. CAREER: 1890-95, practiced medicine, Bay City, Michigan; 1895-1908, ophthalmology and otology faculty, University of Michigan (homeopathic department); 1901-3, mayor, Ann Arbor, Mich.; 1904-5, president, American Ophthalmological and Otological Association; 1908-18, practiced medicine, New York City; 1908, dean, New York Homeopathic Medical College and director, Flower Hospital; 1918-22, commissioner of public health, New York City Department of Health; 1922-38, U.S. senator from N.Y. CONTRIBUTIONS: Early in career, gained prominence as an eye specialist, teacher, and medical writer. Later compiled a mixed record as New York City commissioner of public health: fought vigorously for lower milk prices, increased health department appropriations, and medical responsibility for the treatment of drug addicts but retarded the steady movement toward professionalization in his department by subjecting it to the influence of Tammany Hall politicians. Greatest achievement was the enactment (1938) of the Copeland-Lea Food, Drug, and Cosmetic Bill, after five years of labor as a U.S. senator.

WRITINGS: *Refraction* (1906, with Adolph E. Ibershoff); *The Health Book* (1924); *Dr. Copeland's Home Medical Book* (1934). REFERENCES: *DAB*, Supplement 2: 120-22; John Duffy, *A History of Public Health in New York City* 2 (1974); Charles O. Jackson, *Food and Drug Legislation in the New Deal* (1970); *NCAB*, 15: 358-59; *N.Y. Times*, June 18, 1938; R. J. Potter, "Royal Samuel Copeland, 1868-1938; a Physician in Politics" (Ph.D. thesis, Western Reserve University, 1967).

S. Galishoff

CORDELL, EUGENE FAUNTLEROY (June 25, 1843, Charlestown, Va. [now W.Va.]-August 27, 1913, Baltimore, Md.). *Physician; Medical historian;*

Teacher; Librarian. Son of Levi O'Conner, physician, and Christine (Turner) Cordell. Married Louise Tazewell Southall, 1873; three children. EDUCATION: Charlestown Academy; Episcopal High School, Alexandria, Va.; Virginia Military Institute; 1868, M.D., University of Maryland Medical School, where he was clinical reporter and assistant physician at the hospital (1868-69); 1907, M.A., University of Maryland. CAREER: 1869-72, attending physician, Baltimore General Dispensary; 1870-71, 1880-87, librarian, Medical and Chirurgical Faculty; 1880-82, co-editor, *Maryland Medical Journal*; president: 1884-86, 1899-1901, Medical Society, Woman's Medical College; and 1893-97, Hospital Relief Association of Maryland; 1894-98, editor, *Bulletin of the Medical Society of the Woman's Medical College*; president: 1897-98, Medical Society of the University of Maryland; and 1902-4, Johns Hopkins Historical Club; 1903, elected president, Medical and Chirurgical Faculty at Maryland; 1903-13, professor of the history of medicine, editor of *Old Maryland*, and librarian, Department of Medicine, University of Maryland. CONTRIBUTIONS: Co-founder of Woman's Medical College, Baltimore, where he held chairs in materia medica and therapeutics and in the principles and practice of medicine (1884-1903). A founder of the Hospital of the Good Samaritan and attending physician there (1882-1903). Helped begin the Cottage Convalescent Hospital at St. Lukeland, Home for Incurables in Baltimore, Baltimore General Dispensary, Training School for Nurses of the Woman's Medical College, and Hospital Relief Association of Maryland. Efforts to reform medical education inspired establishment of the Medical College Association at Nashville, Tenn. (May 1890). Created a fund for widows and orphans of Maryland's Medical and Chirurgical Faculty (1903). Helped organize the Home for Widows and Orphans of Physicians.

WRITINGS: *Historical Sketch of the University of Maryland, 1809-90* (1891; 2d ed. in 2 vols., 1907, and extends coverage to 1907); *The Medical Annals of Maryland: 1799-1899* (1903). Writings listed in *Index Catalogue*, 2nd series, 3: 917, and J. R. Quinan, *Medical Annals of Baltimore . . .*, (1884), 84-85. REFERENCES: E. F. Cordell, *Medical Annals of Maryland . . .* (1903), 361-62; Kelly and Burrage (1928), 357-58; *Index Catalogue*, 3rd series, 4: 174; *NCAB*, 19:366. Quinan, *Medical Annals of Baltimore*, pp. 84-85.

C. Donegan

CORI, GERTY THERESA (RADNITZ) (August 16, 1896, Prague, Czechoslovakia-October 26, 1957, St. Louis, Mo.). *Biochemist*. Daughter of Otto and Martha (Neustadt) Radnitz. Married Carl Ferdinand Cori, 1920; one son. EDUCATION: 1920, M.D., German University of Prague. CAREER: 1920-22, internship, Karolinen Children's Hospital, Vienna; 1922-25, assistant pathologist, New York State Institute for the Study of Malignant Diseases (later Roswell Park Memorial Institute); at Washington University School of Medicine: 1925-31, assistant biochemist; 1931-46, research associate, Department of Pharmacology; 1946-47, research associate, Department of Biochemistry; and 1947-57, professor of biochemistry; 1947, Nobel Prize for physiology and medicine, with Carl

Cori and Bernard Houssay; the year she won the Nobel Prize, it was discovered that Cori was suffering from myelofibrosis, a rare blood disease, from which she died in 1957. CONTRIBUTIONS: Despite opposition to her collaborative work with her husband, research with Carl Cori began in 1923 (the year they published their first joint paper) and continued for decades thereafter. The Coris demonstrated (1930s) that the breakdown of glycogen involved the formation of a substance that became known as the "Cori ester" (glucose-1-phosphate). Their subsequent work showed that the metabolic breakdown of glycogen involved an enzymatic mechanism; the Coris later isolated several enzymes involved in this process; made the first synthesis of glycogen in a test tube (1939). In later work, she and colleagues used these enzymes to determine the molecular structure of glycogen; this led (by 1952) to an understanding of the nature of glycogen storage diseases in children, showing that an enzymatic defect can be inherited. The clinical aspects of this work were done at St. Louis Children's Hospital. Continued to be active in the laboratory until shortly before her death.

WRITINGS: "The Formation of Hexosephosphase Esters in Frog Muscle," *J. Biochem.* 116 (1936): 119-28 (with C. F. Cori); "Crystalline Muscle Phosphorylase II Prosthetic Group," *ibid.*, 151 (1943): 31-38 (with C. F. Cori); "The Enzymatic Conversion of Phosphorylase a to b," *ibid.*, 158 (1945): 321-32 (with C. F. Cori and A. A. Green); "Action of Amulo-16-Glycosidase and Phosphorolase on Glycogen and Amylopectin, 17-19," *ibid.*, 199 (1952): 661-67 (with C. F. Cori); "Glucose-6-Phosphatase of the Liver in Glycogen Store Disease," *ibid.*, 199 (1952): 661-67 (with J. Larner); "Glycogen Structure and Enzyme Deficiencies in Glycogen Storage Disease," *Harvey Lectures* 48 (1952-53): 145-71 (with C. F. Cori). REFERENCES: *DAB*, Supp. 6: 126-27; *DSB*, 3: 415-16; E. A. Doisy, obituary, *Am. Philos. Soc. Yearbook* (1958); B. A. Houssay, "Carl F. and Gerty T. Cori," *Biochimica et biophysica acta* 20 (1956): 11-16; *NCAB*, 48: 327-28; S. Ochoa and H. M. Kalckar, "Gerty T. Cori, Biochemist," *Sci.* 128 (1958); Edna Yost, *Women of Modern Sci.* (1964). A personal insight into the Cori collaboration appears in C. F. Cori's autobiographical article, "The Call of Science," *Annual Rev. of Biochem.* 38 (1969): 1-20. See also the essay on Dr. Cori in *Notable Am. Women: The Modern Period* (1980), 165-67.

M. Hunt

COUNCIL, WALTER WOOTEN (May 25, 1882, Council, N.C.-November 13, 1943, Juneau, Alaska). *Physician; Surgeon.* Son of John Pickett and Johanna (Wooten) Council. Married Virginia Scurry, 1907, two children; Jane Murray, 1920; Ruby Allein Apland, 1934. EDUCATION: University of North Carolina, 1897, graduated in premedicine at the age of 15; 1905, University of Virginia, M.D., with honors; 1905-6, interned at Seattle General Hospital. CAREER: surgeon: 1906-11, Ellamar Mining Company, Cordova, Alaska; and 1908-27, Copper River and Northwestern Railway and Kennicott Copper Corp., Cordova; 1916-27, assistant surgeon, U.S. Public Health Service; 1933-43, territorial commissioner of health. CONTRIBUTIONS: During his time in Cordova, served three terms as mayor (1906-27). While commissioner of health, established the Juneau Medical and Surgical Clinic and oversaw the development of a comprehensive health program in the territory. REFERENCES: *Anchorage Times*, November 15, 1943, p. 8; November 17, 1943, p. 1; *Juneau* (Alaska) *Empire*, November 12, 1943, p. 1; letters from acquaintances; personal interviews; *Who Was Who in Am.*, 2: 130.

A.R.C. Helms

COUNCILMAN, WILLIAM THOMAS (January 1, 1854, Pikesville, Md.-May 26, 1933, York Village, Maine). *Physician; Pathology.* Son of John T., physician and farmer, and Christiana Drummond (Mitchell) Councilman. Married Isabella Coolidge, 1894; three children. EDUCATION: St. Johns College (Annapolis, Md.); 1878, M.D., University of Maryland; 1878-80, studied experimental physiology under Henry N. Martin (q.v.), Johns Hopkins; 1880-83, studied pathology in Vienna, Austria; Leipzig, Germany; and Strassburg, France; 1883-86, studied pathology under Martin. CAREER: 1878-80, medical staff, Marine Hospital and Bay View Asylum (Baltimore); pathology faculty: 1886-92, Johns Hopkins Medical School; 1892-1921, Harvard Medical School; and 1923, Union Medical College, Peiping, China. CONTRIBUTIONS: Did significant original research on several diseases including diphtheria, epidemic cerebrospinal meningitis, chronic nephritis, and smallpox. First American to describe and picture the malarial parasite. With H. A. Lafleur, established amoebic dysentery as an independent disease entity. Through his research and teaching, and as founder and first president of the American Association of Pathologists and Bacteriologists, greatly aided in the development of pathology in the United States. Microscopic round bodies seen in certain liver diseases are called Councilman bodies.

WRITINGS: "Amoebic Dysentery," *Johns Hopkins Hosp. Rev.* 2 (1891): 395-548 (with H. A. Lafleur); *Epidemic Cerebrospinal Meningitis and Its Relations with Other Forms of Meningitis* (1898, with F. B. Mallory and J. H. Wright); "A Study of the Bacteriology and Pathology of Two Hundred and Twenty Fatal Cases of Diphtheria," *J. of the Boston Soc. of Med. Sci.* 5 (1900): 139-319 (with F. B. Mallory and R. M. Pearce). A bibliography is in *BMNAS* 18 (1938): 157-74. REFERENCES: *DAB*, Supplement 1: 205-6; *DSB*, 3: 447-48; A. M. Harvey, " . . . The Story of William T. Councilman," *Johns Hopkins Med. J.* 146 (1980): 185-92, 199-201; *Who Was Who in Am.*, 1: 265.

S. Galishoff

COVINGTON, BENJAMIN JESSE (1869, near Marlin, Tex.-July 21, 1961, Houston, Tex.). *Physician; General practice.* Son of former slaves. Married Jennie Belle Murphy, c. 1901; one child. EDUCATION: No college education; 1892, worked way through Hearne Baptist Academy (Tex.); 1895, entered Meharry Medical College after working as schoolteacher and bookkeeper for three years; 1900, M.D., Meharry Medical School; took regular postgraduate courses for 42 years at various institutions, primarily in the South. CAREER: Medical practice: 1900, Wharton, Tex.; 1900-1903, Yoakum, Tex.; and 1903-61, Houston. CONTRIBUTIONS: Established, with four other physicians, Houston Negro Hospital (1925), now Riverside General Hospital. Helped reorganize the Lone Star Medical Association soon after graduation from Meharry; served as its secretary-treasurer for ten years and president (1920). Served Houston black community for 58 years as general practitioner and worker for health improvement and better public facilities. REFERENCES: Howard H. Bell, "Benjamin Jesse Covington, M.D., 1869-1961," *JNMA* 55(1963): 462-63; (also in *Negro Hist. Bull.* 25 [1961]: 5-6); E. P. Perry, "Riverside General Hospital," *JNMA* 57 (1965): 258-63.

T. Savitt

COWIE, DAVID MURRAY (November 19, 1872, Moncton, New Brunswick, Canada-January 27, 1940, Ann Arbor, Mich.). *Physician; Pediatrics.* Son of James Steadman and Isabel Henderson (Harris) Cowie. An early marriage produced one child; second marriage to Anna Marion Cook, M.D., 1908, one child. EDUCATION: Battle Creek College (Mich.); 1896, M.D., University of Michigan; 1908, studied internal medicine, Heidelberg, Germany. CAREER: 1896-1900, medical practice, Ann Arbor; 1896-1940, medical faculty, University of Michigan Medical School, including 1920-40, first professor of pediatrics and infectious diseases; 1912, established Cowie Private Hospital, Ann Arbor; 1912-24, editorial board, *American Journal of Diseases of Children.* CONTRIBUTIONS: Founder of pediatrics, University of Michigan. In a state with extremely high goiter incidence, and with many salt mines, initiated the nation's first iodized-salt goiter-prevention program and convinced manufacturers to market iodized salt (1922-24). Published the first reported use of insulin in juvenile diabetes. First described "Cowie's sign," salivary duct edema characteristic of mumps.

WRITINGS: "Duct Sign in Mumps," *Am. J. of Diseases of Children* 20 (1920): 75-81; "Clinical Observations on the Use of Insulin in the Treatment of Diabetes in Adults and Children," *Trans., Am. Pediat. Soc.* 35 (1923): 217; "A Study of the Effect of the Use of Iodized Salt on the Incidence of Goiter," *Michigan State Med. Soc., J.* 36 (1937): 647-55. REFERENCES: *Am. J. of Diseases of Children* 59 (1940): 853; *Ann Arbor News,* January 27, 1940, p. 1; *JAMA* 114 (1940): 817; *Michigan State Med. Soc., J.* 38 (1939): 897; 39 (1940): 223; *NCAB,* 37: 202; *Who Was Who in Am.,* 1: 267.

M. Pernick

COX, GEORGE WASHINGTON, JR. (September 22, 1879, Gonzales, Tex.-October 29, 1963, Houston, Tex.). *Physician; Public health official.* Son of George W., Sr., physician, and Rachel F. (Roberson) Cox. Married Maude French, October 31, 1906; one son. EDUCATION: 1896-98, pharmacy student, University of Texas, Austin, Tex.; 1906, M.D., Tulane University; 1935, studied public health systems in N.Y., Pa., Ky., and city and state health offices in Tex. CAREER: 1898-1903, practicing pharmacist, Corpus Christi, Tex.; 1906-8, medical practice, Brownsville, Tex., and quarantine officer, Port Isabel, Tex.; practice: 1908-12, Corpus Christi; 1912-14, Moore, Tex.; 1914-18, Ozona, Tex.; and 1919-35, Del Rio, Tex.; 1935, appointed to Texas State Board of Health; 1936-37, elected state health officer; December 1953, resigned, chagrined by curtailment of federal funds for public health. CONTRIBUTIONS: Courageous, organized, imaginative, sometimes controversial public health official. Extended health services throughout Tex.: venereal disease and tuberculosis control, diagnostic laboratories, and U.S.-Mexico border public health conferences. WRITINGS: Major speeches, reports, and programs are described in journals, newspapers, and state documents. REFERENCES: *History of Public Health in Texas* (1950, 1974); *Houston Post*, October 30, 1963; *J. of the Texas Public Health Assoc.* (began Jun. 1949); *Texas Health Bull.* (beginning Oct. 1948).

J. Morris

COXE, JOHN REDMAN (September 16, 1773, Trenton, N.J.-March 22, 1864, Philadelphia, Pa.). *Physician; Pharmacology.* Son of Daniel and Sarah (Redman) Coxe; grandson of John Redman (q.v.). Married Sarah Cox; six children. EDUCATION: 1788-90, studied medicine with Benjamin Rush (q.v.); 1794, M.D., University of Pennsylvania; 1794-96, studied medicine in Europe. CAREER: *Post* 1796, practiced medicine, Philadelphia; 1802-7, medical staff, Pennsylvania Hospital; at University of Pennsylvania: chemistry faculty, 1809-19; and 1819-35, materia medica and pharmacy faculty. CONTRIBUTIONS: An early proponent of vaccination. Wrote *Practical Observations on Vaccination . . .* (1802), which together with his own vaccination and that of his infant son (1801) fostered acceptance of the new practice. Considered the father of pharmacy in Philadelphia; provided the first systematic instruction in the subject and helped found the Chemical Society of Philadelphia (1792) and the Philadelphia College of Pharmacy (1822). Probably introduced the jalap plant into the United States. Devised the compound syrup of squills, described in the U.S. Pharmacopoeia and generally known as Coxe's Hive Syrup, which was used widely for 50 years. A founder of American medical journalism. Edited *Medical Museum* (1805-11), the first uniformly issued periodical in Philadelphia, and *American Dispensatory* (1808) and published a *Medical Dictionary*. Wrote several medical histories. WRITINGS: *An Inquiry into the Claims of Dr. William Harvey to the Discovery of the Circulation of the Blood . . .* (1834). REFERENCES: *DAB*, 4: 486-87; Kelly and Burrage (1928), 262-63; *NCAB*, 22: 151; Miller, *BHM*, p. 23; R. F. Stone, *Biog. of Eminent Am. Physicians and Surgeons* (1894), 101; John H. Talbott, *Biographical History of Med.* (1970), 362-64; *Who Was Who in Am.*, Hist. Vol.: 193.

S. Galishoff

CRAIG, WINCHELL McKENDREE (April 27, 1892, Washington Court House, Ohio-February 12, 1960, Rochester, Minn.). *Physician; Neurosurgery.* Son of Thomas Henry, dry-goods merchant, and Eliza Orlena (Pine) Craig. Married Katherine Fitzgerald, 1928; four children. EDUCATION: 1915, B.A., Ohio Wesleyan University; 1919, M.D., Johns Hopkins University; 1919-21, intern, New Haven (Conn.) and Roosevelt (New York City) hospitals; and resident in surgery, Saint Agnes Hospital (Baltimore); 1921-24, fellow, Mayo Foundation, Graduate School, University of Minnesota; 1930, M.S. (surgery), University of Minnesota. CAREER: 1926-57, surgical staff, Mayo Clinic; 1927-57, neurologic surgery faculty, Mayo Foundation, Graduate School, University of Minnesota; surgical staff: 1941-42, U.S. Naval Hospital, Corona, Calif.; and 1942-45, National Naval Medical Center, Bethesda, Md.; 1945-46, director, Graduate Training Program, Bureau of Medicine and Surgery, Washington, D.C. (is believed to be the first civilian physician to attain the rank of rear admiral); 1959, field representative, Council on Medical Education and Hospitals, American Medical Association; 1959-60, special assistant for health and medical affairs to Arthur S. Flemming, U.S. secretary of health, education and welfare; president: 1946, Society of Neurological Surgeons; 1948, Harvey Cushing Society; and 1953, Association of Military Surgeons of the United States. CONTRIBUTIONS: A pioneer in the modern development of neurosurgery. Distinguished for his works on surgery of the sympathetic nervous system, the surgical treatment of hypertension, and the classification of tumors of the brain and spinal cord. Greatly improved surgical techniques and apparatus in his field. Introduced the Craig headrest (1935), still widely used in ventriculography and other neurological procedures. Helped edit *Journal of Neurosurgery* (1944-57).

WRITINGS: "Treatment of Intractable Cardiospasm by Bilateral Cervicothoracic Sympathetic Ganglionectomy," *Proc. of Staff Meeting, Mayo Clinic* 9 (Dec. 12, 1934): 749-53 (with H. J. Moersch and P. P. Vinson); "Hypertension and Subdiaphragmatic Sympathetic Denervation," *Surgical Clinics of North Am.* 19 (Aug. 1939): 969-80 (with A. W. Adson). Reprints of Craig material published between 1923 and 1958 are in Mayo Clinic Library Collection. REFERENCES: *DAB*, Supplement 6: 130-31; *NCAB*, 46: 54-55; *N.Y. Times*, February 14, 1960; *Who Was Who in Am.*, 3: 191.

S. Galishoff

CRAIK, JAMES (1730, Scotland-February 6, 1814, Fairfax County, Va.). *Physician.* Son of Robert Craik, member of Parliament. Married Marianne Ewell, c. 1760; some children. EDUCATION: Academic and medical training at the University of Edinburgh. CAREER: 1754-58, British colonial surgeon in the French and Indian War; 1758-75, private practice, Port Tobacco, Md.; 1775-81, army assistant director-general of the Hospital of the Middle Department; 1781-83, chief physician and surgeon of the army; 1783-98, private practice, Alexandria, Va.; 1798-1800, physician-general of the army; 1800-1814, semiretired. CONTRIBUTIONS: Successful and esteemed colonial physician, one of the many Scottish physicians who immigrated to America in the eighteenth century. Initially served as an army surgeon during the French and Indian War, treating both George Washington and General Braddock. During the Revolution, served in the medical department of the American army in a number of important positions. After the war, returned to private practice and maintained close friendship with President Washington. One of the attending physicians at Washington's deathbed.

WRITINGS: Only known writing: *Account of the Behavior of Gen. Washington, During His Distressing Illness, Also of the Nature of the Complaint of Which He Died, by Doctors James Craik and Elisha C. Dick, Attending Physicians* (1808). REFERENCES: *BHM* (1964-69), 62; (1980), 11; Wyndham Blanton, *Medicine in Virginia in the Eighteenth Century* (1931); *DAB*, 2, pt. 2: 498-99; Howard Kelly, *Cyclopedia of Am. Med. Biog.* (1912);

NCAB, 7: 494; James Thatcher, *Am. Med. Biog.* (1828); J. M. Toner, *Medical Men of the Revolution* (1876); Charles C. Wall, "His Excellency George Washington to James Craik," *Virginia Mag. of Hist. and Biog.* 55 (1947): 318-28.

P. Addis

CRAMP, ARTHUR JOSEPH (September 10, 1872, London, England-November 25, 1951, Hendersonville, N.C.). *Physician; Investigator and critic of quackery.* Son of Joseph and Mary Ann (Jackson) Cramp. Married Lillian Caroline Torrey, 1897; one daughter. EDUCATION: Maryville (Missouri) Seminary; 1906, M.D., Wisconsin College of Physicians and Surgeons, Milwaukee, Wis. CAREER: 1894-1902, high school science teacher and principal; 1906, medical practice; 1906-36, director, Bureau of Investigation, American Medical Association. CONTRIBUTIONS: The death of his daughter, treated by a man who turned out to be a quack, prompted Cramp to attend medical school and made him a lifelong foe of pseudomedicine. Joining the AMA in the year the Food and Drugs Act was passed, set up that association's bureau to give quackery continuous unrelenting scrutiny and wide exposure and to urge strengthening of regulatory controls. Investigations were ingenious, his key weapon ridicule. Often read a chapter from *Alice in Wonderland* to get into the mood to write his exposures of health deception. Published in the AMA's *Journal* and *Hygeia* and in other magazines, these works were later assembled in pamphlets and books. Also lectured. Burgeoning files aided physicians, journalists, better business bureaus, and health officials across the nation and around the world. Pamphlets mailed out passed the 2 million mark before retirement following a heart attack. Until 1933 only two suits were brought against AMA for antiquackery work; one it won, the other it lost, paying 1 cent in damages.

WRITINGS: Cramp compiled his key articles in three *Nostrums and Quackery* volumes (1912, 1921, 1936). Other representative articles: "Modern Advertising and the Nostrum Evil," *Am. J. of Public Health* 8 (1918): 756-58; "Therapeutic Thaumaturgy," *Am. Mercury* 3 (1924): 423-30; "The Nostrum and the Public Health," *New England J. of Med.* 201 (1929): 1297-1300; "The Work of the Bureau of Investigation," *Law and Contemporary Problems* 1 (1933): 51-54. REFERENCES: AMA archives; *NCAB*, E: 480; obituary, *JAMA* (1951): 1773; James Harvey Young, *The Medical Messiahs* (1967), 129-42.

J. H. Young

CRAWFORD, JOHN (May 3, 1746, north of Ireland-May 9, 1813, Baltimore, Md.). *Physician.* Son of a Protestant clergyman. Married daughter of John and Deborah O'Donnell c. 1778, at least two children; apparently married a second time. EDUCATION: 1763, entered Trinity College, Dublin; M.D., University of Leyden. CAREER: 1772-74, ship's surgeon, East India Company, in which capacity he sailed to Bombay and Bengal; surgeon: 1779-90, British Naval Hospital, Barbados; and 1790-96, Demarara Hospital, Demarara, South America; 1796-1813, practiced in Baltimore; censor, examiner, and orator, Medical and Chirurgical Faculty of Maryland; a founder: 1800, Society for the Promotion of

Useful Knowledge; 1801, Baltimore Dispensary; and 1798, Baltimore Library. CONTRIBUTIONS: Espoused an early germ theory of disease. Believed that disease was caused by minute parasitic organisms that entered the body and reproduced there. Argued that just as a particular vegetable seed gave rise to its respective plant, and to that only, each *contagium vivum* or *animatum* produced its own peculiar disease. Helped promote vaccination in Baltimore.

WRITINGS: "A Series of Observations on the Seats and Causes of Disease," *Baltimore Med. and Physical Recorder* 1 (1809): 40-52, 81-92, 206-21. REFERENCES: *BHM* (1970-74), 43; *DAB*, 4: 521-22; Raymond N. Doetsch, "John Crawford and His Contribution to the Doctrine of Contagium Vivum," *Bacteriological Reviews* 28, no. 1 (Mar. 1964): 87-96; Kelly and Burrage (1928): 266-67; Julia E. Wilson, "An Early Baltimore Physician and His Medical Library," *Annals of Med. Hist.*, 3rd series, 4 (1942): 63-80.

S. Galishoff

CRILE, GEORGE WASHINGTON (November 11, 1864, Chili, Ohio-January 7, 1943, Cleveland, Ohio). *Surgeon; Physiology; Prevention of shock*. Son of Michael, farmer, and Margaret (Dietz) Crile. Married Grace McBride, 1900; four children. EDUCATION: Ohio Northern University: 1884, A.B.; and 1888, M.A.; 1887, M.D., Wooster Medical School (later Western Reserve Medical School); 1887-88, intern, University Hospital (Cleveland); studied: 1893, Vienna; 1895, London; and 1897, Paris. CAREER: At Western Reserve: 1889-90, histology faculty; 1890-93, physiology faculty; and 1893-1924, surgery faculty; 1911-21, visiting surgeon, Lakeside Hospital (Cleveland); at Cleveland Clinic: 1911, founder; *post* 1911, chief surgeon; and 1911-40, president; at American College of Surgeons: 1916-17, founder and president; and 1921-40, member, Board of Regents. CONTRIBUTIONS: Discovered and perfected a method of preventing traumatic shock in surgery, which he called "anoci-association"; method made use of premedication with morphine and atropine, blocking with cocaine the nerve channels between the region of operation and the brain, and anesthesia by inhalation of nitrous oxide and oxygen administered by a team of specialists. Introduced the use of epinephrine and saline solutions for patients in shock. Devised methods for blood transfusion (1905) and pioneered its use in surgery. Popularized the monitoring of blood pressure in surgical procedures. Responsible for many advances in surgical technique, especially in thyroid surgery. Called attention to the effect of emotions on the thyroid and adrenal glands and the importance of the patient's mental state in surgery.

WRITINGS: *On the Blood Pressure in Surgery* (1903); *Hemorrhage and Transfusion* (1909); *Anoci-Association* (1914, with William E. Lower); *The Thyroid Gland* (1922, with others). Major writings are listed in Peter C. English, "George Washington Crile and Surgical Shock: Physiology and Surgery in America, 1888-1918" (Ph.D. diss., Duke University, 1975). REFERENCES: *DAB*, Supplement 3: 200-203; English, *Shock, Physiological Surgery and George Washington Crile* (1980); Miller, *BHM*, p. 24; *NCAB*, C: 72-73; *N.Y. Times*, January 8, 1943; *Who Was Who in Am.*, 2: 134-35.

S. Galishoff

CROSBY, ALPHEUS BENNING (February 22, 1832, Gilmanton, N.H.-August 9, 1877, Hanover, N.H.). *Surgeon*. Son of Dixi (q.v.) and Mary Jane

(Moody) Crosby. Married Mildred Glassel Smith, 1862; three children. EDU-CATION: Moore's Indian Charity School, Hanover; at Dartmouth College: 1853, A.B.; 1856, M.D.; 1855-56, studied with his father and as an intern at U.S. Marine Hospital, Chelsea, Mass. CAREER: 1857 until his death, practiced at Hanover; 1861-62, surgeon, U.S. Army; 1862-77, Dartmouth medical faculty: *post* 1866, professor of surgery; gave lecture courses on surgery at Universities of Michigan and Vermont, Long Island College Medical School, Bowdoin, and Bellevue Hospital Medical College; 1876-77, president, New Hampshire Medical Society. CONTRIBUTIONS: A well-known lecturer, work exemplifies the technical progress of surgery in the middle third of the nineteenth century. "Medical History of New Hampshire" was widely accepted as a prototype of its genre. WRITINGS: "Foreign Bodies in the Knee Joint," *N.H. J. of Med.* 6 (1856): 353-63; "Septicaemia," *Trans., N.H. Med. Soc.* (1867-68): 20-48; "Medical History of New Hampshire," *ibid.* (1870): 46-75; "A Lost Art in Surgery," *Arch. Clin. Surg.* 2 (1877): 41-64. REFERENCES: J. Whitney Barstow, "Obituary Notice of A. B. Crosby," *Trans., N.H. Med. Soc.* (1878): 153-75; Kelly and Burrage, (1928); *NCAB*, 9: 98.

J. W. Estes

CROSBY, DIXI (February 7, 1800, Sandwich, N.H.-September 26, 1873, Hanover, N.H.). *Surgeon; Orthopedics.* Son of Asa and Betsey (Hoit) Crosby. Married Mary Jane Moody, 1827; two children, including Alpheus Benning Crosby (q.v.). EDUCATION: Dartmouth College: 1824, M.D.; and 1867, LL.D. (hon.). CAREER: Practiced in: 1824-34, Gilmanton, N.H.; 1835-38, Laconia, N.H.; and 1838 until death, Hanover; 1838-70, professor of surgery, Dartmouth; 1842-43, 1845-46, president, New Hampshire Medical Society. CONTRIBUTIONS: A careful operator, attempted to improve surgical techniques. Performed what appears to have been the second (he was unaware of the first) one-stage amputation of the clavicle, scapula, and shoulder joint, for an osteosarcoma (1836); although Reuben D. Mussey (q.v.), Amos Twitchell (q.v.), and John C. Warren (q.v.) had refused to attempt the operation, the patient survived for several more months. Also remembered as the defendant in the first malpractice suit against a consulting surgeon, initiated in 1845 but not completed until 1853. The plaintiff was awarded $800 in damages, but the decision was reversed on appeal (1854). WRITINGS: *Report of a Trial for Alleged Mal-Practice* (1854). REFERENCES: A. B. Crosby (q.v.), "Report on the First Recorded Operation Involving the Removal of the Entire Arm, Scapula, and Three-Fourths of the Clavicle, by Dixi Crosby, M.D., LL.D.," *Med. Record* 10 (1875): 753-55; Fielding H. Garrison, *Introduction to the Hist. of Med.*, 4th ed. (1929), 503; Kelly and Burrage (1928); *NCAB*, 9: 97.

J. W. Estes

CROWE, SAMUEL JAMES (April 16, 1883, Washington County, Va.-November 13, 1955, Baltimore, Md.). *Physician; Otolaryngology.* Son of Walter Andrew, physician, and Flora (Thompson) Crowe. Married Susie Childs Barrow, 1908; one child. EDUCATION: 1904, B.A., University of Georgia; 1908, M.D., Johns Hopkins Medical School; 1908-12, surgical intern and resident, Johns

Hopkins Hospital; 1913, studied otolaryngology, Germany. CAREER: 1912-52, otolaryngology faculty, Johns Hopkins Medical School; and otolaryngological staff, Johns Hopkins Hospital; 1952-55, clinical teaching, Europe, Africa, Asia Minor, and Alaska. CONTRIBUTIONS: Established the first modern clinic of otolaryngology in the United States. Did ground-breaking work on the physiology and pathology of hearing. Introduced the audiometer, which had been developed by Bell Laboratories, into clinical otology; made it possible to measure and record accurately the acuity of hearing. Did first important research on deafness in humans by correlating hearing impairments, anatomical defects and injuries in the inner ear. Demonstrated that the growth of lymphoid tissue in and around the eustachian tube was a frequent cause of deafness in children and developed a method of prevention and treatment using radon, a by-product of radium. Recognized that aviators and submariners who were exposed to sudden changes of air pressure experienced symptoms comparable to those of children with blockage of the eustachian tubes and, during World War II, established a course at Johns Hopkins to train medical officers in radon therapy. Developed new techniques of tonsillectomy that greatly minimized the occurrence of postoperative lung abscesses. Demonstrated a relationship between the pituitary and the reproductive system and showed that hypophysectomy caused genital atrophy.

WRITINGS: "Experimental Hypophysectomy," *Johns Hopkins Hosp. Bull.* 21 (1910): 127-69 (with Harvey Cushing [q.v.], and J. Homans); "Correlations of Differences in the Density of Innervation of the Organ of Corti with Differences in the Acuity of Hearing, Including Evidence as to the Location in the Human Cochlea of the Reception for Certain Tones," *Acta Oto-laryngologica* 15 (1931): 269 (with S. R. Guild, C. C. Bunch, and L. M. Polvogt); "Recognition, Treatment, and Prevention of Hearing Impairment in Children," *Annals of Otology, Rhinology and Laryngology* 50 (1941): 15 (with C. F. Burnham); "Irradiation of the Lymphoid Tissue in Diseases of the Upper Respiratory Tract," *Johns Hopkins Hosp. Bull.* 83 (1948): 383. REFERENCES: A. McGehee Harvey, *Research and Discovery in Medicine* (1981), 92-111; *N.Y. Times,* November 14, 1955.

S. *Galishoff*

CRUMBINE, SAMUEL JAY (September 17, 1862, Venango County, Pa.-July 12, 1954, Queens, N.Y.). *Physician; Public health.* Son of Samuel Jacob, blacksmith and farmer, and Sarah (Mully) Krumbine. Married Katherine Zuercher, 1890; two children. EDUCATION: 1878, graduated from Soldiers' Orphan School, Mercer, Pa.; medical preceptorship with Dr. W. E. Lewis, Cincinnati, Ohio; 1889, M.D., Cincinnati College of Medicine and Surgery. CAREER: 1889, private practice, Dodge City, Kans.; on Kansas State Board of Health: 1899, member; and 1904-23, secretary; 1911-19, dean (largely nominal), University of Kansas School of Medicine; 1923-36, secretary and general executive, American Child Health Association. CONTRIBUTIONS: Beginning as a small-town general practitioner, went on to place Kans. among the most enlightened states in the Union in matters of public health. Succeeded largely because of his ability as an educator, by making public health practices as clear and urgent for the citizenry as they were for him. Adept at demonstrating to often-hostile mercantile interests that reforms that might produce short-term economic loss were good business in the long run. Many of his campaigns were quickly emulated by other states —swatting the fly, outlawing the common drinking cup, eliminating roller towels, discouraging spitting on streets and sidewalks, and compulsory reporting of tuberculosis. Important first steps were taken in preventing adulteration of drugs and foodstuffs, regulating sewage and water supplies, and improving vital statistics. Request was granted (1915) to make Kans. the second state in the Union to have a division of child hygiene under the State Board of Health. After being fired by Governor Jonathan Davis (1923), was invited by Herbert Hoover to direct the American Child Health Association. In that position, reputation became international. Has been compared to important public health figures such as James A. Tobey, Thomas Parran (q.v.), William C. Gorgas (q.v.), and Edward L. Trudeau (q.v.).

WRITINGS: *Graded Lessons in Physiology and Hygiene* (1912, with William O. Krohn); *The Most Nearly Perfect Food* (1935, with Dr. J. A. Tobey). REFERENCES: Thomas Bonner, *The Kansas Doctor* (1959); Samuel J. Crumbine, *Frontier Doctor* (1948, autobiography); *DAB*, Supplement 5: 143-44; (1977); Miller, *BMH*, p. 24.

R. Hudson

CULLEN, THOMAS STEPHEN (November 20, 1868, Bridgewater, Ontario, Canada-March 4, 1953, Baltimore, Md.). *Surgeon (abdominal); Gynecologist; Educator*. Son of Thomas, Methodist minister, and Mary (Greene) Cullen. Married Emma Jones Beckwith, 1901; Mary Bartlett Dixon, 1920; no children. EDUCATION: Brighton Public School, Brighton, Ontario; Dufferin School, Toronto, Ontario; 1883, entered Jarvis Collegiate Institute, Toronto; 1890, M.B., University of Toronto; 1890-91, intern, Toronto General Hospital; 1891-92, assisted William Henry Welch (q.v.) and William T. Councilman (q.v.), Johns Hopkins pathology laboratory; 1892-93, intern, 1896, then resident in gynecology under Howard Kelly (q.v.), Johns Hopkins; 1893, studied for six months in Johannes Orth's laboratory, Pathological Institute, University of Göttingen, Germany. CAREER: 1893-96, in charge of gynecological pathology, Welch's laboratory; 1895-96, instructor in gynecology, Johns Hopkins; 1897, entered private practice, Baltimore, although maintained his connections with Hopkins; carried on most of his surgical and gynecological work at the Cambridge-Maryland Hospital in Cambridge, Md.; 1908, became chairman, Church Home and Infirmary and Episcopal Hospital medical board; became gynecologist-in-chief there and established highly regarded surgical clinic, open to "all reputable physicians and surgeons;" 1914, chairman, AMA's newly established Cancer Campaign Committee; 1916, president, Southern Surgical and Gynecological Association; 1919-39, professor of clinical gynecology, Johns Hopkins (title changed to professor of gynecology in 1932); 1927, president, Medical and Chirurgical Faculty of Maryland; 1929-53, Maryland State Board of Health. CONTRIBUTIONS: First to publish on the use of formalin in the development of a "rapid method of making permanent specimens from frozen sections" of tissue

(1895). Recognized "diffuse adenomyoma of the uterus" (adenomyosis), and published his exemplary *Adenomyoma of the Uterus* (1897-1908). Persuaded Henry Walters, Baltimore, to endow permanently at Johns Hopkins School of Medicine the world's first department of art as applied to medicine (1910); department headed by Max Brödel (q.v.). Described the "blue navel" (umbilicus) or "Cullen's Sign" for diagnosis of ruptured ectopic (extrauterine) pregnancy (1919)—published in *Contributions to Medical and Biological Research, Dedicated to Sir William Osler.* . . . Established a "laboratory in Gynecological Pathology which became the mother of many of the gynecological laboratories in this country."

WRITINGS: *Cancer of the Uterus: Its Pathology, Symptomatology, Diagnosis and Treatment* (1900); *Adenomyoma of the Uterus* (1908); *Myomata of the Uterus* (1909, ostensibly with Howard Kelly); *Embryology, Anatomy, and Diseases of the Umbilicus* (1916). Writings listed comprehensively in Judith Robinson, *Tom Cullen of Baltimore* (1949), 413-19. REFERENCES: Alan M. Chesney, *The Johns Hopkins Hospital and The Johns Hopkins University School of Medicine*, vols. 1 and 2; *DAB*, Supplement 5 (1951-55): 146-48; A. McGehee Harvey, *Adventures in Medical Research*. . . (1976), 173-83; *JAMA* 151, no. 14 (Apr. 4, 1953): 1218; Karl H. Martzloff, "Thomas Stephen Cullen," *Am. J. Obstet. Gynecol.* (Presidential Address, American Gynecological Society) 80, no. 5 (Nov. 1960); 833-43; *Index Catalogue*, 3rd series, 4: 302; 4th series, 3: 1023; 5th series, 2: 169; Richard W. TeLinde, "In Memoriam: Thomas Stephen Cullen," *Am. J. Obstet. Gynecol.*, 66, no. 2 (Aug. 1953): 462-64; Thomas B. Turner, *Heritage of Excellence* . . . (1974), 117, 118, 431-35; *Who Was Who in Am.*, 3: 200.

C. Donegan

CURTIS, ALVA (June 3, 1797, Columbia, N.H.-1881, Cincinnati?, Ohio). *Unorthodox practitioner; Botanics.* Personal biographical information not located. CAREER: 1825-31, language teacher in girl's school, Richmond, Va.; 1831-34, Thomsonian practitioner, agent, and infirmary operator, Richmond, Va.; 1835-52, editor of *Thomsonian Recorder* (Columbus, Ohio) and its successor, the *Botanico-Medical Recorder*; 1836-c. 80, president and professor, Botanico-Medical College and its successors (located in Columbus, 1839-41; Cincinnati, after 1841); 1836-81, botanic practitioner, Cincinnati. CONTRIBUTIONS: As leader of the "Independent Thomsonians" he split (1836-38) with Samuel Thomson (q.v.) over establishment of medical schools and infirmaries. His group, the Physio-Medicals, founded schools primarily in the Midwest and South. Following the split, Thomsonianism disintegrated, leaving several botanic sects, strongest of which were the Eclectics and Curtis's Physio-Medicals. Led this group for many years as editor of the leading journal and president of the leading school.

WRITINGS: *Discussions Between Several Members of the Regular Medical Faculty and the Thomsonian Botanic Physicians, on the Comparative Merits of Their Respective Systems* (1836); *Lectures on Midwifery and the Forms of Disease Peculiar to Women and Children* (1841); *A Fair Examination and Criticism of All the Medical Systems in Vogue* (1855). REFERENCES: *Appleton's CAB* 2: 35; Alex Berman, "Neo-Thomsonianism in the United States," *Jour. Hist. Med.* 11 (1956): 133-155; James O. Breeden, "Thomsonianism in Virginia," *Virginia Magazine of Hist. and Biog.* 82 (1974): 150-180; Jonathan Forman, "Dr. Alva Curtis in Columbus," *Ohio State Archaeological and Historical Quarterly* 51 (1942): 332-40; Kelly and Burrage (1928), 275.

T. L. Savitt

CURTIS, AUSTIN MAURICE (January 15, 1868, Raleigh, N.C.-July 13, 1939, Washington, D.C.). *Surgeon.* Son of Alexander W. and Eleanora Patilla (Smith) Curtis. Married Namoyoka Gertrude Sockum, 1891; four children. ED-UCATION: 1888, A.B., Lincoln University (Pa.); 1891, M.D., Northwestern University; 1891-92, intern, Provident Hospital, Chicago, Ill. (first intern) (worked closely with Daniel Hale Williams [q.v.] there). CAREER: 1892-98, private surgical practice, Chicago; 1892-98, visiting staff surgeon, Provident Hospital; 1896-98, staff surgeon, Cook County Hospital; 1898-1902, surgeon-in-chief, Freedmen's Hospital, Washington, D.C.; 1898-1938, surgery faculty and eventually head of department, Howard University; 1902-38, private surgical practice, Washington, D.C. CONTRIBUTIONS: First black physician to receive a regular staff appointment at a "white" hospital (Cook County Hospital, 1896), when the County Commission opened a slot for a black physician and the dozen black physicians and surgeons who attended a meeting chose Curtis. Considered the leading black surgeon in Washington. President, NMA (1911-12). Students regarded him highly for teaching skills at bedside and in operating room. Held numerous surgical demonstration clinics at black hospitals and medical schools throughout the South. Operated, with one of his three physician sons, a surgical hospital for black private patients (1925-33) in Washington, a city without such private facilities.

WRITINGS: "Medical and Surgical Treatment of Appendicitis," *JNMA* 2 (1910): 161-67; "A Symposium on Chronic Appendicitis," *Freedmen's Hosp. Bull.* 1 (1932): 5-7 (with Robert S. Jason et al.). Writings listed in *JNMA* 46 (1954): 298. REFERENCES: W. Montague Cobb, "Austin Maurice Curtis, 1868-1939," *JNMA* 46 (1954): 294-98; John A. Kenney, *The Negro in Medicine* (1912), 20; *WWICA* 6 (1941-43): 141.

T. Savitt

CUSHING, HARVEY WILLIAMS (April 8, 1869, Cleveland, Ohio-October 7, 1939, New Haven, Conn.). *Physician; Neurosurgery; Neurophysiology; Endocrinology.* Son of Henry Kirke, physician, and Betsey Maria (Williams) Cushing. Married Katherine Stone Crowell, 1902; five children. EDUCATION: 1891, A.B., Yale University; 1895, M.A., M.D., Harvard University; 1895-96, house officer, Massachusetts General Hospital; 1896-1900, resident, Johns Hopkins Hospital; 1900-1901, studied in Berne under Theodor Kocher. CAREER: Surgery faculty: 1902-12, Johns Hopkins Medical School; and 1912-32, Harvard University; 1913-32, surgery staff, Peter Bent Brigham Hospital; 1933-37, neurology faculty, Yale University. CONTRIBUTIONS: A pioneer of neurosurgery. Developed many of the basic techniques and procedures used in surgery of the brain and spinal cord; brought the sphygmomanometer into the operating room, devised silver clips for the control of bleeding, and introduced electrocautery in brain surgery. Developed methods for operating on intracranial tumors of the acoustic nerve (1917) and blood-vessel tumors of the central nervous system (gliomas and meningiomas, 1920s, 1930s). Reduced his own operating mortality from nearly 100 percent when he began to less than 10 percent. With his classmate E. A. Codman (q.v.), devised an ether chart for the operating room on which pulse, respiration, blood pressure, and other vital signs could be recorded (late 1890s). Made fundamental discoveries about the pituitary gland; theorized correctly that it influences the secretion of other ductless glands in addition to controlling specific bodily processes. Demonstrated and described the effects of hyperpituitarism and hypopituitarism (1909-12). Recognized a new disease, Cushing's disease, in which there is over-stimulation of the basophil cells of the pituitary (1931). Had a profound impact on the training of young surgeons. Established the Hunterian Laboratory of Experimental Medicine at Johns Hopkins (1905) and the Laboratory of Surgical Research at Harvard. Wrote a Pulitzer prize-winning biography of William Osler (q.v., 1925).

WRITINGS: *The Pituitary Body and Its Disorders* (1912); *Intracranial Tumors . . .* (1932); *Papers Relating to the Pituitary Body, Hypothalamus and Parasympathetic Nervous System* (1932). Writings are listed in *A Bibliography of the Writings of Harvey Cushing . . . Harvey Cushing Society* (1939). REFERENCES: *BHM* (1964-69), 64; (1970-74), 44; (1975-79), 32; (1980), 11; *DAB*, Supplement 2: 137-40; *DSB*, 3: 516-19; John F. Fulton, *Harvey Cushing: A Biography* (1946); Miller, *BHM*, p. 25; *NCAB*, 32: 402-3; E.. H. Thomson, *Harvey Cushing* (1950); *Who Was Who in Am.*, 1: 288.

S. Galishoff

CUSHNY, ARTHUR ROBERTSON (March 6, 1866, Fochabers, Scotland-February 25, 1926, Edinburgh, Scotland). *Pharmacologist; Educator.* Son of Rev. John and Catherine Ogilvie (Brown) Cushny. Married Sarah Fairbank, 1895; one daughter. EDUCATION: 1886, M.A., University of Aberdeen; 1889, M.B., C.M., Marischal College, Aberdeen; 1892, M.D., University of Aberdeen; 1892-93, post-graduate study at Strassburg and Berne. CAREER: 1893, assistant to Professor Oswald Schmiedeberg at the University of Strassburg; 1893-1905, professor of pharmacology at the University of Michigan; 1905-18, chair of pharmacology at University College, London; 1918-26, chair of pharmacology, University of Edinburgh. CONTRIBUTIONS: Completed the first controlled experimental analysis of the action of digitalis on warm-blooded animals (1897), thereby demonstrating its effects and increasing the therapeutic uses of the drug. First to recognize the similarity between clinical and experimental auricular fibrillation. Did pioneering research on the mechanism of kidney secretion (1901-4, 1917) and on the physiological action of optical isomers (1926).

WRITINGS: *Text-Book of Pharmacology and Therapeutics* (1899); *The Secretion of Urine* (1917); *The Action and Uses in Medicine of Digitalis and Its Allies* (1925); *The Biological Relation of Optically Isometric Substances* (1926). REFERENCES: *DAB*, 3, pt. 1:6-7; *DSB*, 15, Supplement 1: 99-104; Kelly and Burrage (1928), 280-81; H. MacGillivray, "A Personal Biography of Arthur Robertson Cushny, (1866-1926)," *Annual*

Rev. of Pharmacology 8 (1968): 1-24; J. Parascandola, "Arthur Cushny, Optical Isomerism, and the Mechanism of Drug Action," *J. of the Hist. of Biol.* 8 (1975): 145-65.

M. Kaufman

CUTLER, ELLIOTT CARR (July 30, 1888, Bangor, Maine-August 16, 1947, Brookline, Mass.). *Physician*; *Surgery*. Son of George Chalmers, lumber merchant, and Mary Franklin (Wilson) Cutler. Married Caroline Pollard Parker, 1919; five children. EDUCATION: 1909, B.A., Harvard University; 1913, M.D., Harvard Medical School; summer 1913, studied pathology, Heidelberg, Germany; 1913-15, interned under Harvey Cushing (q.v.), Peter Bent Brigham Hospital; 1915, surgical staff, Harvard Unit, American Ambulance Hospital, Paris; 1915-16, resident surgeon, Massachusetts General Hospital; 1916-17, studied immunology with Simon Flexner (q.v.) at Rockefeller Institute for Medical Research; 1917-18, attached to Harvard Unit Base Hospital No. 5, American Expeditionary Forces; 1919-21, resident surgeon, Peter Bent Brigham Hospital. CAREER: 1921-24, surgery faculty and director of laboratory for surgical research, Harvard Medical School; and surgical staff, Peter Bent Brigham Hospital; 1924-31, surgery faculty, Western Reserve University Medical School; and surgical staff, Lakeside Hospital, Cleveland; 1932-47, surgical faculty, Harvard Medical School; and surgical staff, Peter Bent Brigham Hospital; 1942-45, chief surgical consultant, European Theater of Operations, U.S. Army; 1945, chief, Professional Services Division, Veterans Administration; 1946-47, civilian consultant to secretary of war; 1947, acting assistant medical director, Veterans Administration; president: 1941-46, Society for Clinical Surgery; and 1947, American Surgical Association. CONTRIBUTIONS: Pioneered in thoracic and cardiac surgery. First American to operate successfully on a heart valve in a patient (1923). First person in the United States to resection successfully the pericardium for constrictive pericarditis. Announced (1934) that he had achieved permanent relief from angina pectoris through excision of normal thyroid glands; operation was soon abandoned because of resulting athyroidism. On the eve of World War II, developed a plan of medical disaster care in Mass. that served as a model for the nation. During World War II, was responsible for many organizational improvements in military surgery. After World War II, effected an improvement in Veterans Administration hospitals by arranging for affiliations with nearby university teaching hospitals and by integrating the house and senior staffs. Trained his students in surgical research methods, many of whom became leaders in their profession. With Robert Zollinger, wrote *Atlas of Surgical Operations* (1939), still perennially reedited. Helped edit several journals, including *American Heart Journal, Journal of Clinical Investigation, Surgery, American Journal of Surgery,* and *British Journal of Surgery.*

WRITINGS: "Cardiotomy and Valvulotomy for Mitral Stenosis. Experimental Observations and Clinical Notes Concerning an Operated Case with Recovery," *Boston Med. and Surg. J.* 188 (1923): 1023-27 (with Samuel Albert Levine); "Total Thyroidectomy for Angina Pectoris," *Trans., Am. Surg. Assoc.* 52 (1934): 18-38 (with Max T. Schnitker);

"Civilian Medical Defense in Massachusetts," *New England J. of Med.* 227 (1940): 7-
10. REFERENCES: David Cheever, "Elliott Carr Cutler," *Trans., Am. Surg. Assoc.* 66
(1948): 565-68; *DAB*, Supplement 4: 208-10; Miller, *BHM*, p. 26; *NCAB*, 36: 327-28;
N.Y. Times, August 17, 1947; Mark M. Ravitch, *A Century of Surgery*, 2 vols. (1981);
Frederick P. Ross, "Master Surgeon, Teacher, Soldier, and Friend: Elliott Carr Cutler,
M.D. (1888-1947)," *Am. J. of Surg.* 137, no. 4 (Apr. 1979): 428-32; *Who Was Who in
Am.*, 2: 141.

S. Galishoff

CUTTER, AMMI RUHAMAH (March 4, 1735, North Yarmouth, Maine-
December 8, 1820, Portsmouth, N.H.). *Physician.* Son of Rev. Ammi Ruhamah
and Dorothy (Bradbury) Cutter. Married Hannah Treadwell, 1758; ten children.
EDUCATION: Cambridge Latin School; 1752, A.B., Harvard College; c. 1752-
55, pupil of Dr. Clement Jackson, Portsmouth; 1792, M.D. (hon.), Harvard.
CAREER: 1755-58, 1775-76, regimental surgeon; 1777-78 physician-general,
Eastern Department, Continental Army; practiced in Portsmouth until his death;
1773, justice of the peace; 1774, Governor's Council; New Hampshire Medical
Society: 1791, charter member; and 1799-1811, president. CONTRIBUTIONS: Although not an innovator in medical science or practice, was an opinion leader
in New England, as recognized by his honorary degrees and his honorary fellowship in the Massachusetts Medical Society (1783). Name appears frequently
in the correspondence of New England physicians of his era. REFERENCES: Kelly
and Burrage (1928); *Sibley's Harvard Graduates* 13: (1965): 220-25.

J. W. Estes

D

DaCOSTA, JACOB MENDEZ (February 7, 1833, Island of St. Thomas, West Indies-September 11, 1900, Villanova, Pa.). *Physician: Internal medicine.* Son of John Mendez DaCosta, gentleman. Married Sarah Frederica Brinton, 1860; two sons. EDUCATION: Gymnasium, Dresden, Germany; 1849-52, apprenticed to Thomas D. Mütter; 1852, M.D., Jefferson Medical College; 1852-53, 18 months postgraduate training in Europe, principally Paris, but also in Vienna and other cities. CAREER: 1853-61, physician, Moyamensing Dispensary; 1861-65, acting assistant surgeon, U.S. Army; and physician at Turner's Lane Hospital, Philadelphia, Pa.; 1865-1900, visiting physician, Pennsylvania Hospital; at Jefferson Medical College, Philadelphia: 1866-72, lecturer on clinical medicine; 1872-91, professor of theory and practice of medicine; and 1891-1900, professor emeritus. CONTRIBUTIONS: By research, writings, and teaching, was influential in the emergence of internal medicine as a specialty. Earliest research was on the pathological anatomy of pneumonia (1855) and pancreatic cancer (1857, 1858). Also made important clinical investigations on typhus (1866), lithemia (1881), the relationship of disease of the kidneys and heart disease (1888), and typhoid fever (1898). Instrumental in resolving the confusion surrounding J. J. Woodward's (q.v.) concept of typhomalarial fever, publishing on the subject repeatedly after 1878. Most enduring clinical contribution was Civil War research on the irritable heart, or neurocirculatory asthenia, in soldiers (published 1871). Greatest contribution to American medicine was clinical instruction; began private teaching of clinical medicine (1853), particularly physical diagnosis, and exerted an increasing influence until retirement (1891). Continued limited ward teaching at the Pennsylvania Hospital until his death. Among many published clinical lectures, perhaps the best known is his description of phantom tumors (1871). His monograph *Medical Diagnosis* (1864) was the first complete guide of its kind and went through nine editions in his lifetime. Instrumental in the founding of the Pathological Society of Philadelphia (1857). In retirement, served as a consultant and supporter of the reform of medical education at the University of Pennsylvania, becoming a trustee of the University (1899).

WRITINGS: *Medical Diagnosis, with Special Reference to Practical Medicine* (1864); "On Irritable Heart; a Clinical Study of a Form of Functional Cardiac Disorder and Its Consequences," *Am. J. of Med. Sci.* 61 (1871): 17-52; "Clinical Lecture on Spurious or 'Phantom' Tumors of the Abdomen," *Phila. Med. Times* 1 (1871): 449-51. Many of DaCosta's lectures and papers are listed in the *Index Catalogue*, 1st and 2nd series, but there is no complete bibliography. REFERENCES: H. M. Beumen, "Medizingeschichte des hyperventilations-syndroms," *Med. Welt* (Stuttgart, Germany) 25 (1974): 471-73; Mary A. Clarke, "Memoir of J. M. DaCosta, M.D.," *Am. J. of Med. Sci.* 125 (1903): 318-29; *DAB*, 5: 24-25; "Jacob Mendez DaCosta (1833-1900), Clinician of Jefferson Medical College," *JAMA* 202 (1967): 837-38; S. Jarcho, "Functional Heart Disease in the Civil War," *Am. J. of Cardiology* 4 (1979): 809-17; Kelly and Burrage (1920), 277-78; *NCAB*, 9: 342; J. C. Wilson, "Memoir of J. M. DaCosta, M.D.," *Trans., Coll. of Physicians of Phila.* 24 (1902): lxxxi-xcii.

D. C. Smith

DAILEY, ULYSSES GRANT (August 3, 1885, Donaldsonville, La.-April 22, 1961, Chicago, Ill.). *Surgeon.* Son of Tony Hanna and Missouri (Johnson) Dailey. Married Eleanor Jane Curtis, 1916; two children. EDUCATION: Straight College (now Dillard University); 1906, M.D., Northwestern University; 1906-8, intern, Provident Hospital, Chicago; 1912, 1925-26, postgraduate study, European medical centers. CAREER: 1906-8, assistant demonstrator in anatomy, Northwestern University Medical School; 1907-8, ambulance surgeon, Chicago civil service; at Provident Hospital Dispensary, Chicago: 1907-12, gynecologist; and 1910-12, associate surgeon; 1912-26, attending surgeon, Provident Hospital; 1916-18, instructor, clinical surgery, Chicago Medical College; 1920-26, attending surgeon, Fort Dearborn Hospital, Chicago; 1926-32, founder and surgeon-in-chief, Dailey Hospital and Sanitarium, Chicago; 1932-61, senior attending surgeon, Provident Hospital. CONTRIBUTIONS: An important, long-time leader in black organized medicine. Associated with *JNMA* in various editorial capacities (1910-61). Served NMA as president (1915-16). A founder-member, John A. Andrew Clinical Society, Tuskegee, Ala. Gave lectures and clinics to black physicians around the country. Did health organizational work in Pakistan and Haiti (1950s).

WRITINGS: Some 60 publications, in *JNMA* and other journals. "Total Congenital Absence of the Vermiform Appendix," *J. Surg., Gynecol. and Obstet.* 11 (1910): 413-16; "A Safe and Efficient Plan of Surgical Treatment for Prostatic Obstruction," *JNMA* 12 (1920): 3-8; "Recent Trends in World Medicine," *JNMA* 47 (1955): 367. Writings listed in *JNMA* 28 (1936): 94; *Index Medicus*, 3rd series, 2 (1922): 561, 913. REFERENCES: *Am. Men of Med.* (1961), 157; "Dr. Ulysses Grant Dailey Receives Distinguished Service Award for 1949," *JNMA* 42 (1950): 39-40; *JNMA* 7, (1915): 290; 52 (1960): 309-10; 53 (1961): 432; John A. Kenney, *The Negro in Medicine* (1912), 22-23; *WWAPS* (1938), 274; *WWICA*, 7 (1950): 132.

T. Savitt

DALTON, JOHN CALL (February 2, 1825, Chelmsford, Mass.-February 12, 1889, New York, N.Y. *Physician; Physiologist.* Son of John Call, physician, and Julia Ann (Spalding) Dalton. Never married. EDUCATION: 1844, A.B., Harvard College; 1847, M.D., Harvard Medical School; 1847-50, study and practice, Boston, Mass.; 1850, studied in Paris under Claude Bernard. CAREER: 1851-54, professor of physiology and morbid anatomy, University of Buffalo; 1854-56, professor of physiology, Vermont College of Medicine; at College of Physicians and Surgeons, N.Y.: 1855-89, professor of physiology; and 1883-89, president; 1859-61, professor of physiology, Long Island College Hospital; 1861-64, brigade surgeon, Seventh New York Volunteers, U.S. Army. CONTRIBUTIONS: The first full-time professor of physiology in an American medical school, introduced Claude Bernard's methods of research and teaching to the United States. After returning from Paris, where he worked on the secretion of bile and the fermentation of sugar by the liver, essay "The Corpus Luteum of Pregnancy" won a prize offered by the American Medical Association (1851). The same year, at Buffalo, delivered the first lectures in the United States during which experiments on animals were performed. At the College of Physicians and Surgeons, organized what was called the "first permanent physiological laboratory in the United States" which evolved into a modern research laboratory (by the 1880s). Textbook *Treatise on Human Physiology* (1859) was used by most American medical schools and had seven editions (by 1882). Active in campaigns to legalize the use of animals in experiments. According to Dr. S. Weir Mitchell (q.v.), had the "rare gift of making those who listened desire to become investigators."

WRITINGS: In addition to writing textbook for medical students, wrote a *Treatise on Physiology and Hygiene for Schools* (1868), which was translated into French. Other books include *The Experimental Method in Medicine and Science* (1882), *Doctrines of the Circulation* (1884), and *The Topographical Anatomy of the Brain* (1885). The best list of his writings is in the *Author Catalogue*, New York Academy of Medicine. REFERENCES: William B. Atkinson, *Physicians and Surgeons of the U.S.* (1878); *DAB* 5: 40; *DSB*, 15, Supplement 1 (1978): 107-10; Kelly and Burrage (1928), 287-88; Walter J. Meek, "The Beginnings of American Physiology," *Annals of Med. Hist.* 10 (1928): 111-25; "MD Remembers: A Pioneer Physiologist," *MD Medical Newsmagazine* 19 (1975): 76; S. Weir Mitchell, "Memoir of John Call Dalton," *BMNAS* 3 (1895): 177-85; *NCAB*, 10: 500; Byron Stookey, "A Lost Neurological Society with Great Expectations," *J. Hist. Med. & Allied Sci.* 16 (1961): 280-91.

D. M. Fox

DAMESHEK, WILLIAM (May 22, 1900, Semlianski, Russia-October 7, 1969, New York, N.Y.). *Physician; Hematology.* Son of Isadore, hatmaker, and Bessie Dameshek. Family immigrated to the United States, 1903. Married Rose Thurman, 1923; one child. EDUCATION: Entered Harvard Medical School after two years at Harvard College, M.D., 1923; 1923-25, intern, Boston City Hospital, where he worked under R. C. Larrabee in one of first "blood" laboratories. CAREER: 1926-27, 1939-66, medicine faculty, Tufts Medical School; 1928-39: established and directed Hematology Laboratory, Beth Israel Hospital, Brookline, Mass.; director, Blood Research Laboratory, and chief of hematology, Pratt Diagnostic Hospital (later New England Medical Center); and hematologist-in-chief, Boston Dispensary and Boston Floating Hospital; 1966-69, attending

178

DANA, CHARLES LOOMIS

hematologist, Mt. Sinai Hospital, New York City; and professor of medicine emeritus, Mt. Sinai Hospital Medical School; died unexpectedly while undergoing surgery for a ruptured aneurism of the aorta. CONTRIBUTIONS: Honored as "the father of hematology." Through his research, teaching, as founding editor of *Blood* (1946), and prime mover in American Society of Hematology (1956), contributed greatly to transforming the scientific study of blood from its emphasis on morphology to a biomedical discipline based on physiology, biochemistry, and nuclear physics. From his first hematology paper on the clinical significance of reticulated blood cells (1926) to his later research on auto-immune disorders, challenged established views and championed innovation. Advocacy of bone marrow aspiration contributed to making this a standard diagnostic procedure. Early studies of agranulocytosis and of hemolytic syndromes led to fruitful research and publication throughout his life, most often in collaboration with his students. Opposing total body radiation as a means of combatting rejection of bone marrow transplants, with R. Schwartz, demonstrated the potential of antimetabolites to inhibit antibody formation (1959). A colorful lecturer of international reputation, coined words such as "hypersplenism" and "auto-immunity" that are now part of our medical vocabulary. Was suspicious of public health involvement in cancer control, which he termed a pernicious forerunner of "State Medicine" (1931).

WRITINGS: "Acute Hemolytic Anemia (Acquired Hemolytic Icterus, Acute Type)," *Medicine* 19 (1940): 231 (with S. O. Schwartz); "Hemolytic Mechanisms," *Annals, N.Y. Acad. of Sci.* 77 (1959): 589. Six books including *The Hemorrhagic Disorders* (1955) and *Leukemia* (1958; 3rd ed., 1970; with Frederick W. Gunz). Bibliography for 1922-60 in *Blood* 15 (May 1960): 585-95. REFERENCES: *Blood* 35 (1970): 577-82; William H. Crosby, "A Biographical Comment," *Blood* 15 (1960): 580-84, an issue honoring Dameshek's 60th birthday; *Who Was Who in Am.*, 5: 168.

B. G. Rosenkrantz

DANA, CHARLES LOOMIS (March 25, 1852, Woodstock, Vt.-December 12, 1935, Harmon, N.Y.). *Physician; Neurology.* Son of Charles and Charitie Scott (Loomis) Dana. Married Lillian Gray Farlee, 1882; three children. EDUCATION: 1872, A.B., Dartmouth College; 1873, apprenticed to Dr. Boynton, Woodstock; 1876, M.D., National Medical College (later Columbian University Medical College, now George Washington University Medical School); 1877, M.D., College of Physicians and Surgeons, N.Y. CAREER: 1872-73, private secretary to Senator Justin Morrill and then to Spencer Fullerton Baird (secretary, Smithsonian Institution); 1877-78, house staff, Bellevue Hospital, N.Y.; 1879, assistant surgeon, U.S. Marine Hospital Corps, N.Y.; 1880-87, professor of physiology, Women's Medical College, N.Y.; 1883-98, professor of diseases of the mind and nervous system, New York Post-Graduate Medical School; 1898-1933, professor of diseases of the nervous system, Cornell University Medical College, N.Y.; president: 1892, American Neurological Association; and 1905-6, 1914-16, New York Academy of Medicine. CONTRIBUTIONS: Among the first neurologists to apply to his field of interest, in his teaching and practice, the results of investigations in general pathology. Carried out extensive studies in pathological neurology, investigating (among other topics) scleroses of the spinal cord. Advised at the trial of assassin Charles J. Guiteau. Studied neurology of alcoholism.

WRITINGS: *Text Book of Nervous Diseases: Being a Compendium for the Use of Students and Practitioners of Medicine* (1892; 10th ed., 1925); *The Peaks of Medical History: An Outline of the Evolution of Medicine for the Use of Medical Students and Practitioners* (1926; 2nd ed., 1928). REFERENCES: *DAB*, Supplement 1: 220-21; bibliography, *J. of Nervous and Mental Diseases* (1936); *NCAB*, 13: 528; *NUC Pre-1956 Imprints*, 132: 162-63; *N.Y. Times*, December 13, 1935, p. 25; Philip Van Ingen, *The New York Academy of Medicine: Its First Hundred Years* (1949).

M. M. Sokal

DANA, ISRAEL THORNDIKE (June 6, 1827, Marblehead, Mass.-April 13, 1904, Portland, Maine). *Physician; Heart and lung diseases.* Son of Samuel, Congregational minister, and Henrietta (Bridge) Dana. Married Carrie Jane Starr, 1854, nine children; Carolina Peck Lyman, 1876, one child. EDUCATION: After graduating from Marblehead Academy, spent two years in a Boston business office; 1847, began the study of medicine in Boston and entered Tremont Medical School; 1850, received a degree from Harvard Medical School after having taken his first, third, and fourth courses of lectures there and his second course at the College of Physicians and Surgeons in N.Y.; two years postgraduate study in Paris, and in Dublin, served as resident assistant physician, Rotunda Lying-in Hospital. CAREER: 1852, opened practice, Portland; 1860, appointed professor of materia medica, Maine Medical School; 1862, volunteer assistant surgeon, Armory Square Hospital, Washington, D.C.; 1862-70, 1880-92, professor of theory and practice, Maine Medical School; for years, attending physician, Maine General Hospital, Portland, and taught physiology, pathology, and practice, Portland Medical School for Preparatory Instruction. CONTRIBUTIONS: A founder and first president, Portland Clinical Society. A founder, Portland Dispensary for the treatment of the poor. Helped create the Portland Medical School for Preparatory Instruction (1856). A founder, Maine General Hospital (1875). President, Cumberland County Medical Society and Maine Medical Society.

WRITINGS: "Renewal or Restorative Principle in the Treatment of Disease," *Maine Med. Assoc. Trans.* (1867): 120-27; "Defective Drainage and Sewerage as a Source of Disease," *ibid.* (1871): 157-75; *History of the Portland School for Medical Instruction* (1874); "The Pathology of Pulmonary Phthisis," Maine Med. Assoc. Trans. (1880): 132-47; "The Treatment of Chronic Bright's Disease," *ibid.* (1885): 546-54; "Apoplectiform Seizures; Diagnosis of Different Forms and Their Treatment" (1889); "The Sequelae of Pneumonia" (1893). Wrote an article about dropsy that was published in the *Reference Handbook of the Medical Sciences*. REFERENCES: Bowdoin College Obituary Record (1904), 281-83; Richard Herndon, *Men of Progress* (1897), 20-21; Howard Kelly, *Cyclopedia of Am. Med. Biog.* 1 (1912): 223-24; Maine Historical Society Collection #85, Records of the Portland School for Medical Instruction, 1871-1904; Maine

Historical Society Collection #513, Maine Physicians, compiled by James Spalding; Maine Historical Society Obituary Scrapbook, 1: 59; 6: 8; Maine Historical Society Post Scrapbook, 4: 210; 5: 6-8; *Maine Med. Soc. Trans.* (1904): 194-96; *Who Was Who in Am.,* 1: 292.

B. Lister

DANDY, WALTER EDWARD (April 6, 1886, Sedalia, Mo.-April 19, 1946, Baltimore, Md.). *Physician*; *Neurosurgery*. Son of John, railroad engineer, and Rachel (Kilpatrick) Dandy. Married Sadie Estelle Martin, 1924; four children. EDUCATION: 1907, A.B., University of Missouri; at Johns Hopkins: 1910, M.D.; and 1911, M.A.; 1911-12, studied under Harvey Cushing (q.v.), Johns Hopkins. CAREER: 1914-46, surgery faculty, Johns Hopkins Medical School; 1911-46, surgery staff, Johns Hopkins Hospital. CONTRIBUTIONS: Considered by many to have been the greatest neurosurgeon of his time. With Kenneth Blackfan (q.v.), elucidated the pathophysiology of hydrocephalus and its diagnosis and treatment by surgery (1913). Introduced air contrast ventriculography for the diagnosis and localization of brain tumors (1918); has been called the single greatest advance in brain surgery. Developed pneumoencephalography for X-raying the subarachnoid space, which is sometimes affected by brain lesions (1918). Devised a procedure for the total removal of tumors of the acoustic nerve (1922). Introduced surgical procedures for the treatment of painful facial neuralgias (1925). Developed an operation that was highly successful in the treatment of Ménière's disease, an affliction that causes extreme dizziness, nausea, and deafness in one ear (1928). Found surgical cures for intracranial aneurysms. Demonstrated that a ruptured vertebral disk is often the cause of low backaches and sciaticas and devised tests and operations for this ailment. Designed a protective helmet for professional baseball players (1941).

WRITINGS: "An Experimental and Clinical Study of Internal Hydrocephalus," *JAMA* 61 (1913): 2216-17 (with K. D. Blackfan); "Ventriculography Following the Injection of Air into the Cerebral Ventricles," *Annals of Surg.* 68 (Jul. 1918): 5; "An Operation for the Total Extirpation of Tumors in the Cerebello-pontine Angle . . . ," *Johns Hopkins Hosp. Bull.* 33 (Sept. 1922): 344; "Ménière's Disease: Its Diagnosis and a Method of Treatment," *Arch. of Surg.* 16 (Jun. 1928): 1127-52. Most important professional papers are published in Charles E. Troland and Frank J. Otenasek, eds., *Selected Writings of Walter E. Dandy* (1957). REFERENCES: *BHM* (1970-74), 45; (1975-79), 33; (1980), 11; *DAB*, Supplement 4: 213-15; A. M. Harvey, in *Johns Hopkins Med. J.* 135 (1974): 358-68; Miller, *BHM*, p. 27; *NCAB*, 35: 8-9; *N.Y. Times*, April 20, 1946; *Who Was Who in Am.,* 2: 143.

S. Galishoff

DANIEL, RICHARD POTTS (August 19, 1828, Pineville, Charleston District, S.C.-April 10, 1915, Jacksonville, Fla.). *Physician*; *General practice*. Son of James Madison and Jaqueline (Smith) Daniel. Married Isabel Fernandez, one son; Evalina Fernandez, sister of first wife; Ella G. Christopher, 1886. EDUCATION: Columbia, S.C., public schools; read medicine under preceptorate of

Dr. H. D. Holland, Jacksonville; 1848-49, student, Medical College of South Carolina; 1851, M.D., University of Pennsylvania. CAREER: 1851-54, general practice, Jacksonville; 1854-59, commissioned and served as assistant surgeon, U.S. Navy; returned to practice in Jacksonville; 1862-65, surgeon, Eighth Florida Regiment, Confederate Army; with General Lee in Army of Northern Virginia until surrender at Appomattox; for remainder of life, general practice, Jacksonville. CONTRIBUTIONS: Close observer of yellow fever while on naval duty, St. Thomas Island (1855), and aboard ship, having himself survived an attack of the disease. Made careful study of yellow fever; was regarded as a leading authority on its treatment. Among first to shun traditional use of phlebotomy and large dosages of calomel and other debilitating procedures. Became a local hero for unselfish and indefatigable attention to yellow-fever victims in Jacksonville epidemic of 1888. A founder of Florida Medical Association (1874), becoming its president (1879). Joined Drs. John P. Wall (q.v.) and Joseph Y. Porter (q.v.) in pressing for legislative enactment creating a State Board of Health (1889), a measure long delayed by a parsimonious Fla. legislature. First president, State Board of Health. President and chief of staff, St. Luke's Hospital, Jacksonville. A founder and sometime president, Duval County Medical Society.

WRITINGS: Several papers read before members of Fla. Med. Assoc., published in *Proc.*: "Cutaneous Diseases" (1880); "Presidential Address" (1880); "Yellow Fever Epidemic in Jacksonville" (1888); "A Plea for Professional Unity" (1902). Also, Daniel's "Journal," a detailed medical record, kept while he was navy surgeon aboard the *San Jacinto*, 1 vol. (1855-58), microfilm, 164 pp., Southern Historical Collection, item M-1871, Library, University of North Carolina, Chapel Hill, N.C. REFERENCES: Webster Merritt, *A Century of Medicine in Jacksonville and Duval County* (1949), 45-49; obituary notice, *Florida Times-Union* (Jacksonville), April 12, 1915; *Proc., Fla. Med. Assoc.* (1874-1902); Rowland P. Rerick, *Memoirs of Florida* 1 (1902): 503-4.

E. A. Hammond

DARLINGTON, WILLIAM (April 28, 1782, Dilworthtown, Pa.-April 23, 1863, West Chester, Pa.). *Physician; Scientist; Politician.* Son of Edward, farmer, road surveyor, and state representative, and Rachael (Townsend) Darlington. Married Katharine Lacey; five surviving children. EDUCATION: Studied with Dr. John Vaughan, Wilmington, Del.; 1804, M.D., University of Pennsylvania. CAREER: 1806-8, ship surgeon; medical practice for 35 years although often diverted by political activities; member: 1815-22, U.S. House of Representatives; and 1826-27, Pennsylvania Canal Commission; 1830-32, designed and engineered road from the Delaware River to the Susquehanna River; 1830-63, president, Bank of Chester County; 1828-63, founder and president, Chester County Cabinet of Natural Science (now West Chester State College); 1855, founder, Teacher's Institute; 1830-44, founder and president, West Chester Railroad; 1814-28, organizer and officer, West Chester Grays, an official militia organization that became the Republican Artillerists. CONTRIBUTIONS: Aside from extensive political and civic responsibilities, practiced medicine for 35 years in

West Chester. Botanical studies of local plant life and weed introduction (1826-53); assessed the medicinal value of botanical remedies (1854). Helped organize the Pennsylvania State Medical Society and served as delegate to the AMA convention of 1851. A well-known public speaker, advocated prison reform (with Dorothea Dix [q.v.]) and women in medicine (with Ann Preston [q.v.]). WRITINGS: *Florula Cestrica* (1826); *Agricultural Botany* (1847); "Medical Botany," *Chester (Del.) Med. Recorder* (1854). Works listed in J. S. Futhey and G. Cope, *Hist. of Chester County, Pa.* (1881); H. S. Pleasants, *Three Scientists from Chester County* (1936); Hugh Stone, *The Flora of Chester County* (1936). REFERENCES: *DAB*, 5:78-79; *DSB*, 3: 562-63; Futhey and Cope, *History of Chester County*; T. P. James, *Memorial of William Darlington* (1853); Kelly and Burrage (1920); D. I. Lansing, *William Darlington* (1965); D. I. Lansing et al., *William Darlington: A Commemorative* (1965); Pleasants, *Three Scientists*; W. Townsend, *Memoir of Dr. William Darlington* (1853).

D. I. Lansing

DARROW, EDWARD McLAREN (January 15, 1855, Neenah, Wis.-November 25, 1919, Fargo, N. Dak.). *Physician; Surgeon.* Son of Daniel C., farmer and contractor, and Isabelle (Murray) Darrow. Married Clara Dillon, 1879; six children. EDUCATION: 1874-75, medical study with Dr. Thomas Russell, Oshkosh, Wis.; 1878, M.D., Rush Medical College. CAREER: 1878-1919, physician and surgeon, Fargo, Dak. Territory, and N.Dak.; 1878, founder, first hospital, Cass County (now St. John's Hospital); 1880, charter member, Red River Medical Association (now Cass County Medical Association); 1885-87, first superintendent of public health, Dak. Territory; 1887, organizational member, North Dakota Medical Association; 1891-92, 1905-6, 1907-12, surgeon-general, N.Dak.; 1919, co-founder, Dakota Clinic, Fargo. CONTRIBUTIONS: Led campaign against typhoid in frontier Red River Valley. Instigator of movement to improve municipal water supplies. As first superintendent of public health for Dak. Territory, instituted medical licensing practices and was issued one of the first licenses. Leader in N.Dak. work to improve care for mentally ill. Eminent physician, surgeon, and diagnostician. At time of death, was hailed as "the prince of general practitioners." REFERENCES: *Compendium of Hist. and Biog. of North Dakota* (1900), 484; *Fargo Forum*, November 25, 1919, p.1; February 24, 1963, p. B-10; March 3, 1963, p. C-8.

L. Remele

DAVIDGE, JOHN BEALE (1768, Annapolis, Md.-August 23, 1829, Baltimore, Md.). *Physician; Surgeon; Teacher.* Son of Capt. Henry, British army, and Honor (Howard) Davidge. Married Wilhelmina Stuart, 1793, one son; after her death, Rebecca Troup Polk, three daughters. EDUCATION: 1789, A.M., St. John's College, Annapolis; studied under Drs. James and William Murray, Annapolis; then attended lectures, Philadelphia, Edinburgh, and Glasgow; 1793, M.D., Glasgow (with a specialty in anatomy). CAREER: After graduation from Glasgow, practiced medicine briefly, Birmingham, England, before moving to Baltimore; 1801, attending physician, Baltimore General Dispensary; 1802-7, offered private lectures in anatomy, surgery, obstetrics, and physiology, Baltimore; 1807, with the aid of Drs. James Cocke and John Shaw, obtained a charter for his school, which then became the College of Medicine of Maryland; 1813, by an 1812 charter, the state legislature established the University of Maryland, and Davidge's school became the medical department; 1805, orator, Medical and Chirurgical Faculty of Maryland (delivered the society's first annual oration); 1807-29, chair of anatomy and surgery, University of Maryland (where he provided, as a gift, an anatomical theater that was subsequently demolished by an antivivisectionist mob); 1807-11, 1813, 1814, 1821, dean, College of Medicine of Maryland; 1823, editor, *Baltimore Philosophical Journal and Review* (the journal survived only one year). CONTRIBUTIONS: Made major contribution to public discussion (lay and professional) on causes of yellow fever (1797-98)—this in response to epidemic that ravaged Baltimore and other Atlantic Seaboard cities in 1797. In surgery, noted for his amputation at the shoulder joint (1792). Credited as being the first to ligate the gluteal artery, which he did for aneurysm. Also ligated the carotid artery for "fungus of the antrum." Perhaps the first to achieve complete surgical removal of the parotid gland (1823); most importantly, is considered the inventor of the "American method" of amputation. With Drs. James Cocke and John Shaw, founded the College of Medicine of Maryland (1807).

WRITINGS: *De Causis Catameniorum* (1794); *A Treatise on the Autumnal Endemial Epidemick of Tropical Climates, Vulgarly Called the Yellow Fever . . . with a Few Reflections on the Proximate Cause of the Diseases* (1798); *Physical Sketches or Outlines of Correctives, Applied to Certain Modern Errours in Physick*, 2 vols. (1814-16). Edited Edward Nathaniel Bancroft's *An Essay on the Disease Called Yellow Fever* (1821). Writings listed in the *Index Catalogue*, 1st series, 3; 604, and J. R. Quinan, *Medical Annals of Baltimore . . .* (1884), 90. REFERENCES: George H. Callcott, *History of the University of Maryland* (1982), 19-21, 108-12; E. F. Cordell, *Historical Sketch of the University of Maryland* (1891); idem, *The Medical Annals of Maryland* (1903), 371; *DAB*, 5: 91; John Duffy, *The Healers . . .* (1976), 170; Kelly and Burrage (1928), 928; *NCAB*, 22: 330-31; Quinan, *Medical Annals of Baltimore*, pp. 89-90; *Who Was Who in Am.*, Hist. Vol.: 205.

C. Donegan

DAVIDSON, HENRY ALEXANDER (May 27, 1905, Newark, N. J.-August 23, 1973, East Orange, N.J.). *Physician*; *Psychiatrist*; *Medical editor*. Son of Louis L., physician, and May (Tannenbaum) Davidson. Married Adelaide Heyman, 1936; two children. EDUCATION: 1925, A.B., Columbia University; 1928, M.D., Jefferson Medical College; 1931, M.S. (neuropsychiatry), University of Pennsylvania; 1929-31, intern, Beth Israel Hospital, Newark; resident physician, Orthopedic Hospital and Infirmary for Nerve Disease, Philadelphia, Pa. CAREER: 1931-42, private practice, Newark; lecturer on law and psychiatry, Columbia University; lecturer on legal medicine, Medical College of Virginia; 1942-47, officer, U.S. Army Medical Corps; 1947-50, chief of psychiatry, Veterans Administration Office for New Jersey; 1950-54, head, Program Development for Psychiatric Services, Veterans Administration, Washington, D.C.; 1957-69, medical director, Essex County (N.J.) Hospital Center; president, New Jersey Medico-Legal Society and New Jersey Psychiatric Association; 1957-72, superintendent, Essex County Overbrook Hospital; died suddenly of coronary arterial occlusion. CONTRIBUTIONS: Leader in forensic psychiatry. Served on editorial boards, *Journal of the American Psychiatric Association* and *Medical Insights*. As editor of the *Journal of the Medical Society of New Jersey* (1939-51), publication was intended to be a "practitioner's book" rather than a "showcase for brilliant research."

WRITINGS: *Forensic Psychiatry* (1952); *Guide to Medical Writing* (1957). REFERENCES: David L. Cowen, *Medicine and Health in New Jersey: A History* (1964), 116; "Henry A. Davidson, M.D., 1905-1973," *J. of the Med. Soc. of New Jersey* 70 (1973): 725, 796-97; *JAMA* 227 (1974): 94; *The Jewish News—New Jersey*, August 30, 1973; *News* (Newark), November 27, 1949; April 25, 1954; *N. Y. Times*, August 24, 1973; "We Point With Pride," *J. of the Med. Soc. of New Jersey* 63 (1966): 185-88; *Who Was Who in Am.*, 6:104.

W. Barlow

DAVIS, ABRAHAM ISAIAH (March 4, 1877, Sturgis, Miss.-October 20, 1973, Oklahoma City, Okla.). *Physician.* Son of Peter Scott, farmer, and Edith (Davis) Davis. Married Nattie Armeade Pegram, 1902 (d. 1944), two children; Lucile Thompson, 1946, no children. EDUCATION: Rust College; 1902, M.D., Meharry Medical College. CAREER: 1902-7, private practice and drug store operator, Wagoner, Indian Territory (Okla.); 1905 (five months), private practice, Coffeyville, Kans.; private practice and drug store operator: 1907-10, Ardmore, Okla.; and 1910-73, Oklahoma City (sold the drug store about 1911 or 1912). CONTRIBUTIONS: One of the first black physicians to settle and practice in the territory and then the new state of Okla. Served the medical needs of black Oklahomans for 70 years, often without payment. REFERENCES: W. Montague Cobb, "Abraham Isaiah Davis, M.D., 1877-1973," *JNMA* 66 (1974): 176-78.

T. Savitt

DAVIS, GEORGE GILBERT (January 4, 1879, Chicago, Ill.-April 21, 1956, Anchorage, Alaska). *Physician; Surgeon; Industrial Medicine.* Son of Charles G. and Isabella (Braden) Davis. Married Mary Nellingham, 1938. EDUCATION: 1901, B.A., University of Chicago; 1904, M.D., Rush Medical College; 1905, interned at Chicago Presbyterian Hospital; 1906-7, pursued postgraduate work in Vienna, Austria, and Berlin. CAREER: 1907-12, private practice; 1913-14, assistant professor of surgery, University of Philippines; 1917-19, colonel, U.S. Army Reserve; 1919-43, private practice, Chicago; surgery faculty, Rush Medical College; 1943, appointed chief of staff, Alaska Railroad base hospital; 1943-56, medical officer, Alaska Native Service; 1943-55, private practice, Anchorage; 1955, retired. CONTRIBUTIONS: Wrote extensively on industrial medicine, particularly pneumonokonioses and injuries. Moved to Alaska late in life, where he provided care to native population.

WRITINGS: Two books and 28 articles in medical journals; "Lever Action in the Production of Traumatic Dislocation," *Surg., Gynec., and Obst.* 15 (1912): 273; *The Pneumonokonioses: Literature and Laws* (1934); "Gas Bacillus Infection," *Indust. Med.* 5 (1936): 234 (with H. A. Hanelin); "Torsion of Undescended Testicle," *ibid.*: 66. REFERENCES: *Anchorage Times*, April 21, 1956, p. 1; April 23, 1956, p. 1; *Who's Important in Medicine* (1952).

A. R. C. Helms

DAVIS, HENRY GASSETT (November 4, 1807, Trenton, Me.-November 18, 1896, Everett, Mass.). *Orthopedic surgeon.* Son of Isaac, manufacturer, and Polly (Rice) Davis. Married Ellen W. Deering, 1856; three children. ED-UCATION: 1839, M.D., Yale Medical School, with clinical training at Bellevue Hospital, New York City. CAREER: 1839-c. 1854, general medical and surgical practice at Millbury and Worcester, Mass.; *post* 1854, moved to New York City where he specialized in orthopedic surgery. CONTRIBUTIONS: Pioneering orthopedic surgeon and founder of the "traction school" of conservative orthopedic surgery. Used weights and pulleys for traction treatment of fractures. Opened a private hospital in New York City for his patients who came from around the globe. First to devise a splint for traction and the protection of the hipjoint. Followers included Lewis A. Sayre (q.v.), Charles Fayette Taylor (q.v.), and Edward Hickling Bradford (q.v.), who developed orthopedic surgery in America.
WRITINGS: "On the Effect of Pressure upon Ulcerated Vertebrae," *N.Y. J. of Med.* (1859); "On the Pathological Basis of the Treatment of Joint Disease," *Am. Med. Monthly* (1862); "The American Method of Treating Joint Diseases and Deformities," *Trans. of the AMA* (1863); *Surgery, as Exhibited in Remedying Some of the Mechanical Causes that Operate Injuriously Both in Health and Disease* (1867). REFERENCES: *DAB*, 3, pt. 1: 118-19; Kelly and Burrage (1928), 301-2. *Med. Record* 68 (1905): 298-302, 868-69; A. R. Shands, "Henry Gasset Davis, A Founder of American Orthopedic Surgery, (1807-1896)," *Current Pract. in Orthopedic Surg.* 4 (1969): 3-21.

M. Kaufman

DAVIS, JOHN STAIGE (January 15, 1872, Norfolk, Va.-December 23, 1946, Baltimore, Md.). *Plastic surgeon.* Son of William Blackford, physician, and Mary Jane (Howland) Davis. Married Kathleen Gordon Bowdoin, 1907; three children. EDUCATION: 1895, Ph.B., Yale University; 1899, M.D., Johns Hopkins University; 1899-1900, house officer, Johns Hopkins Hospital. CAREER: 1900-1903, medical staff, Union Protestant Infirmary; *post* 1903, practiced medicine, Baltimore; 1909-46, surgical faculty, Johns Hopkins Medical School; surgical staff, Johns Hopkins Hospital; 1937, vice-president, American Surgical Association; 1945, president, American Association of Plastic Surgeons. CONTRI-BUTIONS: Developed the field of plastic and reconstructive surgery; introduced many of its basic principles and techniques; perfected the "Davis graft," in which small sections of full-thickness skin are transplanted to raw areas and allowed to grow together and cover the denuded sections; developed technique of local skin flaps for repairing deformities and blemishes around the face and jaws. Studied the physiology of circulation in skin transplantation. Summarized his work in *Plastic Surgery: Its Principles and Practice* (1919), a pioneering classic that was widely used for many years. Helped found and was active in the American Association of Plastic Surgeons, American Board of Plastic Surgery, and American College of Surgeons.

WRITINGS: "A Method of Splinting Skin Grafts," *Annals of Surg.* 49 (1909): 416-48. REFERENCES: *BHM* (1978), 9; *DAB*, Supplement 4: 220-21; *NCAB*, 36: 374-75; *N.Y. Times*, December 25, 1946; *Who Was Who in Am.*, 2: 146.

S. Galishoff

DAVIS, MICHAEL MARKS (November 19, 1879, New York, N.Y.-August 19, 1971, Sherbrooke, Quebec, Canada). *Medical economist.* Son of Michael, merchant, and Miriam Maduro (Peixotto) Davis. Married Janet Hayes, 1907, three children; Alice L. Taylor, 1951. EDUCATION: Columbia University: 1900, A.B.; and 1906, Ph.D. CAREER: 1904-9, secretary, People's Institute (N.Y.); 1910-20, director, Boston Dispensary; 1913, organizer of pay clinic for persons of modest means, Boston, Mass.; 1920-27, secretary, Committee on Dispensary Development, New York City; 1920-71, consultant in hospital organization and medical administration; 1921, organizer of pay clinic, Cornell Medical College (N.Y.); 1928-36, director of medical services, Julius Rosenwald Foundation; 1932-36, lecturer, University of Chicago; 1937-51, chairman, Committee for Research in Medical Economics. CONTRIBUTIONS: Made pioneering studies of the economic and administrative aspects of health care; one of the first persons to recognize that further improvements in the health of the American people would depend at least as much on improvements in the organization and financing of health services as on medical science itself. Revamped the Boston Dispensary; introduced scientific management into its business operations; increased the number of social workers and enhanced their patient-care responsibilities; affiliated the dispensary with local medical schools and hospitals; opened evening and children's preventive health-care clinics; developed evaluative instruments derived from the social sciences for measuring the clinic's administrative and clinical effectiveness. Established pay clinics in Boston (1913) and New York City (1921) for middle-class patients who were ineligible for charity medicine but who could not afford private care. Campaigned for health insurance and group medical practice; supported and directed studies of the costs of medical care that spurred the creation of the Blue Cross system of hospitalization insurance. Founded and edited *Medical Care*, the first American journal concerned solely with the economic and social aspects of health care.

WRITINGS: *Dispensaries* (1917, with A. R. Warner); *Immigrant Health and the Community* (1921); *Public Medical Services* (1937); *America Organizes Medicine* (1941). REFERENCES: *BHM* (1970-74), 47; *N.Y. Times*, August 27, 1971; Ralph E. Pumphrey, "Michael Davis and the Transformation of the Boston Dispensary, 1910-1920," *Bull. Hist. Med.* 49 (Winter 1975): 451-65; idem, "Michael M. Davis and the Development of the Health Care Movement, 1900-1928," *Societas* 2 (Winter 1972): 27-41; George

Rosen, "Michael M. Davis . . . Pioneer in Medical Care," *Am. J. Of Public Health* 62 (Mar. 1972): 321-23; *Who Was Who in Am.*, 5: 173.

S. *Galishoff*

DAVIS, NATHAN SMITH (January 9, 1817, Greene, N.Y.-June 16, 1904, Chicago, Ill.). *Physician; Educator; Medical statesman.* Son of Dow, farmer, and Eleanor (Smith) Davis. Married Anna Maria Parker, 1838; three children. EDUCATION: 1835-37, apprentice to Dr. Thomas Jackson, Binghamton, N.Y.; 1837, M.D., College of Physicians and Surgeons of the Western District of New York (Fairfield). CAREER: 1837-47, practiced medicine, N.Y. State; 1847-49, anatomy, medical jurisprudence faculties, College of Physicians and Surgeons (Columbia); 1849-59, physiology, general pathology, and medicine faculties, Rush Medical College; at Lind University (Chicago Medical College; Northwestern University Medical School): 1859-92, principles and practice of medicine faculty; 1866-70, president; and 1870-98, dean. CONTRIBUTIONS: Founder, American Medical Association (1847). Pioneer for the graded curriculum in medical education and a founder, medical department, Lind University (1859). A founder, Illinois General Hospital of the Lakes, first voluntary hospital in Chicago (1850), Chicago Medical Society (1850), and Illinois State Medical Society (1850). First editor, *Journal of the American Medical Association* (1883-88). Founder and first editor, *Chicago Medical Examiner* (1860-73). President, International Medical Congress (1887).

WRITINGS: *History of Medical Education and Institutions in the United States* (1851); *History of the American Medical Association from its Organization up to January, 1855* (1855); *Lectures on the Principles and Practice of Medicine* (1884; 2nd ed., 1886); *History of Medicine* (1903). Writings listed in I. N. Danforth, *The Life of Nathan Smith Davis* (1907), 88-102. REFERENCES: *BHM* (1975-79), 34; (1980), 12; *DAB* 3, pt. 1: 139; Danforth, *The Life of Nathan Smith Davis*; James B. Herrick, *Bull. of the Soc. of Med. Hist., Chicago* 4 (1928-35): 403-13; Otto Frederic Kampmeier, *J. of Med. Ed.* 34 (1959): 496-508; Kelly and Burrage (1920), 292-93; Miller, *BHM*, p. 27; *NCAB*, 35: 25-26.

W. K. *Beatty*

DAVISON, WILBURT CORNELL (April 28, 1892, Grand Rapids, Mich.-June 26, 1972, Durham, N.C.). *Physician; Medical educator; Pediatrics.* Son of William L., minister, and Mattie E. (Cornell) Davison. Married Atala Thayer Scudder, 1917; three children. EDUCATION: 1913, B.A., Princeton; 1917, M.D., Johns Hopkins; 1919-21, resident, Johns Hopkins Hospital; at Oxford University, England: 1915, A.B.; 1916, B.Sc.; and 1919, M.A. CAREER: 1914, American Red Cross, France and Serbia; 1917-19, Army Medical Corps in American Expeditionary Forces, France; 1921-27, associate professor and acting head, Department of Pediatrics, and assistant dean, Johns Hopkins University Medical School; 1927-61, dean, professor of pediatrics, Duke University School of Medicine; chairman, Duke University Medical Center. CONTRIBUTIONS: As first dean of Duke University School of Medicine, built it from a fledgling institution to a medical center of world renown (1927-61). Helped establish (1932, 1935) two of the earliest prepaid medical-care plans (Blue Cross) in the nation. Held several posts, including editor, on staff of *Bulletin of the Johns Hopkins Hospital* (1919-27). Served on numerous local, state, and national committees, panels, and advisory boards.

WRITINGS: *Pediatric Notes* (1925); *The Complete Pediatrician* (1927, and subsequent editions to 1961); numerous articles. REFERENCES: Obituary, *N.C. Med. J.* 34 (1973): 143-44; William S. Powell, *North Carolina Lives* (1962), 347-48; *Who Was Who in Am.*, 5: 174.

T. Savitt

DEAN, LEE WALLACE (March 28, 1873, Muscatine, Ia.-February 9, 1944, St. Louis, Mo.). *Physician; Otolaryngology.* Son of Henry Munson, physician, and Emma (Johnson) Dean. Married Ella May Bailey, 1904; one child. EDU-CATION: State University of Iowa: 1894, B.S.; and 1896, M.A., M.D.; 1896-97 postgraduate work, Vienna and London. CAREER: At State University of Iowa: 1898-1900, anatomy and physiology faculties; 1900-1927, otolaryngology and oral surgery faculty; and 1912-27, dean; 1917-18, U.S. Army Medical Officers' Reserves Corps, commanding officer, general hospital no. 54, Iowa City; 1927-40, otolaryngology faculty, Washington University; otolaryngology staff: Barnes, St. Louis Children's, and Jewish hospitals; McMillan Eye, Ear, Nose, and Throat Hospital; and Oscar Johnson Research Institute of St. Louis; president: 1922, American Otological Society; 1924, American Laryngological Association; and American Academy of Ophthalmology and Otolaryngology and American Laryngological, Rhinological and Otological Society. CONTRIBUTIONS: Did important research in allergy and sinus disease in children. Built strong otolaryngology departments at both the State University of Iowa and Washington University. Edited *Annals of Otology, Rhinology and Laryngology* (1927-44). Helped secure legislation in Ia. providing free medical treatment for indigent children and adults.

REFERENCES: "In Memoriam. Lee Wallace Dean," *Laryngoscope* 54 (1944): 159-63; Miller, *BHM*, p. 28; *NCAB*, 32: 511; Arthur W. Proetz, "Lee Wallace Dean, Sr., a Personal Appreciation," *Annals of Otology, Rhinology, and Laryngology* 53 (1944): 619-24; *Who Was Who in Am.*, 2: 149.

S. Galishoff

DEARHOLT, HOYT E. (March 2, 1879, Reedsburg, Wis.-July 12, 1939, Milwaukee, Wis.). *Physician; Orthopedic surgeon.* Son of Sylvester J., dry goods merchant, and Adelaide (Mackey) Dearholt. Married Edith Tweeden, 1907; two children. EDUCATION: 1900, M.D., Rush Medical College, Chicago, Ill.; 1900-1901, extended education in a N.Y. clinic; 1902, studied at the Vienna clinic of Dr. Adolf Lorenz. CAREER: 1902, began practice, Milwaukee; 1905-7, orthopedic surgeon on staff, Milwaukee County Hospital; 1906-10, staff, Milwaukee Children's Hospital; 1906, co-founder with Thomas H. Hay, River Pines Tuberculosis Sanatorium near Stevens Point, Wis.; 1910-39, executive secretary, Wisconsin Anti-Tuberculosis Association, and editor of its publication, *The Crusader*; 1913-20, associate professor and chief, Health Institute Bureau, University of Wisconsin Extension Division. CONTRIBUTIONS: A founder of the *Wisconsin Medical Journal* (1903) and managing editor (1903-10). Vice-chairman and secretary of the Wisconsin Committee of the International Congress of Tuberculosis (1907-8). A founder of the Wisconsin Anti-Tuberculosis Association (1908). Member of the Board of Directors or chairman of one of the standing committees, National Tuberculosis Association (1910-39). President of the board, Milwaukee County Tuberculosis Sanatorium (1912-15). A founder, Mississippi Valley Conference on Tuberculosis (1914), its secretary-treasurer (1919-1920), and its president (1925). President, Wisconsin State Medical Society (1916-17). Dedicated to education and dissemination of knowledge concerning the causes, treatment, and prevention of tuberculosis. Believed that tuberculosis could be cured if detected early enough and that it could be prevented by proper public health measures. Was instrumental in starting the Christmas Seal Campaign in Wis., passing the legislation enabling counties to hire public health nurses, and directing the Wisconsin Anti-Tuberculosis Association to set up clinics for the detection of tuberculosis. Encouraged the establishment of sanatoria, hospitals, and dispensaries to deal with the disease.

WRITINGS: As editor, wrote extensively for *The Crusader*; published Executive Committee reports and special studies. "The Relation of the Physician to the Public Campaign Against Tuberculosis," *Wisconsin Med. J.* 10 (1911): 65-84; "A Survey of Dunn County, Wisconsin, an Investigation of Tuberculosis in Rural Districts," *The Crusader*, no. 23 (Feb. 1912): 15-21; "Are Physicians Square with Their Tuberculosis Patients?" *Wisconsin Med. J.* 13 (1915): 333-45. REFERENCES: Louise Fenton Brand, "Beloved Chief, We Salute You!" *The Crusader* (Sept. 1939): 4-12; State Historical Society of Wisconsin, *Dict. of Wisconsin Biog.* (1960), 97-98; *Who's Who in Am.* 20 (1938-39), 721; *WWAPS* 1 (1938), 291.

M. V. H. Jones

DEAVER, JOHN BLAIR (July 25, 1855, Lancaster County, Pa.-September 25, 1931, Wyncote, Pa.). *Surgeon*. Son of Joshua Montgomery, physician, and Elizabeth (Moore) Deaver. Married Caroline Randall, 1889; four children. EDUCATION: 1878, M.D., University of Pennsylvania; intern: 1878-79, Germantown Hospital; and 1879-80, Children's Hospital. CAREER: *Post* 1880, practiced medicine, Philadelphia, Pa.; at University of Pennsylvania: 1880-99, anatomy faculty; and 1911-22, surgery faculty; 1886-1931, surgery staff, German Hospital (later Lankenau Hospital); president: 1921-22, American College of Surgeons; and 1928, Inter-State Post Graduate Medical Association of North America. CONTRIBUTIONS: Internationally known for his surgery of the head, neck, breast, and abdomen. Pioneered in the operation for appendicitis and educated physicians about the importance of early recognition and prompt surgical intervention. Made many advances in surgery of the gallbladder and biliary passages. With the Mayos (q.v.), helped move surgery from the periphery to the forefront of medical practice. A tireless operator and an outstanding teacher whose books were used in medical schools throughout the world.

WRITINGS: *A Treatise on Appendicitis* (1896); *Surgical Anatomy* (1899-1903); *Enlargement of the Prostate* (1905, with A. P. C. Ashhurst); *Surgery of the Upper Abdomen* (1909-13, with A. P. C. Ashhurst). REFERENCES: *DAB*, Supplement 1: 235-36; Miller *BHM*, p. 28; *NCAB*, 22:7; *N.Y. Times*, September 26, 1931; *Who Was Who in Am.*, 1: 308.

S. Galishoff

DeKRUIF, PAUL HENRY (March 2, 1890, Zeeland, Mich.-February 28, 1971, Holland, Mich.). *Bacteriologist; Author*. Son of Hendrik, businessman, and Hendrika J. (Kremer) DeKruif. First marriage ended in divorce; married Rhea E. Barbarin, 1922 (d. 1957), two children; Eleanor Lappage, 1959. EDUCATION: University of Michigan: 1912, B.S.; and 1916, Ph.D. CAREER: 1912-17, bacteriology faculty, University of Michigan; 1917-19, Sanitary Corps, U.S. Army; 1920-22, pathology faculty, Rockefeller Institute for Medical Research; *post* 1922, freelance writer; 1940-71, contributing editor, *Reader's Digest*. CONTRIBUTIONS: Trained as a bacteriologist. Won fame as a popular writer on medical science; authored more than a dozen books, including several best-sellers and over 200 magazine articles; three of the books made into motion pictures. During World War I, developed an antitoxin for gas gangrene. At Rockefeller Institute, did important research on hemolytic streptococcus. Published *Our Medicine Men* (1922), a book whose characters resembled those of his colleagues at the Institute. Resigned from the Institute shortly thereafter and took up writing full time. Collaborated with Sinclair Lewis on the medical aspects of his novel *Arrowsmith* (1925). Wrote *Microbe Hunters* (1926), a highly dramatized account of the lives of 14 pioneers of bacteriology, which sold more than a million copies and was translated into 18 languages. With Sidney Howard, co-authored *Yellow Jack!*— a Broadway play that depicted Walter Reed's battle against yellow fever. Worked on a 24-hour treatment for early syphilis involving the artificial inducement of fever and the use of arsenicals and bismuth (1930s).

WRITINGS: *Men Against Death* (1932); *The Fight for Life* (1938). Nonscientific writings are briefly described in *Contemporary Authors*, 9-12: 222. REFERENCES: *BHM* (1975-79), 34; *Contemporary Authors*, 9-12: 222; *Current Biog.* (1942): 186-88 (1963): 104-6; *N.Y. Times*, March 2, 1971; *Who Was Who in Am.*, 5: 178.

S. Galishoff

DELAFIELD, EDWARD (May 7, 1794, New York, N.Y.-February 13, 1875, New York). *Physician; Ophthalmology*. Third son of 11 children of John, merchant, and Ann (Hallett) Delafield. Married Eliva E. Langdon Elwyn, 1821, six children; Julie Floyd, 1839, one son, the physician Francis Delafield (q.v.). EDUCATION: Private tutoring and Union Hall Academy (Md.); 1812, A.B., Yale College; 1816, M.D., College of Physicians and Surgeons (N.Y.), after an apprenticeship with Dr. Samuel Borrowe and writing a thesis on "Pulmonary

Consumption''; 1815, assistant house surgeon, New York Hospital; 1816-18, studied in London with Sir Astley Cooper, John Richard Farr, Sir William Lawrence, and Benjamin Travers and trained at the London Infirmary for Curing Diseases of the Eye. CAREER: With Dr. John Kearny Rogers, planned and opened the New York Eye Infirmary (1818), which he served as visiting surgeon for 30 years; professor of obstetrics and diseases of women and children (1825-38) and president (1858-75), College of Physicians and Surgeons, N.Y.; founded the first society for the relief of widows and children of deceased doctors (1842). First president of the American Ophthalmological Society (1864). CONTRIBU-TIONS: Conducted the first study of the incidence of eye diseases in N.Y. and founded the first permanent outpatient clinic and hospital in the United States dedicated to their treatment. With Rogers, founded the New York Eye Infirmary ''on their own private responsibility.'' Subsequently received generous support from philanthropists and the state of N.Y. An active leader in the organization of his specialty and the medical policy of N.Y. for half a century.

WRITINGS: Not a prolific writer. Most of his few papers in medical journals are listed in the *Author Catalogue* of the New York Academy of Medicine. His influence as a teacher and medical leader is evident in Edward Delafield, *Notes of Lectures on Diseases of the Eye and on Obstetrics in the Hand of Henry S. Downs, 1832-33* (MSS. in the New York Academy of Medicine [NYAM], New York City) and idem, *Biographical Sketch of J. Kearny Rodgers, M.D.* (1852). The thoroughness with which he studied anatomy and surgery in London is evident in Edward Delafield, *Notes on Abernathy's Lectures on Anatomy* (1818; 2 vols., NYAM) and *Notes on a Course of Lectures on Surgery by Astley Cooper* (3 vols., NYAM). REFERENCES: *BHM* (1970-74), 48; *DAB* 5: 207-8; Gerald B. Kara, "History of the New York Eye and Ear Infirmary," *N.Y. State J. of Med.* 73 (1973): 2801-8; Kelly and Burrage (1928), 314-15; Miller, *BHM*, p. 28; *NCAB*, 10: 278; George Rosen, "Social Factors in the Development of Medical Specialization," *Ciba Symposium* 11 (1949): 1135-56; B. Samuels, "The Foundation of the New York Eye and Ear Infirmary," *Arch. Ophthal.* 7 (1932): 681-99.

D. M. Fox

DELAFIELD, FRANCIS (August 3, 1841, New York, N.Y.-July 17, 1915, Stamford, Conn.). *Physician; Pathology; Histology.* Son of Edward (q.v.), physician, and Julia (Floyd) Delafield. Married Katherine van Rennsselaer, 1870; three children. EDUCATION: 1860, A.B., Yale University; 1863, M.D., College of Physicians and Surgeons (Columbia); studied in London and Paris. CAREER: Post c.1864, practiced medicine, New York City; 1875-1901, pathology faculty, College of Physicians and Surgeons; 1871, pathology staff, Roosevelt Hospital; 1874, post 1885, medical staff, Bellevue Hospital; surgery staff, New York Eye and Ear Infirmary; first president, Association of American Physicians and Pathologists; consulting physician at the illness of President McKinley following assassination attempt. CONTRIBUTIONS: A prominent pathological investigator whose writings in that field were authoritative sources. Book *Studies in Pathological Anatomy* (1882) was the result of ten years of research. Other work for which he is best known, *A Handbook of Pathological Anatomy and Histology*

(1885, with T. M. Prudden [q.v.]), was used as a textbook in the great majority of American medical colleges. One of the first physicians to distinguish between acute lobar pneumonia and broncho-pneumonia (1882). Classified the diseases of the kidneys and the colon based on their pathologies and clinical features.

WRITINGS: *Manual of Physical Diagnosis* (1878); *Diseases of the Kidneys* (1895). REFERENCES: Kelly and Burrage (1928), 315-16; *DAB*, 5:208; *NCAB*, 10: 278-79; *N.Y. Times*, July 18, 1915; *Who Was Who in Am.*, 1: 311.

S. Galishoff

DELAMATER, JOHN (April 18, 1787, Chatham, N.Y.-March 28, 1867, Cleveland, Ohio). *Physician; Medical education.* Son of Jacob, farmer, and Elizabeth (Dorr) Delamater. Married; at least two children. EDUCATION: 1804-7, apprenticed to his uncle Dr. Russell Dorr, in Chatham; 1807, medical license, Medical Society of Otsego County, N.Y. CAREER: 1807-15, in private practice with various relatives in Chatham, Florida (in Montgomery County), N.Y., and Albany, N.Y.; 1815-25, practiced medicine, Sheffield, Mass.; at Berkshire Medical Institution, Pittsfield, Mass.: 1823-26, materia medica and pharmacy faculty; and 1826, obstetrics faculty; at College of Physicians and Surgeons of the Western District of New York at Fairfield: 1827-c. 1837, surgery faculty; 1837-39, physic and female diseases faculties; and 1839-40, physic and midwifery faculties; 1829-41, lecturer: 1829-34, 1840-41, Bowdoin College, Maine; 1836-40, Dartmouth Medical School; 1838-39, University of Vermont and Medical College of Ohio, Cincinnati, Ohio; and 1838-43, Medical Department of Willoughby University, Willoughby, Ohio; 1840-43, pathology and materia medica faculty, Medical Institution of Geneva, Geneva, N.Y.; 1842-44, taught at Franklin Medical College, St. Charles, Ill.; *post* 1842, lived and practiced medicine in Cleveland; at Cleveland Medical College (medical department, Western Reserve College): 1844-61, founder, dean, and pathology and obstetrics and gynecology faculties. CONTRIBUTIONS: Assisted his pupil Horace A. Ackley in the founding of Cleveland Medical College (1844). A brilliant, peripatetic lecturer on medicine who held professorships in nine medical colleges in seven states. Taught hundreds of physicians who practiced on the N.Y., New England, and Old Northwest frontiers. One of the nation's leading authorities on surgery and on obstetrics and gynecology. Performed the first excision of the scapula in the United States.

WRITINGS: "Dr. Fisher's Case [Inversion of the Womb]," *Cleveland Med. Gazette* 1 (1860): 285-300, 353-69; 2 (1861): 91-101, 138-51, 273-82, 321-29; 3 (1862): 113-14. REFERENCES: Kelly and Burrage (1928), 316-17; Miller, *BHM*, p. 28; Genevieve Miller, "Dr. John Delamater, 'True Physician,' " *J. of Med. Ed.* 34 (1959): 24-31.

S. Galishoff

DELANO, JANE ARMINDA (March 12, 1862, Townsend, N.Y.-April 15, 1919, Savenay, France). *Nurse.* Daughter of George and Mary Ann (Wright) Delano. Never married. EDUCATION: Cook Academy, Montour Falls, N.Y.; 1884-86, student, Bellevue Hospital Training School for Nurses, graduated 1886;

1896, medical studies, University of Buffalo. CAREER: 1887, private duty nurse, New York City; 1888, superintendent of nurses, Sandhills Emergency Center, near Jacksonville, Fla., during yellow-fever epidemic; 1889, superintendent of nurses, Copper Queen Mining Company Hospital, Bisbee, Ariz.; 1890-95, instructor and assistant superintendent of nurses, University of Pennsylvania nurse training school; 1900-1902, superintendent, Girls' department, New York City House of Refuge; 1902-6, superintendent, training schools, Bellevue and allied hospitals, New York City; 1906-8, resigned to care for her dying mother; 1909-19, chair, National Committee on Red Cross Nursing Service; 1909-12, superintendent, Army Nurse Corps. Died while inspecting facilities in France. CONTRIBUTIONS: As superintendent, Army Nurse Corps, replaced the Army Nursing Reserves with a Red Cross nursing service, increasing pay to attract a better quality of nursing graduate; established a nurses' aides training program. Helped supply 20,000 Red Cross nurses during World War I. President, Nurses' Associated Alumnae (1909-11); Board of Directors, *American Journal of Nursing* (1908-11); and American Nurses' Association (1909-12).

WRITINGS: *American Red Cross Textbook on Elementary Hygiene and Home Care of the Sick* (1913, with Isabel McIsaac). REFERENCES: *BHM* (1980), 12; *DAB*, 5: 218-19; L. L. Dock, *History of American Red Cross Nursing* (1922); M. E. Gladwin, *The Red Cross and J.A. Delano* (1931); P. B. Kernodle, *Red Cross Nurse in Action* (1949); Miller, *BHM*, p. 28; *NCAB*, 19: 31; *Notable Am. Women*, 1: 456-57; *N.Y. Times*, April 17, May 4, and 21, 1919.

M. Kaufman

DELANY, MARTIN ROBISON (May 6, 1812, Charles Town, (West) Va.- January 24, 1885, Xenia, Ohio). *Physician*. Son of Samuel, slave and then paper-mill worker, and Pati (Peace) Delany. Married Catherine A. Richards, 1843; 11 children. EDUCATION: Early 1830s, basic education, Rev. Lewis Woodson's school (informal), Pittsburgh, Pa.; 1836-37, apprentice to Dr. Andrew McDowell, Pittsburgh; October 1846-March 1848, read medicine under Dr. Joseph Gazzam, Pittsburgh; 1849-50, read medicine under Dr. Francis J. LeMoyne, Pittsburgh; November 1850-March 1851, Harvard University Medical College, after being refused entrance to several medical schools in Pa. and N.Y.; he and two other black students were barred, because of their race, from continuing their medical studies after the 1850-51 winter term. CAREER: 1836-39, cupper and bleeder, Pittsburgh; 1840s, writer and antislavery activist, including a newspaper and work with Frederick Douglass (1847-49) in publishing the *North Star*; 1851-56, medical practice and writing on racial policy and black reform in Pittsburgh and Old Northwest; 1856-59, medical practice and writing, Chatham, Ontario, Canada; 1859-64, travel in Africa, Europe, and England; 1861-65, Union Army recruiter; 1865, commissioned a major, U.S. Army; 1865-68, Freedmen's Bureau agent, Hilton Head, S.C.; 1868-80, black rights activist and politician, Charleston, S.C.; 1873-74, custom-house inspector, Charleston; 1875-78, trial justice (justice of the peace), Charleston; 1878-80, medical practice, Charleston. CONTRIBUTIONS: One of earliest black physicians in United States and a leader in nineteenth century Negro rights movement. Had regular practice in Pittsburgh and then in Chatham. Because of his heavy involvement in advancing the Negro cause, did not use his medical skills regularly to earn a living after 1859. Scientific background aided him in pursuing lecturing and writing for black reform. Edited and founded one of first black weeklies, the *Mystery*, in Pittsburgh (1843-46).

WRITINGS: *The Condition, Elevation, Emigration, and Destiny of the Colored People of the United States, Politically Considered* (1852); *Principia of Ethnology: The Origin of Races and Color* (1879). Writings listed in *DAB*, 5: 219-20; *JNMA* 44 (1952): 232-38. REFERENCES: Philip Cash, "Pride, Prejudice, and Politics," *Harvard Med. Alumni Bull.* 54 (1980): 20-25; W. Montague Cobb, "Martin Robison Delany," *JNMA* 44 (1952): 232-38; *DAB*, 3: 219-20; *Encycl. of Am. Biog.* (1934): 270-71; Leslie Falk and Samuel Cameron, "Dr. Martin R. Delany's Canadian Years as Medical Practitioner and Abolitionist (1856-64)," *Congress international d'histoire de la medecine, XXVe, Quebec, 1976, Actes*: (1977): 537-45; Frank A. Rollin, *Life and Public Services of Martin R. Delany* (1868); Dorothy Sterling, *The Making of an Afro-American: Martin Robison Delany* (1971); *Webster's Am. Biographies* (1974), 267-78; Delany Papers are at Countway Library, Harvard Medical School, Cambridge, Mass.; *Who Was Who in Am.*, Hist. Vol.: 144.

                                                                                    T. Savitt

DE LEE, JOSEPH BOLIVAR (October 28, 1869, Cold Spring, N.Y.-April 2, 1942, Chicago, Ill.). *Obstetrician*. Son of Morris, dry goods merchant, and Dora (Tobias) De Lee. Never married. EDUCATION: 1888, South Division High School (Chicago); 1891, M.D., Chicago Medical College; 1892-93, intern, Cook County Hospital; 1893-94, studied in Vienna, Berlin, and Paris. CAREER: 1894-1929, obstetrics faculty, Northwestern University Medical School; 1895-1942, director, Chicago Lying-in Dispensary; 1917-39, medical staff, Chicago Lying-in Hospital; 1929-34, obstetrics and gynecology faculty, University of Chicago. CONTRIBUTIONS: Crusader for maternal welfare. Founder, Chicago Lying-in Dispensary (1895), first institution in Ill. devoted to maternal welfare. Founder, Chicago Lying-in Hospital (1899) and Chicago Maternity Center (1932). Pioneer in developing modern techniques for caesarean section (especially the low cervical) and in making and using sound moving pictures for obstetric education. Devised many instruments and made major improvements in stethoscope and forceps.

WRITINGS: *Obstetrics for Nurses* (1904; 12th ed., 1941); *Yearbook of Obstetrics* (1904-41, editor); *The Principles and Practice of Obstetrics* (1913; 7th ed., 1938); "The Newer Methods of Caesarean Section, Report of Forty Cases," *JAMA* 73 (1919): 91-95; "An Illustrated History of the Low or Cervical Caesarean Sections," *Am. J. Obstet. Gynecol.* 10 (1925): 503-20; "Low, or Cervical, Caesarean Section (Laparotrachelotomy), Three Hundred and Thirty Operations, with Two Deaths," *JAMA* 84 (1925): 791-98. REFERENCES: Leslie B. Arey, *Northwestern University Medical School, 1859-1959* (1959), 388-93; *BHM* (1964-69), 70; (1970-74), 48; *DAB*, Supplement 3: 222-23; Morris Fishbein with Sol Theron De Lee, *Joseph Bolivar De Lee, Crusading Obstetrician* (1949); Chassar Moir, *J. Obstet. Gynecol., Brit. Emp.* 49 (1942): 444-46.

W. K. Beatty

DEN, RICHARD SOMERSET (1821, County Kilkenny, Ireland-July 20, 1895, Los Angeles, Calif.). *Surgeon.* Son of Emanuel and Catherine Den. Never married. EDUCATION: 1842, graduated from the medical department, Trinity College, Dublin, Ireland. CAREER: 1842, sailed as a ship surgeon to Australia from London, continued to Mexico, and joined his brother in Santa Barbara, Calif., on September 1, 1843; 1844, practiced surgery, Los Angeles, under a special license to practice from the Mexican government; 1848-50, practice, Mother Lode country, northern Calif.; 1850-54, 1862-95, surgical practice, Los Angeles; 1854-66, rancher on his brother's property, Santa Barbara. CONTRIBUTIONS: First foreign physician possessing a medical degree in Calif. Chief physician and surgeon, Mexican forces facing the U.S. Army and Navy, southern Calif. (1846, 1847). Last surgeon-general of the Mexican Army in Calif. REFERENCES: Henry Harris, *California's Medical Story* (1932), 54-57.

Y. V. O'Neill

DENISON, CHARLES (November 1, 1845, Royalton, Vt.-January 10, 1909, Denver, Colo.). *Physician; Pulmonary Medicine.* Son of Joseph Adams, physician, and Eliza (Skinner) Denison. Married Ella Strong, 1878; three children. EDUCATION: Diploma, Kimball Union Academy (Meriden, N.H.); 1867, A.B., Williams College; 1869, M.D., University of Vermont. CAREER: Until 1873, practiced in Hartford, Conn.; 1873, following a pulmonary hemorrhage, moved to Denver; 1881-95, professor of diseases of the chest and climatology, University of Denver. CONTRIBUTIONS: More than any other person, promoted Colo.'s climate and altitude as a cure for tuberculosis; believed the beneficial effects were due to low humidity, "diathermacy" of the air, atmospheric electricity, increased ozone, and lessened atmospheric pressure; said that the "altitude of approximate immunity from phthisis" was 6,000 feet. To the Colorado Medical Society, gave a report on Koch's discovery of the tubercle bacillus two months after the news was published in Berlin (1882), and six months after Koch's report on tuberculin, gave a comprehensive report on 19 cases he had treated with the new substance (1891). Developed a dozen new variants on old instruments: a stethoscope, spirometer, valvular empyema drainage tube, tuberculin syringe. His "sanitary cement-block house," exhibited as a model at the International Congress on Tuberculosis (1908), was designed for optimal ventilation; his "Denison sleeping-canopy" was popular for a time. President, Denver Medical Society (1879). Specialized in tuberculosis, attracted many patients from the eastern seaboard, and compiled data on over 700 cases (by 1884). Charter member, American Climatological Association, and its president (1890). The medical library of the University of Colorado now bears his name.

WRITINGS: Bibliography of 77 items in *Medical Coloradoana* (1922). *Rocky Mountain Health Resorts* (1880); *Pocket Atlas of Denison's Annual and Seasonal Climatic Maps of the U.S.* (1885). REFERENCES: Kelly and Burrage (1920), 305; *NCAB*, 17: 281; F. B. Rogers, "The Rise and Decline of the Altitude Therapy of Tuberculosis," *Bull. Hist. Med.* 63: (1969) 1-16; James J. Waring, "Charles Denison," *J. of the Outdoor Life* (Summer 1932): 349-51,419.

F. B. Rogers

DENNIS, FREDERIC SHEPARD (April 17, 1850, Newark, N.J.-March 8, 1934, New York, N.Y.). *Physician; Surgery.* Son of Alfred Lewis, railroad executive, and Eliza (Shepard) Dennis. Married Fannie (Rockwell) Carhart, 1880. EDUCATION: 1872, B.A., Yale University; 1874, M.D., Bellevue Hospital Medical School; 1876, went with his friend William H. Welch (q.v.) to Europe to study in the universities of France, Germany, and Scotland. CAREER: *Post* 1878, practiced medicine, New York City; at Bellevue Hospital Medical School: 1879-82, anatomy faculty; and 1883-98, surgery faculty; 1882-1934, surgical staff, St. Vincent's Hospital; 1894, president, American Surgical Association; 1898-1910, clinical surgery faculty, Cornell University Medical School; surgical staff: Montefiore Home (N.Y.), Bellevue, St. Joseph's (Yonkers) and Litchfield County (Winsted, Conn.) hospitals. CONTRIBUTIONS: Introduced Listerian antiseptic methods in the United States. Achieved outstanding success in his radical operations for breast cancer, in his suprapubic cystotomy, and in his treatment of compound fractures. Persuaded Andrew Carnegie (1884) to endow a laboratory of medical research bearing his name at Bellevue Hospital Medical School in an unsuccessful attempt to keep William H. Welch from leaving Bellevue to accept an appointment at Johns Hopkins. Founded Harlem Hospital, New York City.

WRITINGS: "Suprapubic Cystotomy. Its Techniques Illustrated by Anatomical Preparations," *Trans., Am. Surg. Assoc.* 5 (1887): 9-28; "Recurrence of Carcinoma of the Breast," *ibid.*, 60 (1891): 219-45; *System of Surgery*, 4 vols. (1895-96); *Selected Surgical Papers*, 2 vols. (1934). REFERENCES: *DAB*, Supplement 1: 239-40; *NCAB*, 13: 601; Mark M. Ravitch, *A Century of Surgery*, 2 vols. (1981); *Who Was Who in Am.*, 1: 315.

S. Galishoff

DE SCHWEINITZ, GEORGE EDMUND (October 26, 1858, Philadelphia, Pa.-August 22, 1938, Philadelphia). *Physician; Ophthalmology.* Son of Edmund Alexander, Moravian bishop, and Lydia Joanna (de Tschirschky) de Schweinitz. Never married. EDUCATION: 1876, A.B., Moravian College; 1881, M.D., University of Pennsylvania; 1881-83, intern, Children's and University of Pennsylvania hospitals. CAREER: 1876-78, taught at Nazareth Hall, Nazareth, Pa.; *post* 1883, practiced medicine, Philadelphia, Pa., specializing exclusively in ophthalmology after 1887; 1882-87, quizmaster in therapeutics, Medical Institute of Philadelphia; 1883-88, prosector in anatomy, University of Pennsylvania; ophthalmic surgical staff: *post* 1885, Children's Hospital; *post* 1886, Orthopedic Hospital and Infirmary for Nervous Diseases; and *post* 1887, Philadelphia General Hospital; ophthalmology faculty: 1891-92, Philadelphia Polyclinic and College for Graduates in Medicine; 1892-1902, Jefferson Medical College; and *post* 1924, School of Medicine, University of Pennsylvania; president: 1910-13, College of Physicians of Philadelphia; 1916, American Ophthalmological Society; 1922, American Medical Association; and 1922, International Congress of Ophthalmology; 1917-18, U.S. Army Medical Reserve Corps, in charge of ophthalmology, Surgeon General's Office; and founder and director, army's school of ophthalmology, Camp Greenleaf, Fort Oglethorpe, Ga. CONTRIBUTIONS: Leading American authority on ophthalmology. Advanced knowledge of toxic amblyopias, pathogenesis of iridocyclitis, mechanism of papilledema, effect of intraocular injections of antiseptic substances, and pathology of the eye. Principal work was *Diseases of the Eye* (1892), which for over 32 years (in ten revised editions and five reprints) was the most respected work in its field.

WRITINGS: *Toxic Amblyopias* (1896); *An American Textbook of Diseases of the Eye, Ear, Nose and Throat* (1899, edited with B. Alexander Randall); *Pulsating Exophthalmos* (1908, with T. B. Holloway). REFERENCES: *BHM* (1980), 12; *DAB*, Supplement 2: 603-5; *NCAB*, C: 144; *Who Was Who in Am.*, 1: 1093.

S. Galishoff

DEWEES, WILLIAM POTTS (May 5, 1768, Pottsgrove [Pottstown], Pa.-May 20, 1841, Philadelphia, Pa.). *Physician; Obstetrics; Medical education.* Married Martha Rogers, c. 1791; Mary Lorrain, 1802; eight children. EDUCATION: Apprentice to Dr. Phyle and Dr. William Smith (1787-89), Philadelphia; University of Pennsylvania: 1789, M.B.; and 1806, M.D. CAREER: 1789-93, practiced in Abington, Pa; 1793-1812, 1817-35, practiced in Philadelphia; 1805-12, 1817-35, faculty, University of Pennsylvania. CONTRIBUTIONS: Contributed to evolution of obstetrics from midwifery and its establishment as an academic discipline. Wrote first systematic textbook of obstetrics in America. Through his prolific writings, exerted a wide influence on obstetrics and pediatrics. Advocated more radical teachings of Baudelocque and the French school than those of the English school. Incorrectly held that pelvic contracture was rare and advocated blood letting along lines of Benjamin Rush (q.v.).

WRITINGS: *An Essay on the Means of Lessening Pain and Facilitating Certain Cases of Difficult Parturition* (1806); *A Compendious System of Midwifery* . . . (1824); *A Treatise on the Physical and Medical Treatment of Children*, 10 eds. (1825); *A Treatise on the Diseases of Females*, 10 eds. (1826); *A Practice of Physic* . . . (1830). REFERENCES: *DAB*, 3, pt.1: 267; Hugh L. Hodge, *An Eulogium on William P. Dewees, M.D.* . . . (1842); Kelly and Burrage (1920), 309; Herbert Thoms, "William Potts Dewees and the First System of Obstetrics," in *Chapters in American Obstetrics*, 2nd ed. (1961), 53-58; John Whitridge Williams, "William Potts Dewees (1768-1841)," in "A Sketch of the History of Obstetrics in the United States up to 1860," *Am. Gynecol.* 3 (1903): 33-38.

L. D. Longo

DE WITT, LYDIA MARIA (ADAMS) (February 1, 1859, Flint, Mich.-March 10, 1928, Winter, Tex.). *Physician; Pathology; Pharmacology.* Daughter of Oscar, attorney, and Elizabeth (Walton) Adams. Married Alton De Witt, 1878; separated 1904; two children. EDUCATION: Michigan State Normal College; at University of Michigan: 1899, B.S.; 1898, M.D.; and 1914, A.M.; 1906, studied in Berlin. CAREER: 1877-95 schoolteacher; 1898-1910, instructor of histology, University of Michigan medical department; 1910-12, assistant city pathologist and bacteriologist, St. Louis; and instructor of pathology, Washington University Medical School; 1912-28, assistant, then associate, professor of pathology, University of Chicago. CONTRIBUTIONS: Among first women to hold regular faculty appointment in the medical school, University of Michigan (Eliza Mosher, a physician, was the first woman on the undergraduate faculty). At Chicago, pioneered the attempt to apply Paul Ehrlich's "magic bullet" chemotherapeutic methods to the treatment of tuberculosis by compounding poisonous heavy metals with various dyes that were specifically attracted to the T.B. bacillus. Eminent researcher.

WRITINGS: "The Chemotherapy of Tuberculosis," in *The Chemistry of Tuberculosis* (1923). REFERENCES: *NCAB*, B: 457-58; *Notable Am. Women*, 1: 468; *Who Was Who in Am.*, 1: 320.

M. Pernick

DEXTER, AARON (November 11, 1750, Malden, Mass.-February 28, 1829, Cambridge, Mass.). *Physician; Medical educator.* Son of Richard, a prosperous farmer, and Rebecca (Peabody) Dexter. Married Rebecca Amory, 1787; 12 children. EDUCATION: 1776, A.B., Harvard University; studied medicine with Dr. Samuel Danforth, Boston's leading student of chemistry. CAREER: Ship's surgeon during the Revolution; was captured, taken to Halifax, and later exchanged; 1783-1816, member, original faculty, Harvard Medical School, and first Erving professor of chemistry and materia medica; at Massachusetts General Hospital: 1816-29, emeritus; and 1820-29, medical staff; 1824-28, on Board of Consulting Physicians, Boston. CONTRIBUTIONS: Although he had received only apprenticeship training supplemented by wartime experience as a ship's surgeon, was elected to the original faculty of the Harvard Medical School, where he served as a balance wheel between the more expansive egos of John Warren (q.v.) and Benjamin Waterhouse (q.v.). A poor classroom teacher, was an early and perceptive supporter of the revolutionary advances in chemistry then being made in England and especially France. Lectures were the first systematic teaching of chemistry at Harvard. Friendship with William Erving, a retired major in the British army and Harvard graduate (1753), influenced the latter to leave £1,000 in his will to endow the Erving chair of chemistry and materia medica (1791). Played a role in the early history of the Massachusetts Medical Society, being an incorporator and its first librarian (1782-92). Because he was basically a quiet and pleasant man in a society with more than its share of charismatic and combative personalities, importance to the medical and public life of Boston during the Revolutionary and Federalist eras has been seriously underestimated.

REFERENCES: H. W. Foote, *Annals of King's Chapel from the Puritan Age to the Present*

Day, 3 vols. (1882-1940), 2: 480; Kelly and Burrage (1920), 312; T. E. Moore, "Early Years of the Harvard Medical School, 1782-1810," *Bull Hist. Med.* 27 (1953): 530-61; *NCAB*, 19: 345; C. C. Smith, "Notice of Aaron Dexter, M.D.," Mass. Hist. Soc., *Proceedings* 1 (1791-1835): 421-23. For a more complete discussion of Dexter's role, see Moore's "The Early Years of the Harvard Medical School: Its Founding and Curriculum, 1782-1810" (Honors thesis, Harvard University, 1952).

P. Cash

DIBBLE, EUGENE HERIOT (August 14, 1893, Camden, S.C.-June 2, 1968, Tuskegee, Ala.). *Physician.* Son of Eugene Heriot and Sally (Lee) Dibble. Married Helen A. Taylor, 1926; five children. EDUCATION: 1915, A.B., Atlanta University; 1919, M.D., Howard University; 1919-20, intern, Freedmen's Hospital, Washington, D.C.; surgical resident, John A. Andrew Hospital, Tuskegee. CAREER: 1920-23, assistant medical director, John A. Andrew Memorial Hospital; 1923-25, first surgeon-in-chief, Veteran's Administration Hospital, Tuskegee; 1925-36, medical director, John A. Andrew Memorial Hospital; 1936-46, manager and medical director, Veteran's Administration Hospital, Tuskegee; 1946-65, medical director, John A. Andrew Memorial Hospital. CONTRIBUTIONS: A long-time leader in the drive to improve medical care of blacks and the professional status of black physicians. The prime moving spirit of the John A. Andrew Clinical Society, Tuskegee (1925-65), a vital component of postgraduate education efforts for black physicians before the end of segregation in the medical profession. Served on Editorial Board, *JNMA*, and on the Board of Trustees, Meharry Medical College. REFERENCES: W. Montague Cobb, "Eugene Heriot Dibble, M.D., Perspective and Profile," *JNMA* 57 (1965): 435-37; Fred C. Collier, "Eugene Heriot Dibble, M.D., 1893-1968," *JNMA* 60 (1968): 446; "Dr. Eugene Heriot Dibble, Jr., Distinguished Service Medalist for 1962," *JNMA* 54 (1962): 711-12; J. A. Kenney, "Eugene Heriot Dibble," *JNMA* 35 (1943): 175.

T. Savitt

DIBRELL, JAMES ANTHONY (August 14, 1817, Nashville, Tenn.-February 23, 1897, Van Buren, Ark.). *Physician.* Son of Edwin, city clerk and recorder, and Martha (Shrewsbury) Dibrell. Married Ann Eliza Pryor, 1841, three children, including James A., Jr. (q.v.); Jane Emily Pryor, 1855, four children. EDUCATION: 1836-39, University of Nashville; 1838-39, apprentice to Dr. Thomas R. Jennings; 1839, M.D., University of Pennsylvania Medical School. CAREER: Private practice: 1840-62, 1866-97, Van Buren, Ark.; and 1862-66, Little Rock, Ark. CONTRIBUTIONS: Mainly responsible for organizing the Crawford County Medical Society (1845), the earliest medical society in Ark. Helped organize a second Crawford County Medical Society (1871)—the first one failed after two years— and provided additional leadership as its first president. President, Little Rock and Pulaski County Medical Society (1866). Vice-president, Arkansas State Medical Association (1874) and Arkansas Medical Society (1882). President, Arkansas Medical Society (1886). Served as first chairman, Crawford County Medical Examiners Board, after its establishment under the state medical licensing law of 1881. Acquired the reputation in his later years as west Ark.'s finest example of the family physician ideal. REFER-ENCES: Auxiliary to Sebastian County Medical Society, *Physicians and Medicine: Crawford and Sebastian Counties* (1977), 304-6; *History of Crawford County* (1961), 900; *NCAB*, 12: 82.

D. Konold

DIBRELL, JAMES ANTHONY, JR. (August 20, 1846, Van Buren, Ark.-November 11, 1904, Little Rock, Ark.). *Physician; Surgery.* Son of James A., physician, and Ann Eliza (Pryor) Dibrell. Married Lillie Reardon, 1876; two sons. EDUCATION: 1865, apprentice to James A. Dibrell (q.v.); 1867-68, St. Louis Medical College; 1870, M.D., University of Pennsylvania Medical School; 1890, two postgraduate terms, New York Polyclinic. CAREER: 1870-1904, private practice, Little Rock; 1879-1904, medical faculty, Medical Department of Arkansas Industrial University. CONTRIBUTIONS: Helped Arkansas guard against a yellow-fever epidemic (1879-81) while secretary of a temporary State Board of Health. Strongly supported professional organizations: as a charter member, Arkansas State Medical Association (1870), its recording secretary (1873-74), and its delegate to the American Medical Association (1875) to defend it against charges of unprofessionalism; as president, Arkansas Medical Society (1891-1892) and vice-president, American Medical Association (1902-3). Helped educate Ark. physicians, as the state's most celebrated surgeon, with frequent descriptions of unusual surgical cases in the surgical sessions and *Journal* of the state medical society. Made a major contribution to the medical department, Arkansas Industrial University, as a co-founder and later as dean, by securing funds for new buildings and for the establishment of the Logan A. Roots Memorial Hospital and the Isaac Folsom Clinic as integral parts of the medical school. REFERENCES: W. David Baird, *Medical Education in Arkansas* (1979), 29; Nolie Mumey, *University of Arkansas School of Medicine* (1975), 66-68; *Who Was Who in Am.*, 1 (1942): 321.

D. Konold

DICK, GEORGE FREDERICK (July 21, 1881, Fort Wayne, Ind.-October 12, 1967, Palo Alto, Calif.). *Physician; Microbiology.* Son of Daniel, railroad engineer, and Elizabeth (King) Dick. Married Gladys Rowena Henry, 1914 (d. 1963), two children; Kathryn Davis, 1965. EDUCATION: 1900-1901, Indiana University; 1905, M.D., Rush Medical College; 1905-6, intern, Cook County Hospital; 1908, studied in Vienna and Munich. CAREER: 1909-18, pathology faculty, University of Chicago; medicine faculty: 1919-33, Rush Medical College; and 1933-46, University of Chicago; 1910-24, staff, McCormick Institute for Infectious Diseases. CONTRIBUTIONS: Developed a skin test for susceptibility to scarlet fever (the "Dick Test"), proved that the disease is caused by a streptococcus, and developed an antitoxin against it—all three were done with Gladys Henry Dick, (q.v.).
WRITINGS: With Gladys Henry Dick: "The Etiology of Scarlet Fever," *JAMA* 82

(1924): 301-2; "A Scarlet Fever Antitoxin," *JAMA* 82 (1924): 1246-47; "A Skin Test for Susceptibility to Scarlet Fever," *JAMA* 82 (1924): 265-66; *Scarlet Fever* (1938). REFERENCES: *NCAB*, 54:240.

W. K. Beatty

DICK, GLADYS ROWENA (HENRY) (December 18, 1881, Pawnee City, Nebr.-August 21, 1963, Palo Alto, Calif.). *Physician; Microbiology.* Daughter of William Chester, army officer, and Azelia H. (Edson) Henry. Married George Frederick Dick, 1914; two children. EDUCATION: 1900, B.S., University of Nebraska; 1907, M.D., Johns Hopkins University; 1908, studied in Berlin; 1908-9, intern, Johns Hopkins Hospital. CAREER: 1914, practiced medicine, Evanston, Ill.; and pathologist, Evanston Hospital; 1914-53, staff, McCormick Institute for Infectious Diseases, Chicago, Ill.; 1917-19, medical staff, St. Luke's Hospital. CONTRIBUTIONS: Developed a skin test for susceptibility to scarlet fever (the "Dick Test"), proved that the disease is caused by a streptococcus, and developed an antitoxin against it—all three done with George Dick (q.v.).

WRITINGS: With George Frederick Dick: "The Etiology of Scarlet Fever," *JAMA* 82 (1924): 301-2; "A Scarlet Fever Antitoxin," *JAMA* 82 (1924): 1246-47; "A Skin Test for Susceptibility to Scarlet Fever," *JAMA* 82 (1924): 265-66; *Scarlet Fever* (1938). REFERENCES: *NCAB*, 51: 107; *Who Was Who in Am.*, 4: 248.

W. K. Beatty

DICKERSON, SPENCER CORNELIUS (December 1, 1871, Austin, Tex.-February 25, 1948, Chicago, Ill.). *Ophthalmologist; Otolaryngologist.* Son of Patrick and Eliza (Robinson) Dickerson. Married Daisy Hunter, 1910. EDUCATION: 1897, B.S., University of Chicago; 1901, M.D., Rush Medical College; 1901-2, intern, Freedmen's Hospital, Washington, D.C. CAREER: 1902-7, private practice, New Bedford, Mass.; 1907-48, on staff of Provident Hospital, Chicago: 1907-12, pathology; and 1920-48, ophthalmology and otolaryngology: 1930-37, chair of department; 1937-48, emeritus; 1943-46, chair of Executive Committee; 1914-c.1920, assistant in EENT, Rush Medical College. CONTRIBUTIONS: First black pathologist at Provident (a black) Hospital (1907). Trained a generation of black EENT specialists at Provident Hospital. Achieved brigadier general status in the military. Universally acclaimed by colleagues and students to be a giving, selfless person.

WRITINGS: "Etiology of Diabetes," *Detroit Med. J.* 5 (1904): 150-55; "The Defensive Properties of the Organism," *Boston Med. and Surg. J.* 154 (1906): 405-8. REFERENCES: U.G. Dailey, "Brig. General Spencer C. Dickerson, B.S., M.D., 1871-1948," *JNMA* 40 (1948): 165-66; Carl G. Roberts, *ibid.*, p. 166; *WWAPS* 1 (1938): 303.

T. Savitt

DICKINSON, JONATHAN (April 22, 1688, Hatfield, Mass.-October 7, 1747, Elizabeth, N.J.). *Minister; Physician.* Son of Hezekiah, merchant, and Abigail (Blakeman) Dickinson. Married Joanna Melyen, 1708, nine children; Mary Crane, 1747, no children. EDUCATION: Tutored privately by the Rev. John Hart and the

Rev. Abraham Pierson; 1706, A.B., Yale College; studied theology with the Rev. Thomas Ingersoll. CAREER: 1709-47, pastor, Presbyterian Church, Elizabeth; 1747, first president, College of New Jersey (now Princeton University). Died from a sudden attack of pleurisy. CONTRIBUTIONS: For 38 years, practiced "the healing arts" and gained a widespread reputation in the medical profession. Authored the first professional medical work by a New Jerseyite, a description of an epidemic (probably diphtheria); it appeared initially in Peter Zenger's *New York Weekly Journal* (February 16, 1735-36) and was published in book form (1740).

WRITINGS: *Observations on That Terrible Disease, Vulgarly Called the Throat Distemper, with Advices as to the Method of Cure* (1740). REFERENCES: Henry C. Cameron, *Jonathan Dickinson and the College of New Jersey* (1880), 1-37; *DAB*, 5: 301-2; Frederick B. Dexter, ed., *Biographical Sketches of Yale Graduates* (1885) 1: 45-52; Edwin F. Hatfield, *History of Elizabeth, New Jersey* (1868), 326-54; John McLean, *History of the College of New Jersey* (1879), 117-26; *NCAB*, 5: 463; Stephen Wickes, *History of Medicine in New Jersey, and of Its Medical Men, from the Settlement of the Province to A.D. 1800* (1879), 34.

W. Barlow

DICKINSON, ROBERT LATOU (February 21, 1861, Jersey City, N.J.-November 20, 1950, Amherst, Mass.). *Physician; Gynecology.* Son of Horace, hat manufacturer, and Jeannette (Latou) Dickinson. Married Sarah Truslow, 1890; three children. EDUCATION: Brooklyn Polytechnic Institute and studied for four years in Germany and Switzerland; 1882, M.D., Long Island College Hospital, Brooklyn, N.Y. (later Long Island College of Medicine); intern, Williamsburg Hospital and Long Island College Hospital. CAREER: 1883-1921, practiced medicine, Brooklyn, N.Y.; at Long Island College Hospital: 1883-86, chest department dispensary staff; 1884-1910, obstetrics staff; 1886-1918, obstetrics faculty; and *post* 1918, gynecology and obstetrics faculty; 1894-99, obstetrics staff, King's County Hospital (Brooklyn); at Brooklyn Hospital: 1897-1910, gynecological surgery staff; and 1910-35, gynecology staff; 1905-11, obstetrics staff, Methodist Episcopal Hospital (Brooklyn); 1917, assistant chief, medical section, Council of National Defense; 1918-19, Medical Corps, U.S. Army; 1919, 1926, headed missions to China for U.S. Public Health Service; at National Committee on Maternal Health: 1923, founder; 1923-37, secretary; and 1937-50, chairman; president: 1920, American Gynecological Society; and 1946-49, Euthanasia Society. CONTRIBUTIONS: One of the leading American gynecologists of his time. Introduced several new surgical procedures, including the use of electric cauterization in the treatment of cervicitis and in intrauterine sterilizations. Devised improved methods for controlling postpartum hemorrhage and infection. Gained widespread prominence for his innovative teaching methods. Used rubber models to teach female anatomy and sculpted life-size models to show fetal growth from fertilization to birth, which were published as *Birth Atlas* (1941). Co-edited *American Textbook of Obstetrics* (1895). Supported several feminist causes, including dress reform, sex education, and, especially, birth control. The most prominent physician associated with the early birth-control movement. Founded the Committee on Maternal Health (1923; in 1930 it became the National Committee) to compile data on contraception. Publications under the auspices of the National Committee on Maternal Health—particularly *Control of Conception* (1931) and, with Woodbridge Edward Morris, *Techniques of Conception Control* (1941)—were instrumental in gaining physician support for birth control. Did pioneering studies of the sexual behavior of ordinary people.

WRITINGS: *A Thousand Marriages* (1931, with Laura Beam); *Atlas of Human Sex Anatomy* (1933); *The Single Woman: A Medical Study in Sex Education* (1934, with Laura Beam). REFERENCES: *Current Biography* (1950), 120-21; *DAB*, Supplement 4: 230-32; David M. Kennedy, *Birth Control in America: The Career of Margaret Sanger* (1970), ch. vii; *NCAB*, 39: 485-86; *N.Y. Times*, November 30, 1950; *Who Was Who in Am.*, 3: 227.

S. Galishoff

DICKSON, SAMUEL HENRY (September 20, 1798, Charleston, S.C.-March 31, 1872, Philadelphia, Pa.). *Physician; Medical education.* Son of Samuel, schoolmaster, and Mary (Neilson) Dickson. Married Elizabeth B. Robertson, 1832; Jane R. Robertson, 1834; Marie S. DuPré, 1845; at least four children. EDUCATION: 1814, A.B., Yale University; 1814-19, studied medicine with Philip G. Prioleau, Charleston; 1819, M.D., University of Pennsylvania. CAREER: 1817-47, 1850-58, practiced medicine, Charleston; at Charleston Medical College: 1824, founder; and 1824-32, institutes and practice of medicine faculty; at Medical College of South Carolina: 1833, founder, and 1833-47, 1850-58, institutes and practice of medicine faculty; 1847-50, medical faculty, University of the City of New York; 1858-72, institutes and practice of medicine faculty, Jefferson Medical College (Philadelphia). CONTRIBUTIONS: Played a leading role in the establishment of the Medical College of South Carolina. Gave an accurate description of dengue, a hitherto new and obscure disease. Writings on medicine went through several editions and were adopted as textbooks in the schools in which he taught. Claimed to have been one of the first American physicians to have substituted stimulants and anodynes for heroic remedies in the treatment of fevers. An early writer on racial anthropometry.

WRITINGS: *On Dengue; Its History, Pathology, and Treatment* (1839); *Manual of Pathology and Practice* (1839); *Elements of Medicine* (1855); *Studies in Pathology and Therapeutics* (1867). REFERENCES: *DAB*, 5: 305-6; Kelly and Burrage (1928), 327-28; *NCAB*, 10: 285; S. X. Radbill, "Samuel H. Dickson...," *Annals of Med. Hist.*, 3rd series, 4 (1942): 382-89.

S. Galishoff

DILLEHUNT, RICHARD BENJAMIN (July 12, 1886, Decatur, Ill.-October 31, 1953, Portland, Oreg.). *Surgeon; Orthopedist; Medical educator.* Son of Benjamin Webster, hardware merchant, and Augusta (Buchert) Dillehunt. Never married. EDUCATION: 1904-6, University of Illinois; 1910, M.D., Rush Medical

College; 1910-11, intern, Cook County Hospital; 1915, postgraduate study, orthopedic clinics in Boston, Mass.; Chicago, Ill.; New York, N.Y.; and Philadelphia, Pa. CAREER: 1911, practice, Portland; 1912-20, medical faculty, University of Oregon; 1917-19, U.S. Army Medical Corps; 1920-43, dean, University of Oregon Medical School; 1924-43, surgeon-in-chief, Shriner's Hospital for Crippled Children, Portland; 1935, member, Advisory Committee of Orthopedic Surgeons to Georgia Warm Springs Foundation. CONTRIBUTIONS: As dean, made many contributions to the University of Oregon Medical School. An addition to the medical science building was completed (1922). The Multnomah County Hospital was opened on the Medical School campus (1923). Persuaded the Doernbecher family to contribute a children's hospital (1926). A library auditorium and a tuberculosis hospital were built (1939). The Portland Medical Hospital was purchased and converted to a nurses' dormitory. One of the great orthopedic surgeons of the American West.

WRITINGS: "Physical Therapy in Deformities of the Spine," in H. E. Mock, *Principles and Practices of Physical Therapy* (1933), 1-73; "Melorheostosis Leri: A Case Report," *J. of Bone and Joint Surg.* 18 (1936): 991-96 (with E. G. Chuinard); "Giant-Cell Tumor of the Patella: A Case Report," *Western J. of Surg., Obstet. and Gynec.* 46 (1938): 525-27. REFERENCES: *Encyclopedia of Northwest Biog.* (1943): 195-97; Multnomah County Medical Society, *Bull.* 10 (1946): 5, 10; *Who's Who in Am.* (1952-53).

G. B. Dodds

DIMOCK, SUSAN (April 24, 1847, Washington, N.C.-May 7, 1875, Scilly Islands, England). *Physician; Surgeon.* Daughter of Henry, teacher, lawyer, and newspaper editor, and Mary Malvina (Owens) Dimock, teacher. Never married. EDUCATION: 1860, Washington Academy; 1866-68, entered New England Hospital for Women and Children as student of Dr. Marie Zakrzewska (q.v.) and Dr. Lucy Sewall; 1871, M.D., University of Zurich; 1872, further medical study, Vienna and Paris. CAREER: 1872-75, resident physician, New England Hospital; 1872-75, private practice, Boston, Mass.; 1872-75, honorary member of North Carolina Medical Society. CONTRIBUTIONS: Considered one of the most brilliant, most promising, and best educated of pioneer women physicians. Particularly impressed contemporaries, because her surgical skill and incisive intellect were accompanied by a strikingly feminine manner and physical appearance. Tragic and untimely death on the shipwrecked steamer *Schiller* while returning from an European study sojourn created a martyr to the cause of women in medicine.

WRITINGS: *Ueber die verschiedenen Formen des Puerperalfiebers* (1871). REFERENCES: Ednah Dow Cheney, *Memoir of Susan Dimock* (1875); Shirley Phillips Ingegritsen, "Susan Dimock," *Notable Am. Women* 1 (1971): 483-84; *NCAB*, 19: 30; Kelly and Burrage (1920), 315.

R. M. Morantz

DIX, DOROTHEA LYNDE (April 4, 1802, Hampden, Maine-July 17, 1887, Trenton, N.J.). *Humanitarian; Philanthropist.* Daughter of Joseph, merchant and itinerant Methodist minister, and Mary (Bigelow) Dix. Never married. ED-

UCATION: Largely self-educated. CAREER: 1821-24, teacher in a "dame school," Boston, Mass.; 1824-31, rest due to exhaustion and incipient tuberculosis, worked as a governess during summers, wrote during this time; 1831-36, opened a school in Boston, eventually suffering a nervous collapse; 1836-37, rested in England; 1837-41, lived in semi-retirement, New England; 1841-61, reformer, exposing and correcting conditions of the insane and handicapped; 1861-66, superintendent, Union army nurses; 1866-81, continued to expose prison and asylum conditions; raised funds for orphans' homes, disaster victims, public drinking fountains in Boston, and so forth; 1881-85, retirement at the Trenton state hospital. CONTRIBUTIONS: Played a direct role in developing state mental hospitals in 20 states. By publicizing the inhumane conditions of the insane, helped provide the basis for advances in the care and treatment of the mentally ill.

WRITINGS: Wrote a number of books, listed in the *DAB* biography, but most important were her reports on conditions for prisoners and the insane presented to various state legislatures. Papers are in the Houghton Library, Harvard University, Cambridge, Mass. REFERENCES: *BHM* (1964-69), 73; (1970-74), 51; (1975-79),36; Gladys Brooks, *Three Wise Virgins* (1957); *DAB*, 5: 323-25; Helen E. Marshall, *Dorothea Dix* (1937); Robin McKown, *Pioneers in Mental Health* (1961); Miller, *BHM*, p. 29; *NCAB*, 3: 438; *Notable Am. Women*, 1 (1971): 486-89.

M. Kaufman

DOCHEZ, ALPHONSE RAYMOND (April 21, 1882, San Francisco, Calif.-June 30, 1964, New York, N.Y.). *Physician; Microbiology*. Son of Louis and Josephine (Dietrich) Dochez. Never married. EDUCATION: Johns Hopkins University: 1903, A.B.; and 1907, M.D.; 1907-10, fellowship in pathology, Rockefeller Institute for Medical Research. CAREER: 1910-19, bacteriologist, Rockefeller Institute for Medical Research; 1917-18, Medical Corps, U.S. Army; 1919-21, medicine faculty, Johns Hopkins Medical School; at College of Physicians and Surgeons (Columbia): 1921-49, medicine faculty; and 1940-49, bacteriology faculty; *post* 1921, visiting physician, Presbyterian Hospital. CONTRIBUTIONS: Made important investigations of pneumonia, scarlet fever, and the common cold. With Rufus Cole (q.v.), devised a simple method for typing the pneumococci responsible for lobar pneumonia and then developed a serum treatment for one of the most common kinds of lobar pneumonia, type 1 (1910-17); type-specific antisera soon became the standard treatment for pneumococcal pneumonia and was widely used until the introduction of the sulfa drugs and penicillin. Demonstrated that there was a direct relationship between streptococcal pharyngitis and scarlet fever and developed an antitoxin effective against the disease (1921-26); similar investigations had been completed about the same time by George F. and Gladys H. Dick (q.v.), who were awarded patent rights to the development of the scarlatinal toxin. Did last major research on the common cold; using first chimpanzees and later humans as experimental animals, showed that common colds (common upper respiratory infections) were caused by filterable viruses (1930s).

WRITINGS: *Acute Lobar Pneumonia; Prevention and Serum Treatment. Monographs of the Rockefeller Institute for Medical Research, No. 7* (1917, with O. T. Avery [q.v.], H. T. Chickering, and R. Cole); "The Significance of Streptococcus Hemolyticus in Scarlet Fever and the Preparation of a Specific Anti-Scarlatinal Serum . . . ," *JAMA* 82 (1924): 542-44 (with Lillian Sherman); "Studies in the Common Cold . . . ," *J. of Experimental Med.*, 52 (1930): 701-16 (with Gerald S. Shibley and K. C. Mills). A bibliography is in *BMNAS*. REFERENCES: Saul Benison, "Oral History—New Technique in Medical Historiography," *Ohio State Med. J.* 68 (Aug. 1972): 770-73; *BMNAS* 42 (1971): 29-46; *NCAB*, E: 325-26; *N.Y. Times*, July 1, 1964; *Who Was Who in Am.*, 4: 254.

                                                                                          S. Galishoff

DOCK, GEORGE (April 1, 1860, Hopewell, Pa.-May 30, 1951, Altadena, Calif.). *Physician; Internal medicine*. Son of Gilliard, landowner, and Lavinia Lloyd (Bombaugh) Dock. Married Laura McLemore, 1892, two children; Miriam Gould, 1925, no children. EDUCATION: Harrisburg (Pa.) Academy; 1884, M.D., University of Pennsylvania; 1884-85, intern, St. Mary's Hospital (Philadelphia, Pa.); 1885-87, 1893, 1897, studied in Leipzig, Berlin, and Frankfurt, Germany; and Vienna, Austria. CAREER: 1887-88, assistant in clinical pathology laboratory, University of Pennsylvania; 1888-91, professor of pathology and clinical medicine, Texas Medical College and Hospital (Galveston); 1891-1908, professor of the theory and practice of medicine and clinical medicine, University of Michigan; 1908-10, professor of theory and practice of medicine, Tulane University; 1910-22, professor of medicine, Washington University; 1916-17, president, Association of American Physicians; 1922-51, practice of internal medicine and writing of medical history, Pasadena, Calif.; 1923, president, American Society of Tropical Medicine. CONTRIBUTIONS: Finally disproved existence of supposed disease entity "typho-malarial fever" and established the "camp fever" of the Spanish-American War as typhoid (1898). An early advocate of the controversial full-time plan of clinical teaching; established the first permanent teaching clinics at the University of Michigan (1891, 1898). Contributed the first American description of coronary thrombosis to be diagnosed before death (preceded by Adam Hammer of Austria).

WRITINGS: "Some Notes on the Coronary Arteries," *Med. & Surg. Reporter* (Philadelphia) 75 (1896): 1-7; "Typho-malarial Fever, So-Called," *N.Y. Med. J.* 69 (1899): 253-58; *Hookworm Disease* (1940, with C. C. Bass). Writings listed in *Bibliography of the Writings of Dr. George Dock* (1950). REFERENCES: *Annals of Internal Med.* 35 (1951): 761; Burke Hinsdale, *History of the University of Michigan* (1906), 289; *JAMA* 146 (1951): 335; Martin Kaufman, *American Medical Education: The Formative Years* (1976), 176; *Michigan State Med. Soc., J.* 39 (1940): 961; 50 (1951): 1286; *NCAB*, C: 360; *Who Was Who in Am.*, 3: 230.

                                                                                          M. Pernick

DOCK, LAVINIA LLOYD (February 26, 1858, Harrisburg, Pa.-April 17, 1956, Chambersburg, Pa.). *Professional nursing organizer; Author; Nurse*.

Daughter of Gilliard, landowner, and Lavinia Lloyd (Bombaugh) Dock. Never married. EDUCATION: 1886, graduate, Bellevue Hospital Training School, N.Y. CAREER: 1890-93, assistant superintendent of nurses, Johns Hopkins Hospital; 1893-96, superintendent of nurses, Illinois Training School of the Cook County Hospital, Chicago, Ill.; 1898-1915, resident member, Nurses' Henry Street Settlement, N.Y.; secretary: 1893-1901, American Society of Superintendents of Training Schools for Nurses; and 1899-1922, International Council of Nurses; 1900-1923, contributing editor, *American Journal of Nursing*; leader in the struggle for woman's suffrage and birth control and active in the crusade against venereal disease and prostitution. CONTRIBUTIONS: Instrumental in helping to found the first professional nursing association in the United States (1893) and co-founder, International Council of Nurses (1900). Author of the first manual of drugs designed for nurses and an authoritative and comprehensive history of the nursing profession.

WRITINGS: *Textbook of Materia Medica for Nurses* (1889); *History of Nursing* (1907-12, with M. Adelaide Nutting [q.v.]); *Hygiene and Morality* (1910); *History of Red Cross Nursing* (1922, co-author). REFERENCES: T. E. Christy, "Portrait of a Leader," *Nursing Outlook* 17 (1969): 72-75; *DAB* (1980), Supplement 6: 166-68; Miller, *BHM*, p. 29; *Notable Am. Women* 4 (1980): 195-98.

N. Gevitz

DODD, WALTER JAMES (April 22, 1869, London, England-December 13, 1916, Boston, Mass.). *Physician; Radiologist.* Parents died when he was young. Married Margaret Lea, 1910; no surviving children. EDUCATION: Studied pharmacy while employed as assistant apothecary, Massachusetts General Hospital, Boston; 1894, was licensed in Mass.; 1900, Harvard Medical School; 1908, M.D., University of Vermont. CAREER: 1887-92, janitor, Boylston Chemical Laboratory, Harvard; at Massachusetts General Hospital: 1892-94, assistant apothecary; 1894-98, apothecary and photographer; and 1896-1916, radiologist; 1909-1916, instructor of radiology, Harvard. CONTRIBUTIONS: While working as pharmacist and photographer at Massachusetts General Hospital, read reports of Roentgen's discovery of X-rays (1895) and within months began to experiment with them using borrowed electrical apparatus. Soon was able to produce medically useful plates and to interpret them for the staff. Realizing the need for a medical degree, attended Harvard Medical School for a year but was still in demand at the hospital. Accordingly, went to the University of Vermont in Burlington, Vt., for a degree and while there established the Department of Radiology, Mary Fletcher Hospital. Returned to Boston as a radiologist. Went to France (1915) with the first Harvard Medical Unit to set up its military X-ray unit, returning to his work in Boston later that year. Incurred X-ray dermatitis (1897), which (by 1902) became carcinomatous. Continued professional activity in spite of pain and disability until he died with metastatic disease (1916). Name is included in the "Memorial to X-ray Martyrs" at the Roentgen Institute in Hamburg, Germany.

WRITINGS: "The Diagnosis of Stone in the Pelvic Portion of the Ureter . . . ," *Boston Med. and Surg. J.* 163 (1910): 85 (with Hugh Cabot); "The Treatment of Acute Roentgen Ray Dermatitis," *Am. J. Roentgenol.* 1 (1914): 430. REFERENCES: *Walter James Dodd, a Biographical Sketch* (1918); Kelly and Burrage (1920), 317; *Am. J. Roentgenol.* (Jan. 1917).

L. J. Wallman

DOLLEY, SARAH READ (ADAMSON) (March 11, 1829, Schuylkill Meeting, Pa.-December 27, 1909, Rochester, N.Y.). *Physician.* Daughter of Charles and Mary (Corson) Adamson, farmers and country store operators. Married Dr. Lester S. Dolley, 1853; one surviving child. EDUCATION: Studied at the Friends' School, Philadelphia, Pa.; apprentice to her uncle, Dr. Hiram Corson, of Philadelphia; 1851, M.D., Central Medical College (eclectic) of Rochester; 1851-53, unpaid internship, Blockley Hospital, Philadelphia; 1869-70, 1875, postgraduate work, Paris, Prague, and Vienna. CAREER: 1853-72, *post* 1874, practice, Rochester; 1873-74, after death of her husband in 1872, went to Philadelphia as professor of obstetrics, Woman's Medical College of Pennsylvania. CONTRIBUTIONS: Third American woman medical college graduate. Helped establish Rochester's first dispensary for the care of needy women and children (1886), the Provident Dispensary, of which she was president. Helped organize the Practitioner's Society, a medical society for women (1887), which met annually on her birthday in Rochester. This society changed its name to the Blackwell Society (1906), and the following year, organized the Women's Medical Society of the State of New York. REFERENCES: Kelly and Burrage (1920), 317-18; *Notable Am. Women*, 1: 497-99.

M. Kaufman

DONAHOE, WILLIAM E. (May 18, 1886, Sioux Falls, S. Dak.-December 23, 1975, Sioux Falls). *Physician.* Son of Dennis and Cora (Muench) Donahoe. Married Florence Flemming, 1917; two children. EDUCATION: 1908, College of St. Thomas, St. Paul, Minn.; 1912, M.D., University of Illinois; 1919, postgraduate study, University of Iowa (pediatrics). CAREER: *Post* 1913, began general practice, Sioux Falls; 1917-18, U.S. Army Medical Corps; 1920-36, school physician, Sioux Falls; 1925-36, city health officer, Sioux Falls; 1936-40, superintendent, Minnehaha County Board of Health; 1944-52, commander, U.S. Public Health Service, Armed Forces Reserve. CONTRIBUTIONS: Made significant contributions to public health programs in S.D. Introduced the area's first diphtheria immunization program and established the first public health clinic for well children in the state (1921). Consolidated two organizations to form the South Dakota Public Health and Tuberculosis Association. A founder, American Academy of Pediatrics. Founded the University of South Dakota School of Medicine's pediatrics department (1942). Received the South Dakota Medical Association's Distinguished Service Award (1957). Nominated for U.S. Pediatrician of the Year (1969).

WRITINGS: "Medicine in South Dakota, 1870-1950," *J.-Lancet* 70: (1950): 43-45.
REFERENCES: *American Men of Med.* (1961), p. 180; Sioux Falls Town Records.

D. W. Boilard and P. W. Brennen

DONALDSON, HENRY HERBERT (May 12, 1857, Yonkers, N.Y.-January 23, 1938, Philadelphia, Pa.). *Neurologist.* Son of John Joseph, banker, and Louisa Goddard (McGowan) Donaldson. Married Julia Desboro Vaux, 1884, two children; Emma Brace, 1907. EDUCATION: 1879, A.B., Yale University; 1880, College of Physicians and Surgeons (Columbia); 1885, Ph.D., Johns Hopkins University; 1886-87, studied in Munich and Zurich. CAREER: At Johns Hopkins University: 1883-84, biology faculty; and 1887-89, psychology faculty; 1889-92, neurology faculty, Clark University; at University of Chicago: 1892-1906, neurology faculty; and 1892-98, dean, Ogden (graduate) School of Science; 1906-36, head, Wistar Institute of Anatomy and Biology (Philadelphia). CONTRIBUTIONS: One of the world's foremost authorities on the brain and nervous system. Made a detailed anatomical study (1889-92) of the brain of Laura Bridgman, a blind, deaf mute who nonetheless had developed considerable mental ability; one of the most exhaustive studies of its type. Determined the main theme of his life's work: the study of the development of the human brain from birth to maturity. Studies primarily quantitative: size and weight of divisions, rate of growth, relationship of weight and length to that of the entire body, and the number of cells. First major monograph *The Growth of the Brain: A Study of the Nervous System in Relation to Education* (1895) went through three editions and was long used as a reference book. Determined that the rat was the most suitable mammal for laboratory research in problems of growth. Correlated the equivalence in age between man and rodent and developed a pure strain of white rats that has since been used in countless research projects. Book *The Rat: Reference Tables and Data* (1915) made the albino rat one of the world's best studied animals, further enhancing its laboratory value.

WRITINGS: "The Physiology of the Central Nervous System," in *An American Textbook of Physiology* (1898). Writings are listed in *BMNAS*. REFERENCES: *BMNAS*, 20 (1939): 229-43; *DAB*, Supp. 2: 156-57; *DSB*, 4: 160-61; *N.Y. Times*, January 24, 1938; *Who Was Who in Am.*, 1: 331.

S. Galishoff

DONALDSON, MARY ELIZABETH (January 12, 1851, Reedsburg, Wis.-1930, location unknown). *Physician.* Daughter of Zechariah, farmer, and Elizabeth (Delia) Craker. Married Mr. Hesford, 1871, divorced, one child; Thomas L. Johnston, no children; Gilbert Donaldson, 1912, no children. EDUCATION: 1892, M.D., Wooster College. CAREER: 1898, after establishing sanitaria at Boise, Idaho; Milton, Oreg.; and Portland, Oreg., moved to Boise. CONTRIBUTIONS: Early female physician in Idaho. Founder of the Idaho Sanitarium Institute. Charter member of the American Woman's League. Founded and edited the *Idaho Magazine* (1903). Active in temperance movement; led local forces

seeking prohibition, organizing a group known as the Prohibition Alliance. REF-
ERENCES: H. T. French, *History of Idaho* 3 (1914): 1134; J. H. Hawley, *History of Idaho* 2 (1920): 286.

A. A.Hart

DONNELL, CLYDE HENRY (August 4, 1890, Greensboro, N.C.-October 10, 1971, Durham, N.C.). *Physician.* Son of Smith, real estate agent, and Lula Jane (Ingold) Donnell. Married Martha Merrick, 1919; no children. EDUCATION: 1907, B.S., North Carolina A & T College (Greensboro); 1911, A.B., Howard University; 1915, M.D., Harvard University Medical School; 1915, stood third in exam for interns, Boston City Hospital but was not offered position because of race; Dr. Richard C. Cabot (q.v.) arranged for Donnell to work as junior house officer on medical service of Boston City Hospital under auspices of Harvard Graduate School; 1915-16, spent one year as junior house officer; during part of 1918-22, 1924, 1932, did postgraduate study at Harvard in internal medicine, roentgenology, and physical therapy. CAREER: 1917-71, medical prac-tice (1917-20, general medicine; 1920-71, X-ray, physical therapy, and internal medicine); 1917-59, on medical staff, North Carolina Mutual Life Insurance Company, Durham: 1920-59, medical director; 1934-54, vice-president; 1954-60, senior vice-president; and 1960-67, board chairman. CONTRIBUTIONS: Held important position as first full-time medical director of the largest black-owned life insurance company in United States. Served on North Carolina Mutual's Board of Directors (1920-67). Established Life Extension Department at North Carolina Mutual (1925) that sought to improve black health through publications, letters, and lectures to policyholders and examining physicians and through provision of medical care at a hospital in the Durham headquarters. Worked to improve medical knowledge of black physicians by encouraging attendance at and sponsoring medical meetings and postgraduate seminars and clinics with help of President Frank Graham of University of North Carolina. Organized Durham Academy of Medicine (1918). Served 32 years as secretary-treasurer of the Old North State Medical Society. General secretary of National Medical Association and business manager of *JNMA* (1924-28). President (1952-71) and board chairman of Lincoln Hospital, Durham. Involved in many black business and civic affairs of Durham and N.C. Invested in improved housing for Durham blacks and in black hotel and drug stores. Provided a stable cohesive force for black Durham community during his many years of practice. REFERENCES: W. Montague Cobb, "Clyde Donnell, M.D., 1890-," *JNMA* 52 (1960): 382; *NCAB*, 57: 379; Charles D. Watts and Frank W. Scott, "Lincoln Hospital of Durham, North Carolina, A Short History," *JNMA* 57 (1965): 178-79; Walter B. Weare, *Black Business in the New South* (1973), 111, 128; *WWAPS* 1 (1938): 314; *WWICA* 7 (1950): 158.

T. Savitt

DOOLEY, THOMAS ANTHONY, III (January 17, 1927, St. Louis, Mo.-January 18, 1961, New York, N.Y.). *Physician; Author; Medical missionary.*

Son of Thomas Anthony, Jr., business executive, and Agnes Wise (Manzelman) Dooley. Never married. EDUCATION: 1944-45, *post* 1948, completed premedical training, Notre Dame University; 1953, M.D., St. Louis University School of Medicine; 1953-54, intern, Medical Corps, U.S. Naval Reserve, stationed at hospitals in Camp Pendleton, Calif., and Yokosuka, Japan. CAREER: At U.S. Navy Medical Corps: 1944-46, enlisted man; and 1953-56, officer; 1956-61, author and medical missionary. CONTRIBUTIONS: Organized medical relief work in Southeast Asia. Ran refugee camps in Haiphong (1954) servicing more than 600,000 Vietnamese refugees following the Communist victory at Dienbienphu. Described his experiences in a book, *Deliver Us from Evil* (1956), whose proceeds he used to establish a private medical mission in Laos (1956). With Peter D. Comanduras, organized Medico (1957), an international medical-aid mission sponsored by private subscription. Subsequently, returned to Southeast Asia, where he established several hospitals.

WRITINGS: *The Edge of Tomorrow* (1958); *The Night They Burned the Mountain* (1960). REFERENCES: *Current Biog.* (1961), 140-41; *DAB*, Supp. 7: 190-91; Charles L. Van Doren and Robert McHenry, *Webster's Am. Biographies* (1974), 284.

S. Galishoff

DORSETTE, CORNELIUS NATHANIEL (1851, 1852, or 1859, Davidson County, N.C.-December 7, 1897, Montgomery, Ala.). *Physician.* Born a slave. Son of David, farmer, and Lucinda Dorsette. Married Sarah Hale, no children; Lula Harper, 1886; two children. EDUCATION: 1878, A.B., Hampton Institute; 1878-81, studied Latin, N.Y.; served Dr. Vosburgh of Syracuse, N.Y. (as driver and handyman), who inspired and encouraged him to study medicine; attended Medical College of Syracuse (but dropped out because of bad health) and University of Buffalo Medical School; 1882, M.D., University of Buffalo Medical School. CAREER: 1882-84, assistant physician, Wayne County, N.Y., almshouse and insane asylum and part-time general practice in Lyons, N.Y.; 1884-97, general practice, Montgomery. CONTRIBUTIONS: Ala.'s first licensed black physician (1884). Founded Hale Infirmary (Montgomery), the first hospital in Alabama for blacks (1890-1958). A Hampton classmate and lifelong friend of Booker T. Washington. Helped Washington's Tuskegee Institute in numerous ways, including financial and medical; served on its Board of Trustees (1883-97). Influential in attracting black physicians and other black professionals to Montgomery. Active in Montgomery and state Republican party affairs, as well as in civic matters. REFERENCES: Brief biographical sketch (II, 220) and some Dorsette letters published in Louis R. Harlan, ed., *The Booker T. Washington Papers* (1972-81); W. Montague Cobb, "Cornelius Nathaniel Dorsette, M.D., 1852-1897," *JNMA* 52 (1960): 456-59; other Dorsette letters, Booker T. Washington Papers, Library of Congress, Washington, D.C.

T. Savitt

DORSEY, JOHN SYNG (December 23, 1783, Philadelphia, Pa.-November 12, 1818, Philadelphia). *Physician; Surgery.* Son of Leonard Dorsey, merchant;

nephew of Philip Syng Physick (q.v.). Married Maria Ralston, 1807; three children. EDUCATION: 1798-c. 1802, studied medicine with Philip Syng Physick; 1802, M.D., University of Pennsylvania; 1803-4, studied medicine in London and Paris. CAREER: *Post* 1804, practiced medicine, Philadelphia; at Pennsylvania Hospital: 1807-10, dispensary staff; and 1810-18, surgical staff; at University of Pennsylvania: *post* 1807, adjunct surgery faculty; 1816-18, materia medica faculty; and 1818, anatomy faculty. CONTRIBUTIONS: A renowned surgeon who performed the first successful ligation of the external iliac artery in the United States (1811). Wrote *The Elements of Surgery* (1813), the first American textbook of surgery, which went through three editions and was well received in both Europe and America.

WRITINGS: "Inguinal Aneurism Cured by Tying the External Iliac Artery in the Pelvis," *Eclectic Repertory and Analytical Review* 2 (1811): 111-15. REFERENCES: *DAB*, 5: 385-86; Kelly and Burrage (1928): 336-37; Miller, *BHM*, p. 29; *NCAB*, 10: 279.

S. Galishoff

DOUGLASS, WILLIAM (c. 1691, Gifford, Haddington County, Scotland-October 21, 1752, Boston, Mass.). *Physician.* Son of George, "portioner" of Gifford and factor for the Marquis of Tweeddale, Douglass. Never married. EDUCATION: 1705, M.A., Edinburgh; 1712, M.D., Utrecht; studied medicine in Paris and under Pitcairn in Scotland and Boerhaave at Leyden. CAREER: 1718-52, Medical Practice, Boston; 1728-52, president, Scotch Charitable Society. CONTRIBUTIONS: Best known for bitter opposition to the introduction of inoculation in Boston by Cotton Mather (q.v.) and Zabdiel Boylston (q.v.) during the smallpox epidemic of 1721. Although motivated in part by vanity and an instinctive combativeness, did have some valid grounds for opposition. Inoculation was a new and highly dangerous practice that had not been carefully evaluated by competent physicians. Furthermore, Boylston conducted his inoculation in the heart of a city, albeit a smallpox-ridden one, and in defiance of the orders of the Boston selectmen. Douglass soon came to accept inoculation but remained hostile to Mather and Boylston. The most professionally conscious physician of his era in Boston, played the leading role in founding the city's first medical society (1735), which lasted about a decade. His *Practical History of A New Epidemical Eruptive Miliary Fever* was an outstanding study of the Boston scarlet-fever epidemic of 1735-36 and the first adequate description of that disease in English, antedating John Fothergill's study by 12 years. A product of the Scottish Enlightenment, exhibited an interest in botany and is said to have collected more than 1,100 plants from the Boston area. Also recorded observations on the weather, calculated eclipses, and published an almanac under the pseudonym "William Nadir." Possessing a fine library, wrote important works on history (*A Summary, Historical and Political of the First Planting, Progressive Improvement and Present State of the British Settlements in North America,* 2 vols [1749-51]) and economics (*A Discourse Concerning the Currencies of the British Plantations in America . . .* [1739]).

WRITINGS: *A Dissertation Concerning Inoculation of the Small-Pox* (1730); *Practical Essay Concerning the Small Pox* (1730); *The Practical History of a New Eruptive Miliary Fever . . . in Boston in New England in the Years 1735 and 1736* (1736); "Letters from Wm. Douglass to Cadwallader Colden of New York, 1721-1736," *Mass. Hist. Soc., Collections*, 4th series, 2 (1854): 164-89. REFERENCES: *BHM* (1964-69), 75; (1975-79), 37; *DAB*, 5: 407-8; B. Hindle, *The Pursuit of Science in Revolutionary America, 1735-1789* (1956), 48-50; T. L. Jennings, "A Brief Memoir of William Douglass, M.D.," *Mass. Med. Soc., Communications* 5 (1836): 195-235; Kelly and Burrage (1920), 326; Miller, *BHM*, p. 30; G. H. Weaver, "Life and Writings of William Douglass, M.D., 1691-1752," *Bull. of the Soc. of Med. Hist., Chicago* 2 (1921): 229-59.

P. Cash

DOWNEY, HAL (October 4, 1877, State College, Pa.-January 9, 1959). *Hematologist.* Son of John F., math professor and dean of the college at Penn State, and Stella (Osborn) Downey. Married Iva Mitchell, 1905; three children. EDUCATION: University of Minnesota: 1903, B.A.; 1904, M.A.; and 1909, Ph.D.; postgraduate study: 1910, University of Berlin; and 1911, University of Strassbourg. CAREER: At the University of Minnesota: 1903-29, staff member of the Department of Zoology; and 1929-46, professor of anatomy. CONTRIBUTIONS: Pioneer studies of the hematology of infectious mononucleosis (1921-23); certain characteristic cells have been named "Downey Cells."

WRITINGS: American editor, *Folia Hematologica*, (1923-41); editor of the four-volume *Handbook of Hematology* (1938). REFERENCES: *BHM*, (1970-74), 53; *J. Hist. Med.* 27 (Apr. 1972): 173-86; J. A. Myers, *Masters of Medicine* (1968); Miller, *BHM*, p. 30; *Sci.* 30 (1959): 778-79; *Who Was Who in Am.*, 3: 236.

R. Rosenthal

DRAGSTEDT, LESTER REYNOLD (October 2, 1893, Anaconda, Mont.-July 16, 1975, Wabigama, Mich.). *Physician; Surgery; Physiology.* Son of John A. and Caroline (Selene) Dragstedt. Married Gladys Shoesmith, 1922; four children. EDUCATION: University of Chicago: 1915, B.S.; 1916, M.S.; and 1920, Ph.D.; 1921, M.D., Rush Medical College; 1925, studied surgery in Europe. CAREER: 1916, physiology faculty, University of Chicago; at State University of Iowa: 1916-17, pharmacology faculty; and 1917-19, physiology faculty; 1918-19, medical corps, U.S. Army; 1920-23, physiology faculty, University of Chicago; 1923-25, physiology and pharmacology faculty, Northwestern University; 1925-59, surgery faculty, University of Chicago; and surgical staff, Billings Hospital; 1959-75, research faculty, University of Florida. CONTRIBUTIONS: One of the leading surgeons of the alimentary tract in his generation. Found that removal of the duodenum is compatible with life (1918). Demonstrated that dogs undergoing total parathyroidectomy could be kept alive indefinitely and free from parathyroid tetany if placed on a milk diet fortified with lactose. Isolated a fat-utilizing hormone, lipocaic, secreted by the pancreas (1936-46). Made important contributions to the physiological understanding of pancreatic function and gastric secretion and advanced knowledge of the cause of gastric and duodenal ulcer.

Reintroduced and established the value of vagotomy combined with gastroen-
terostomy for the treatment of peptic ulcers (1943); replaced the more hazardous
operation of gastric resection.
WRITINGS: "Studies on the Pathogenesis of Tetany. I. The Control and Cure of
Parathyroid Tetany by Diet," *Am. J. of Physiology* 64 (1923): 424-34 (with S. C.
Peacock); "Observations on a Substance in Pancreas (a Fat Metabolizing Hormone) Which
Permits Survival and Prevents Liver Changes in Depancreatized Dogs," *ibid.*, 117 (1936):
175-81 (with J. Van Prohaska and H. P. Harms); "Supra-Diaphragmatic Section of the
Vagus Nerves in Treatment of Duodenal Ulcer," *Proc., Soc. Exp. Biol. Med.* 53 (1943):
152-54 (with F. M. Owens, Jr.); "Experimental Gastrojejunal Ulcers Due to Antrum
Hyperfunction," *Arch. of Surg.* 63 (1951): 298-302. A selected bibliography is in *BMNAS*.
REFERENCES: *BMNAS* 51 (1976): 63-95; *McGraw-Hill Modern Men of Sci.* 2 (1966):
126-28; *N. Y. Times*, July 17, 1975; Mark M. Ravitch, *A Century of Surgery*, 2 vols.
(1981); *Who Was Who in Am.*, 6: 118.

S. Galishoff

DRAKE, DANIEL (October 20, 1785, near Scotch Plains, Essex County, N.J.-
November 5, 1852, Cincinnati, Ohio). *Physician; Educator*. Son of Isaac, farmer
and miller, and Elizabeth (Shotwell) Drake. Married Harriet Sisson, December
20, 1807; five children. EDUCATION: 1800-1805, study of medicine under William
Goforth, Cincinnati; 1805-6, 1815-16, attended lectures, University of Pennsylvania School of Medicine, Philadelphia, Pa.; 1816, M.D., University of
Pennsylvania. CAREER: 1804-6, 1807-23, 1827-30, 1831-39 practice, Cincinnati;
1806-7, practice, May's Lick, Ky.; 1817-18, first medical lecturer in Cincinnati
with Coleman Rogers and Elijah Slack; at Medical College of Ohio: 1819,
founder and first president; 1820-22, professor of institutes and practice of medicine; and 1831-32, professor of clinical medicine; 1817-18, 1823-24, professor
of materia medica and medical botany, Transylvania University medical department, Lexington; 1824-27, professor of theory and practice of medicine and
dean of the faculty, Transylvania; 1827, in Cincinnati, co-founder *Western Medical and Physical Journal*; 1828, founder and editor, *Western Journal of the
Medical and Physical Sciences* (Cincinnati); 1830-31, professor of theory and
practice of medicine, Jefferson Medical College, Philadelphia; 1835, organized
medical department, Cincinnati College, and was professor of theory and practice
there (1835-39); 1839-49, associated with Louisville Medical Institute (which
in 1846 became the University of Louisville medical department); 1839-44,
professor of clinical medicine and pathological anatomy; and 1844-49, professor
of medicine; co-founder and co-editor with L. P. Yandell (q.v.) of *Western
Journal of Medicine and Surgery*; 1849-50, Medical College of Ohio, professor
of special pathology, practice, and clinical medicine; 1850-52, the University
of Louisville medical department; spring 1852, returned to Cincinnati to finish
writing the second volume of *Systematic Treatise* . . . and accepted his old chair
at the Medical College of Ohio; died of "congestion of the brain." CONTRI-
BUTIONS: Foremost physician and medical educator of the old Northwest. Author
of classic *Systematic Treatise on the Principal Diseases of the Interior Valley*

. . . , 2 vols. (1850, 1854). In addition to undertaking faculty duties and practice, was instrumental in founding schools for the blind in Cincinnati (1835) and Louisville (1842). Founded medical journals, schools, societies, teaching hospital, museum, and circulating library. Dr. Drake was considered by many to be the most indefatigable professor and practitioner to grace the profession in the United States.

WRITINGS: A bibliography of 692 entries of his publications and manuscripts has been published by H. D. Shapiro and Z. L. Miller in *Physician to the West* . . . (1970). Most representative publications are *Notices Concerning Cincinnati* (1810); *Natural & Statistical View, or Picture of Cincinnati* . . . (1815); *An Inaugural Discourse on Medical Education* . . . (1820; rep., 1951); *Practical Essays on Medical Education and the Medical Profession in the United States* (1832); *A Practical Treatise on* . . . *the Cholera* (1832). REFERENCES: *BHM* (1964-69), 74; (1970-74), 53; (1975-79), 37; *DAB*, 3, pt. 1: 426-27; S. D. Gross, "Daniel Drake," in S. D. Gross, ed., *Lives of Eminent American Physicians and Surgeons* (1861), 614-62; E. F. Horine, *Daniel Drake (1785-1852) Pioneer Physician of the Midwest* (1961); Kelly and Burrage (1920), 328-29; Miller, *BHM*, p. 30; *NCAB*, 5: 110; Shapiro and Miller, *Physician to the West* (1970).

E. H. Conner

DREW, CHARLES RICHARD (June 3, 1904, Washington, D.C.-April 1, 1950, Burlington, N.C.). *Surgeon; Blood preservation.* Son of Richard T., carpet layer, and Nora (Burrell) Drew. Married Minnie Lenore Robbins, September 23, 1939; four children. EDUCATION: 1926, A.B., Amherst College; 1933, M.D., C.M. (master of surgery), McGill University; 1933-35, intern and resident, Montreal General Hospital; 1934, diplomate, National Board of Medical Examiners; 1936-37, resident in surgery, Freedmen's Hospital, Washington, D.C.; 1938-40, resident in surgery, Presbyterian Hospital, N.Y., and graduate student at Columbia University; 1940, Sc.D., Columbia University. CAREER: At Howard University Medical School: 1935-36, instructor in pathology; 1936-50, surgical faculty; and 1941-50, head of the department at Freedmen's Hospital: 1942, chief surgeon; 1944-46, chief of staff; and 1946-48, medical director. CONTRIBUTIONS: Major work in blood research, especially blood preservation. Worked with Dr. John Scudder (q.v.) at Presbyterian Hospital on problems of fluid balance, blood chemistry, and blood transfusion, and established the hospital's first blood bank (1939). When World War II began, chosen by the board of the Blood Transfusion Association in N.Y. to be the medical supervisor of the "Blood for Britain" project. He and colleagues established uniform procedures for procuring and processing blood and for shipping the plasma. Appointed medical director, American Red Cross blood bank program, and assistant director, blood procurement, for the National Research Council (February 1941), which was in charge of collecting blood for use by the American armed forces. But a few weeks later, an official directive from the armed forces to segregate Caucasian blood from the rest, and the acceptance of that directive by the Red Cross over the objections of Drew and other scientists, led him to resign. Certified as diplomate, American Board of Surgery (1941). Received the Spingarn Medal of the National Association for the Advancement of Colored People (1944) for his work on blood banks. Fellow, International College of Surgery (1946). WRITINGS: A list of publications is at the end of the obituary by W. Montague Cobb in *JNMA* 42 (1950): 245-46. Most important work was "Banked Blood: A Study in Blood Preservation" (Doctoral thesis, Columbia University, June 1940). REFERENCES: W. Montague Cobb, "Charles Richard Drew, M.D., 1904-1950," *JNMA* 42 (1950): 239-46; *DAB*, Supplement 4: 242-43; *Encyclopedia of Am. Biog.* (1974), 296-97; Richard Hardwick, *Charles Richard Drew, Pioneer in Blood Research* (1967); Herbert M. Morais, *History of the Negro in Medicine* (1967), 107-9; *Who Was Who in Am.*, 3: 237-38.

R. Kondratas

DuBOIS, EUGENE FLOYD (June 4, 1882, West New Brighton, Staten Island, N.Y.-February 12, 1959, New York, N.Y.). *Physician; Physiology.* Son of Eugene, import-export broker, and Anna Greenleaf (Brooks) DuBois. Married Rebeckah Rutter, 1910; four children. EDUCATION: 1902, A.B., Harvard University; 1906, M.D., College of Physicians and Surgeons (Columbia); 1906, studied pathology in Germany; 1907-8, intern, Presbyterian Hospital (New York City); 1908, studied metabolism in Germany. CAREER: 1909, pathology staff, Presbyterian Hospital; at Cornell University Medical College: 1910-18, clinical medicine and applied pharmacology faculty; 1910-40, medicine faculty; and 1941-50, physiology faculty; 1913-50, medical director, Russell Sage Institute of Pathology, Cornell Medical Division, Bellevue Hospital (moved in 1932 to New York Hospital); 1917-18, medical corps, U.S. Navy Reserve; 1919-32, visiting physician and director, Second Medical Division, Bellevue Hospital; 1932-41, physician-in-chief, New York Hospital; 1942-45, medical corps, U.S. Navy Reserve, on active duty for three months each year; *post* 1947, member, National Research Council Committee on Undersea Warfare; 1947-50, member, Cornell Committee Air Safety Research; 1948-52, chairman, Research and Development Board Panel on Shipboard and Submarine Medicine; president: 1927, American Society for Clinical Investigation; 1939, Association of American Physicians; and 1923-25, Harvey Society. CONTRIBUTIONS: Made experimental studies of human metabolism, especially heat loss and temperature regulation. Developed a technique for determining the surface areas of humans and established normal basal metabolic rates related to surface area. Discovered that the body could give off as much heat through a cool skin as through a warm one, and that body vasoconstriction could change the skin and subcutaneous tissue into a "suit of clothes" and so regulate heat loss. Recognized the first case of hyperparathyroidism in America and showed how calorimetry could be used in the diagnosis and treatment of thyroid diseases. Book *Basal Metabolism in Heath and Disease* (published in 1924 and again in 1927 and 1936) popularized the metabolic effects of fever, chills, and infections. One of the leading authorities on the health hazards encountered in deep-sea diving, submarines, aviation, and gas warfare.

WRITINGS: "The Measurement of the Surface Area of Man," *Arch. of Internal Med.* 15, pt. 2 (1915): 868; "The Respiration Calorimeter in Clinical Medicine," *Harvey*

Lectures 11 (1915-16): 101; "A Case of Osteitis Fibrosa Cystica (Osteomalacia?) with Evidence of Hyperactivity of the Parathyroid Bodies. Metabolic Study No. 1," *J. Clin. Invest.* 8 (1930): 215 (with R. R. Hannon, E. Shorr, and U. S. McClellan); *The Mechanism of Heat Loss and Temperature* (1948). A bibliography is in *BMNAS* 36 (1962): 125-45. REFERENCES: *BHM* (1975-79), 38; D. B. Dill, "Eugene F. DuBois, Environmental Physiologist," *Sci.* 130 (1959): 1746-47; A. McGehee Harvey, *Science at the Bedside* (1981), 230-34, 237, 244; *NCAB*, 54: 467-68; *Who Was Who in Am.*, 3: 239.

S. Galishoff

DUDLEY, BENJAMIN WINSLOW (April 12, 1785, Spotsylvania County, Va.-January 20, 1870, Lexington, Ky.). *Surgeon; Lithotomist; Teacher.* Son of Ambrose, Baptist minister, and Annie (Parker) Dudley. Married Anna Maria Short, 1821; three children. EDUCATION: Early schooling, local schools, Lexington; medical training under Frederick Ridgely (q.v.), Lexington; 1806, M.D., University of Pennsylvania medical department; 1810-14, studied in Paris and London; 1814, admitted by exam to Royal College of Surgeons, London. CAREER: 1805, practice, Lexington, with Dr. James Fishback between sessions at the University of Pennsylvania; 1809, professor of anatomy and physiology, Transylvania University medical department, Lexington, but classes did not convene; 1817-44, professor of anatomy and surgery, Transylvania University medical department, Lexington; 1844-50, professor of principles and practices of surgery; 1850, retired to his estate "Fairlawn" outside Lexington. CONTRIBUTIONS: Established an enviable reputation as a surgeon throughout Ky. and adjoining states. A popular teacher at Transylvania University throughout his career. Lectures were dynamic and he prided himself on independence from authorities. Strongly opposed the practice of bleeding. Fame as a lithotomist was based upon 225 lithotomies with but three or four deaths. Used the gorget of Cline and the lateral approach that had been abandoned by others as too dangerous. Pioneering effort in the surgical treatment of epilepsy by removing depressed skull fragments was attended with modest success and was the subject of one of his few publications.

WRITINGS: "Observations on Injuries of the Head," *Transylv. J. Med.* 1 (1828); *Observations on the Nature and Treatment of Calculous Diseases* (1836); *Observations on the Operations of Lithotomy* (n.d., with J. M. Bush). REFERENCES: A. H. Barkley, *Kentucky's Pioneer Lithotomists* (1913); W. O. Bullock, "Dr. Benjamin Winslow Dudley," *Annals of Med. Hist.*, n.s., 7 (1935): 201; *DAB*, 3, pt. 1: 478-79; Kelly and Burrage (1920), 338-39; Miller, *BHM*, p. 31; *NCAB*, 11: 60; L. P. Yandell, Sr., "A Memoir of the Life and Writings of Dr. Benjamin W. Dudley," *Am. Practitioner* 1 (1870): 150, reprinted in *J. Ky. Med. Assoc.* 15 (1917): 56.

E. H. Conner

DUGAS, LOUIS ALEXANDER (January 3, 1806, Washington, Ga.-October 19, 1884, Augusta, Ga.). *Physician; Surgeon.* Son of Louis Rene Adrien and Mary Pauline (Bellemeau) de la Vincendire Dugas. Married Mary C. Barnes,

1833; Louisa V. Harris, 1840, five children. EDUCATION: Private tutors and the Academy of Richmond County; studied medicine under Charles Lambert de Beauregard and John Dent; 1827, M.D., University of Maryland; postgraduate work, Paris hospitals; 1831, returned to America. CAREER: At Medical College of Georgia: 1832, a founder and professor of anatomy and physiology during the early years; later took the chair of physiology and pathological anatomy, which he held until 1855; and 1855-83, professor of principles and practice of surgery; 1861-76, dean; 1834, returned to France to buy Medical College of Georgia's library and museum; at *Southern Medical and Surgical Journal*: 1851-54, editor; and 1855-56, 1866-67, co-editor; three times president of the Medical Association of Georgia. CONTRIBUTIONS: Author of roughly 130 papers and a number of translations in medical literature. Did important work in treatment of penetrating wounds to the abdomen. Experimented successfully with hypnotism in surgery. Best remembered for a test (called Dugas's Test or Dugas's Sign) devised to determine shoulder dislocation. Term as dean, Medical College of Georgia, coming in the critical period following the Civil War, was decisive in mandating that the school would survive the hostilities that Dugas, as a foe of secession, had most heartily opposed.

WRITINGS: Of his body of articles, roughly two-thirds are in the *Southern Med. and Surg. J*. His "Report on a New Principle of Diagnosis in Dislocation of the Shoulder-Joint" is in *TAMA* 10 (1857): 175-79. REFERENCES: William B. Atkinson, *Physicians and Surgeons of the U. S.* (1878), 10; William H. Goodrich, *History of the Medical Department of the University of Georgia* (1928); Kelly and Burrage (1920), 340; *Memoirs of Georgia* 2 (1895): 190-99; George A. Traylor, "Master Surgeons of America. Louis Alexander Dugas," *Surg. Gyn. & Obst.* 64 (1937): 714-17. For listings of his articles see George T. McCutchen, "Louis Alexander Dugas," *The Recorder* (1965), 14-20, and particularly Eugene Foster, "In Memoriam. L. A. Dugas, M.D., LL.D.," *Atlanta Med. and Surg. J.*, o.s., 25 (1886): 768-81, esp. 772-74.

P. Spalding

DUHRING, LOUIS ADOLPHUS (December 23, 1845, Philadelphia, Pa.-May 8, 1913, Philadelphia). *Dermatology*. Son of Henry, merchant, and Caroline (Oberteuffer) Duhring. Never married. EDUCATION: 1861-63, attended University of Pennsylvania; 1863, enlisted in the 32nd Regiment, Penn. Volunteers and served 3 months in the Civil War, honorably discharged; 1867, M.D., University of Pennsylvania; 1867-68, resident physician, Blockley Hospital; 1868-70, postgraduate study in Europe where he came under the influence of Ferdinand Hebra who developed dermatology into a distinct specialty. CAREER: 1870, practice of dermatology in Philadelphia, opening the Dispensary for Skin Diseases and remaining on the staff as director until 1880 and as consultant until 1890; University of Pennsylvania: 1871-76, lecturer on skin diseases; 1876-90, clinical professor of skin diseases; 1890, full professor; 1876-87, visiting dermatologist to the Philadelphia Hospital. CONTRIBUTIONS: Pioneering dermatologist, author of the first American textbook on the subject (1877). Demonstrated that dermatitis herpetiformis (known as Duhring's Disease) was a specific clinical entity.

WRITINGS: *Atlas of Skin Diseases* (1876); *Practical Treatise on Diseases of the Skin* (1877); *Cutaneous Medicine* (2 volumes, 1895, 1898). REFERENCES: *DAB*, 3, pt. 1: 494-95; Kelly and Burrage (1928), 355-56; *NCAB*, 20: 351; L. C. Parish, *Louis A. Duhring, M.D.: Pathfinder for Dermatology* (1967).

M. Kaufman

DUNGLISON, ROBLEY (January 4, 1798, Keswick, England-April 1, 1869, Philadelphia, Pa.). *Physician*; *Medical education*; *Physiology*. Son of William, wool manufacturer, and Elizabeth (Jackson) Dunglison. Married Harriet Leadam, 1824; seven children. EDUCATION: Apprenticed to surgeon in Keswick; studied medicine, Edinburgh, Paris, and London; 1818, medical degree, Royal College of Surgeons (London); diploma, Society of Apothecaries; 1823, M.D., University of Erlangen (Germany). CAREER: 1819-25, practiced medicine, London, and appointed physician-accoucheur, Eastern Dispensary; medicine faculty: 1825-33, University of Virginia; and 1833-36, University of Maryland; 1836-68, institutes of medicine faculty and sometimes dean, Jefferson Medical College (Philadelphia). CONTRIBUTIONS: Through writings and teaching, played a prominent role in American medical education. Took a leading part in the early development of the medical school at the University of Virginia and largely responsible for the early success of Jefferson Medical School. At Virginia, first full-time professor of medicine in the United States. Wrote the first American textbook on physiology and pioneered in its teaching. Assisted William Beaumont (q.v.) in his investigations of the physiology of digestion. Wrote a medical dictionary that was known throughout the world and by 1897 had gone through 23 editions. Authored books on numerous medical subjects, derived largely from the works of others, which made available to Americans the most current scientific thought. Edited several medical journals in the United States and England and translated and edited a number of foreign-language works. Promoted the development of raised type for the blind and was active in bettering the care of the insane poor.

WRITINGS: *Commentaries on the Diseases of the Stomach and Bowels of Children* (1824); *Syllabus of Lectures on Medical Jurisprudence, and on the Treatment of Poisoning and Suspended Animation* (1827); *Human Physiology* (1832); *A New Dictionary of Medical Science and Literature* (1833); *General Therapeutics, or Principles of Medical Practice* (1836). A bibliography is in *Trans., Am. Philos. Soc.*, n.s., 53, pt. 8 (Dec. 1963). REFERENCES: *BHM* (1964-69), 77; (1970-74), 54; (1975-79), 15; Jerome J. Bylebyl, "William Beaumont, Robley Dunglison, and the 'Philadelphia Physiologists,' " *J. Hist. Med. & Allied Sci.* 25 (1970): 3-21; *DAB*, 5: 512-13; *DSB*, 4: 251-53; Clark A. Elliott, *Biographical Dict. of Am. Sci.* (1979), 80; Kelly and Burrage (1928), 357; Miller, *BHM*, p. 31.

S. Galishoff

DUNLAP, LIVINGSTON (1799, Cherry Valley, N.Y.-1862, Indianapolis, Ind.). *Physician*. Three sons. EDUCATION: Apprenticeship; attended course of lectures, Transylvania University, Lexington, Ky. CAREER: 1821, settled in Indianapolis and began medical practice; 1845-49, postmaster, also serving as city councilman; 1845-48, served (with Dr. John Evans [q.v.] and Dr. John Bobbs [q.v.]) as commissioner in erecting the state's first mental hospital; 1849, elected first president, Indiana State Medical Society; 1849, helped organize the first medical college in Indianapolis, Central Medical College, and served as professor of theory and practice of medicine. CONTRIBUTIONS: A founder of the Indiana State Medical Society, Central Medical College (Indianapolis), and City Hospital (Indianapolis), the latter of which continues as the Wishard Memorial Hospital, the oldest hospital on the Indiana University Medical Center campus. Remembered as a pioneer in organizing Ind. medicine and medical education. REFERENCES: G. W. H. Kemper, *Medical History of the State of Indiana* (1911); Miller, *BHM*, p. 31; J. H. B. Nowland, *Sketches of Prominent Citizens* (1877).

C. A. Bonsett

DURHAM, JAMES (b. May 1, 1762, Philadelphia, Pa.). *Physician*. Married; no children. CAREER: Learned as a child and slave to compound medicines while helping his owner, Dr. John A. Kearsley (q.v.), Philadelphia; c. 1777-81, after death of Kearsley, did menial medical work as slave of Dr. George (or Gregory) West, surgeon of 16th British Regiment; 1781-83, assistant to Dr. Robert Dow, New Orleans, La., his next owner; 1783-1802, practiced medicine as a free man (purchased freedom, 1783) in New Orleans, often under the patronage of Dow; even before city authorities restricted his practice to throat diseases only (1801), because he had no formal training, Durham contemplated leaving; appears to have left New Orleans by 1802. CONTRIBUTIONS: One of earliest known free black healers in America. Appears to have been a successful practitioner who was well respected in New Orleans and by Benjamin Rush (q.v.) with whom he corresponded (1789-1802) after their meeting in Philadelphia (fall 1788).

WRITINGS: Correspondence with Rush is in Rush papers, Historical Society of Pennsylvania, Philadelphia. REFERENCES: Lyman H. Butterfield, ed., *Letters of Benjamin Rush* 1 (1951): 497-98; Henry M. Morais, *The History of the Afro-American in Medicine* (1976), 8-10; C. E. Wines, "Dr. James Durham . . . " *Pa. Mag. of Hist. and Biog.* 103 (1979): 325-33. Correspondence with Rush is reproduced in Betty L. Plummer, "Letters of James Durham to Benjamin Rush," *J. of Negro Hist.* 65 (1980): 261-69.

T. Savitt

DYER, ISADORE (November 2, 1865, Galveston, Tex.-October 12, 1920, New Orleans, La.). *Physician; Dermatology; Leprosy*. Son of Isadore and Amelia Ann (Lewis) Dyer. Married Mercedes Louise Perceval, 1905. EDUCATION: 1887, Ph. B., Sheffield Scientific School (Yale); 1889, M.D., Tulane University; 1890-92, intern, New York Skin and Cancer Hospital; 1902, did graduate study in Paris and London. CAREER: 1891-92, lecturer, New York Post Graduate Medical School; 1892-1908, diseases of the skin faculty, New Orleans Polyclinic; at Tulane University School of Medicine: 1892-1920, diseases of the skin faculty; and 1908-20, dean; visiting and consulting dermatologist to many New Orleans hospitals; 1908-20, officer, U.S. Army Medical Reserve Corps, rising in rank from lieutenant to colonel; president: 1899-1900, Orleans Parish Medical Society; 1902-3, Louisiana State Medical Society; 1910-11, Southern Medical Association; 1912-13, American Dermatological Association; 1913-14, New Orleans Academy of Science; and 1915-16, Association of American Medical Colleges. CONTRIBUTIONS: One of the nation's leading authorities on leprosy. Improved medical treatment of the disease and was instrumental in obtaining proper care for its victims. Established and became president of the first Board of Control of the Louisiana Leper Home (1894); subsequently induced the federal government to operate the institution as a national lepers' home, later renamed the National Leprosarium. Edited *New Orleans Medical and Surgical Journal* (1896 until death) and co-edited *American Journal of Tropical Diseases and Preventive Medicine* (1914-16). Helped organize and played an active role in the National Board of Medical Examiners (1915-20).

WRITINGS: *Report on the Leprosy Question in Louisiana* (1894); "The History of the Louisiana Leper Home," *New Orleans Med. and Surg. J.* 54 (1901-2): 714-37; *The Art of Medicine and Other Addresses, Papers, etc.* (1913). REFERENCES: *DAB*, 5: 582; Kelly and Burrage (1928), 363; *Who Was Who in Am.*, 1: 352.

S. Galishoff

DYOTT, THOMAS W. (c. 1777, England-January 17, 1861, Philadelphia, Pa.). *Proprietary medicine manufacturer and marketer; Glass manufacturer.* Married c. 1816; at least two sons. EDUCATION: Perhaps an apothecary's apprenticeship in England; dubious claim of M.D. from Marischal College and University of Aberdeen. CAREER: 1804 or 1805, went to Philadelphia from England or West Indies; 1806-39, made and marketed patent medicines; 1809-c. 1819, treated patients for sexual ailments; 1815, began to acquire interest in glass factories near Philadelphia that (by 1831) were largest and producing best quality glassware in the nation, underselling imports; c. 1833-38, operated Dyottsville as a self-contained paternalistic glassworks community with rules of decorum and temperance for apprentices; 1835-38, established Manual Labor Bank; 1838-41, bankruptcy during depression; conviction for fraudulent insolvency; one and one-half years in jail; 1841-61, resumed patent-medicine business. CONTRIBUTIONS: Brought formulas from England for stomachic elixir of health, vegetable nervous cordial, gout and rheumatic drops, worm-destroying lozenges, numerous other nostrums. Developed marketing system (by early 1810s) using Conestoga wagons with agents in all major cities of West and South. Has been called America's first drug price cutter. Pioneered aggressive newspaper advertising throughout nation, using testimonials and stressing merit of self-dosage proprietaries as against learned physicians. Also marketed drugs, dry stuffs, paints, snuff, spices, garden seeds, coonskin whips, and produce secured by barter for fabricated wares. Got into glass manufacturing because of need for patent medicine bottles. Noted for making historical portrait flasks, one showing himself and Franklin on its two faces. At height as America's nostrum king, lived extravagantly, dressed eccentrically, and drove about in an elegant English coach drawn by four horses.

WRITINGS: *Approved Patent and Family Medicines* (1814); *An Exposition of the System of Moral and Mental Labor, Established at the Glass Factory of Dyottsville* (1833). REFERENCES: *DAB*, 3, pt. 1: 586-87; Helen McKearin, *Bottles, Flasks and Dr. Dyott* (1970); various newspapers and Philadelphia city directories; M. I. Wilbert, "America's First Cutter," *Bull. Pharm.* 18 (1904): 237-38; J. H. Young, "Thomas W. Dyott," *J. of the Am. Pharmacy Assoc. (Practical Ph. Ed.)*, n.s., 1 (1961): 290-91, 294; idem, *The Toadstool Millionaires* (1961), 31-43.

J. H. Young

E

EAGLESON, JAMES BEATY (August 30, 1862, Chillicothe, Ohio-January 26, 1928, Seattle, Wash.). *General surgeon.* Son of William and Elizabeth W. (Hodsden) Eagleson. Married Blanche Mills, 1889; four children. EDUCATION: Dagues' Collegiate Institute, Chillicothe; North Indiana Normal School, Valparaiso, Ind.; 1885, M.D., College of Physicians and Surgeons, Chicago, Ill. CAREER: 1885-86, U.S. Marine Hospital, Chicago; 1886-87, private practice, Port Townsend, Wash.; 1887-98, U.S. Marine Hospital Service, Seattle; 1899-1925, general surgery, Seattle; numerous hospital appointments in Seattle; 1891-96, surgeon-general, National Guard, Washington; 1911-19, medical officer, U.S. Army. CONTRIBUTIONS: Organized and served as commanding officer and director of Base Hospital No. 50, and U.S. General Hospital No. 50 (1917-25). Co-founder and associate editor, *Northwest Medicine* (1917). Co-founder and regent, American College of Surgeons. President, State Board of Health, Wash. (1891), and State Board of Medical Examiners, Wash. (1898). REFERENCES: C. B. Bagley, *History of Seattle* 3 (1916): 497-98; *Who Was Who in Am.*, 1: 352; *Who's Who in Am. Med.* (1925), 436.

T. Savitt

EARLE, PLINY (December 31, 1809, Leicester, Mass.-May 17, 1892, Northampton, Mass.). *Physician; Psychiatry.* Son of Pliny, textile manufacturer, and Patience (Buffum) Earle. Bachelor. EDUCATION: 1820-24, Leicester Academy; 1826-28, Friends' School, Providence, R.I.; 1837, M.D., University of Pennsylvania. CAREER: 1828-35, taught at the Friends' School, rising from assistant teacher to principal; 1837-39, after receiving medical degree, continued studies in Europe and visited a number of European insane asylums; 1840, appointed superintendent, Friends' Asylum for the Insane (Frankford, Pa.); 1844-49, superintendent, Bloomingdale Asylum for the Insane (New York, N.Y.); 1849-64, lived for the most part in Leicester, with the exception of 1852-54, when he opened an office in New York City and served as a member of the

Board of Visiting Physicians to the New York City Lunatic Asylum on Black-well's Island; 1862-64, worked at the Government Hospital for the Insane, Washington, D.C.; 1864-85, superintendent, State Lunatic Asylum in Northamp-ton, Mass. CONTRIBUTIONS: Wrote extensively on mental hospitals and was one of the 13 original founders (1844) of the Association of Medical Superintendents of American Institutions for the Insane (now the American Psychiatric Associ-ation). Among the earliest to analyze mentally ill institutional populations and outcomes in a statistical manner. Published a number of studies (1870s and 1880s) designed to discredit the curability claims made by mental hospital su-perintendents in the 1830s and 1840s. Reorganized the Northampton State Lu-natic Asylum, where he was noted for an efficient and economical administration.

WRITINGS: *History, Description, and Statistics of the Bloomingdale Asylum for the Insane* (1848); "Historical Sketch of the Institutions for the Insane in the United States of America," N.Y. Acad. of Med., *Trans.* 1, pt. 1 (1851); *Institutions for the Insane, in Prussia, Austria and Germany* (1854); *The Curability of Insanity: A Series of Studies* (1887). Writings listed in Franklin B. Sanborn, ed., *Memoirs of Pliny Earle, M.D.* (1898), 317-20. REFERENCES: E. T. Carlson and L. Peters, "Dr. Pliny Earle (1809-1892)," *Am. J. of Psychiatry* 116 (1959): 557-58; *DAB*, 3, pt. 1: 595-96; Gerald N. Grob, *Mental Institutions in America* (1973); Kelly and Burrage (1920), 349-50; *NCAB*, 11: 146; Sanborn, *Memoirs of Pliny Earle*.

G. Grob

EASTMAN, JOSEPH (January 29, 1842, Fulton County, N.Y.-June 5, 1902, Marion County, Ind.). *Physician; Surgeon; Obstetrics and Gynecology.* Son of Rufus, justice of the peace, and Catherine (Jipson) Eastman. Married Mary Katherine Barker, 1868; three children. EDUCATION: Public schools; 1858-61, apprentice to a blacksmith; 1865, M.D., University of Georgetown; 1871, M.D., Bellevue Hospital Medical College. CAREER: Served in the infantry in the Civil War; suffered from typho-malaria; while recuperating at the Mount Pleasant Hospital, Washington, D.C., assigned to serving as a male nurse and then reassigned as hospital steward; while in military service, attended three sessions at Georgetown medical school; commissioned first lieutenant and assistant sur-geon, U.S. volunteers; *post* 1866, medical practice, Clermont, Brownsburg, and then Indianapolis, Ind.; 1875, demonstrator of anatomy, College of Physicians and Surgeons (Indianapolis); 1875, established own hospital and limited practice to diseases of women and abdominal surgery; 1879, professor of anatomy and clinical surgery and diseases of women, Central College of Physicians and Sur-geons. CONTRIBUTIONS: An innovator in surgical technique and inventor of sur-gical instruments, the latter being facilitated by his early machine and blacksmithing experience. First American surgeon to operate successfully for extrauterine preg-nancy by dissecting out the sac containing the fetus, thereby saving the life of both mother and infant (1888). Delegate to the International Medical Congress in Berlin (1890), which he addressed on his method of hysterectomy, using his hysterectomy staff and Eastman clamp, both examples of his mechanical ingenuity and both of which came into wide international usage. The first abdominal surgeon in Ind. to operate "in doubtful cases," to do exploratory procedures as life-saving measures in selected situations. A founder and surgical editor, *Medical and Surgical Monitor* (1898).

WRITINGS: Numerous contributions to the medical literature of the day. Most appeared in *Trans., Indiana State Med. Soc.* and *Med. and Surg. Monitor.* Article on extrauterine pregnancy appeared in *Am. J. of Obstetrics* 21 (1888): 929-31. REFERENCES: G. W. H. Kemper, *Medical History of the State of Indiana* (1911), 264-66; J. D. MacDougall, *Indiana Med. Hist. Q.* 1 (1974): 26-30; *NCAB*, 7: 46; R. F. Stone, *Biog. of Eminent Physicians and Surgeons* (1894), 150-51; *Who Was Who in Am.*, 1: 35.

C. A. Bonsett

EBERLE, JOHN (December 10, 1787, Lancaster, Pa.-February 2, 1838, Cincinnati, Ohio). *Physician; Educator; Medical editor.* EDUCATION: Studied medicine with Abraham Carpenter of Lancaster; 1809, M.D., University of Pennsylvania. CAREER: 1809-14, began medical practice, Lancaster; 1814-15, surgeon in War of 1812; 1815-30, medical practice, Philadelphia, Pa.; 1818-30, established and edited *American Medical Recorder*; at Jefferson Medical College: 1825-31, member, founding faculty; and professor of theory and practice of medicine; 1830-37, faculty, Medical College of Ohio; 1837, professor of theory and practice of medicine, Transylvania University; 1832, established the *Western Medical Gazette*; 1837, editor, *Transylvania Medical Journal.* CONTRIBUTIONS: Brilliant Pa. Dutchman who combined American and Germanic trends in medical education in Philadelphia, Lexington, Ky., and Cincinnati. Founded important medical journals and author of texts on materia medica and practice.

WRITINGS: *Treatise on the Materia Medica and Therapeutics* (1823); *Treatise on Diseases and Physical Education of Children* (1833); *Notes of Lectures on the Theory and Practice of Medicine* (1834); *Treatise on the Practice of Medicine* (1838). Writings listed in Kelly and Burrage (1920), 351. REFERENCES: *Appleton's CAB* (1888); *DAB*, 5: 615-16; S. D. Gross, *Lives of Eminent Physicians* (1861); F. P. Henry, *Standard Hist. of the Medical Profession in Philadelphia* (1877); Kelly and Burrage (1920); *NCAB*, 11: 423.

D. I. Lansing

EDDY, HARRISON PRESCOTT (April 29, 1870, Millbury, Mass.-June 15, 1937, Montreal, Canada). *Sanitary engineer.* Son of William Justus, treasurer of a textile mill, and Martha Augusta (Prescott) Eddy. Married Minnie Locke Jones, 1892; four children. EDUCATION: 1891, B.S., Worcester Polytechnic Institute. CAREER: Sewerage department, City of Worcester, Mass.: 1891, chemist and superintendent of the sewerage treatment works; 1892-1907, superintendent; 1907-37, partner in the engineering firm of Metcalf and Eddy; active in the American Society of Civil Engineers and helped enact the Federal Emergency Relief Act of 1933 which made possible a huge construction program under the Public Works Administration. CONTRIBUTIONS: One of the nation's foremost authorities on sewage treatment and disposal. In 1907 became partners with

Leonard Metcalf, a distinguished waterworks engineer; firm of Metcalf and Eddy served as consultants on water purification and sewage treatment for more than 125 cities and towns leading to a marked reduction in deaths from typhoid fever.

WRITINGS: With Metcalf, wrote the standard three-volume study, *American Sewerage Practice* (1914-1915), and a widely-used text entitled *Sewerage and Sewage Disposal* (1922). REFERENCES: *DAB*, Supplement 2: 169-70; *NCAB*, 28: 265; *Who Was Who in Am.*, 1: 357.

S. Galishoff

EDDY, MARY A. (BAKER) (July 21, 1821, Bow near Concord, N.H.-December 3, 1910, District Hill near Boston, Mass.). *Founder of Christian Science.* Daughter of Mark and Abigail (Ambroise) Baker. Married George W. Glover 1843, (d. 1844), one son; Dr. Daniel Patterson, June 21, 1853 (deserted 1862); Asa G. Eddy, January 1, 1877 (d. 1882). EDUCATION: As a child, was in "delicate" health and was educated privately; 1862, consulted with Dr. Phineas P. Quimby, who treated her diseases by mental methods; formulation of her theories are dated from 1866; 1879, ordained a minister and received a charter for "Church of Christ, Scientist"; 1881, received charter from Mass. for a Metaphysical College of Boston; 1883, established the *Christian Science Journal*; 1889, due to church dissension, "Mother Eddy" moved to Concord; 1889, invited to become a member of Victoria Philosophical Institute of London, England. CONTRIBUTIONS: Founder of Christian Science. "Mind is divine, mind is all." Sin and sickness are delusions of the mortal mind, and sickness is therefore not a reality. Taught not to brood over the ills of life. A faith healer relying on meditation, not on drugs or paraphernalia of any type.

WRITINGS: *Science and Health* (1875); *Science of Man . . .* (1876). REFERENCES: *DAB*, 6:7-15; *NCAB*, 3: 80-81; *Notable Am. Women*, 1:551-61; Edwin Franden Oakin, *Mrs. Eddy* (1929; rev., 1968); Robert Peel, *Mary Baker Eddy, The Years of Discovery* (1966).

R. Edwards

EDSALL, DAVID LINN (July 6, 1869, Hamburg, N.J.-August 12, 1945, Cambridge, Mass.). *Physician; Medical educator; Industrial hygiene.* Son of Richard E., merchant, and Emma Everett (Linn) Edsall. Married Margaret Harding Tileston, 1899, three children; Elizabeth Pendleton Kennedy, 1915; Louisa Cabot Richardson, 1930. EDUCATION: 1890, A.B., Princeton University; 1893, M.D., University of Pennsylvania; 1893-94, intern, Mercy Hospital (Pittsburgh); 1894-95, studied in London, England, and Graz and Vienna, Austria. CAREER: 1896-1922, practiced medicine, first in Philadelphia, Pa., and then in Boston; 1896-1910, clinical medicine faculty, University of Pennsylvania; 1911-12, preventive medicine faculty, Washington University School of Medicine (St. Louis); at Harvard University: 1912-23, clinical medicine faculty; 1918-35, dean of the medical school; and 1921-35, dean of the school of public health; 1912-22, medical staff, Massachusetts General Hospital; 1927-35, trustee, Rockefeller

Foundation. CONTRIBUTIONS: Made basic biochemical investigations of nutritional diseases, metabolic disorders of children, and industrial sicknesses. Described "heat cramps," a severe disorder that struck workers who had been exposed to intense heat (1908); sometimes called "Edsalls's disease," ailment was later revealed to be caused by salt depletion. Identified occupations in which there was a high risk of chronic metallic poisoning and aroused the medical profession to the importance of industrial medicine generally. One of the original members, Interurban Clinical Club (1905), and co-founder of the American Society for Clinical Investigation (1908). Played a major role in the movements to reform medical education in three universities following the publication of the Flexner Report in 1910. Most successful at Harvard, where he assembled an outstanding staff, modernized the curriculum, and stimulated research. Helped establish and edit *Journal of Industrial Hygiene and Toxicology* (1919).

WRITINGS: "Diseases Due to Chemical Agents," in William Osler (q.v.), ed., *Modern Medicine* . . . (1907); "The Bearing of Metabolism Studies on Clinical Medicine," *Trans., Assoc. of Am. Physicians*, 22 (1907): 667-82; "A Disorder Due to Exposure to Intense Heat: Characterized Clinically Chiefly by Violent Muscular Spasms and Excessive Irritability of the Muscles. Preliminary Note," *JAMA* 51 (1908): 1969-71. A bibliography is in Joseph C. Aub and Ruth K. Hapgood, *Pioneer in Modern Medicine: David Linn Edsall of Harvard* (1970). REFERENCES: *DAB*, Supplement 3: 243-44; Miller, *BHM*, p. 32; *N.Y. Times*, August 13, 1945; *Who Was Who in Am.*, 2: 170.

S. Galishoff

EINHORN, MAX (January 10, 1862, Grodno, Russia-September 25, 1953, New York, N.Y.). *Physician; Gastroenterology.* Son of Abraham and Sara Einhorn. Married Flora Strauss, 1892. EDUCATION: 1879, A.B., Gymnasium, Riga, Russia; 1884, M.D., University of Berlin; 1888, studied in Berlin. Came to the United States in 1885. CAREER: *Post* 1885, practiced medicine in New York City; *post* 1885, internal medicine staff, German Hospital (later Lenox Hill Hospital); 1889-1922, internal medicine faculty, Post-Graduate Medical School and Hospital. CONTRIBUTIONS: Invented many devices used in the diagnosis and treatment of intestinal diseases including transillumination of the stomach, pyloric dilators, and stomach and duodenal buckets. Pioneered in the use of radium for making X-ray photographs of the stomach. A benefactor of Lenox Hill Hospital. Shared responsibility for the section on "Progress in Gastroenterology" in the *American Journal of Gastroenterology* (1911-14). A director of *Archiv für Verdauungs-Krankheiten* (Berlin). *Post* 1905, associate editor of *Medicinische Monatschrift* (New York).

WRITINGS: *Diseases of the Stomach* (1896); *Diseases of the Intestines* (1900); *Practical Problems of Diet and Nutrition* (1905); *Lectures on Dietetics* (1914); *The Duodenal Tube and Its Possibilities* (1920). A bibliography is contained in *Die Medizin Der Gegenwart in Selbstdarstellungen*, 8 (1929): 1-24. REFERENCES: Hyman I. Goldstein, "Max Einhorn, M.D.," *J. of the Internat. Coll. of Surgeons* 5(1942): 343-46; *N.Y. Times*, September 26, 1953; *Who Was Who in Am.*, 4: 282.

S. Galishoff

ELIOT, CHARLES WILLIAM (March 20, 1834, Boston, Mass.-August 22, 1926, Northeast Harbor, Maine). *University president.* Son of Samuel Atkins and Mary (Lyman) Eliot. Married Ellen Derby Peabody, 1858, two children; Grace Mellen Hopkinson, 1877. EDUCATION: 1853, A.B., Harvard University; 1863-65, studied chemistry and investigated educational methods in Europe. CAREER: At Harvard University: 1854-63, chemistry and mathematics faculties; 1869-1909, president; and 1910-16, overseer; 1865-69, analytical chemistry faculty, Massachusetts Institute of Technology; at National Education Association: 1890-92, chairman, Committee of Ten; and 1903, president; 1908, president, National Civil Service Reform League; *post* 1909, editor, Harvard Classics; 1908-17, member, International Health Board; trustee, Carnegie Foundation for the Advancement of Teaching. CONTRIBUTIONS: Transformed Harvard from an undistinguished, provincial college with a few professional schools into a great university. Remodeled the medical school along German lines so that medical education was placed on a scientific basis within the framework of a university. Established a three-year graded curriculum (1871), later lengthened to four years (1892); a full academic year divided into two sections; laboratory work in the basic sciences; clinical instruction and internship at local hospitals; the free elective system in the fourth year; and an admission examination for all applicants. Ended the school's proprietary era by transferring its finances to the university. Led to similar reforms in several of the nation's other better medical colleges, thereby preparing the way for the additional reforms inaugurated at Johns Hopkins (1893). Fought to secure a place for preventive medicine in the medical curriculum, which culminated in the establishment of the pioneering Harvard Medical School and Massachusetts Institute of Technology School of Public Health (1913-22). Active in the movement to introduce Western medicine into China; participated in the establishment of the Harvard Medical School of China (1912-16) and the Peking Union Medical College (1917-World War II).

WRITINGS: *Reports of the President of Harvard College* (1869-1910); *Educational Reform* (1898). REFERENCES: John Z. Bowers, "The Influence of Charles W. Eliot on Medical Education," *Pharos Alpha Omega Alpha* 35 (1972): 156-59; Jean A. Curran, "Charles William Eliot, Medical Messiah," *Harvard Medical Alumni Bulletin*, 45 (Mar.-Apr. 1971): 6-12; *DAB*, 6: 71-78; Henry James, *Charles W. Eliot, President of Harvard University, 1869-1909* (1930); Samuel E. Morison, *The Development of Harvard University Since the Inauguration of President Eliot, 1869-1929* (1930); *Who Was Who in Am.*, 1: 364.

S. Galishoff

ELLETT, EDWARD COLEMAN (December 18, 1869, Memphis, Tenn.-June 8, 1947, Atlantic City, N.J.). *Physician; Ophthalmology.* Son of Henry T., lawyer and chancery court judge, and Katherine (Coleman) Ellett. Married

Nina Polk Martin, 1896; no children. EDUCATION:1888, A.B., University of the South, Sewanee, Tenn.; 1891, M.D., University of Pennsylvania; house surgeon at Will's Eye Hospital, Philadelphia. CAREER: 1893-1947, private practice in ophthalmology, Memphis; professor of ophthalmology: 1906-11, Memphis College of Physicians and Surgeons; and 1911-22, University of Tennessee College of Medicine; 1926-47, chief of staff, Memphis Eye, Ear, Nose and Throat Hospital; in World War I, served as a lieutenant colonel, U.S. Army Medical Corps, and commanded a base hospital in France; president: 1926, American Academy of Ophthalmology and Oto-Laryngology; 1932, American Ophthalmological Association. CONTRIBUTIONS: Internationally known as an ophthalmologist, attracted patients from Europe as well as the United States. Recognized as a skillful surgeon who introduced into the United States innovations in cataract surgery such as the corneoscleral stitch and intracapsular extraction of the cataract. Involved in the organization of the American Board of Ophthalmology (1916) and conducted the board's first examination in Memphis for specialty certification, marking the start of the concept of specialty boards in the United States. Exercised great influence on the development of ophthalmology, especially in the South, by his great talent and skill as well as by his kindly interest in his patients and the wise counsel he offered his colleagues.

WRITINGS: Contributed over 125 papers to the medical literature, mainly clinical subjects with emphasis on diseases of the eye. Wrote the chapter on "Lacrimal Diseases" in Conrad Berens, *The Eye and Its Diseases* (1936). REFERENCES: *Trans., Am. Acad. of Ophthal. & Otol.* 51 (1947): 548-50; *Who Was Who in Am.*, 2: 172.

                                                                              S. R. Bruesch

ELMER, JONATHAN (November 29, 1745, Cedarville, N.J.-September 3, 1817, Bridgeton, N.J.). *Physician: Statesman.* Son of Daniel, farmer, and Abigail (Lawrence) Elmer. Married Mary Seeley, 1769; eight children. EDUCATION: Tutored privately; apprentice to Dr. John Morgan (Philadelphia); at University of Pennsylvania Medical School: 1768, B.M.; and 1771, M.D. CAREER: Private practice: 1768-71, Roadstown, N.J.; and 1771-1817, Bridgeton; 1772-74, sheriff, Cumberland County, N.J.; 1775, member, Provincial Congress of New Jersey; 1776-78, 1781, 1786-89, clerk, Cumberland County; member: 1776-78, 1781-84, 1787, 1788, Continental Congress; and 1780, 1784, New Jersey Council; 1784-1802, 1813-14, surrogate, Cumberland County; 1789-91, member, U.S. Senate; 1787, president, Medical Society of New Jersey. Although Elmer preferred "political and judicial business," Dr. Benjamin Rush (q.v.) said that he was "exceeded by no physician in the United States." CONTRIBUTIONS: The first New Jerseyite to receive (1771) an M.D. from an American medical school. As a member of Congress during the Revolutionary War, served on the medical committee and investigated hospitals. Instrumental in procuring legal recognition (1790) of the Medical Society of New Jersey from the state legislature. REFERENCES: *Biog. Directory of the Am. Congress, 1774-1949*, p. 1130; *Biog. Encyclopaedia of N.J.* (1877), 279; *DAB*, 6: 116-17; Lucius Q. C. Elmer, *Genealogy and*

Biography of the Elmer Family, 34-44; *NCAB*, 11: 538; Kelly and Burrage (1928), 516-17; *N.J. Med. Rep.* 1 (1848): 133-36; Fred B. Rogers, "Jonathan Elmer: Medical Progenitor," *J. of the Med. Soc. of New Jersey* 62 (1965): 576.

W. Barlow

ELVEHJEM, CONRAD ARNOLD (May 27, 1901, McFarland, Wis.-July 27, 1962, Madison, Wis.). *Biochemist; Nutrition.* Son of Ole Johnson, farmer, and Christine (Lewis) Elvehjem. Married Constance Waltz, 1926; two children. EDUCATION: University of Wisconsin: 1923, B.S.; 1924, M.S.; and 1927, Ph.D.; 1929-30, postgraduate study, Cambridge, England. CAREER: At University of Wisconsin: 1925-62, biochemistry faculty; 1944-58, chairman of Department of Biochemistry; 1946-58, dean of Graduate School; and 1958-62, president. CONTRIBUTIONS: Career devoted to study of animal nutrition and especially the role of trace elements and vitamins. In association with Harry Steenbock (q.v.) and E. B. Hart, established importance of traces of copper for iron uptake in hemoglobin formation. Showed that nicotinic acid cures canine black tongue, thus paving way for its use in treatment of pellagra. Carried out extensive researches on role of biotin, pantothenic acid, paraaminobenzoic acid, folic acid, and inositol in animal nutrition and on action of intestinal bacteria in synthesizing trace nutrients. As president, University of Wisconsin, noted especially for encouraging growth of humanities and social sciences.

WRITINGS: "Iron in Nutrition, VIII. Copper as a Supplement to Iron for Hemoglobin Building in the Rat," *J. of Biol. Chem.* 77 (1928): 797-812 (with E. B. Hart, H. Steenbock, and J. Waddell); "Mineral Metabolism," *Annual Rev. of Biochem.* 5 (1936): 271-94 (with E. B. Hart); "The Isolation and Identification of the Anti-Black Tongue Factor," *J. Biol. Chem.* 123 (1938): 137-47 (with R. J. Madden, F. M. Strong, and D. W. Woolley); *The Vitamin Content of Meat* (1941, with Harry A. Waisman); "Factors Affecting the Dietary Niacin and Tryptophane Requirement of the Growing Rat," *J. of Nutrition* 31 (1946): 85-106. Scientific writings are in *J. of Biol. Chem., J. of Nutrition, Am. J. of Physiol.,* and *Proc., Soc. for Experimental Biol. & Med.* REFERENCES: *Current Biog.* (1948), 188-90; *DAB*, Supp. 7: 223-24; *DSB*, 4: 357-59; *NCAB*, 52: 23; *N.Y. Times*, July 28, 1962; *Who Was Who in Am.*, 4: 286-87.

W. J. Orr, Jr.

ELWELL, JOHN JOHNSON (June 22, 1820, near Warren, Ohio-March 13, 1900, Cleveland, Ohio). *Lawyer; Physician; Medical jurisprudence.* Son of a farmer. Married Nancy Chittenden; four children. EDUCATION: 1846, M.D., Cleveland Medical College; 1852-54, studied law, admitted to the bar in 1854. CAREER: 1846-c.1852, practiced medicine; 1854-61, practiced law, specializing in the medico-legal area; lectured on medical jurisprudence at Ohio University (Athens), the Union Law College, and the medical department of Western Reserve; 1853-54, member of the Ohio Legislature from Ashtabula County; founder, *Western Law Monthly*, 1857, editor, 1857-61; 1861-65, served with Quartermaster's Corps, U.S. Army, rising to the rank of brigadier general; *post* 1865, practiced law in Cleveland. CONTRIBUTIONS: Wrote *A Medico-Legal Trea-*

tise on Malpractice and Medical Evidence, Comprising the Elements of Medical Jurisprudence (1860), the first treatise on medical malpractice; went through four editions and was the standard work in the English-speaking world on medical malpractice. REFERENCES: *DAB*, 6: 122; Kelly and Burrage (1928), 378-79; *Who Was Who in Am.*, Hist. Vol.: 238-39.

S. Galishoff

EMERSON, HAVEN (October 19, 1874, New York, N.Y.-May 21, 1957, Greenport, N.Y.). *Physician; Health officer.* Son of John Haven, physician, and Susan (Tompkins) Emerson. Married Grace Parrish, 1901; five children. EDU-CATION: 1896, A.B., Harvard University; 1899, M.D., College of Physicians and Surgeons; intern, Bellevue Hospital. CAREER: 1899-1913, private practice, New York City; 1902-14, associate in physiology and medicine, College of Physicians and Surgeons; 1906-14, medical staff, Bellevue Hospital; at New York City Department of Public Health: 1914-15, deputy commissioner of health; 1915-17, commissioner of health; and 1937-57, Board of Health; 1918-19, chief epidemiologist, American Expeditionary Force; 1921-40, professor and head, Columbia University School of Public Health; 1933-34, president, American Public Health Association. CONTRIBUTIONS: Made significant contributions to epidemiology and vital statistics. Developed a uniform system of disease no-menclature and of reporting and classifying causes of morbidity and mortality. Expanded public health to include alcoholism, heart disease, and mental hygiene. Advocated mass inoculations to control communicable diseases. Conducted health surveys in major American cities and abroad. Investigation of N.Y. hospitals led to the formation of the Hospital Council of Greater New York.

WRITINGS: *Control of Communicable Disease in Man*, 8 eds. (1917-55); *A General Survey of Communicable Diseases in the A.E.F.* (1919); *Standard Classified Nomenclature of Disease* (1932); *Local Health Units for the Nation* (1945); *Selected Papers of Haven Emerson* (1949). REFERENCES: *Am. J. of Public Health* 40 (1950): 1-4; 47 (1957): 1009-11; *DAB*, Supplement 6: 142-43; *JAMA* 164 (1957): 898; Miller, *BHM*, p. 32; *NCAB*, 43: 330-31; *N.Y. State J. of Med.* 57 (1957): 2269-70; *N.Y. Times*, May 22, 1957.

D. O. Powell

ENGSTAD, JOHN EDWARD (May 4, 1858, Oslo, Norway-February 19, 1937, Grand Forks, N.D.). *Physician; Surgeon.* Son of Evan O., farmer, and Elsa (Wallen) Engstad. Married Mathilda; two children. EDUCATION: 1885, M.D., Rush Medical College (Chicago, Ill.); postgraduate study, Europe and the United States. CAREER: 1885-1935, physician and surgeon, Grand Forks, N.Dak.; in North Dakota Medical Association: 1887, charter member; and 1888-89, secretary; 1890-91, founder, St. Luke's Hospital, Grand Forks (now United Hospital). CONTRIBUTIONS: Medical scholar and writer (honorary member, Medical Writers and Authors Society of New York). Developed several operating techniques for abdominal surgery. Leader in local and state medical associations.

WRITINGS: "Hernia Through the Foramen of Winslow," *JAMA* 72 (1919); "Sinus

Pericranii," *ibid.*, 87 (1926); "Spastic Paralysis of Jejunem," *ibid.*, 90 (1928); "Treatment of Gastric and Duodenal Ulcers with special reference to the use of Barium," *Clin. Med. and Surg.* 38 (1930); "Foreign Bodies in the Appendix," *Minnesota Med.* 15 (1932). REFERENCES: *Grand Forks* (N.Dak.) *Herald*, February 20, 1937.

L. Remele

ERLANGER, JOSEPH (January 5, 1874, San Francisco, Calif.-December 15, 1965, St. Louis, Mo.). *Physiologist; Neurophysiology; Circulatory physiology.* Son of Herman, merchant, and Sarah (Galinger) Erlanger. Married Aimée Hirstel, 1906; three children. EDUCATION: 1895, B.S., University of California; 1899, M.D., Johns Hopkins University; 1899-1900, resident house officer, Johns Hopkins Hospital. CAREER: Physiology faculty: 1900-1906, Johns Hopkins Medical School; 1906-10, University of Wisconsin; and 1910-46, Washington University. CONTRIBUTIONS: Best known for his pioneering electrophysiological studies of nerve impulses, he and his student Herbert Gasser (q.v.) were awarded the 1944 Nobel Prize in medicine or physiology for their discoveries regarding the highly differentiated functions of single nerve fibers. Adapted the cathode-ray oscillograph, coupled with amplifying vacuum tubes, to study the transmission of nerve impulses through muscle fibers (1921-37). Discovered that the speed with which an impulse is transmitted is a function of the diameter of the fiber, being faster in thicker fibers. Work done with Gasser and other associates constitutes the fundamentals of neurophysiology. Made major contributions to the study of circulation and cardiac physiology. Devised an improved sphygmomanometer that allowed him to demonstrate that the output of the kidneys in persons affected by albuminuria depends primarily upon the pulse pressure (1904). Device bearing his name was manufactured, and the principle on which it was based was adopted in the models that superceded it. Showed that the fainting spells that characterize Stokes-Adams syndrome occur when the conduction between the atria and ventricles becomes momentarily blocked. Experiments on the auriculoventricular bundle (His's bundle—the muscle fiber connecting the atria with the ventricles of the heart) established that it alone makes auriculoventricular conduction possible in the mammalian heart (1905-6). Also contributed to the treatment of wound shock (1917-18).

WRITINGS: "On the Physiology of Heart-Block in Mammals, with Especial Reference to the Causation of Stokes-Adams Disease," *J. of Experimental Med.* 7 (1905): 675-724; 8 (1906):8-58; "The Compound Nature of the Action Current of Nerve as Disclosed by the Cathode Ray Oscillograph," *Am. J. of Physiol.* 70 (1924): 624-66 (with Herbert S. Gasser); *Electrical Signs of Nervous Activity* (1937). Writings are listed in *BMNAS*. REFERENCES: *BMNAS* 41 (1970): 111-39; *DAB*, Supp. 7:225-27; *DSB*, 4: 397-99; Joseph Erlanger, "A Physiologist Reminisces," *Am. Rev. of Physiol.* 26 (1964): 1-14; *McGraw-Hill Modern Men of Sci.* 1 (1966): 55-56; *NCAB*, 51: 547; *Who Was Who in Am.*, 4: 291.

S. Galishoff

ESPINOSA, TOBÍAS (January 2, 1879, Del Norte, Colo.-July 7, 1964, Española, N.Mex.). *General practitioner.* Son of Celso, rancher and later em-

ployee, University of Colorado, and Rafaela (Martinez) Espinosa. Married
Celestina Sanchez, 1924; one daughter. EDUCATION: Del Norte High School (Rio
Grande County), Colo.; 1902, M.D., University of Colorado School of Medicine. CAREER: 1902-8, physician for Denver and Rio Grande Railroad, Chama,
N.Mex.; 1908-12, chief steward, U.S. Navy Submarine Service, Mare Island,
Calif.; 1912-14, medical practice in Albuquerque, N. Mex.; 1914-26, moved
practice to Belen, N. Mex., since most of his patients were from there (during
this period, accepted as colleagues a number of Mexican doctors, refugees of
the Mexican revolution); 1926-64, general practice, Española; 1924-27, state
senator from Valencia County; 1927-33, mayor of Española; member of the
Española School Board for 20 years and served on the Board of New Mexico
State Medical Examiners for many years, being its chairman at one time. CON-
TRIBUTIONS: A skillful diagnostician, did minor surgery and was greatly interested
in pediatrics. Large home served as office for consultation and hospital for minor
cases. Assisted at approximately 6,000 home births. Essentially a rural doctor
with an interest in community life. Was named General Practitioner of the Year
by the New Mexico Medical Society (1954). In a remote area to which other
doctors had come and gone, Espinosa remained for 38 years, gaining the trust
of his mostly Spanish-speaking patients to whom he could easily relate both
culturally and linguistically. REFERENCES: Albert Rosenfeld, "Modern Medicine:
Where the Clock Walks," *Collier's Magazine* (Feb. 3, 1956): 24-28; interviews with
Gilberto Espinosa and Felice Espinosa, brother and daughter of Tobías, and interview
with patients and colleagues from the Espanola area.

C. Cutter

EVANS, GEORGE (June 14, 1900, St Mary's, Ontario, Canada-August 25,
1976, Morgantown, W. Va.). *Physician; Internal medicine.* Son of James William, merchant, and Sarah Agnes (Claw) Evans. Married Elah Pettit Evans, June
18, 1936. EDUCATION: University of Toronto and McGill Medical School, M.D.,
1923; 1923-25, internship in City Hospital, Binghamton, N.Y. CAREER: 1924-
33, practice, Hopemont Hospital and Sanitarium, Preston County, W.Va.; 1934-
76, private practice, Clarksburg, W. Va.; 1952-76, editor, *West Virginia Medical
Journal.* CONTRIBUTIONS: As editor, *West Virginia Medical Journal,* made changes
that kept it abreast of the times. Served the state as member (1949-66) and
chairman (1963) of the Medical Licensing Board. REFERENCES: *History of Medicine
in Harrison County* (1978), 331-34; *West Virginia Med. J.* (Oct. 1976).

K. Nodyne and R. Murphy

EVANS, JOHN (March 19, 1814, Waynesville, Ohio-July 3, 1897, Denver,
Colo.). *Physician; Businessman; Politician.* Son of David, toolmaker, and Rachel
(Burnet) Evans. Married Hannah Canby, 1838, one surviving child; Margaret
Gray, 1853, three children. EDUCATION: 1838, M.D., Cincinnati Medical Col-
lege. CAREER: 1839-43, medical practice, Ind.; 1844-47, superintendent, Indiana
Hospital for the Insane; 1845-57, professor of obstetrics, Rush Medical College;

1848-52, proprietor and editor, *Northwestern Medical and Surgical Journal* (which he traded for five acres on Chicago, Ill.'s west side); 1862, appointed by President Lincoln as territorial governor of Colo., serving three years. CONTRIBUTIONS: Instrumental in legislation for, construction of, and management of the first hospital for the insane in Ind. A founder: Chicago Medical Society (1850), Illinois State Medical Society (1850), Illinois General Hospital of the Lakes (1850), and Northwestern University (1851). Moved to Evanston, Ill. (1855), to be near Northwestern University, and Evanston was named in his honor. President, Board of Trustees, Northwestern University (until 1894). As governor of Colo., resigned after three years under criticism for his handling of Indian affairs. Founder of Colorado Seminary (1864), which became the University of Denver (1879), and was president, Board of Trustees, until death.

WRITINGS: "Observations upon the Spread of Asiatic Cholera, and Its Communicable Nature," *North-Western Med. and Surg. J.* 7 (1850-51): 53-62. REFERENCES: Elizabeth F. Carr, "Dr. John Evans: The Medical Career of the Founder of Northwestern University," *Q. Bull., Northwestern Univ. Med. School* 25 (1951): 113-17; Kelly and Burrage (1920), 370-71; Harry E. Kelsey, Jr., *Frontier Capitalist: The Life of John Evans* (1969); *Who Was Who in Am.*, Hist. Vol.: 173.

> F. B. Rogers,
> W. K. Beatty, and
> C. A. Bonsett

EVANS, MATILDA ARABELLE (May 13, 1872, Aiken County, S.C.-November 17, 1935, Columbia, S.C.). *Physician.* Daughter of Harriet and Anderson Evans. Never married; adopted and reared several children. EDUCATION: 1887-91, preparatory department, Oberlin College; 1897, M.D., Woman's Medical College of Pennsylvania. CAREER: 1898, returned to S.C. and began practice, Columbia; there, opened Taylor Lane Hospital and Nurses' Training School and, after it was destroyed by fire, built a second hospital, St. Luke; conducted a clinic where economically deprived black children received free medical treatment; both medical and surgical practices were reportedly successful from the beginning and patients were composed of "both races"; particular interest was the health care of women and children. CONTRIBUTIONS: First black woman physician in Columbia. Opened the first black hospital in Columbia (a nurses' training hospital) and three clinics. Provided health care and facilities for the medical treatment of black women and children and for the clinical training of black physicians. Organized the Negro Health Association of South Carolina to promote sanitation. Introduced medical examinations into the public schools of Columbia.

WRITINGS: Issued several numbers of *Negro Health J.* in 1916. Wrote a biography of Martha Schofield, founder, Schofield Industrial School, Aiken, which Evans attended in her youth. REFERENCES: History of her life by Dr. G. S. Dickerman (n.d.). Brief data on her education in the Archives, Oberlin College, Oberlin, Ohio, and in the Archives and Special Collections on Women in Medicine, The Medical College of Pennsylvania,

Philadelphia, Pa. Obituaries on file in the South Caroliniana Library, University of South Carolina, Columbia.

S. L. Chaff

EVANS, WILLIAM AUGUSTUS, JR. (August 5, 1865, Marion, Ala.-November 8, 1948, Aberdeen, Miss.). *Hygienist; Public health reformer.* Son of William Augustus and Julia Josephine (Wyatt) Evans. Married Ida May Wildberger, 1907; no children. EDUCATION: 1883, B.S., Agricultural College of Mississippi; 1885, M.D., Tulane University School of Medicine; 1895, M.S., Agricultural College of Mississippi; 1899, M.D., University of Illinois. CAREER: 1885-91, began practice of medicine with father, W. A. Evans, Sr., in Aberdeen; 1888, worked with Mississippi State Board of Health to keep the state free of yellow fever during the Jacksonville (Fla.) epidemic; 1891-1908, professor of pathology, Medical School of the University of Illinois; erected first pathological laboratory, Chicago, Ill.; 1907-11, commissioner of health, Chicago; 1908-28, professor of public health, Northwestern University Medical School; member: Board of Health Advisers, Health Commission of Chicago; and Board of Health Advisers, Health Commission, Cook County, Ill.; Health editor of column "How to Keep Well," which appeared in Chicago *Tribune* for many years; 1928-48, professor emeritus; Health column in Memphis *Commercial Appeal.* CONTRIBUTIONS: Outstanding educator and spokesman for public health. Meritorious service as commissioner of health for Chicago. Recognized importance of chemical, bacteriological, and pathological studies in medicine.

WRITINGS: *Notes on Pathology for Students' Use* (1897); *Disease and Health* (1917); *Dr. Evans' How to Keep Well: A Health Book for the Home* (1917); *Health and Success* (co-author, 1925); *Health and Good Citizenship* (1933, co-author); "Jefferson Davis, His Diseases and His Doctors," *The Mississippi Doctor* (1942); numerous articles in medical journals, historical journals, and newspapers. Writings listed in the Evans Collection, Evans Memorial Library, Aberdeen. REFERENCES: Dorothy Nell Phillips, *William Augustus Evans: Statesman of Public Health*, Social Science Research Center of Mississippi State College, Historical Series Number 5 (Sept. 1956), 65; *Who Was Who in Am.*, 2: 179.

M. S. Legan

EVE, PAUL FITZSIMMONS (June 27, 1806, Forest Hall, Richmond County, Ga.-November 3, 1877, Nashville, Tenn.). *Physician; Surgery.* Son of Oswell, captain of a Pa. company before the Revolutionary War and manufacturer of gunpowder, and Aphra Ann (Prichard) Eve. Married Sarah Louisa Twiggs, 1832, two children; Sarah Ann Duncan, 1852, three children. EDUCATION: Private tutors at home; Richmond Academy (Augusta, Ga.) and Mount Zion (Hancock County, Ga.); 1826, A.B., Franklin College (now the literary department, University of Georgia); later received A.M. and LL.D., Franklin College; 1826, began study of medicine under Dr. Charles D. Meigs (q.v.), in Philadelphia, Pa.; 1828, M.D., University of Pennsylvania; 1829-30, European study, London and Paris; 1831-32, reached Poland and served as field surgeon in General Turno's division;

taken prisoner by the Russians and imprisoned 30 days; received the Golden Cross of Honor from the Polish government. CAREER: 1828-29, began practice of medicine, Augusta; professor of surgery: 1832-48, Medical College of Georgia; 1849-50, University of Louisville; and 1851-76, University of Nashville, except for 1862-66 and 1868-70; during Civil War, chief surgeon to Gen. J. E. Johnston's army and president, Army Medical Board to examine qualifications of surgeons seeking appointment to the Confederate States Army; professor of surgery: 1868-70, Missouri Medical College, St. Louis, Mo.; and 1877, Nashville Medical College; 1857-58, 11th president, American Medical Association; 1876, Medical Commission of the Centennial selected him to represent medicine. CONTRIBUTIONS: Internationally known as a surgeon, especially as lithotomist. Did 238 operations of lithotomy with 11 deaths. Also pioneered in improved methods of amputation, ligature, and other preantiseptic innovations. Outstanding teacher of surgery, having given 43 courses of lectures on surgery.

WRITINGS: According to T. Chalmers Dow (1878) Eve published 625 articles, but the list compiled by Robert A. Halley (1904) contains 436 entries. *A Collection of Remarkable Cases in Surgery* (1857). REFERENCES: *Am. Hist. Mag.* 9 (1904): 281-324; *BHM* (1964-69), 83; (1975-79), 42; *DAB*, 3, pt. 2: 219-20; *NCAB*, 1: 30; *Surg., Gyn., & Obst.* 46 (1928) : 582-86; *TAMA* (1878): 641-46; *Trans., Med. Soc. of Tenn.* (1878): 83-88.

S. R. Bruesch

EWELL, JAMES (February 16, 1773, near Dumfries, Va.-November 2, 1832, Covington, La.). *Physician; Author; Medical handbooks for the layman.* Son of Jesse, planter, and Charlotte (Ewell) Ewell. Married Margaret Robertson, 1794. EDUCATION: Early 1790s, studied medicine with Dr. James Craik (q.v.), Alexandria, Va., and Dr. Stevenson, Baltimore, Md. CAREER: Practiced medicine: c. 1795-c. 1802, Lancaster County, Va., and at Dumfries; c. 1802-c. 1809, Savannah, Ga.; c. 1810-c. 1829, Washington, D.C.; and c. 1830-c. 1832, New Orleans, La. CONTRIBUTIONS: A prominent southern physician, introduced vaccination in Savannah and wrote one of the most popular manuals on domestic medicine in the early nineteenth century. *The Planter's and Mariner's Medical Companion* (1807) went through ten editions and was widely used by planters in the South and West. Handbook offered sound, practical advice on the prevention and treatment of disease presented in a "pleasant mingling of poetical quotations, anecdotes, [and] sentiment."

WRITINGS: *The Planter's and Mariner's Medical Companion* (1807). REFERENCES: *DAB*, 6: 229; *Who Was Who in Am.*, Hist. Vol.: 243.

S. Galishoff

EWING, JAMES (December 25, 1866, Pittsburgh, Pa.-May 16, 1943, New York, N.Y.). *Pathologist; Oncology.* Son of Thomas, lawyer, and Julia R. (Hufnagel) Ewing. Married Catherine Crane Halsted, 1900; one child. EDUCATION: Amherst College: 1888, A.B.; and 1891, A.M.; 1891, M.D., College of Physicians and Surgeons (Columbia); 1892, intern, Roosevelt Hospital (N.Y.).

CAREER: 1893-98, histology and pathology faculties, College of Physicians and Surgeons (Columbia); at Medical College of Cornell University: 1899-1932, pathology faculty; and 1932-39, oncology faculty; at Memorial Hospital (later, part of the Memorial Sloan-Kettering Cancer Center): 1919-39, pathology staff; and 1932-39, director. CONTRIBUTIONS: One of the first full-time oncology specialists in the United States, played a prominent role in early cancer research and helped establish several of the leading institutions involved in its treatment and prevention. Did important work in the early 1900s on the transmission of lymphosarcoma in dogs. Desirous of studying neoplastic diseases in man, raised money to have Memorial Hospital (originally founded as the New York Cancer Hospital) made an affiliate of Cornell Medical College (1913). Under Ewing's direction, hospital became one of the world's leading centers for cancer diagnosis, treatment, and research. Book *Neoplastic Diseases: A Textbook on Tumors* (1919) became the standard reference work in its field and was translated into several languages. Co-founder and first president (1907-9), American Association for Cancer Research, and charter member and active figure, American Society for the Control of Cancer (later, American Cancer Society). Did significant pathological research on other diseases as well, including diseases of the blood, ganglion cells, malaria, smallpox, and the toxemia of pregnancy; investigations of hematological disorders summarized in *Clinical Pathology of the Blood* (1901-3). Contributed several articles to textbooks on legal medicine and toxicology.

WRITINGS: *Causation, Diagnosis, and Treatment of Cancer* (1931). A bibliography is in *BMNAS*. REFERENCES: *BHM* (1977), 11; *BMNAS* 26 (1951); 45-60; *DAB*, 6: 257-58; *DSB*, 4: 498-500; Miller, *BHM*, p. 33; *Who Was Who in Am.*, 2: 180.

S. Galishoff

F

FABRIQUE, ANDREW HINSDALE (September 9, 1842, Vt.-May 10, 1928, Wichita, Kans.). *Physician.* Son of Henry Lewis, miller, and Louise (Hinsdale) Fabrique. Married Sarah Philler, 1866; one child. EDUCATION: Read medicine with Dr. Mitchel, Corydan, Ind.; thereafter, story is not clear; 1860, apparently enrolled in Tulane University Medical School but fled to escape Confederate military service; 1866-69, while living in Aurora, Ill., reportedly attended lectures, Rush Medical College; *American Medical Directory* of 1907 lists Fabrique as a 1905 graduate of the College of Physicians and Surgeons of Indiana, but Howard Clark stated that Fabrique's 1905 medical degree was "arranged" through Northwestern University, although it was a regular and not honorary degree. CAREER: 1869-1928, practice, Wichita. CONTRIBUTIONS: In the late nineteenth century, it was not unusual for a single individual to distinguish himself by improving the general level of medical practice in a given region. Not infrequently this was done without benefit of outside financial support and in the absence of a medical school. For south Kans., that person was Fabrique. When he arrived in Wichita in September 1869, was only the third physician in the community. Gradually, became the focus of an effort to improve the medical profession in his region. Organized the Wichita Pathological Society (1888), first local medical society to function in his city. Society organized the Wichita Medical College (1889), which closed its doors in 1890, having issued no diplomas. Induced the local Roman Catholics to open a hospital (1887). Initial venture failed, but two years later, it was revived, and St. Francis Hospital began its still-uninterrupted existence. Went to Chicago, Ill., to study surgery (c. 1887) and was befriended by Nicholas Senn (q.v.). Result was a long-standing arrangement that brought interns from Northwestern to Wichita for a part of their training. From among these young men, who came to be called "Fab's Boys," were many of the better trained physicians of Wichita. As a nucleus of excellence, their influence on Wichita medicine cannot be quantified, but it must have been considerable.

REFERENCE: Howard C. Clark, *A History of the Sedgwick County Medical Society* (privately printed, n.d.).

R. P. Hudson

FAGET, JEAN CHARLES (June 26, 1818, New Orleans, La.-December 7, 1884, New Orleans). *Physician.* Son of Jean Baptiste and ? (LeMormand) Faget. Married Glady Ligeret de Chazet; many children. EDUCATION: Received early education from Jesuits in La.; 1830-37, College Rolin (Paris); 1837-44, intern, Paris hospitals; 1844, M.D., Faculté de Paris. CAREER: 1845-65, practice, New Orleans; member: Louisiana State Board of Health; and 1864, Sanitary Commission (appointed by Gen. Nathaniel Banks); 1865-67, resided in Paris; 1867-84, practice, New Orleans. CONTRIBUTIONS: Described Faget's sign (1859) to differentiate between yellow fever and pernicious malaria, allowing an earlier diagnosis and treatment. This became the proof of the existence of yellow fever. A supporter of the infectious theory of disease, debating with many of his contemporaries on the matter. Had a large practice among the French and Creole population of New Orleans. Paid little attention to the business side of the profession, dying poor. Grandfather of Guy Henry Faget (1891-1947), pioneer in the treatment of leprosy.

WRITINGS: *Etudes sur les Bases de la Science Medicale* (1856); *Memoires et Lettres sur la Fievre Jaune et la Fievre Paludeenne* (1864). REFERENCES: William B. Atkinson, *Phys. and Surg. of the U.S.* (1878); *BHM* (1980), 14; *DAB*, 3, pt. 2: 244-45; John Duffy, *History of Medicine in Louisiana* 2 (1962); Kelly and Burrage (1920), 374-75.

M. Kaufman

FAIRCHILD, DAVID STURGES (September 16, 1847, Fairfield, Vt.-March 22, 1930, Clinton, Ia.). *Physician; Surgery.* Son of Eli, farmer, and Grace Dimond (Sturges) Fairchild. Married Wilhelmina Conrad Tattersall, 1870; three children. EDUCATION: 1865, studied medicine with Dr. J. O. Cramton, Fairfield; 1866-68, student, medical department, University of Michigan; 1868, M.D., Albany Medical College; 1880s, studied surgical techniques with Dr. Christian Fenger (q.v.), Chicago, Ill. CAREER: medical practice: 1869-72, High Forest, Minn.; and 1872-79, Ames, Ia.; 1879-93, professor of physiology, Veterinary Medical School, Iowa State Agricultural College; 1881-92, professor of pathology and professor of surgery, College of Physicians and Surgeons, Des Moines, Ia.; 1903-9, dean, Drake University Medical School; *post* 1893, division surgeon, Chicago and Northwestern Railway Co.; president: 1895-96, Iowa State Medical Society; and 1898, Western Surgical Association; *post* 1900, division surgeon, Chicago Rock Island and Pacific Railway Co.; 1901, president, American Academy of Railway Surgeons; 1905-27, chairman, Commission on Medico-Legal Defense, Iowa State Medical Society; *post* 1910, division surgeon, Chicago Burlington and Quincy Railroad Co.; 1911-28, editor, *Journal of the Iowa State Medical Society*; 1913, charter member and fellow, American College of Surgeons; 1914, president, American Association of Railway Surgeons. CON-

TRIBUTIONS: Helped organize several county medical societies in Ia. and frequently served as a state delegate to national and international medical meetings, actively promoting a broader view for Ia. medicine (1872-1914). Medical educator (1879-1909). Influential in the spread of antiseptic surgical techniques and interest in microscopy in Ia. (1880s). Widely known expertise in personal injury court cases (as railway surgeon in five-state area) enhanced his contributions to Ia. medicine through connection with the state society's committee on physician defense in medico-legal cases (1905-27). Called by his peers the "Nestor" of Ia. medical history, meticulously recorded the early history of medicine in the state (1876-1928).

WRITINGS: Published a number of influential case studies in the *Iowa State Med. Reporter* (1883-85): tuberculosis, nephritis, Addison's disease, actinomycosis, spinal concussion. *History of Iowa Medicine to 1876* (1912); *The History of Medicine in Iowa* (1923). REFERENCES: Walter L. Bierring, "David Sturges Fairchild, M.D., F.A.C.S. A Biography," *J. of the Iowa Med. Soc.* 18 (1928): 347; *NCAB*, 17:189; *One Hundred Years of Iowa Medicine* (1950), 138; *Who Was Who in Am.* 1: 382.

                                                                    R. E. Rakel

FARBER, SIDNEY (September 30, 1903, Buffalo, N.Y.-March 30, 1973, Brookline, Mass.). *Physician; Pediatric pathology.* Son of Simon, in the insurance business, and Matilda (Goldstein) Farber. Married Norma C. Holtzman, 1928; four children. EDUCATION: 1923, A.B., University of Buffalo; began medical education at Universities of Heidelberg and Freiburg; 1927, M.D., Harvard Medical School; 1927-28, intern, Peter Bent Brigham Hospital; 1928-29, University of Munich Pathological Institute; 1935-36, Moseley Traveling Fellow, Ghent, Belgium; student of S. Burt Wolbach (q.v.). CAREER: 1929-70, pathologist, Children's Hospital; and medical faculty, Harvard Medical School; 1967-70, S. Burt Wolbach Professor; 1946, chairman, Staff Planning Committee, Children's Hospital Medical Center (CHMC); 1947-70, chairman, Division of Laboratories and Research, CHMC; 1948, established Children's Cancer Research Foundation (Jimmy Fund); 1970-73, director, Children's Cancer Research Center (after 1973, Sidney Farber Research Center; 1976, in association with Charles A. Dana, Cancer Center became Sidney Farber Research Institute). CONTRIBUTIONS: Research covered many aspects of pathology associated with pediatric disease: called early attention to hyaline membrane disease of newborn and sudden infant death syndrome; identified eastern equine encephalitis in humans; elucidated cystic fibrosis as a generalized disorder and lipid metabolic disorders of children, including ceramide lipidosis, known as Farber's disease. Celebrated for his illuminating descriptions of pathology in children, lectures included a classic history of the autopsy. An early advocate of chemotherapy in cancer, used folic acid antagonists aminopterin and methotrexate to induce complete remission of acute hemolytic anemia (1947); found specificity for Wilms's tumor of the kidney in the antibiotic actinomycin D (1954). To encourage voluntary cooperative research, founded the Cancer Chemotherapy National Committee. An enthusiast of "total care" for patients, saw this outlook endorsed when the National Cancer Institute (NIH) designated Children's and Dana Centers as a Regional Comprehensive Research and Demonstration Center (1971).

WRITINGS: *The Postmortem Examination* (1937); "Temporary Remission in Acute Leukemia in Children Produced by Folic Acid Antagonist, 4-Aminopteroyl-Glutamic Acid," *New England J. of Med.* 238 (1948): 787 (with L. K. Diamond, R. D. Mercer, R. F. Sylvester, J. A. Wolff); "Approaches to the Chemotherapy of Cancer," *Trans. and Studies of the Coll. of Physicians of Phila.* 23 (1955-56): 74. REFERENCES: *Cancer Research* 34 (1974): 659-61; "Memorial Minute," *Harvard Univ. Gazette* 69 (Nov. 9, 1973): 5; Susan Weld Putnam, "Sidney Farber and Cancer in Children" (Senior thesis, Department of the History of Science, Harvard University, 1980).

B. G. Rosenkrantz

FARRAR, BERNARD GAINES (July 4, 1784, Goochland County, Va.-July 1, 1849, St. Louis, Mo.). *Physician; Surgeon.* Son of James Royal and Jane (Ford) Farrar. Married Sarah Christy, 1811, three children; Ann C. Thruston, February 2, 1820, six children. EDUCATION: 1797-1800, literary department, Transylvania University, Lexington, Ky.; 1800, apprentice to Dr. Selmon, Cincinnati, Ohio; 1801-4, apprentice to Dr. Samuel Brown (q.v.), Lexington; 1804-5, medical lectures, University of Pennsylvania; 1806, M.D., Transylvania University. CAREER: Private practice: 1806, Frankfort, Ky.; and 1807-35, St. Louis; 1812-14, surgeon, U.S. Army; 1835, retired from active practice according to one source and died during the cholera epidemic of 1849. CONTRIBUTIONS: First American trained physician to set up permanent residence west of the Mississippi. Helped to found the St. Louis Medical Society (1836) and became its first president. REFERENCES: "Farrar, Bernard G.," *Encyclopedia of the Hist. of St. Louis* (1899), 2: 730; C. A. Pope, "The Life of Dr. B. G. Farrar," *St. Louis Med. and Surg. J.* 8 (1850): 404-14; J. T. Scharf, *History of St. Louis City and County* 2 (1883): 1518-19; "St. Louis Medical Society," *Encyclopedia of the Hist. of St. Louis* 4 (1899): 1968-69.

D. Sneddeker

FAVILL, HENRY BAIRD (August 14, 1860, Madison, Wis.-February 20, 1916, Springfield, Mass.). *Physician; Public Health.* Son of John, physician, and Louisa Sophia (Baird) Favill. Married Susan Cleveland-Pratt, 1885; one child. EDUCATION: 1880, A.B., University of Wisconsin; 1883, M.D., Rush Medical College; 1883, intern, Cook County Hospital, Chicago, Ill. CAREER: 1883-94, physician, Madison; 1890-94, special lecturer on medical jurisprudence, law department, University of Wisconsin; 1894-1916, chair of medicine, Chicago Polyclinic; at Rush Medical College: 1894-98, adjunct chair of medicine; 1898-1900, Ingalls Professor of Preventive Medicine and Therapeutics; 1900-1906, chairman, Department of Therapeutics; and 1906-16, chairman, clinical medicine; 1901, first president, National Committee for Mental Hygiene; 1907-13, president, Chicago Tuberculosis Institute; 1910-16, first chairman, AMA Council on Health and Public Instruction. CONTRIBUTIONS: Attained distinction as a public health reformer in Chicago around the turn of the century. Early recognized that public health reform could only follow political reform and assumed presidency of the Municipal Voter's League (1907-10), committee organized by prominent citizens of Chicago to screen publicly qualifications of candidates for public office. Specialized in the prevention of tuberculosis. Founded an antituberculosis movement (c. 1906), which led to his purchase of a dairy farm in Lake Mills, Wis., where he researched methods to halt the contagion of the disease among dairy cattle.

WRITINGS: Bibliography and selected articles appear in *Henry Baird Favill; A Memorial Volume—Life, Tributes, Writings* (1917). REFERENCES: *Biographical Review of Dane County, Wisconsin* (1893), 521; *Chicago Herald*, February 21, 1916; *DAB*, 3, pt. 2: 301-2; *Henry B. Favill* (1917); Kelly and Burrage (1920), 377-78; *NCAB*, 10: 497; J. Schafer, "Henry Baird Favill: A Wisconsin Gift to Chicago," *Wis. Mag. of Hist.* 24 (1940): 199-227.

R. B. Schoepflin

FAVILL, JOHN (October 10, 1819, Manheim, N.Y.-December 9, 1883, Madison, Wis.). *Physician; General practice.* Son of John, farmer, and Elizabeth (Guile) Favill. Married Louisa Sophia Baird, 1854; four children, including Henry B. (q.v.). EDUCATION: 1847, M.D., Harvard Medical School. CAREER: Physician: 1847-48, Lake Mills, Wis.; and 1848-83, Madison; 1860-61, assistant physician, Mendota State Hospital for the Insane, Madison; 1861-65, examining physician, Dane County, Wis.; in Dane County Medical Society, Wis.: 1850-83, charter member; and 1858, president; in Wisconsin State Medical Society: 1869, vice-president; and 1872, president; on Wisconsin State Board of Health: 1876-82, charter member; and 1876, first chairman. CONTRIBUTIONS: An early, influential leader of organized medicine in Wisconsin and an implacable foe of homeopathy and other medical "irregulars."

WRITINGS: "On the Relation the Profession Holds and Ought to Hold Towards Community," Annual Address of the President, *Trans., Wis. State Med. Soc.* 6 (1872): 25-28; "Mental Hygiene," *Annual Report*, Wisconsin State Board of Health 1 (1876): 45-54. REFERENCES: H. B. Favill, "Sketch of John Favill, M.D., in *Henry Baird Favill: A Memorial Volume—Life, Tributes, Writings* (1917), 577-79; William Snow Miller, "Dane County Medical Society," *Wis. Med. J.* 36 (1937): 929-40.

R. B. Schoepflin

FAYSSOUX, PETER (1745, S.C., probably Charleston-February 1, 1795, Charleston). *Physician.* Son of Daniel and Francis (Dott) Fayssoux, Huguenot emigrés. Married Sarah Wilson, 1772 (d. 1776), 1 child; Ann (Smith) Johnston, 12 children. EDUCATION: 1769, M.D., Edinburgh. CAREER: 1773, curator of the Charleston Museum; being an active patriot, volunteered for medical services before and during Revolution; senior physician, General Hospital, under David Olyphant (q.v.); 1780, physician and surgeon general, Southern Department of the Army; 1780, during the British siege of Charleston, prisoner of war, but remained in charge of the hospital that was then controlled by the British; exchanged to join Greene's army and continued medical applications; 1789, leader in forming Medical Society; 1790-92, president, Medical Society; 1792-95, one of 12 directors, Santee Canal Company; 1784-85, Privy Council; 1786-90, member, South Carolina General Assembly. CONTRIBUTIONS: Volunteered medical efforts before and throughout the American Revolution. Considered by contemporaries as a leading physician in Charleston region.

WRITINGS: Before graduating, wrote a thesis on lockjaw; though some historians believe he authored many other articles anonymously, no evidence exists. REFERENCES: *DAB*, 3: 6: 307; Chalmers G. Davidson, *Friend of the People, The Life of Dr. Peter Fayssoux* (1950); Kelly and Burrage (1920), 379; Joseph Ioor Waring, *History of Medicine in South Carolina, 1670-1825* (1964).

J. P. Dolan

FEARN, THOMAS (November 15, 1789, near Danville, Va.-January 16, 1863, Huntsville, Ala.). *Physician; Surgeon.* Son of Thomas and Mary (Burton) Fearn. Married Sallie Bledsoe Shelby, 1822; seven children. EDUCATION: Early education in Danville; 1806, entered Washington College, Lexington, Va.; 1810, M.D., University of Pennsylvania; 1818, studied surgery, London and Paris. CAREER: 1810-12, 1820-37, practice of medicine, Huntsville; 1812-13, surgeon, British and Creek Wars; 1831, offered chair of surgery: at Transylvania University, Lexington; Center College, Ky.; School of Medicine, Louisville, Ky.; and University of Cincinnati; all of which he refused; 1822-29, Madison County Representative, Ala. State Legislature; 1823-29, member, Ala. Board of Medical Examiners; owner of water supply, Huntsville, until he sold it to the city; 1830-35, built canal from the Tennessee River to Huntsville, which was abandoned when a turnpike was constructed along the same course; member, first Confederate Congress. CONTRIBUTIONS: Said to have been the first in this continent or in Europe to discern the true nature of quinine, to make his own from bark, and to use it accordingly.

WRITINGS: "Sulphate of Quinine in Large Doses," *Transylv. J. Med.* 9 (1836): 705-7. REFERENCE: T. M. Owen, *History of Alabama*, 4 vols. (1978).

S. Eichold

FENGER, CHRISTIAN (November 3, 1840, Breininggard, Breininge Sogn, Denmark-March 7, 1902, Chicago, Ill.). *Surgeon; Pathology.* Son of Hans Fritz, prosperous farmer, and Frederikke Mathilde, (Fjelstrup) Fenger. Married Caroline Sophia Abildgaard, 1878; two children. EDUCATION: 1860-67, University of Copenhagen; 1867-69, intern, Frederik's Hospital; 1871-74, prosector, Kommune Hospital; 1874, M.D., University of Copenhagen. CAREER: Army surgeon: 1864-65, German-Danish War; and 1870-71, Franco-Prussian War; 1875-77, sanitary commission, Egypt; 1878-93, pathologist, Cook County Hospital, Chicago; 1880-92, surgery staff, Cook County Hospital; 1882-85, taught general pathology and pathological anatomy, Chicago Medical College; 1893-99, taught surgery, Northwestern University Medical School; and surgical staff, Mercy Hospital; 1899-1902, taught surgery, Rush Medical College. CONTRIBUTIONS: Ranks as the "father of modern pathological surgery." Demonstrated the ball-valve action of stones in the common bile duct and worked out a classic operation for stenosis of the uretero-pelvic junction (1894). First in North America to demonstrate the bacterial nature of acute endocarditis (1879). First surgeon in Chicago to do a vaginal hysterectomy for cancer. Productively studied advanced abdominal extrauterine pregnancy (1891). Internationally known as a brain surgeon, pioneered in the exploration of the brain with the aspirating needle and in the removal of intramedullary tumors. Made valuable investigations in experimental asepsis.

WRITINGS: "The Total Extirpation of the Uterus Through the Vagina," *Am. J. of Med. Sci.* 83 (1882): 17-47; "Operation for the Relief of Valve Formation and Stricture of the Ureter in Hydro- or Pyo-Nephrosis," *JAMA* 22 (May 10, 1894): 335-43; *The Collected Works of Christian Fenger, 1840-1902* (1912, ed. Ludwig Hektoen and C. G. Buford). REFERENCES: J. C. Bay, *Dr. C. Fenger* (1940); *BHM* (1970-74), 59-60; *DAB*, 6: 320-21; L. Hektoen, "Early Pathology in Chicago and Christian Fenger," *Proc., Inst. Med. Chicago* 11 (1936-37): 258-72; Kelly and Burrage (1928), 403-4; E. R. LeCount, "C. Fenger as Pathologist," *Trans., Chicago Path. Soc.* 6 (1903): 1-20; Miller, *BHM*, p. 33; *NCAB*, 17: 279; George Rosen, "Christian Fenger: Medical Immigrant," *Bull. Hist. Med.* 48 (1974): 129-45; *Who Was Who in Am.*, 1: 391.

W. K. Beatty

FENNER, ERASMUS DARWIN (1807, Franklin County, N.C.-May 4, 1866, New Orleans, La.). *Physician; Editor; Educator; Sanitarian.* Son of N.C. physician. Married Ann Collier, 1832; one child. EDUCATION: Private academy, Raleigh, N.C., and later received private tutoring; read medicine under elder brother, Dr. Robert Fenner, Jackson, Tenn.; 1830, M.D., University of Transylvania. CAREER: 1830-33, practiced medicine with brother, Jackson; 1833-41, private practice, Clinton, Miss.; 1841-66, physician, New Orleans, La.; 1844-48, founder and co-editor, *New Orleans Medical Journal* (later *New Orleans Medical and Surgical Journal*); editor: 1849, *Southern Medical Reports*; and 1853-54, *New Orleans Medical and Surgical Journal*; 1857-60, assistant editor, *New Orleans Medical News and Hospital Gazette*; 1856-62, 1865-66, dean and professor, New Orleans School of Medicine. CONTRIBUTIONS: Best known for his work as editor and educator, founded three significant medical publications and organized the New Orleans School of Medicine. The latter was the first medical school to make clinical training a basic part of the medical curriculum. Within four years of its establishment, the school ranked seventh in the country (1860) in terms of enrollment. A leading sanitarian who constantly campaigned in New Orleans for better health conditions. As with many of his contemporaries, accepted the miasmic theory of disease and was firmly convinced that a sound sanitary program would eliminate disease from New Orleans.

WRITINGS: Much of his work was done as editor, *New Orleans Medical and Surgical Journal, Southern Medical Reports, New Orleans Medical News and Hospital Gazette*, and *Southern Journal of Medical Sciences*. Among the best of his articles are "The Yellow Fever Quarantine at New Orleans," *TAMA* 2 (1849): 623-34; "Remarks on Clinical Medicine," *New Orleans Med. News and Hosp. Gazette* 4 (1857-58): 458-72; "Remarks on the Sanitary Condition of the City of New Orleans During the Period of Federal Military Occupation, from May 1862 to March 1866," *Southern J. of Med. Sci.* 1 (1866): 22-23, 37. REFERENCES: D. Warren Brickell, "Biographical Sketch of Erasmus Darwin Fenner, M.D.," *Southern J. of Med. Sci.* 1 (1866-67): 401-23; John Duffy, "Erasmus Darwin Fenner (1807-66), Journalist, Educator, and Sanitarian," *J. of Med. Ed.* 35 (1960): 819-31; idem, *Rudolph Matas History of Medicine in Louisiana* 2 (1962); Albert E. Fossier, "History of Medical Education in New Orleans . . . ," *Annals of Med. Hist.*, n.s., 6 (1934): 427-47.

J. Duffy

FERGUSON, RICHARD BABBINGTON (1769, Londonderry, Ireland-April 9, 1853, Louisville, Ky.). *Physician; Internal medicine*. Married Elizabeth Aylett Booth, February 3, 1803; seven children. EDUCATION: It is not known at what age he went to the Shenandoah Valley of Va. with his family or where he received his early education or even his medical education. CAREER: 1802, went to Louisville, an experienced practitioner and commenced the practice of medicine, surgery, and midwifery; owned an apothecary shop; 1812, president, Hibernian Society, Louisville; 1817, supervisor, Port of Louisville; 1832-36, Board of Managers, Marine (City) Hospital; 1841, elected first president, Louisville District Medical Society. CONTRIBUTIONS: Trained apprentices: Thomas Booth (1810-15), William Loftus Sutton ([q.v.] 1815-17), James H. Owen (1816), and his son, Richard William Ferguson (1824-27). An attending surgeon at the Marine (City) Hospital (1823-32). Became an auxiliary agent of the National Vaccine Institution (1821) and vaccinated gratis all who came to him. REFERENCES: *History of the Ohio Falls Cities and Their Counties* 1 (1882): 214, 464; obituary, *Louisville Weekly Courier*, October 29, 1853, p. 2, col. 5.

E. H. Conner

FINDLEY, PALMER (April 22, 1868, Lewis, Ia.-November 8, 1964, Omaha, Nebr.). *Physician; Gynecologist; Obstetrician*. Son of David, physician, and Martha Jane (Barr) Findley. Married Lyda M. Hanna, June 3, 1896; four children. EDUCATION: 1886, Atlantic (Ia.) High School; 1890, B.S., University of Iowa; 1893, M.D., Northwestern University; 1893-95, intern, Cook County Hospital, Chicago, Ill.; 1898-99, studied in Berlin, Vienna, and Paris. CAREER: 1900-1906, instructor, Rush Medical College, Chicago; at University of Nebraska College of Medicine: 1906-14, professor of didactic and clinical gynecology; 1914-16, professor of gynecology; and 1916-18, professor of gynecology and operative obstetrics; contributor: 1924, *Abt's Pediatrics*; and 1933, *Sojor's Encyclopedia of Medicine, Obstetrics and Gynecology*; state chairman, American Society for the Control of Cancer; in American Association of Obstetricians, Gynecologists and Abdominal Surgeons: 1925, vice-president; and 1927, president; 1931-32, chairman, obstetric teaching, White House Conference on Child

Welfare and Protection; president, Central Association of Obstetricians and Gynecologists; 1925-26, president, Nebraska State Medical Society; 1932, vice-president, American Gynecological Society; 1922, president, Omaha-Douglas County Medical Society. CONTRIBUTIONS: In addition to very active practice in the field of obstetrics and gynecology, a prolific writer with publications dating from an article on arteriosclerosis of the uterus (1905) to a biography of Ignaz Semmelweis (1947). In addition to being the author of several books on the history of obstetrics and gynecology as well as clinical subjects, was author of over a hundred papers, including subjects of puerperal thrombophlebitis, management of genital tuberculosis, complications of pregnancy, prevention of venereal disease, psychotherapy and disease of women, caesarean section, pelvic inflammation, and use of radium therapy in cancer.

WRITINGS: *Diagnosis of Diseases of Women* (1903; 2d ed., rev. and enl., 1905); *Gonorrhea in Women* (1908); *A Treatise on the Diseases of Women, for Students and Practitioners* (1913); *The Story of Childbirth* (1933); *Priests of Lucina: The Story of Obstetrics* (1939). Writings listed in the University of Nebraska Medical Center Library of Medicine, Omaha. REFERENCES: A. E. Sheldon, *Nebraska the Land and the People* 2 (1931): 472-73; A. T. Tyler and E. F., Auerbach, *History of Medicine in Nebraska* (1977, enlarged by B. M. Hetzner), 116-18; *Who's Who in Nebraska* (1940), 327-28; *Who Was Who in Am.*, 4: 309.

B. M. Hetzner

FINFROCK, JOHN H. (December 9, 1836, Columbia, Ohio-November 11, 1893, Idaho). *Physician; Surgeon.* Son of Jonathan Finfrock. Married Anna Catherine McCullough, 1862; four children. EDUCATION: Richmond College of Ohio, University of Michigan, and Medical College of Ohio (M.D., 1863); interned at Long Island Hospital. CAREER: Captain, 54th Ohio Volunteer Regiment; first assistant surgeon, U.S. Army, Fort Sanders; 1865, established practice, Laramie, Wyo., as the first physician in the city; surgeon, Union Pacific Railroad hospital. CONTRIBUTIONS: Capacity as a surgeon was well known in that he would often attempt surgery when no one else would. One example was the repair of a severed ulnar nerve (c. January 20, 1891). Removed a cancerous breast (April 16, 1885) in which the cancer weighed over three pounds. Served as the medical director of the Grand Army of the Republic. Also served on the first Board of Trustees, University of Wyoming. REFERENCES: Numerous citations in *The Laramie Daily Boomerang* and the *Laramie Republican*; statement by Finfrock on file, American Heritage Center, University of Wyoming, Laramie; A. Palmieri and C. Humberson, "Medical Incidents in the Life of Dr. John H. Finfrock," *Annals of Wyoming* 55, pt. 2 (1981): 64; *Trans. Colorado St. Med. Soc.* (1898-99): 509.

A. Palmieri

FINNEY, JOHN MILLER TURPIN (June 20, 1863, Natchez, Miss.-May 30, 1942, Baltimore, Md.). *Surgeon.* Son of Ebenezer Dickey, Presbyterian minister, and Annie Louise (Parker) Finney. Married Mary E. Gross, 1892; four children. EDUCATION: 1884, A.B., Princeton University; 1889, M.D., Harvard

University; 1888-89, intern, Massachusetts General Hospital; 1889-90, resident, Johns Hopkins Hospital. CAREER: *Post* 1890, practiced medicine, Baltimore; 1893-1933, surgery faculty, Johns Hopkins Medical School; surgery staff: *post* 1893, Johns Hopkins Hospital; and *post* 1895, Union Protestant Infirmary (later Union Memorial Hospital); 1913-16, first president, American College of Surgeons; 1921, president, American Surgical Association. CONTRIBUTIONS: Leading American surgeon, particularly renowned for gastric surgery. Developed the standard operating procedure for the relief of duodenal ulcer (1902-27). Enlarged and transformed Union Protestant Infirmary into a modern hospital. Helped establish Provident Hospital, a medical facility for blacks.

WRITINGS: "A New Method of Gastroduodenostomy, End-to-Side. . .," *Trans., Southern Surg. Assoc.* 26 (1923): 576-87; "A New Method of Pyloroplasty," *Trans., Am. Surg. Assoc.* 20 (1902): 165-77; "The Surgery of Gastric and Duodenal Ulcer," *Am. J. Surg.*, n.s., 1 (1926): 323-43. REFERENCES: *DAB*, Supplement 3: 270-71; John Staige Davis (q.v.), "John Miller Turpin Finney, 1863-1942," *Annals of Surg.* 119 (1944): 616-21; Miller, *BHM*, p. 34; *N.Y. Times*, May 31, 1932; *Who Was Who in Am.*, 2: 187.

S. Galishoff

FISHBEIN, MORRIS (July 22, 1889, St. Louis, Mo.-September 27, 1976, Chicago, Ill.). *Physician; Medical writer and editor.* Son of Benjamin, merchant, and Fanny (Gluck) Fishbein. Married Anna Mantel, 1914; four children. EDUCATION: 1910, B.S., University of Chicago; at Rush Medical College: 1912, M.D.; and 1912-13, fellow in pathology. CAREER: 1913, medical staff, Durand Hospital, McCormick Institute for Infectious Diseases; *Journal of the American Medical Association*: 1913-24, assistant editor; and 1924-49, editor; 1924-49, editor, *Hygeia*; managing editor, numerous specialized medical journals published by the AMA; chief editor, *Quarterly Cumulative Index Medicus*. CONTRIBUTIONS: Voice of the AMA for many years. Championed the traditional fee-for-service medical practice of the ordinary American physician and vigorously opposed government aid in medical care and prepaid, group practice, both of which he denounced as "socialized medicine"; believed that to shift the financial responsibility for health care from the individual to the state would weaken the self-reliance and initiative of the American people and would lead to time serving on the part of physicians who were paid a fixed salary; argued further that the involvement of government or other nonmedical third parties would interfere with the physician-patient relationship, bring about commercialization in medicine, and result in incompetent medical control by nonphysicians. Contributed articles and editorials to medical and popular journals and had a syndicated daily column that appeared in 200 newspapers. Improved the quality and status of the *Journal of the American Medical Association*. Edited the *Modern Home Medical Adviser* (1935), which went through many editions and sold more than 4 million copies.

WRITINGS: *The Medical Follies* (1925); *The Art and Practice of Medical Writing* (1925, with George H. Simmons [q.v.]); *New Medical Follies* (1928). REFERENCES:

BHM (1964-69), 87; (1976), 11; James G. Burrow, *AMA, Voice of American Medicine* (1963); *Current Biog.* (1940), 297-99; M. Fishbein, *An Autobiography* (1969); F. J. Inglefinger, "Morris Fishbein, M.D.," *New England J. of Med.* 295 (Nov. 11, 1976): 1134-35; *N.Y. Times*, September 28, 1976.

S. Galishoff

FISHER, JOHN DIX (March 27, 1797, Needham, Mass.-March 3, 1850, Boston, Mass.). *Physician.* Son of Aaron and Lucy (Stedman) Fisher. EDUCATION: 1820, graduated from Brown University; 1825, M.D., Harvard Medical School; 1825-27, studied medicine in Paris with Laënnec, Andral, and Velpeau. CAREER: *Post* 1827, praticed medicine, Boston; *post* 1829, vice-president and physician, New England Asylum (later the Perkins Institution and Massachusetts School for the Blind); shortly before his death, acting physician, Massachusetts General Hospital. CONTRIBUTIONS: Largely responsible for the establishment of the Perkins Institution and Massachusetts School for the Blind (1829) and served as its vice-president and physician until his death. Pioneered in the use of ether in childbirth. One of the first in America to use auscultation, which he had studied with Laënnec in Paris, and extend its application to diseases other than those of the chest. Wrote an illustrated book, *Description of the Distinct, Confluent, and Inoculated Smallpox. . .*(1829), which was well received. REFERENCES: Walter Channing, *Sketch of the Life and Character of John D. Fisher, M.D.* (1850); *DAB*, 6: 409; Kelly and Burrage (1920), 386-87.

S. Galishoff

FITE, FRANCIS BARTOW (October 17, 1861, near Cartersville, Ga.-August 15, 1938, Muskogee, Okla.). *Physician; Surgeon.* Son of Henderson Wesley, Civil War surgeon, and Sarah Turney (Denman) Fite. Married Julia Patton, November 13, 1889; five children. EDUCATION: Pine Log Academy and Johnstone Academy, Ga.; at age 19 moved to Tahlequah, Indian Territory, to study medicine under his brother and half-brother; attended Cherokee Norman Academy and taught school for one year and then enrolled at Southern Medical College (now Emory University), M.D., 1886. CAREER: 1886-88, practice with Dr. R. L. Fite, his brother, in Tahlequah; 1888-89, attended New York Polyclinic Medical School, as first assistant to Dr. John A. Wyeth; 1889-1938, practice, Muskogee, Indian Territory. CONTRIBUTIONS: Because much of his surgery had to be performed in homes or in his office, established a sanitarium that later became Martha Robb Hospital, first such institution in Muskogee. A founder of the Indian Territory Medical Association, which later merged into the Oklahoma Medical Association. Served as secretary, Board of Health,, Cherokee Nation, and mayor, Muskogee; ran for governor, Okla., immediately after it was admitted to the Union. REFERENCES: Mark R. Everett, *Medical Education in Oklahoma: The University of Oklahoma School of Medicine and Medical Center 1900-1931* (1972); "F. B. Fite" file, History of Medicine Collection, University of Oklahoma Health Sciences Center Library, Oklahoma City, Okla.; R. Palmer Howard, and Richard E. Martin, "The

Contributions of B. F. Fortner, LeRoy Long, and Other Early Surgeons in Oklahoma,'' *Journal of the Oklahoma State Medical Association* (November 1968): 541-49; *Indian Territory Biographical Data* (1901), 248-50; *JAMA*, 78: 1738; *NCAB*, 27: 465; *Oklahoma State Med. J.* 31 (Sept. 1938).

V. Allen

FITZ, REGINALD HEBER (May 5, 1843, Chelsea, Mass.-September 30, 1913, Brookline, Mass.). *Physician; Intestinal surgery; Pathology.* Son of Albert, U.S. consul, and Eliza Roberts (Nye) Fitz. Married Elizabeth Loring Clarke, 1879; four children. EDUCATION: Harvard University: 1864, A.B.; 1867, A.M.; and 1868, M.D.; 1867-68, intern, Boston City Hospital; 1868-70, studied in Europe. CAREER: At Harvard Medical School: 1870-92, pathological anatomy faculty; and 1892-1908, theory and practice of physic faculty; at Massachusetts General Hospital: *post* 1871, pathology staff; and 1887-1908, visiting physician; 1897, 1903, president, Congress of American Physicians and Surgeons. CONTRIBUTIONS: Established the diagnosis and a method of treatment of appendicitis and acute pancreatitis. Demonstrated that a perforating inflammation of the appendix was a frequent cause of death from peritonitis; convinced physicians of the need to remove the appendix immediately if threatening symptoms did not subside within 24 hours (1886). Distinguished the hemorrhagic, suppurative, and gangrenous forms of acute pancreatitis; suggested that fat necrosis results from a lesion of the pancreas (1889). Stressed the need for surgery in many cases of intestinal obstruction (1889). Brought Rudolph Virchow's creation of a cellular pathology to the United States. A strong and influential supporter of the reforms instituted at Harvard Medical School by Charles W. Eliot (q.v.).

WRITINGS: "Perforating Inflammation of the Vermiform Appendix; with Special Reference to Its Early Diagnosis and Treatment," *Trans., Assoc. of Am. Physicians* 1 (1886): 107-44; "Acute Intestinal Obstruction," *Trans., Coll. of Am. Physicians & Surgeons* 1 (1888): 1-42; "Acute Pancreatitis. . .," *Boston Med. and Surg. J.* 120 (1889): 181-87, 205-7, 229-35; *The Practice of Medicine* (1897, with Horatio C. Wood [q. v.]). REFERENCES: *DAB*, 6: 433-34; Kelly and Burrage (1928): 411-13; Hyman Morrison, articles on Fitz and ". . .Acute Pancreatitis. . .," *Bull. Hist. Med.* 22 (1948): 263-72; ". . .Appendicitis. . .," *ibid.*, 20 (1946): 256-69; ". . .The Borderland of Medicine and Surgery. . .," *ibid.*, 22 (1948): 680-84; ". . .Development of Medical Education. . .," *ibid.*, 25 (1951): 60-65; *NCAB*, 10: 456; *Who Was Who in Am.*, 1: 403.

S. Galishoff

FITZBUTLER, (WILLIAM) HENRY (December 22, 1842, Amherstburg, Ontario, Canada-December 28, 1901, Louisville, Ky.). *Physician; Education.* Son of William Butler, farmer and escaped slave coachman and indentured white English immigrant to Va. Dropped his first name and added "Fitz" to his last name. Married Sarah Helen McCurdy, 1866; six children. EDUCATION: 1864-c.1866, Adrian College, Adrian, Mich.; 1867-71, apprentice to Dr. William C. Lundy (white), perhaps to Dr. Daniel Pearson (black), both in Amherstburg; January-June 1871, Detroit Medical College (first black student); 1872, M.D.,

University of Michigan (first black student and graduate). CAREER: 1872-1901, medical practice, Louisville; 1888-1901, affiliated with Louisville National Medical College as co-founder (1888), dean, and faculty member; editor and financial manager, *The Planet* (black newspaper); 1879-c.1901, editor, *Ohio Falls Express*, weekly newspaper (both published in Louisville). CONTRIBUTIONS: The first black regular physician to practice in Ky. (1872). Co-founded and operated the Louisville National Medical College (1888-1912), a school that trained about 110-20 black physicians before it closed (1912). Established Auxiliary Hospital (1895), which treated black patients, in connection with medical school. Central figure in the functioning of the school and hospital. Before the school's founding, took black students as apprentice physicians. As editor of a weekly black newspaper, *Ohio Falls Express*, was an outspoken critic of racial discrimination and outrages. Involved in local and state politics on behalf of blacks. REFERENCES: W. Montague Cobb, "Henry Fitzbutler," *JNMA* 44 (1952): 403-7; Leslie L. Hanawalt, "Henry Fitzbutler: Detroit's First Black Medical Student," *Detroit in Perspective* 1 (1973): 126-40; *NCAB*, 14: 317; obituary, Louisville National Medical College, *Catalog, 1901-1902*, p. 32; H. C. Weeden, ed., *Weeden's History of the Colored People of Louisville* (1897), 26, 44, 57.

T. Savitt

FLEXNER, ABRAHAM (November 13, 1866, Louisville, Ky.-September 21, 1959, Falls Church, Va.). *Educator*. Son of Morris, merchant, and Esther (Abraham) Flexner; brother of Simon Flexner (q.v.). Married Anne Laziere Crawford, 1898; two children. EDUCATION: 1886, A.B., Johns Hopkins University; 1906, A.M., Harvard University; 1907, A.M., University of Berlin. CAREER: 1886-91, teacher, Louisville Male High School; 1891-1905, founder, owner, and director, Mr. Flexner's School (Louisville); 1908-12, staff member, Carnegie Foundation for Advancement of Teaching; at General Education Board, Rockefeller Foundation: 1913-17, assistant secretary; 1917-25, secretary; and 1925-28, director, Division of Studies and Medical Education; 1930-39, founder and director, Institute for Advanced Study (Princeton). CONTRIBUTIONS: Fathered a revolution in American medical education. Asked by the Carnegie Foundation for the Advancement of Teaching to conduct a study of medical schools; report *Medical Education in the United States and Canada* (1910) castigated medical schools for turning out large numbers of poorly trained physicians; resulted mainly from the existence of commercial schools that accepted inadequately prepared students; furthermore, schools were not equipped with laboratories to train students in medical science or to provide research facilities for faculty members. Obtained $50 million from John D. Rockefeller to upgrade the nation's better medical schools and persuaded other philanthropists to donate lesser sums. These and other pressures to reform medical education led to a more than 50 percent reduction in the number of American medical schools from the 148 Flexner had studied to 60 to 70 superior institutions in 1930.

WRITINGS: *The American College* (1908); *Medical Education in Europe* (1912); *Medical Education, A Comparative Study* (1925). REFERENCES: *Autobiography* (1960); *BHM* (1964-69), 88; (1970-74), 61; *Current Biog.* (1941): 289-91; *DAB*, Supp. 6: 207-9; R. Hudson, "A. Flexner in Perspective," *Bull. Hist. Med.* 46 (1972): 545-61; Miller, *BHM*, p. 35; *NCAB*, 52: 320-21; *N.Y. Times*, September 22, 1959; *Who Was Who in Am.*, 3: 288.

S. Galishoff

FLEXNER, SIMON (March 25, 1863, Louisville, Ky.-May 2, 1946, New York, N.Y.). *Physician; Medical administrator; Pathology; Microbiology.* Son of Morris, merchant, and Esther (Abraham) Flexner; brother of Abraham Flexner (q.v.). Married Helen Whitall Thomas, 1903; two children. EDUCATION: 1882, graduated from Louisville College of Pharmacy; 1899, M.D., University of Louisville; 1890-92, studied under William H. Welch (q.v.), Johns Hopkins; 1893, studied in Prague, Czechoslovakia, and Strassburg, France. CAREER: Pathology faculty: 1892-98, Johns Hopkins; and 1899-1903, University of Pennsylvania; at Rockefeller Institute for Medical Research (later Rockefeller University): 1901-35, director of laboratories and unofficial director (made official in 1924); 1937-38, Eastman professor, Oxford University; trustee: 1913-28, Rockefeller Foundation; and 1937-42, Johns Hopkins University. CONTRIBUTIONS: Made the Rockefeller Institute one of the world's foremost centers for medical research; determined that the institute would devote itself to all areas of medical science and not limit itself to one branch as European research institutes did; assembled a distinguished staff of investigators that he directed with great skill. Isolated *Shigella dysenteriae*, frequently referred to as the "Flexner bacillus," a common cause of dysentery (1899). Headed a governmental commission that confirmed the existence of bubonic plague in San Francisco, Calif. (1901). Helped develop a serum treatment for epidemic spinal meningitis (1907). Transferred poliomyelitis from monkey to monkey and determined that the causative agent of the disease was a filterable virus (1908). Did important research on experimental dysentery, experimental pancreatitis, and immunological problems. Principal or sole editor, *Journal of Experimental Medicine*, for nearly two decades after Welch stepped down from the job (1902). Responsible for getting the Rockefeller Foundation to support National Research Council postdoctoral fellowships in physics, chemistry, and the biological sciences. WRITINGS: "On the Etiology of Tropical Dysentery. . .," *Johns Hopkins Hosp. Bull.* 11 (1900): 231-42 and *Phila. Med. J.* 6 (1900): 414; *Report of the Commission. . .for the Investigation of Plague in San Francisco. . .*(1901, with F. G. Novy [q.v.] and L. F. Barker [q.v.]); "Serum Treatment of Epidemic Cerebrospinal Meningitis," *J. of Experimental Med.* 10 (1908): 141-203 (with J. W. Jobling); "The Transmission of Acute Poliomyelitis to Monkeys," *JAMA* 53 (1909): 1639 (with P. A. Lewis); *William Henry Welch and the Heroic Age of American Medicine* (1941, with James T. Flexner). A bibliography is in *Obituary Notices, Fellows of the Royal Society* 6 (1948-49): 409-45. REFERENCES: *BHM* (1970-74), 61; (1975-79), 44; *DAB*, Supplement 4: 286-89; *DSB*,

5: 39-41; Miller, *BHM*, p. 35; *NCAB*, 52: 319-20; E: 22-23; *Who Was Who in Am.*, 2: 191.

S. Galishoff

FLICK, LAWRENCE FRANCIS (August 10, 1856, Carrolltown, Pa.-July 7, 1938, Philadelphia, Pa.). *Physician; Tuberculosis*. Son of John and Elizabeth (Sharbaugh) Flick. Married Ella Josephine Stone, 1885; seven children. EDU-CATION: Studied at St. Vincent College (Pa.); 1879, M.D., Jefferson Medical College; 1879-80, intern, Philadelphia General Hospital. CAREER: *Post* 1879, practiced medicine, Philadelphia, specializing in tuberculosis; 1881, orange packer in Calif., where he sought to cure himself of tuberculosis; 1884, helped found American Catholic Historical Society; 1895-1935, director, Free Hospital for Poor Consumptives; 1901-35, president, White Haven Sanatorium, Luzerne County, Pa.; 1903-10, medical director, Henry Phipps Institute for the Study, Prevention, and Treatment of Tuberculosis. CONTRIBUTIONS: Helped establish sanatoriums, voluntary public health organizations, and a prominent research center to combat tuberculosis. Evolved a method of treatment for tuberculosis based on rest, fresh air, and nutritious diet. Conducted a study of tuberculosis in Philadelphia's fifth ward that demonstrated that the disease was contagious rather than hereditary as was commonly believed (1889). Campaigned for the isolation of tuberculosis victims; led to the founding of Rush Hospital for Consumption and Allied Diseases (1890), Free Hospital for Poor Consumptives (1895), and White Haven Sanatorium (1901). Established the Pennsylvania Society for the Prevention of Tuberculosis, a pioneer association of physicians and laymen that educated the public in preventive methods and the importance of early diagnosis. Helped create the National Tuberculosis Association (1904), which became the prototype of the many national, voluntary public health organizations that were subsequently created. Persuaded Henry Phipps to endow an institute for the study of tuberculosis which became renowned throughout the world (1903).

WRITINGS: *Consumption, a Curable and Preventable Disease, What the Layman Should Know About It* (1903); *Development of Our Knowledge of Tuberculosis* (1925); *Tuberculosis—A Book of Practical Knowledge to Guide the General Practitioner of Medicine* (1937). A bibliography is in Ella M. E. Flick, *Dr. Lawrence F. Flick, 1856-1938* (1940). REFERENCES: *DAB*, Supplement 2: 196-97; Miller, *BHM*, p. 35; *NCAB*, 28: 434-35; *N.Y. Times*, July 8, 1938; *Who Was Who in Am.*, 1: 406.

S. Galishoff

FLINT, AUSTIN (October 20, 1812, Petersham, Mass.-March 13, 1886, New York, N.Y.). *Physician*. Son of Joseph Henshaw, physician, and Hannah (Reed) Flint. Married Anne Skillings, 1835; one child, Austin, Jr. (q.v.). EDUCATION: Amherst and Harvard Colleges; 1833, M.D., Harvard Medical School; private pupil of James Jackson, Sr.; studied under Jacob Bigelow and John C. Warren (qq.v.) at Harvard. CAREER: 1833-44, practice of medicine, Boston and Northampton, Mass., and Buffalo, N.Y.; 1844-45, professor of the institutes and practice of medicine, Rush Medical College, Chicago, Ill.; 1845, founder and editor, *Buffalo Medical Journal*; 1846-52, professor of principles and practice of medicine and clinical medicine and a founder, University of Buffalo; 1852-56, professor of principles and practice of medicine and clinical medicine, University of Louisville; 1856-59, professor of pathology and clinical medicine, University of Buffalo; 1858-61 (winters), professor of clinical medicine, New Orleans School of Medicine; 1861-68, professor of pathology and practical medicine, Long Island College Hospital; 1861-86, professor of the principles and practice of medicine and clinical medicine and a founder, Bellevue Hospital Medical College. CONTRIBUTIONS: Educator of physicians—possibly the most influential and distinguished American physician of the midnineteenth century. Made a sustained effort to elevate the standards of teaching and practice of American physicians. Greatly influenced medical education in N.Y. State by the founding of University of Buffalo Medical School, Bellevue Hospital Medical College, and the *Buffalo Medical Journal*. Critical observer who refined and extended the art of percussion and auscultation of the heart and lungs that was initiated by Auenbrugger and Laennec. Lifelong interest in infectious diseases and author of articles on almost every aspect of internal medicine.

WRITINGS: "Account of an Epidemic Fever Which Occurred at North Boston, Erie County, New York, During the Months of October and November, 1843," *Am. J. of Med. Sci.* 10 (1845): 21; "On Variations of Pitch in Percussion and Respiratory Sounds, and Their Application in Physical Diagnosis," *TAMA* 5 (1852): 75; "On Cardiac Murmurs," *ibid.*, 44 (1862): 29; *A Treatise on the Principles and Practice of Medicine* (1866, 1867, 1868, 1873, 1881, 1886). Writings listed in *Medical Classics* 4 (1940): 842, compiled by Emerson Crosby Kelly. REFERENCES: *BHM* (1964-69), 88; (1970-74), 62; (1975-79), 44; *DAB*, 6: 471-72; Alfred S. Evans, "Austin Flint and His Contributions to Medicine," *Bull. Hist. Med.* 32 (1958): 224-41; Oliver P. Jones, "Our First Professor of Medicine, Austin Flint (1812-1886)," *The Buffalo Physician* 7 (1973): 54-61; Miller, *BHM*, p. 35; Norman Shaftel, "Austin Flint, Sr. (1812-1886): Educator of Physicians," *J. of Med. Ed.* 35 (1960): 1122-35; Dale C. Smith, "Austin Flint and Auscultation in America," *J. Hist. Med.* 33 (1978): 129-49.

R. Batt

FLINT, AUSTIN, JR. (March 28, 1836, Northampton, Mass.-September 22, 1915, New York, N.Y.). *Physician; Physiologist*. Son of Austin (q.v.), physician, and Anne (Skillings) Flint. Married Elizabeth McMaster, 1862; four children. EDUCATION: Private schools, Buffalo, N.Y.; 1851-52, Academy of Leicester, Mass.; 1852-53, Harvard College; 1853-54, worked in engineering department, Louisville and Nashville Railroad; spring 1854, medical department, University of Buffalo; autumn 1854, apprentice to Frank H. Hamilton, M.D., Buffalo, N.Y.; 1854-56, medical department, University of Kentucky; summer 1855, assistant to John Call Dalton (q.v.), M.D., Woodstock Medical College, Vt.; 1856-57, M.D., Jefferson Medical College, Philadelphia, Pa. CAREER: 1857, practice of medicine with Austin Flint, Sr., Buffalo; 1858-60, editor, *Buffalo*

Medical Journal; professor of physiology: 1858-59, University of Buffalo; 1859-60, New York Medical College; and 1860-61, New Orleans School of Medicine; 1861, several months in Paris studying physiology with Claude Bernard and histology with Charles Robin; 1861-98, professor of physiology and a founder, Bellevue Hospital Medical College; professor of physiology: 1862-68, Long Island College Hospital; and 1898-1906, Cornell University Medical College. CONTRIBUTIONS: Pioneer American professor of physiology whose experiments spanned the entire field in the era before specialized systematic laboratory investigations. Teaching and writings helped to establish the discipline of physiology in American medical schools. By repeating and confirming crucial experiments of other investigators as demonstrations before his medical students, prepared for his great work—the synthesis of the whole of human physiology—*The Physiology of Man*, 5 vols. (1866-75). Subsequently applied his physiological knowledge to psychiatry, criminology, and forensic medicine.

WRITINGS: *The Physiology of Man*, 5 vols (1866-75); "Experimental Researches into a New Excretory Function of the Liver; Consisting in the Removal of Cholesterin from the Blood, and Its Discharge from the Body in the Form of Stercorin," *Am. J. of Med. Sci.* 44 (1862): 305-65. Writings listed in Austin Flint, *Collected Essays and Articles of Physiology and Medicine*, 2 vols. (1903). REFERENCES: *DAB* 3 , pt. 2 (1964): 472-73; Kelly and Burrage (1920), 395-96; *NCAB* 9 (1907): 360-61.

R. Batt

FLOCKS, RUBIN HYMAN (May 7, 1906, New York, N.Y.-May 17, 1975, Iowa City, Ia.). *Physician; Urology*. Son of Morris, tailor, and Rose (Blackman) Flocks. Never married. EDUCATION: Johns Hopkins University: 1926, A.B.; and 1930, M.D. CAREER: 1930-31, resident house officer (orthopedics), Johns Hopkins Hospital; 1931-75, medical faculty, Department of Urology, University of Iowa College of Medicine (1949-75, professor and head); urologist-in-chief, university hospitals; in AMA: 1954, Urology Section secretary; and 1957, president; in American Urology Association: 1954, president, North Central Section; 1962, secretary; and 1968-69, president; on American Board of Urology: *post* 1952, member, Board of Trustees; and 1963, president; *post* 1965, member, National Research Council and National Advisory Cancer Council. CONTRIBUTIONS: Nationally known for pioneering work in prostatic diseases (especially cancer), urinary stones, and transurethral prostatic resection, was instrumental in the development of urology as a specialty. Contributed significantly to knowledge of the blood supply of the prostate (1937), as anatomical study necessary for the advancement of transurethral prostatic resection. Early laboratory studies (1939) on urinary calculi were landmark observations and measurements of calcium excretion have long been routine in the investigation of patients with urinary stones. Initiated the successful, if controversial, treatment of locally advanced but not metastatic prostatic cancer by irradiation with gold isotopes (1952). Also interested in cryosurgery as a new technique offering hope for these patients (1972).

WRITINGS: Published over 150 journal articles. "Arterial Distribution within the Prostate Gland. Its Role in Transurethral Prostatic Resection," *J. Urol.* 37 (1937): 524; "Calcium and Phosphorus Excretion in Urine of Patients with Renal or Ureteral Calculi," *JAMA* 113 (1939): 1466; "Treatment of Carcinoma of the Prostate by Interstitial Radiation with Radioactive Gold (Au198): Preliminary Report," *J. Urol.* 68 (1952): 510; *Surgical Urology*, 4 eds. (1954-75, with David A. Culp); *Radiation Therapy of Early Prostatic Cancer* (1960, with David A. Culp); "Perineal Cryosurgery for Prostatic Carcinoma," *J. Urol.* 108 (1972): 933 (with C. M. Nelson and D. L. Boatman). REFERENCES: *JAMA* 234 (1975): 546; Hugh J. Jewett, "Rubin H. Flocks and the Prostatic Disease Center," *J. Iowa Med. Soc.* 62 (1972): 572; University of Iowa Archives, Iowa City; University of Iowa News Service, release dated 5/21/74; *Who's Who in Am., 1974-1975*.

R. E. Rakel

FLOWER, BENJAMIN ORANGE (October 19, 1858, Albion, Ill.-December 24, 1918, Boston, Mass.). *Journalist; Critic of medicine.* Son of Alfred, minister, and Elizabeth (Orange) Flower. Married Hattie Cloud, 1855; no children. EDUCATION: c. 1878, Kentucky University. CAREER: 1880-1918, editor of several national magazines (most notably *Arena*, 1889-96, 1904-9) and author of numerous books advocating a broad range of social reform projects. In later years, became fanatically anti-Catholic, venting his hatred in the magazine *Menace*. CONTRIBUTIONS: President, National League for Medical Freedom (c.1910) which resisted the efforts of the orthodox medical profession to inhibit the growth of alternative medical systems (homeopathy, eclecticism, osteopathy, and so on), opposed compulsory vaccination, and fought against the establishment of a national department of health. Defended Christian Science from medical ridicule. Urged female dress reform as part of his support for women's suffrage. Promoted psychical research and argued science would eventually demonstrate the existence of an afterlife.

WRITINGS: *Christian Science, as a Religious Belief and a Therapeutic Agent* (1909); "National Health and Medical Freedom," *Century Mag.* 85 (1912-13): 512-13; *Progressive Men, Women, and Movements of the Past Twenty-Five Years* (1914). REFERENCES: *DAB*, 3, pt. 2: 477-78; Hamlin Garland, "Roadside Meetings of a Literary Nomad," *The Bookman* 70 (1929-30): 514-28; Allen Matusow, "The Mind of B. O. Flower," *New Eng. Q.* 34 (1961): 492-509; *NCAB*, 9: 228.

J. C. Whorton

FOLEY, FREDERICK EUGENE BASIL (April 5, 1891, St. Cloud, Minn.-March 24, 1966, St. Paul, Minn.). *Urologist.* Son of Thomas and Jenny Ann (Craig) Foley. Married Elizabeth Doran Dearth, 1914. EDUCATION: Studied at Yale University (1913), Johns Hopkins University (MD., 1918), and the University of Minnesota; interned at Peter Bent Brigham Hospital, Boston, Mass. CAREER: Worked with Dr. Harvey Cushing (q.v.) in surgical research; 1922-60, practiced urology, St. Paul; professor of urology, University of Minnesota. CONTRIBUTIONS: Inventor of the inflatable Foley Catheter. Developed the Foley urological operating table (1961). Established the urological department at the

Ancker Hospital in St. Paul (1929). Developed the Foley Y Plasty for stricture of the kidney pelvis (1929). REFERENCES: *JAMA* 197 (1966): 235; A. W. Zorgniotti, "Frederick E. B. Foley. Early Development of Balloon Catheter," *Urology* 1 (Jan. 1973): 75-80; *Who's Who in America* (1968).

R. Rosenthal

FOLIN, OTTO KNUT OLOF (April 4, 1867, Asheda, Sweden-October 25, 1934, Brookline, Mass.). *Biochemist.* Son of Nils Magnus, tanner, and Eva (Olson), midwife, Folin; 12th of 13 children. Followed older brother to the United States, 1882. Married Laura Churchill Grant, September 11, 1899; three children. EDUCATION: 1892, B.S., University of Minnesota; Ph.D., 1898, University of Chicago; studied physiological chemistry with Olaf Hammerstein, Uppsala, Sweden; Albrecht Kossel, Marburg, Germany; and E. L. Salkowski, Berlin, Germany. CAREER: 1899-1900, assistant professor of chemistry, University of West Virginia; 1900-1908, research biochemist, McLean Hospital (Waverly, Mass.); at Harvard Medical School: 1907-9, associate professor of biochemistry; and 1909-34, Hamilton Kuhn professor; 1903, surgical removal of a parotid tumor affected the left side of face but continued active research and teaching until death. CONTRIBUTIONS: A pioneer in biological chemistry that led him to the development of practical colorimetric methods for quantitative microanalysis of body fluids. In his first medical investigation, recognized that it was useless to search for "toxins" in the urine of insane patients without reliable criteria for normal protein metabolism. The ingenious methods he subsequently devised for identifying and measuring the chemistry of urine (1900-1904) were adapted (after 1912) to the study of blood and tissues. With Hsien Wu, developed a simple laboratory procedure (1920) for separating a nonprotein filtrate from whole blood, enormously facilitating determination of glucose and other important constituents of portal blood. Was attracted to the "puzzle aspect" of laboratory work and established methods through which the color reactions of different chemical reagents were measured and used as the foundation of quantitative clinical biochemistry in the first half of the twentieth century. Charter member, American Society of Biological Chemists (1906) and founder, *Journal of Biological Chemistry* (1905).

WRITINGS: "Laws Governing the Chemical Composition of Urine," *Am. J. of Physiol.* 13 (1905): 66; "Protein Metabolism from the Standpoint of Blood and Tissue Analysis I-VII," *J. Biol. Chem.* 11-17 (1912-14, with W. Denis); *A Laboratory Manual of Biological Chemistry* (1916; 5th ed., 1934); "A System of Blood Analysis," *J. Biol. Chem.* 38 (1919): 81 (with Hsien Wu). *BMNAS* 27 (1952): 47 lists writings. REFERENCES: R. H. Chittenden, *The Development of Physiological Chemistry in the United States* (1930), 79-82; *DAB*, Supplement 1: 306-8; *DSB*, 5: 53; William H. Forbes, "Recollections of Otto Folin," *Harvard Med. Alumni Bull.* 46 (Sept.-Oct. 1971): 8-10; *NCAB* 25: 197.

B. G. Rosenkrantz

FOLKS, HOMER (February 18, 1867, Hanover, Mich.-February 13, 1963, Riverdale, N.Y.). *Public health; Child welfare.* Son of James, farmer, and Esther

(Woodliff) Folks. Married Maud Beard, 1891; three children. EDUCATION: 1889, graduated from Albion College (Michigan); 1890, graduated from Harvard University. CAREER: 1890-93, general superintendent of the Children's Aid Society of Pennsylvania; 1893-1902, 1903-17, 1919-47, executive secretary, New York State Charities Aid Assoc.; 1902-3, commissioner of public charities of New York City; 1917-18, director of the Department of Civil Affairs, American Red Cross, France. CONTRIBUTIONS: (1890-93) Introduced home care of delinquent, orphaned, and neglected children, Philadelphia. Credited with playing a major role in the public health movement of the early 20th century. Founded America's first municipal tuberculosis hospital. Helped to conduct the first analysis of the "white plague" in the U.S. (1903). Helped create the National Association for the Study and Prevention of Tuberculosis (1904) serving on its board; elected president (1912). Conducted an anti-tuberculosis campaign leading to laws governing the reporting and treatment of all cases, as well as the construction of public institutions. Helped establish juvenile courts in New York State, and created the nation's first state probation commission (1907), serving as chairman for ten years. Founder and chairman (1935-44) of the National Child Labor Committee. Helped introduce widows' pensions to New York State (1915). A founder, American Association for the Study and Prevention of Infant Mortality (1909); president (1915). President, National Conference of Social Work (1911 and 1923). Drafted the bill creating the New York Public Health Council, the first in the nation to separate public health administration from politics; served as vice-chairman, 1913-55. After suffering a stroke in 1946, retired the following year.

WRITINGS: *The Care of the Destitute, Neglected and Delinquent Children* (1902); *The Human Costs of the War* (1920); *Public Health and Welfare: The Citizens' Responsibility* (1958). REFERENCES: *DAB*, Supplement 7: 250-52; Introduction to Folks, *Public Health and Welfare*; *N. Y. Times*, February 14, 1963; W. I. Trattner, *Homer Folks: Pioneer in Social Welfare* (1968).

M. Kaufman

FORBES, ALEXANDER (May 14, 1882, Milton, Mass.-March 27, 1965, Milton). *Physiologist; Neurophysiology*. Son of William Hathaway, telephone company executive, and Edith (Emerson) Forbes. Married Charlotte Irving Grinell, 1910; four children. EDUCATION: Harvard University: 1904, B.A.; 1905, M.A.; and 1910, M.D.; 1911-12, studied with Charles S. Sherrington, Liverpool, England, and, briefly in 1912, with Keith Lucas, Cambridge, England. CAREER: 1911-48, physiology faculty, Harvard University; 1917-19, U.S. Navy Reserve; 1941-45, Medical Corps; after retiring in 1948, continued to do research, Harvard Biological Laboratories and Veterans Administration Hospital, Boston, Mass.; was equally known for his work as a geographer and was actively associated with the George Junior Republic Association for troubled adolescents, Freeville, N.Y. CONTRIBUTIONS: Developed new methods for the investigation of nerve functions, especially in the recording of electric responses of nerve and muscle.

Installed what was probably the first string galvanometer in New England to record electrically central reflex phenomena (c. 1912). First person to report the use of an electronic tube amplifier in a physiological experiment (1920). Turned American neurophysiology in the direction of the study of the transmission of impulses through reflex centers of the spinal cord and brain in terms of what was known concerning the physiology of isolated nerves. Reaffirmed the all-or-none law of nerve conduction in his work on the effect of ether anesthesia on sensory impulses entering the brain. Showed that the strength of a nerve impulse as it passes through a uniformly narcotized stretch of nerve is reduced but of uniform electrical intensity and velocity and does not undergo progressive diminution as was previously taught. An early advocate of the use of microelectrodes and electroencephalography to study the brain. Did pioneering studies of the electrical responses of the brain under Nembutal narcosis.

WRITINGS: "Electrical Studies in Mammalian Reflexes. I. The Flexion Reflex," *Am. J. of Physiol.* 37 (1915): 118-76 (with A. Gregg); "Amplification of Action Currents with the Electron Tube in Recording with the String Galvanometer," *J. of Physiol.* 52 (1920): 409-71 (with C. Thacher); "The All-or-Nothing Response of Sensory Nerve Fibres," *ibid.*, 56 (1922): 301-30 (with E. Adrian); "The Interpretation of Spinal Reflexes in Terms of Present Knowledge of Nerve Conduction," *Physiological Reviews* 2 (1922): 361-414; "Studies of the Nerve Impulse. II. The Question of Decrement," *Am. J. of Physiol.* 66 (1923): 553-617 (with H. Davis, D. Brunswick, and A. McH. Hopkins). A bibliography is in *BMNAS*. REFERENCES: *BHM* (1970-74), 62; (1975-79), 45; *BMNAS* 40 (1969): 113-41; *DSB*, 5: 64-66; *NCAB*, 52: 528-29.

S. Galishoff

FORD, LEWIS DeSAUSSURE (December 30, 1801, Morristown, N.J.-August 21, 1883, Augusta, Ga.). *Physician; Educator.* Son of Gabriel H. Ford, judge of superior court of state of N.J. Married Frances Emily Chiles, 1828; six children. EDUCATION: Studied medicine with a Dr. Jones, Morristown; 1822, M.D., New York College of Physicians and Surgeons. CAREER: At Medical College of Georgia: first professor of chemistry and first dean; and until retirement in 1881, professor of institutes and practice of medicine; twice mayor of Augusta; president, Augusta Board of Health; frequently member, Augusta City Council; Civil War surgeon: First Georgia Hospital, Richmond, Va.; and staff, Dr. Humphrey Marshall and later in charge of the Third Georgia Hospital, Richmond. CONTRIBUTIONS: As first dean of the Medical College of Georgia, was instrumental in introducing a six-month course. Also signed and is, presumably, author of the circular letter sent (1835) to 15 medical schools suggesting "a Convention of Representatives" be called where medical schools could create "a uniform system of requisitions" for the M.D. degree, length of study, entry requirements, and so on. On the state level, a founder of the Medical Association of Georgia and that group's first president (1849).

WRITINGS: Concentrated in the area of pathology and therapeutics of malarial fevers. A number of his articles can be found in the *Southern Med. and Surg. J.* (1837-39, 1845). For text of 1835 circular letter, see *J. of the Assoc. of Am. Med. Colleges* 14 (1939):

120. REFERENCES: Eugene Foster, "Lewis DeSaussure Ford," *Trans., Med. Assoc. of Georgia* (1884): 425-41; William H. Goodrich, *History of the Medical Department of the University of Georgia* (1928); *Memoirs of Georgia* 2 (1895): 201-7; William F. Norwood, *Medical Education in the United States Before the Civil War* (1944); George A. Traylor, "Lewis DeSaussure Ford, M.D., " *J. Med. Assoc. of Georgia* 30 (1941): 179-81; George H. Yeager, "Medical Schools of [the] Southern United States, 1779-1830," *Annals of Surg.* 171 (1970): 623-40.

P. Spalding

FORDYCE, JOHN ADDISON (February 16, 1858, Guernsey County, Ohio-June 4, 1925, New York City). *Dermatologist; Syphilologist; Educator.* Son of John and Mary (Houseman) Fordyce. Married Alice Dean Smith, 1886; two children. EDUCATION: 1878, B.A., Adrian College (Michigan); 1881; M.D., Chicago Medical College (Northwestern University); 1881-83, intern at Cook County Hospital; 1886-88, postgraduate study in Berlin, Paris, and Vienna; 1888, M.D., University of Berlin. CAREER: 1883-86, medical practice in Hot Springs, Ark.; 1888-1925, practice in dermatology and genito-urinary diseases, New York City; 1889-93, instructor and lecturer in the New York Polyclinic Hospital; 1893-98, professor of dermatology, Bellevue Hospital Medical College; 1898-1911 (after merger of Bellevue and New York University), professor of dermatology and syphilology at New York University; 1912-25, professor of dermatology and syphilology, College of Physicians and Surgeons, Columbia University; medical and surgical staff of various hospitals, including City Hospital, Presbyterian Hospital, Fifth Avenue Hospital, Woman's Hospital, and New York Infirmary for Women and Children. CONTRIBUTIONS: Demonstrated the value of having dermatologists treat cases of syphilis. Editor (1889-97) of the *Journal of Cutaneous and Genito-urinary Diseases* (now the *Archives of Dermatology*). Organized one of the best teaching centers of dermatology in America training over 150 specialists in the new field. President, American Dermatological Association, 1899. Among the first to receive samples of Paul Ehrlich's "606" (salvarsan) and advocated its use in syphilis. REFERENCES: *Arch. of Dermatology and Syphilology*, August 1925; *DAB*, 6: 521-22; Kelly and Burrage (1928), 424; *NCAB*, 20: 165; *N.Y. Times*, June 5, 1925.

M. Kaufman

FORTNER, BENJAMIN FRANKLIN (August 15, 1847, near Dallas, Tex.-September 23, 1917, Vinita, Okla.). *Physician.* Married Lucy Jennie Gunter of the Cherokee Nation. EDUCATION: After returning from Civil War service, enrolled in the medical department, University of Nashville (now University of Tennessee Medical School), M.D., 1872. CAREER: Began medical practice, western Ark.; 1879-82, first entered Indian Territory with Cherokee wife and practiced medicine, Claremore (now in Okla.); 1884-1917, practice, Vinita, except 1907-11, when he was physician in charge of Frisco Railroad Hospital, Springfield, Mo. CONTRIBUTIONS: Major organizer and guiding spirit of the Indian Territory Medical Association, serving as president three times and as a member of the Judicial Council (1891-1906). Played a leading role in developing affiliation of the Indian Territory Medical Association with the American Medical Association and constantly upheld principles of the AMA code of ethics. Leading figure in efforts to improve health care in Indian Territory and persuaded officials of the Five Civilized Tribes to elevate standards for doctors practicing there, while still allowing for native practice by and for Indians. When statehood came, was first president of the combined Indian Territory and Oklahoma Territory Medical Associations. Served as railway surgeon, general surgeon, and medical consultant.

WRITINGS: Read many papers at state association meetings. Some are listed in Howard and Martin, "Contributions." REFERENCES: Mark R. Everett, *Medical Education in Oklahoma: The University of Oklahoma School of Medicine and Medical Center 1900-1931* (1972); "B. F. Fortner" file, History of Medicine Collection, University of Oklahoma Health Sciences Center Library, Oklahoma City, Okla.; R. Palmer Howard, "Nominations for the All American Medical Hall of Fame," *Journal of the Oklahoma State Medical Association* 72, (Mar. 1979): 202-5; R. Palmer Howard and Richard E. Martin, "The Contributions of B. F. Fortner, Leroy Long, and Other Early Surgeons in Oklahoma," *Journal of the Oklahoma State Medical Association* (Nov. 1968): 541-49.

V. Allen

FOSTER, EUGENE (April 7, 1850, Augusta, Ga.-January 23, 1903, Augusta). *Physician; Educator; Sanitarian.* Son of John and Jane E. M. (Zinn) Foster. EDUCATION: General Capers' Academy, Augusta; studied medicine under his brother Dr. W. H. Foster; 1872, M.D., Medical College of Georgia; 1872, postgraduate work, University Medical College, New York City. CAREER: 1873, upon return to Augusta, put in charge of the Augusta and Richmond County smallpox hospital; 1880, president, Augusta Board of Health, reelected 1884, 1888, 1892; 1880-1903, professor of the principles and practice of medicine and sanitary science and professor of the principles and practice of medicine and state medicine, Medical College of Georgia; 1884-85, president, Medical Association of Georgia; 1889-1903, chairman and member, Board of Trustees, State of Georgia Lunatic Asylum; active in the American Public Health Association. CONTRIBUTIONS: An early advocate of proper municipal sanitation in Ga. During his long tenure on the Augusta Board of Health, Augusta secured its first real sewerage system, improved the quality of its water supply dramatically, and saw its death rate fall as a result of these—and other—reforms backed by Foster. As dean, Medical College of Georgia, pushed for an extended term, an expanded curriculum, and improved standards for entry and graduation. Wrote a pioneering section in the cooperative *Memoirs of Georgia* that dealt with the early history of medicine and public health in the state. An "exceedingly able expounder of the germ theory of disease" when such a position indicated a "radical new standpoint."

WRITINGS: "Report of the Committee on Compulsory Vaccination," *Public Health Papers and Reports* 9 (1884): 238-89; authored some of the most important chapters in Albert H. Buck, ed., *Reference Hand-book of Med. Sci.* (1886-89). His extensive section in *Memoirs of Georgia* 2 (1893) provides information on questions relating to the history of the public health movement in Ga. REFERENCES: *Augusta Chronicle*, January 24, 1903, p. 4; *NCAB* 6: 393-94; Irving A. Watson, *Physicians and Surgeons of Am.* (1896): 615-16.

P. Spalding

FOWLER, GEORGE RYERSON (December 25, 1848, New York, N.Y.-February 6, 1906, Albany, N.Y.). *Surgeon*. Son of Thomas W., railroad machinist, and Sarah Jane Fowler. Married Louise R. Wells, 1873; four children. EDUCATION: Public Schools, Jamaica, Long Island, N.Y.; 1871, M.D., Bellevue Hospital Medical College. CAREER: From age 13 to 20, was railroad telegrapher and machinist; entered general, and later surgical, practice; gradually appointed attending or consulting surgeon to 11 N.Y. hospitals, including King's County, Nassau, Saint John's; 1896-1906, chief of surgery, Brooklyn Hospital; 1890-1906, examiner in surgery, New York State Board of Medical Examiners; Spanish-American War: division surgeon, consultant, and corps surgeon; captain (1877) to brigadier general (1903), Medical Corps, New York National Guard; 1896-1906, professor of surgery, New York Polyclinic Postgraduate School. CONTRIBUTIONS: An early advocate of Listerism and antiseptic surgery and an early operator for appendicitis. Fowler's Position (semisitting, to drain peritonitis), Fowler's Operation (pleurectomy for chronic empyema), and Fowler's Dredger (iodoform) and Bougies (ENT) are also named for him. Author of over 100 case reports and clinical papers in surgery as well as widely used textbooks. Founder and first president (1884), Brooklyn Red Cross. Introduced first-aid and ambulance drill in New York National Guard. Associate editor, *Annals of Anatomy and Surgery*. President, officer, or member of many local and national clinical societies. Delegate to international congresses. Fellow, American Surgical Society.

WRITINGS: *A Treatise on Appendicitis* (1894); *A Treatise on Surgery* (1906). Writings listed in *Med. Classics* 4 (1940): 531-48. REFERENCES: *Brooklyn Med. J.* 20 (1906): 114-22, 268-71; *DAB*, 3, pt. 2: 563-64; Russell S. Fowler, "George Ryerson Fowler," *Med. Times* 72 (1944): 61-70; *Med. Classics* 4 (1940): 531-48; *NCAB*, 4: 194; Lewis S. Pilcher, "Master Surgeons of America," *Surg. Gyn & Obst.* 38 (1925): 564-67.

R. J. T. Joy

FRANCIS, GROSSI HAMILTON (November 29, 1885, St. Christopher, British West Indies-May 5, 1963, Norfolk, Va.). *Physician*. Son of Barnabus and Mary C. (Hamilton) Francis. Married Nevada C. Burrows, 1913; two children. EDUCATION: 1904-7, Berkeley Institute (no degrees given at this school), Hamilton, Bermuda; 1911, M.D., Meharry Medical College; 1910-11, intern, Hubbard Hospital, Nashville, Tenn.; postgraduate study in internal medicine: 1924-37, 1943, Columbia University College of Physicians and Surgeons; 1944-45, University of Buffalo; and 1949, Cook County Post-Graduate School of Medicine. CAREER: 1911-63, private practice, Norfolk, Va. CONTRIBUTIONS: First intern, Hubbard Hospital (1910-11). Served black medical profession locally in Old Dominion Medical Society (as president and other offices) and Tidewater Medical Society and nationally in NMA (as assistant secretary, member of executive board, and president, 1933-34). Founded and organized the NMA House of Delegates (1935) and served as its speaker (until 1947). Considered the elder statesman and patriarch of the NMA in his later years owing to the long service he devoted to it. Strong advocate of and participant in public health programs and education. REFERENCES: W. Montague Cobb, "Dr. G. Hamilton Francis Received Distinguished Service Award for 1953," *JNMA* 45 (1953): 433-34; *WWICA* 6 (1941-43): 191.

T. Savitt

FRANCIS, JOHN WAKEFIELD (November 17, 1789, New York, N.Y.-February 8, 1861, New York). *Physician*. Son of Melchior Francis, German immigrant. Married Mary Eliza McAlister, 1829; one child. EDUCATION: Columbia College: 1809, B.A.; and 1812, M.A.; apprentice to Dr. David Hosack (q.v.); M.D., College of Physicians and Surgeons (N.Y.); studied with Dr. Abernathy, London, and attended lectures of Brande and Pearson. CAREER: Until 1820, partnership with Dr. Hosack; 1820-26, medical faculty, College of Physicians and Surgeons, in obstetrics and diseases of women and children; 1826, helped organize the medical department of Rutgers; 1810-14, co-editor, *American Medical and Philosophical Register*; 1830, retired from teaching. CONTRIBUTIONS: A founder, New York Academy of Medicine (1846). First to call attention to the use of croton oil, elaterium, and iodine. Largely responsible for the founding of the State Inebriate Asylum, Binghamton, N.Y.

WRITINGS: *Old New York* (1858); *Introduction to the Practice of Midwifery* (1825). Others mentioned in *NCAB*, 1: 393. REFERENCES: *BHM* (1970-74), 63; *DAB*, 3, pt. 2: 581; Kelly and Burrage (1920), 409; "List of Founders of the N.Y. Academy of Medicine, with Biographical notes . . .," ms., New York City; Miller, *BHM*, p. 36; obituaries on file at the New York Academy of Medicine, New York City; *NCAB*, 1: 393.

D. Rosner

FRANCIS, THOMAS, JR. (June 15, 1900, Gas City, Ind.-October 1, 1969, Ann Arbor, Mich.). *Physician; Epidemiology; Virology*. Son of Thomas, Methodist lay preacher and steel worker, and Elizabeth Ann (Cadogan), Salvation Army worker, Francis. Married Dorothy Packard Otton, 1933; two children. EDUCATION: 1921, B.S., Allegheny College; 1925, M.D., Yale University; at New Haven Hospital: 1925-26, medical intern; and 1926-27, resident physician. CAREER: 1927-28, instructor of medicine, Yale University; 1928-36, researcher, Rockefeller Institute for Medical Research; 1938-41, professor of bacteriology, New York University; 1941-69, professor of epidemiology, University of Michigan medical and public health schools, including 1947-69, Henry Sewall University Professor of Epidemiology; 1941-55, director, Commission on Influenza; president: 1958-60, Armed Forces Epidemiology Board; 1945-46, American

Society for Clinical Investigation; 1947, Society of American Bacteriologists; 1949-50, American Association of Immunologists; and 1954-55, American Epidemiological Society; 1948, elected to National Academy of Sciences. CON-TRIBUTIONS: First in the United States to isolate Type A influenza virus (1934, with Thomas Magill); first to isolate Type B influenza virus (1941); developed and field tested first effective influenza vaccine (1943); first to discover antigenic variability of influenza (1936). Designed and conducted historic field trials of Salk polio vaccine (1953-55), the largest ever double-blind controlled study. Developed early test for pneumonia immunity. Initiated Tecumseh, Mich., long-range prospective, community-health statistical project.

WRITINGS: "Transmission of Influenza by a Filterable Virus," *Sci.* 80 (1934): 457-59; "A New Type of Virus from Epidemic Influenza," *ibid.*, 92 (1940): 405-8; "A Clinical Evaluation of Vaccination Against Influenza," *JAMA* 124 (1944): 982; *Evaluation of the 1954 Field Trial of Poliomyelitis Vaccine: Final Report* (1957). Writings listed in *BMNAS* 44 (1974): 92-110; *Arch. of Environmental Health* 21 (1970): 237-46. REFER-ENCES: *Arch. of Environmental Health* 21 (1970): 226-74; *BMNAS* 44 (1974): 57-110; *Michigan Med.* 68 (1969): 1204, 1238; *NCAB*, I: 432; *Who Was Who in Am.*, 5: 246.

M. Pernick

FREDERICK, RIVERS (May 22, 1873, Pointe Coupee Parish, La.-September 9, 1954, New Orleans, La.). *Physician; Surgeon.* Son of George S. and Armintine (Dalcourt) Frederick. Married Arcina Boris, 1906, two children; Eloise Clark, one child. EDUCATION: 1893, completed English course, New Orleans University; 1897, M.D., University of Illinois College of Medicine (Chicago, Ill.). CAREER: 1897-99, worked in surgical clinic of Dr. John B. Murphy (q.v.), Chicago; 1899-1901, 1904-54, private practice, New Orleans; 1901-4, surgeon-in-chief, Government Hospital, El Roi Tan, Spanish Honduras; 1907-11, faculty member (physical diagnosis), Flint Medical School, New Orleans; 1904-53, surgeon, Flint Goodrich Hospital (at first called Sarah Goodrich Hospital), New Orleans; 1913-32, surgeon, Southern Pacific Railroad. CONTRIBUTIONS: Served the medical needs of many black New Orleans residents for almost 50 years. A well-known medical and community figure in New Orleans owing to professional skills and involvement in important local activities both medical and general. Worked to improve health and living conditions of blacks. Was deeply involved in teaching and improving the facilities and services offered at Flint-Goodrich Hospital.

WRITINGS: "Acute Intestinal Obstruction," *JNMA* 27 (1935): 68; "Primitive Surgeons in Modern Medicine," *ibid.*, 38 (1946): 206; "The Treatment of Toxic Goiter," *ibid.*, 43 (1951): 25 (with U. G. Dailey [q. v.]). REFERENCES: "Dr. Rivers Frederick Receives Distinguished Service Award for 1951," *JNMA* 43 (1951): 400; obituary, *ibid.*, 46 (1954): 434-35; obituary notice, *Time*, September 13, 1954, p. 104; *WWICA* 6 (1941-43): 195. Some of his private papers are housed at the Amistad Research Center, New Orleans.

T. Savitt

FREEDLANDER, SAMUEL OSCAR (July 30, 1893, Wooster, Ohio-January 4, 1971, Cleveland, Ohio). *Surgeon (thoracic and general).* Son of David, retail merchant, and Anna (Arnson) Freedlander. Married Adeline Kaden, 1931, two children; Edith Einstein, 1960. EDUCATION: 1915, A.B., Adelbert College, Western Reserve University; 1918, M.D., Western Reserve School of Medicine; 1918-1921, intern and resident, Cleveland City Hospital; 1921-22, pathology training, Vienna. CAREER: *Post* 1920, surgery faculty, Western Reserve University Medical School; at Cleveland City Hospital: 1924-29, resident surgeon-in-charge; 1930-32, surgeon-in-charge; and 1932-53, chief of Surgical Division and chief of thoracic surgery; 1945-59, director of surgery, Mt. Sinai Hospital; 1932-59, chief of surgery, Sunny Acres Sanitarium; 1945-59, director, Katz-Sanders Laboratory for Surgical Research; postretirement consultant, Mt. Sinai Hospital, St. Luke's, Metropolitan, Forest City Hospital, and the Community Health Foundation; 1964-66, member, National Advisory Council for the Health Professions; maintained a private practice. CONTRIBUTIONS: Began the modern era in lung resection for tuberculosis; performed the first planned lobectomy for pulmonary tuberculosis. Pioneered treatment of tetanus with antitoxin. A founding member, Forest City Hospital. Drafted legislation for organizing the Community Health Foundation (forerunner of the Kaiser Foundation).

WRITINGS: Author of 35 articles in medical journals. "Treatment of Tetanus," *Am. J. of Med. Sci.* 161 (Jun. 1921): 819; "The Surgical Treatment of Pulmonary Tuberculosis," *Ohio St. Med. J.* (Apr. 1929); "Lobectomy in Pulmonary Tuberculosis," *J. Thor. Surg.* 5 (Dec. 1935): 132-42; "Surgical Lesions of the Chest," *Postgrad. Med.* 2 (Aug. 1947): 93. REFERENCE: *NCAB*, 56: 230.

G. Jenkins

FREEMAN, JOHN WILLIAM (December 13, 1853, Virden, Ill.-February 2, 1926, Lead, S. Dak.). *Physician; Surgery.* Son of Peter S., farmer, and Elizabeth Pierce (Warrimer) Freeman. Married Hattie V. Dickinson, 1885; four children. EDUCATION: Blackburn Academy, Carlinville, Ill.; 1876-78, Miami Medical College, Cincinnati; 1879, M.D., University Medical College, now New York University; worked at New York Polyclinic. CAREER: c. 1879-81, practiced with Dr. David Prince and assistant, Sanitarium, Jacksonville, Ill.; 1881-83, assistant surgeon, U.S. Army, Ft. Meade, Dakota Territory; 1884-1918, practicing physician and chief surgeon for the Homestake Mining Company, Lead, S. Dak. CONTRIBUTIONS: Pioneer physician and skilled microscopist. Performed earliest known appendectomy in the Midwest (1884). Lectured on treatment for scalpings. President, State Medical Association (1890) and State Medical Board of Examiners (1920). REFERENCES: George W. Kingsbury, *History of Dakota Territory*; *Memorial and Biographical Record-The Black Hills Region* (1898), 340-43; George Martin Smith, *South Dakota, Its History and Its People: Biographical* 4 (1915): 40; *Who Was Who in Am.*, 1: 425.

D. W. Boilard and P. W. Brennen

FRENCH, HARLEY ELLSWORTH (December 7, 1873, Delphi, Ind.-February 4, 1961, Grand Forks, N.Dak.). *Physician; Medical educator.* Son of

Charles A., farmer, and Mina (Fischer) French. Married Mabel Townsley, 1910; two children. EDUCATION: 1902, B.A., State College of Washington, Pullman, Wash.; 1907, M.D., Northwestern University; 1911, M.S., University of Chicago. CAREER: 1893-1900, 1902-3, public schoolteacher; 1907-11, professor of anatomy and physiology, University of South Dakota School of Medicine (Vermillion, S. Dak.); 1911-47, professor of anatomy and dean, School of Medicine, University of North Dakota; 1921-22, president, North Dakota Medical Association; 1921-23, secretary, North Dakota State Board of Health; 1925-26, assistant professor of anatomy (on leave of absence), University of Pennsylvania; 1947-52, professor and dean emeritus, University of North Dakota School of Medicine. CONTRIBUTIONS: Responsible for the N.Dak. movement that resulted in establishment of full-time Department of Health (1921). N.Dak.'s first full-time state health officer. Maintained the School of Medicine, University of North Dakota, during the Great Depression of the 1930s (the Medical Library, University of North Dakota, was posthumously named in his honor). Among the leading medical scholars and educators in the history of N.Dak.

WRITINGS: "Production of Hydrochloric Acid in the Stomach," *J.-Lancet* 38 (1918); "Medicine and Society: A Few General Relationships," *ibid.*, 42 (1922); (with W. H. McShan), "Chemistry of Lactogenic Hormone Extracts," *J. Biol. Chem.* 117 (1938); "North Dakota Medicine: A 70-Year Span," *J.-Lancet* 71 (1951). Writings listed in the Harley E. French Medical Library, University of North Dakota, Grand Forks. REFERENCES: *Grand Forks Herald*, February 5, 1961, p.1; James Grassick, *North Dakota Medicine: Sketches and Abstracts* (1926), 127-29; *Who Was Who in Am.*, 5: 251.

L. *Remele*

FRISBIE, EVELYN (FISHER) (September 15, 1873, Grinnell, Ia.-April 22, 1965, Albuquerque, N. Mex.). *Physician*; *Obstetrics*. Daughter of Josiah Fisher, banker. Married to and divorced from Charles Frisbie, some time between 1902 and 1908; no children. EDUCATION: 1898, Ph. B., Grinnell College; 1902, M.D., Physician's and Surgeon's College (University of Illinois); internship, Chicago Maternity Hospital. CAREER: 1902-8, staff, Drake University Medical College, Des Moines, Ia.; 1909-12, practiced, Ocate, N. Mex., having homesteaded at nearby Wagon Mound, N.Mex.; 1912-58, practice, Albuquerque, and staff of St. Joseph's and Presbyterian hospitals; 1962, retired. CONTRIBUTIONS: Under auspices of the Congregational Church, established small medical clinics (1920s) at isolated communities in N. Mex. (Cubero, San Mateo, and Blue Water) to which she made monthly rounds. Often worked in association with a dentist and was supported by the Shrine crippled children's program. Called N. Mex.'s "horse and buggy doctor," this reflected her practice while still at Ocate. In Albuquerque, was the only woman doctor, had her own small lying-in hospital, and was readily accepted. Delivered thousands of babies, second only to Dr. Meldrum Wylder (q.v.). Elected president, New Mexico Medical Society (1915), first woman to become president of a state medical society.

WRITINGS: Does not appear to have done any professional writing but is known to have given paper "Gastric and Duodenal Ulcers with Especial Reference to Their Nonsurgical Treatment" (indicating her interests were not confined to obstetrics and gynecology). REFERENCES: Judith DeMark, "Evelyn Fisher Frisbie: Pioneer New Mexico Doctor," Seminar paper, Univ. of New Mexico; interview with Mrs. Joe Miller, Albuquerque, N.Mex. (patient and friend of Frisbie); news clippings in the Special Collections Library, Coronado Room, Zimmerman Library, Univ. of New Mexico, Albuquerque, N.Mex.

C. Cutter

FRISSELL, JOHN (March 8, 1810-1893). *Surgeon.* Son of Amasa, farmer, and ? (Wilcox) Frissell. EDUCATION: 1831, B.A., Williams College; 1834, M.D., Berkshire Medical College; 1834, M.A., Williams College. CAREER: Surgeon, W.Va. CONTRIBUTIONS: Pioneering surgeon, W.Va., performing first operations for hare lip with deformed upper jaw (1838), club foot (1839), strabismus (1841), stone in bladder (1846). Introduced into Wheeling, W.Va., the use of chloroform in operations (1853). First operation for vesico-vaginal fistula (1856) and extensive reconstructive surgery of the face (1871). Appointed by Governor Pierpont as medical superintendent of military prisoners and soldiers at Wheeling during Civil War. Twenty-five years surgeon for marine patients at Wheeling. First president, West Virginia Medical Society. REFERENCE: *West Virginia Heritage Encyclopedia.*

K. Nodyne and R. Murphy

FROST, WADE HAMPTON (March 3, 1880, Marshall, Va.-April 30, 1938, Baltimore, Md.). *Physician; Epidemiology.* Son of Henry, physician, and Sabra J. (Walker) Frost. Married Susan Noland Haxall, 1915; one child. EDUCATION: University of Virginia: 1901, A.B.; and 1903, M.D.; 1903-4, intern, St. Vincent's Hospital (Norfolk, Va.). CAREER: 1905-28, U.S. Public Health Service: assigned to posts combating yellow fever, examining immigrants, and attached to the Coast Guard; 1905-8, Hygienic Laboratory, Washington, D.C.; 1908-13, head, stream pollution studies, Cincinnati, Ohio; 1917, director, Bureau of Sanitary Service, American Red Cross; and 1918-19, director, statistical studies of influenza epidemic; at Johns Hopkins School of Hygiene and Public Health: 1921-34, epidemiology faculty; and 1931-34, dean. CONTRIBUTIONS: Through use of quantitative methods, transformed epidemiology from a descriptive to an analytical science closely integrated with other fields of medical science and biology. With V. P. Sydenstricker, developed a method of epidemiological investigation based on family studies. Made basic discoveries about the epidemiology of poliomyelitis (1916). With Sydenstricker, described the epidemiological characteristics of influenza (1918-19). Supervised important studies of the pollution and purification of streams (1913-28).

WRITINGS: *Epidemiologic Studies of Acute Anterior Poliomyelitis,* U.S. Public Health Service, *Hygienic Laboratory Bull. No. 90* (1913): 9-105, 234-52; "Some Considerations in Estimating the Sanitary Quality of Water Supplies," *J. of the Am. Water Works Assoc.,*

2 (1915): 712-22; "The Epidemiology of Influenza," *JAMA* 73 (1919): 313-18; "Risk of Persons in Familial Contact with Pulmonary Tuberculosis," *Nation's Health* 23 (1933): 426-32. A bibliography is in Kenneth F. Maxcy (q.v.), ed., *Papers of Wade Hampton Frost* (1941). REFERENCES: *BHM* (1970-74), 68; (1975-79), 48; *DAB*, Supplement 2: 211-12; *N.Y. Times*, May 2, 1938; *Who Was Who in Am.*, 1: 429.

S. Galishoff

FULLER, SOLOMON CARTER (August 11, 1872, Monrovia, Liberia-January 16, 1953, Framingham, Mass.). *Neuropathologist; Psychiatry*. Son of Solomon, coffee planter and government official, and Anna U. (James) Fuller. Married Meta Vaux Warrick, 1909; three children. EDUCATION: Liberia College, Monrovia, Liberia; 1893, A.B., Livingstone College; 1893, Long Island College Hospital; 1897, M.D., Boston University Medical School; 1897-99, intern, Westborough State Hospital (Mass.), in pathology; 1904-5, studied at Psychiatric Clinic and Pathology Institute, University of Munich, Germany, under Kraepelin and Alzheimer. CAREER: 1889, came to United States and enrolled at Livingstone College; 1898-1922, pathologist, Westborough State Hospital; 1899-1933, faculty member, Boston University School of Medicine, in pathology (1899-1909), neurology instructor, (1909-53); neuropathology (1919-21); for long periods during his career, on neurology staffs: Westborough State Hospital, Massachusetts Memorial Hospital, Framingham Union Hospital, Marlboro (Mass.) General Hospital, and Allentown (Pa.) State Hospital. CONTRIBUTIONS: One of the first black physicians to serve on faculty of American medical school other than Meharry or Howard. Studied dementias and Alzheimer's Disease. Suggested (1911), in reporting the ninth known case of Alzheimer's Disease, that the condition was not caused by arteriosclerosis, a view later upheld (1953). Edited, for several years, *Westborough State Hospital Papers*.

WRITINGS: Numerous publications, including "A Statistical Study of 109 Cases of Dementia Praecox," *J. Am. Inst. of Homeopathy* 1 (1909): 322-37; "An Examination of 3,140 Admissions to Westborough State Hospital with Reference to the Frequency of Involution Melancholia (Kraepelin's Melancholia)," *ibid.*, 4 (1911-12): 855-59 (with H. I. Klopp); "Alzheimer's Disease (Senilium Praecox): The Report of a Case and Review of Published Cases," *J. of Nervous and Mental Disorders* 39 (1912): 440, 536; "Further Observations on Alzheimer's Disease," *Am. J. of Insanity* 69 (1912-13): 17-29 (with H. I. Klopp). Writings listed in *JNMA* 46 (1954): 371-72; *WWAPS* 1 (1938): 417; *Index Medicus*, 2nd series, 7 (1909): 895; 10 (1912): 186, 1077, 1296, 1333, 1334, 1335, 1338; 12 (1914): 664; 3rd series, 1 (1921): 991; 4 (1924): 505; John A. Kenney, *The Negro in Medicine* (1912), 14-15. REFERENCES: W. Montague Cobb, "Solomon Carter Fuller, 1872-1953," *JNMA* 46 (1954); 37-72; *The Crisis* 6 (May 1913): 18; John A. Kenney, *The Negro in Medicine* (1912), 14-15; *WWAPS* (1938), 417.

T. Savitt

FULTON, JOHN FARQUHAR (November 1, 1899, St. Paul, Minn.-May 28, 1960, New Haven, Conn.). *Neurophysiologist; Medical historian*. Son of John Farquhar, M.D., ophthalmologist, and Edith Stanley (Wheaton) Fulton.

Married Lucia Pickering Wheatland, 1923; no children. EDUCATION: 1917-18, University of Minnesota; 1921, A.B., Harvard University; 1927, M.D., Harvard Medical School; at Magdalen College, Oxford University: Rhodes Scholar for two years and Christopher Welch Scholar and demonstrator in physiology for another two years; 1923, B.A. and 1925, M.A. and D.Phil. CAREER: 1927, associate in neurosurgery under Dr. Harvey Cushing (q.v.), Peter Bent Brigham Hospital; 1928, fellow, Magdalen College; 1929, professor of physiology, Yale Medical School; 1930-51, chairman and Sterling Professor of physiology, Yale Medical School; 1951-60, Sterling Professor of the history of medicine, Yale Medical School. CONTRIBUTIONS: While working with Cushing (with Jaime Pi-Suñer), made the now classical distinction between the in-parallel position of muscle spindles and the in-series position of tendon organs relative to muscle stretch and contraction. Organized the first primate laboratory in America for the purpose of studying the correlations between cerebral physiology in apes and human neurological disorders. With Carlyle Jacobsen, reported on the behavioral effects of extirpation of the anterior association areas of the frontal lobes (1935). Their initial report prompted Egas Moniz of Portugal to develop prefontal lobotomy for relief of psychosis in mental patients, for which Moniz received the Nobel Prize in 1954. Maintained a deep interest in the history of medicine and was inspired to collect his own library in the history of physiology, consisting of more than 7,000 volumes. With the aid of Cushing and Dr. Arnold Klebs, became the motivating force in planning and establishing a historical library in the Yale Medical Library (1941). When Yale established a department in the history of medicine (1951), resigned the chairmanship of physiology to become Sterling Professor of the history of medicine and the first chairman of the new department, the third in the United States.

WRITINGS: *Muscular Contraction and the Reflex Control of Movement* (1926); *Selected Readings in the History of Physiology* (1930); *The Sign of Babinski, A Study of the Evolution of Cortical Dominance in Primates* (1932), with Allen D. Keller; *Physiology of the Nervous System* (1938); *Harvey Cushing, A Biography* (1946). Co-founder, *Journal of Neurophysiology* (1938) and its editor (until 1960). Appointed to the Editorial Board, *Journal of the History of Medicine and Allied Sciences*, at its founding (1946) and became its editor (1952). Bibliography of 520 entries is in the *Yale J. Biol. Med.* 28 (1955-56): 168-84, and *J. Hist. Med.* REFERENCES: *BHM* (1964-69), 97; (1970-74), 68; (1975-79), 48; *DAB*, Supplement 6: 222-24; *DSB*, 5 (1970-78): 207-8; *J. Hist. Med.* 17 (1962): 1-71; Miller, *BHM*, pp. 38-39; *NCAB*, 53: 9; Elizabeth H. Thomson, "John Farquhar Fulton," unpublished ms.

J. W. Ifkovic

FULTON, MARY HANNAH (May 31, 1854, Ashland, Ohio-January 7, 1927, Pasadena, Calif.). *Medical missionary.* Daughter of John S., attorney, and Augusta Louise (Healy) Fulton. Never married. EDUCATION: Ashland public schools; studied at Lawrence University (Wis.); Hillsdale College (Mich.): 1874, B.S.; and 1877, M.S.; 1880-84, Woman's Medical College of Pennsylvania, M.D.,

1884. CAREER: 1884-91, 1893-1903, 1904-18, medical missionary, China, where she joined her brother Rev. Albert A. Fulton; 1891-93, 1903-4, fund raising in America; 1918, retired to Pasadena, Calif. CONTRIBUTIONS: Missionary, Presbyterian Board of Foreign Missions, serving in China for virtually her entire professional career. Established two dispensaries in Canton (1887), another at Fati (where she worked with Dr. Mary Frost Niles, who had been the first Presbyterian medical missionary woman in China). Taught pediatrics, Canton Hospital. Organized the David Gregg Hospital for Women and Children (1902), including the Julia Mather Turner Training School for Nurses. Established the Hackett Medical College for Women (1902), intending to educate at least two women physicians for every city and large town in Kwangsi and Kwangtung provinces.

WRITINGS: Translated into Chinese some of the leading texts on surgery, nursing, gynecology, and diseases of women and children. *Twenty-Five Years of Medical Work in China* (n.d.). REFERENCES: William W. Cadbury and Mary Hoxie Jones, *At the Point of a Lancet* (1935); *Notable Am. Women* 1: 685-86. Fulton's papers are in the United Presbyterian Missionary Library, New York City.

M. Kaufman

FUSSELL, BARTHOLOMEW (January 1, 1794, Chester County, Pa.-January 4, 1871, Chester Springs, Pa.). *Physician; Educator; Reformer*. Son of Bartholomew, farmer and Quaker leader, and Rebecca (Bond) Fussell. Married Lydia Morris, 1826; Rebecca Hewes, 1841, one son. EDUCATION: 1824, M.D., University of Maryland. CAREER: Practice, Baltimore, Md., and then Chester, Pa.; 1840, informal medical school, in his house, for women. CONTRIBUTIONS: The unassuming Quaker lynch-pin in the group of physicians who (1846) founded a medical school for women (Medical College of Pennsylvania). Educated his sister Esther in a medical class for ladies in his house (1840). Reformer involved in abolition movement and other reforms of the age. Refusing recognition and working quietly behind the scenes, was the driving force behind women in medicine while masquerading as a simple religious country physician. REFERENCES: *DAB* 7: 80-81; John S. Futhey and Gilbert Cope, *History of Chester County* (1881); D. I. Lansing, *Chester County in the 19th Century; A List of its Practicing Physicians and Surgeons*, (1977) 418; (1977); Kelly and Burrage (1920) 418.

D. I. Lansing

G

GAGE, EVERETT LYLE (October 22, 1901, Whitehall, Wis.-October 30, 1972, Bluefield, W.Va.). *Neurosurgeon.* Son of Charles Quincy, farmer, and Rosalinda (Wing) Gage. Married Mary Slotman, 1934; five children. EDUCATION: 1921-26, University of Wisconsin; 1928, M.D., University of Pennsylvania; 1931, M.Sc., McGill University; 1928-30, intern, Univ. of Penn. Hospital; 1930-34, fellow and resident, McGill University, Royal Victoria Hospital, and Montreal Neurosurgical Institute. CAREER: 1934-39, associate surgeon, British-American Hospital, Lima, Peru; 1941-48, consultant in neurosurgery, Beckley Hospital, W.Va.; 1941-72, neurosurgeon-in-chief, Bluefield Sanitorium, Bluefield; 1942-46, commander, U.S. Navy, and chief of surgery, U.S. Naval Hospital, Bainbridge, Md. CONTRIBUTIONS: President, West Virginia Medical Association (1958). Director, Bluefield Sanitarium (1966-70).

WRITINGS: *Manual of Technique in Neuropathology* (with Dr. Arthur Elvidge); "Diagnosis of Brain Tumors in Middle Age," *Geriatrics* 22 (Oct. 1967): 150-67; *Rymes of a Restless Man*; "Cerebral Localization of Epileptic Manifestations," *Arch. Neurol. Psychiat.* 30 (1933): 907. REFERENCES: *Am. Men of Med.* (1961), 238; *Leaders in Am. Sci.* 4 (1960-61); *Outstanding West Virginians* (1969); *Who's Who in Am.* (1963), 1093.

K. Nodyne and R. Murphy

GALLAND, ISAAC (1790 or 1792, Chillicothe, Ohio-1858, Ft. Madison, Ia.). *Physician; Adventurer.* Little is known about the background of this early Iowa settler; his daughter Eleanor is said to be the first white child born in Ia. EDUCATION: Acquired a medical background before arrival in Lee County, Ia., in 1827, probably in Fulton Co., Ill. (possibly while serving a term in jail for counterfeiting). CAREER: Fur trader; counterfeiter; land speculator; established first school in Ia. (Lee County); 1829, founded town of Nashville (now Galland, Ia.); 1836, newspaper publisher; said to have been a Mormon elder and secretary to Prophet Joseph Smith (Nauvoo, Ill.); 1833-39, medical practice, Montrose and Nashville, Ia. CONTRIBUTIONS: Reputed to be particularly successful in the treatment of cholera and prevention of epidemics. Placed in homes throughout his field of practice a medicine chest containing the remedies ordinarily used by physicians of the day, each chest labeled "Dr. Isaac Galland's family medicines." WRITINGS: *The Western Adventure* (*post* 1836), the second newspaper published in Ia.); *The Iowa Emigrant* (1840); a history and a map of Iowa. REFERENCES: David S. Fairchild, *History of Medicine in Iowa* (1923), 9-10; *One Hundred Years of Iowa Medicine* (1950), 11.

R. E. Rakel

GALLAUDET, THOMAS HOPKINS (December 10, 1787, Philadelphia, Pa.-September 10, 1851, Hartford, Conn.). *Educator of the Hearing-Impaired.* Son of Peter Wallace, merchant, and Jane (Hopkins) Gallaudet. Married Sophia Fowler, 1821; eight children. EDUCATION: Hopkins Grammar School, Hartford, Conn.; A.B., 1805, Yale College; 1805-6, apprentice in law office of Chauncey Goodrich; 1806-8, studied English literature and composition at Yale; 1808-10, tutor, Yale College; 1812-14, Andover Theological Seminary; 1815-16, studied educational methods for deaf students in England and France. CAREER: 1810-12, worked for a New York City commercial house; 1817-30, principal, Hartford, Conn. School for the Deaf; 1830-51, engaged in philanthropic activities including advocacy and founding of schools for women and blacks. CONTRIBUTIONS: An early leader in movement to provide education for the hearing-impaired. Helped raise money for and found the first free American school for the deaf in Hartford (1817). Trained a number of men in deaf education who then became heads of similar schools. Furthered the cause of deaf education by presenting talks throughout the country and writing articles for national and professional journals. Two of his sons, Thomas (1822-1902) and Edward Miner (1837-1917), became prominent educators of the deaf.

WRITINGS: Writings on deaf education in *American Annals of the Deaf*; edited six volumes of *Annals of the Deaf and Dumb* (Hartford). REFERENCES: *DAB*, 7: 111; E. M. Gallaudet, *Life of Thomas Hopkins Gallaudet* (1888); *NCAB*, 9: 138-40.

T. L. Savitt

GALLUP, JOSEPH ADAMS (March 30, 1769, Stonington, Conn.-October 12, 1849, Woodstock, Vt.). *Physician.* Son of William, a public figure in Windsor County, and Lucy (Denison) Gallup. Married Abigail Willard, 1792; three children. EDUCATION: 1798, B.M., Dartmouth. CAREER: 1791-1800, practice in Bethel, Vt.; 1800, moved to Woodstock, where he became the leading physician of eastern Vt. and a well-known preceptor; 1820-23, professor of theory and practice of medicine and then president, Castleton Medical College; 1823, professor at University of Vermont; 1827, founded the Clinical School of Medicine (later called the Vermont Medical College) at Woodstock at which he was professor until 1834; 1813, charter member, Windsor County Medical Society and Vermont State Medical Society (president, 1818-28). CONTRIBUTIONS: A month after Benjamin Waterhouse (q.v.) published an account of cowpox vaccination, advertised his readiness to perform the operation (1802). As president, Vermont State Medical Society (1825-26), circularized the other state societies, urging the establishment of uniform high standards of medical education. This led to a convention for that purpose held in Northampton, Mass. (1827). WRITINGS: *Sketches of Epidemic Diseases in the State of Vermont—to Which Is Added Remarks on Pulmonary Consumption* (1815); *Pathological Reflections on the Supertonic State of Disease* (1822); *Outlines of the Institutes of Medicine* (1839; 2nd ed., 1845). REFERENCES: *DAB*, 4, pt. 1: 118; Kelly and Burrage (1920), 419-20; *NCAB*, 5: 250; F. C. Waite, *The Story of a Country Medical College* (1945), 44-48, 50-55.

L. J. Wallman

GALT, WILLIAM CRAIG (April 8, 1777, Williamsburg, Va.-October 22, 1853, "Repton," Louisville, Ky.). *Physician.* Son of John Minson, physician, and Judith (Craig) Galt. Married Matilda Booth Beall, May 1802; one son. EDUCATION: Apprentice under his father in Williamsburg. CAREER: 1803, opened an apothecary shop, Louisville, selling drugs, chemicals, paints, varnishes, and spices; continued to operate his apothecary until his practice was sufficient to support his family; 1816, an original incorporator, Louisville Library Company; 1819, a founding member, Louisville Medical Society; 1822, appointed to the first Board of Health. CONTRIBUTIONS: In addition to rendering medical care to the citizens of Louisville, was busy as a preceptor, and several of his apprentices completed their formal medical education elsewhere. Lifelong interest in medical education reached full expression when he and 11 other physicians obtained a charter for the Louisville Medical Institute (February 3, 1833) and he was chosen president of the incorporators. REFERENCES: Obituary, *Louisville Weekly Courier*, October 29, 1853, p. [2], col. [5].

E. H. Conner

GAMBLE, HENRY FLOYD (January 16, 1862, North Garden, Va.-September 1932, Charleston, W.Va.). *Physician; Surgeon.* Son of Henry Harmon, slave and then worker around train station and telegraph office, and Willie Ann (Howard) Gamble. Married Elizabeth Gilmer, 1894, one child; Anna Banks, one child; Nina Hortense Clinton, 1917, two children. EDUCATION: Lincoln University (Pa.): 1882-84, preparatory department; and 1888, A.B.; 1891, M.D., Yale University. CAREER: 1891-92, private general practice, Charlottesville, Va.; 1892-1932, private general practice and then primarily surgical practice, Charleston. CONTRIBUTIONS: A long-time, highly respected practitioner of Charleston, serving especially the black and mining populations of the area. Organized the West Virginia State Medical Association (black). Served the NMA as president (1911-12) and as chair, Committee on Medical Education, during the Flexner era when black medical schools were under close scrutiny. Wrote open honest reports on the state of these schools. Was deeply involved in affairs at Tuskegee Institute (where his friend Booker T. Washington was principal), especially the John A. Andrew Hospital (where his cousin John A. Kenney [q.v.] practiced medicine).

WRITINGS: "Report of a Case of Puerperal Eclampsia; Placenta Praevia, Caesarean Section," *Yale Med. J.* 15 (1908-9): 357-59; "Report of the Committee on Medical Education and Negro Medical Schools," *JNMA* 1 (1909): 257-58; "Report of Committee on Medical Education in Colored Hospitals," *ibid.*, 2 (1910): 283-90; "Report on Medical Education," *ibid.*, 2 (1910): 23-29; "President's Inaugural Address," *ibid.*, 4 (1912): 299; "Case Reports: Thoracic Aneurysms," *ibid.*, 12 (1920): 18-19; "Caesarean Section," *ibid.*, 16 (1924): 189-90. Some of his writings are listed in *JNMA* 64 (1972): 86. REFERENCES: Robert L. Gamble, "Henry Floyd Gamble, M.D., 1862-1932," *JNMA* 64 (1972): 85-86; John A. Kenney, *The Negro in Medicine* (1912), 11-12; *WWCR* 1 (1915): 112.

T. Savitt

GAMBLE, JAMES LAWDER (July 18, 1883, Millersburg, Ky.-May 28, 1959, Boston, Mass.). *Physician; Pediatrics.* Son of Edwin, gentleman farmer, and Elizabeth (Lawder) Gamble. Married Elizabeth Chafee, 1916; five children. EDUCATION: 1906, A.B., Stanford University; 1910, M.D., Harvard University; intern: 1910-12, Massachusetts General Hospital; and 1912-13, Children's Hospital (Boston); 1913, clinical studies, Austria and Germany; 1914, metabolism studies, Massachusetts General Hospital. CAREER: 1915-22, pediatrics faculty, Johns Hopkins Medical School; 1917-19, physician, American Red Cross, France; 1922-50, pediatrics faculty, Harvard Medical School; 1933-53, director, metabolic research laboratory, Children's Hospital; 1945, president, American Pediatric Society. CONTRIBUTIONS: Pioneered in applying quantitative chemical and physiologic methods to the study of disease. Designed a method of studying electrolyte and water metabolism that was widely used; expressed data by simple graphic means, now known as "Gambelian diagrams" or "Gamblegrams." Elucidated the effects of disease upon the volume and composition of the body fluids; forms the basis for modern methods of treatment of dehydration and edema. Syllabus on *Chemical Anatomy, Physiology and Pathology of Extracellular Fluid* (1939) influenced a whole generation of medical investigators and physicians. Made important studies of acidosis (1920s), the provisioning of life rafts for use on the open seas (during World War II), and the chemistry of growth (after World War II). Edited *Journal of Clinical Investigation* (1941-45).
    WRITINGS: "The Metabolism of Fixed Base During Fasting," *J. Biol. Chem.* 57 (1923): 633 (with S. G. Ross and F. F. Tisdall); "Intracellular Fluid Loss in Diarrheal Disease," *J. Pediat.* 3 (1933): 84 (with A. M. Butler and C. F. McKhann); "Extracellular Fluid, and Its Vicissitudes (Thayer Lecture)," *Johns Hopkins Hosp. Bull.* 61 (1937): 131; "Physiological Information from Studies on the Life Raft Ration," *Harvey Lectures* 42 (1946-47): 247; *The Lane Medical Lectures: Companionship of Water and Electrolyte in the Organization of Body Fluids* (1951). A bibliography is in *BMNAS* and *J. Pediat.* REFERENCES: *BHM* (1975-79), 50; *BMNAS* 36 (1962): 145-60; A . McGehee Harvey, *Science at the Bedside* (1981), 163-67; Charles A. Janeway, "Charles Lawder Gamble (1883-1959)," *J. Pediat.* 56 (1960): 701-8; Miller, *BHM*, p. 39; *N.Y. Times*, May 29, 1959; *Who Was Who in Am.*, 3: 310.

S. Galishoff

GANT, HARRIS ALLEN (March 28, 1852, Columbia, Tenn.-May 6, 1941, Columbia). *Physician; Public Health.* Son of John I. and Martha Jane (Cocke)

Gant. Married Mary Loy Rainey, 1888; two children. EDUCATION: Oxford (Miss) High School; attended University of Mississippi for three years; 1874-75, medical lectures, Vanderbilt University; 1876, M.D., University of Pennsylvania; 1892, postgraduate study, New York Polyclinic. CAREER: 1870, schoolteacher, Water Valley, Miss.; 1872-73, prescription clerk, Water Valley drug store; 1876, began practice of medicine, Water Valley; Mississippi State Board of Health: 1890-1901, member; and 1900, president; early 1900s, moved to Jackson, Miss., and became associated with Dr. John Farrar Hunter (q.v.); upon retirement, returned to Columbia. CONTRIBUTIONS: Outstanding work in Miss. was his handling of epidemics of yellow fever at different periods. Principal achievement in connection with yellow fever was during the Orwood, Miss., epidemic in Lafayette County (1898) in collaboration with Dr. H. R. Carter (q.v.), U.S. Public Health Service. They kept an accurate record of the time required by the disease to develop in a person after being infected, this being the first progressive step in what was to be a victorious war on yellow fever. Many of Gant's recommendations, while a member of the Mississippi State Board of Health, laid the foundations for a broad public health program in that state.

WRITINGS: "Yellow Fever in Mississippi, 1878-1905," *The Mississippi Doctor* (1936). REFERENCES: "Autobiography of Harris Allen Gant" appeared serially in *The Mississippi Doctor* (1936); "Death of H. A. Gant," *ibid.*, 19 (Jun. 1941): 40, 42; *Goodspeed's Biographical and Historical Memoirs of Mississippi* 2 (1891): 256; Dunbar Rowland, ed., *Mississippi: Comprising Sketches of Counties, Towns, Events, Institutions, and Persons Arranged in Cyclopedic Form* 3 (1907): 292-94.

M. S. Legan

GARCELON, ALONZO (May 6, 1813, Lewiston, Maine-December 7, 1906, Medford, Mass.). *Physician; Surgeon.* Son of William, noted agriculturist and political activist, and Mary (Davis) Garcelon. Married Ann Waldron, 1841; seven children. EDUCATION: Lewiston private and public schools; attended Monmouth, Waterville, and Newcastle Academies in preparation for Bowdoin College from which he graduated in 1836; summer 1837, brief medical apprenticeship under Dr. Abiel Hall, Jr., of Alfred, Maine; 1837-38, attended Dartmouth Medical College as the private pupil of Dr. Reuben D. Mussey (q.v.); 1838-39, accompanied Mussey to the Medical College of Ohio, Cincinnati, serving as his "Demonstrator of Surgical Anatomy;" 1839, received M.D. CAREER: 1839-1906, practice in Lewiston. CONTRIBUTIONS: Almost immediately, gained renown for successfully fighting a smallpox epidemic. Developed his own vaccine and distributed it to colleagues throughout the state. Treated Irish immigrants during a cholera epidemic (1854). Reported to be the first Maine surgeon to operate for mastoid disease and goiter. Consulting physician and surgeon for Catholic Sisters' Hospital, which he had helped create. Played an important role in securing Central Maine General Hospital for Lewiston and making it a success. Worked for the creation of a state Board of Health and Board of Registration for doctors. With others, incorporated the Lewiston School for Medical Instruction (1879), where he instructed in anatomy, orthopedic surgery, and disease of the joints.

Served as surgeon-general for Maine during the Civil War. Helped organize the Maine Medical Association (1853) and founded the Androscoggin County Chapter. A public spokesman for improved housing for the poor, the importance of public education for preventive medicine, human anatomy and public hygiene, and on "Quackery, Its Causes and Cures." Had numerous business and political involvements; founded the longest lasting newspaper in Maine; first Democrat to serve as mayor of Lewiston; and governor of Maine (1878-79). REFERENCES: Brian Lister, "Alonzo Garcelon, 1813-1906: The Man and His Times" (Ph.D. diss., Orono, Maine, 1975); *DAB*, 4, pt. 1: 131-32; *NCAB*, 6: 316.

B. Lister

GARDEN, ALEXANDER (January 1730, Aberdeenshire, Scotland-April 15, 1791, London, England). *Physician; Naturalist.* Son of Rev. Alexander and Elizabeth (Nicholson) Garden. Married Elizabeth Perronneau, 1755; three surviving children. EDUCATION: 1743-46, studied at the University of Aberdeen, while apprentice to Dr. James Gordon, professor of medicine, who also helped cultivate Garden's botanical interest; 1750, University of Edinburgh; 1751, qualified to graduate from the University of Aberdeen, but did not have the fee until 1754. CAREER: 1748-50, naval surgeon; 1752, arrived in Charlestown, S.C., and began practice with Dr. William Rose; 1754, due to ill health, traveled to New York, N.Y., and Philadelphia, Pa.; returned to S.C. to practice with Dr. David Olyphant (q.v.), who then moved, leaving him a busy practice; 1782, banished as a Loyalist and property confiscated; 1783, moved to England. CONTRIBUTIONS: Experimented with smallpox vaccine, promoted the use of pinkroot as a drug, and treated routine illnesses and fevers of S.C. Studied and collected natural science specimens, which he sent to friends in New York City, Philadelphia, and overseas. Many biological species carry his name: the gardenia that Ellis and Linnaeus named in his honor is the best known.

WRITINGS: *An Account of the Medical Properties of the Virginia Pink-Root* (1756, 1764); *The Effects of the Ashes of Tobacco in the Cure of Dropsy* (1784). REFERENCES: Edmund Berkeley, *Dr. Alexander Garden of Charlestown* (1969); *DAB*, 4, pt. 1: 132-33; P. G. Jenkins, "Alexander Garden, Colonial Physician and Naturalist," *Annals of Med. Hist.* 10 (1928): 149-58; Miller, *BHM*, p. 39; *NCAB*, 23: 361; J. I. Waring, *History of Medicine in S.C., 1670-1825* (1964).

J. P. Dolan

GARDINER, CHARLES FOX (October 12, 1857, New York, N.Y.-July 31, 1947, Colorado Springs, Colo.). *Physician.* Son of James Madison and Mary Louise (Sprague) Gardiner. Married Daisy Monteith, 1884 (d. 1893), two children; Fanny Anderson, 1897. EDUCATION: 1882, M.D., Bellevue Medical College; interned at Charity Hospital, N.Y.; surgeon, prison on Blackwell's Island. CAREER: Mid-1880s, moved to Colo.; practiced medicine among the Indians, trappers, miners, and cowboys at Crested Butte, a mining camp at 9,000 feet elevation, and at Meeker, a new settlement on the White River; 1895, moved to Colorado Springs. CONTRIBUTIONS: Did much to popularize the climatic therapy of tuberculosis. Developed his "Gardiner tent," conical and open at the top like a tepee, to provide continuous fresh air for the invalid. On the first medical staff, Glockner Sanatorium (1905), and vice-president, American Climatological Association (1908).

WRITINGS: *Doctor at Timberline* (1938); *The Care of the Consumptive* (1900). REFERENCES: Lee W. Bortree, *Trans., Clinical and Climatological Assoc.* 59: (1948): 51-52; *N.Y. Times*, Aug. 1, 1947.

F. B. Rogers

GARDNER, LEROY UPSON (December 9, 1888, New Britain, Conn.-October 24, 1946, Saranac Lake, N.Y.). *Physician; Pathology; Industrial medicine.* Son of Irving Isaac, real estate and insurance broker, and Inez Baldwin (Upson) Gardner. Married Carabelle McKenzie, 1915; two children. EDUCATION: Yale University: 1912, B.A.; and 1914, M.D.; 1914-17, intern and postgraduate study, Boston City Hospital and Harvard Medical School. CAREER: 1917, pathology faculty, Yale Medical School; 1917-18, U.S. Army Medical Corps; discharged from duty when it was discovered he had tuberculosis; 1918-38, research pathologist, 1938-46, director, Edward L. Trudeau Foundation, Saranac Lake, N.Y.; at Saranac Laboratory for Tuberculosis: *post* 1927, director. CONTRIBUTIONS: Began an investigation of the role of mineral dusts in tuberculosis after learning that granite cutters had a much higher incidence of tuberculosis than marble cutters. In experiments using guinea pigs, demonstrated that the inhalation of granite dust injured the lungs and accelerated the progress of tuberculosis (1920); later showed that the silica particles in the dust could activate latent infections; led to the introduction and requirement of safety measures for the suppression of dust in mining and quarrying operations. Explored the basic histopathologic mechanisms involved in silicosis and devised ingenious research apparatus and methods for its study. Investigated the pathogenicity of a variety of mineral dusts. Charter member (1946), American Academy of Industrial Medicine. Helped edit *American Review of Tuberculosis* (1938 until death).

WRITINGS: ". . .The Relatively Early Lesions in Experimental Pneumokoniosis Produced by Granite Inhalation and Their Influence on Pulmonary Tuberculosis," *Am. Rev. of Tuberculosis* 4 (1920-21): 734-55; *Tuberculosis: Bacteriology, Pathology and Laboratory Diagnosis* (1927, with Edward R. Baldwin and S. A. Petroff); "Studies on Experimental Pneumonokoniosis; VI. Inhalation of Asbestos Dust: Its Effect upon Primary Tuberculous Infection," *J. of Industrial Hygiene* 13 (Feb. 1931): 65-81; 13 (Mar. 1931): 97-114 (with D. E. Cummings). REFERENCES: *DAB*, Supplement 4: 313-15; *N.Y. Times*, October 25, 1946; *Who Was Who in Am.*, 2: 204.

S. Galishoff

GARLAND, JOSEPH (January 1, 1893, Gloucester, Mass.-May 17, 1973, Chestnut Hill, Mass.). *Physician; Editor; Pediatrics.* Son of Joseph Everett, physician, and Sarah (Rogers) Garland. Married Mira Wellman Crowell, Massachusetts General Hospital nurse, 1921; two children. EDUCATION: 1915, A.B., Harvard College; 1919, M.D., Harvard Medical School; 1919-21, medical house officer, Massachusetts General Hospital. CAREER: 1921-48, pediatric practice; 1923-54, medical staff, Massachusetts General Hospital and Boston City Hospital; instructor in pediatrics, Harvard Medical School; 1922-47, associate editor and member, Editorial Board, *Boston Medical and Surgical Journal* (after 1928, *New England Journal of Medicine*); 1947-67, editor-in-chief, *New England Journal of Medicine*; 1927-29, 1968-71, editor, *Harvard Medical Alumni Bulletin*; 1967-70, president, Boston Medical Library; although he suffered from persistent patent ductus arteriosus, was never incapacitated by his own frail health. CONTRIBUTIONS: After a quarter century of successful pediatric practice combined with service on the Boston Medical Milk Commission and good citizenship in the medical community, assumed full-time responsibility for the *New England Journal of Medicine* (1947). The previous editor had established a national audience with 25,000 subscribers; in the next 20 years (1947-67), that number was quadrupled as regular communications and scientific contributions from at home and abroad were solicited. Benefiting from the support of a rigorous Editorial Board, Garland also faced controversy independently when he opened the debate on informed consent with the publication of H. K. Beecher's (q.v.) "Ethics in Clinical Research" (1966).

WRITINGS: "The Occurrence of Acetonuria in Childhood," *Arch. of Ped.* 36 (1919): 469; *The Youngest of the Family* (1932); *The Road to Adolescence* (1934). Best known for his intelligent use of the blue pencil on articles submitted to *New England J. of Med.* and his own 2,000 editorials. REFERENCES: *Harvard Med. Alumni Bull.* 48 (Sept.-Oct. 1973): 26-27; *New England J. of Med.* 289 (Sept. 20, 1973): 639-42; *Who Was Who in Am.*, 6: 153.

B. G. Rosenkrantz

GARRETSON, JAMES EDMUND (October 18, 1828, Wilmington, Del.-October 26, 1895, Lansdowne, Pa.). *Dentist; Oral surgery*. Son of Jacob M. and Mary A. (Powell) Garretson. Married Beulah Craft, 1859; two children. EDUCATION: 1856, graduated from the Philadelphia College of Dental Surgery; 1859, M.D., University of Pennsylvania. CAREER: Practiced dentistry in Woodbury, N.J.; 1854-64, served as demonstrator and as faculty member, Philadelphia School of Anatomy; *post* 1856, practiced dentistry in Philadelphia; Civil War, military hospital service; *post* 1869, oral surgeon, Hospital of the University of Pennsylvania; Philadelphia Dental College, anatomy and surgery faculty (*post* 1878) dean (1880); clinical surgery faculty, Medico-Chirurgical College of Philadelphia; under the pseudonym of John Darby, wrote several works dealing with philosophical and metaphysical issues. CONTRIBUTIONS: Founded and developed oral surgery as a specialty of dentistry; outstanding feature of his technique was to avoid possible external incisions and consequent scarring of the face; performed extensive operations confined entirely to the interior of the mouth including the removal of the entire superior maxilla. Introduced into oral surgery the modified dental engine for surgical operations.

WRITINGS: *A System of Oral Surgery*, which went through six editions from 1869 to 1895 and was the standard work in its field. REFERENCES: *DAB*, 7: 161-62; Harold L. Faggart, "Dr. James E. Garretson and the First Hospital for Oral Surgery," *Bull. Hist. Med.* 17 (1945): 360-76; Kelly and Burrage (1928), 454-55; *NCAB*, 3: 212-13; *Who Was Who in Am.*, Hist. Vol.: 268.

S. Galishoff

GARRISON, CHARLES WILLIS (July 15, 1879, Bastrop, Tex.-August 26, 1935, Lexington, Ky.). *Physician; Public Health*. Son of Samuel Harvey, farmer, and Hannah (Bogar) Garrison. Married Vinnie A. Middleton, 1906; two adopted children. EDUCATION: Abilene, Tex., public high school; Simmons College; 1903, University of Texas Medical School; 1905, M.D., Memphis Hospital Medical College. CAREER: Private practice: 1905-8, Tuscola, Tex.; and 1908-11, Fort Smith, Ark.; 1911-14, field director, Rockefeller Commission for the Eradication of Hookworm Disease; 1914-33, State Health Officer, Ark.; 1913-18, 1922-31, professor of preventive medicine, University of Arkansas medical department; 1917-18, acting assistant surgeon, U.S. Public Health Service; 1918-23, surgeon, U.S. Public Health Service Reserve; 1934, city health officer, Lexington, Ky., until ill health forced him to retire. CONTRIBUTIONS: Supervised the establishment of county health units in Ark. (1914-17). Policed health and sanitary measures around Camp Pike, near Little Rock (1917-18); established Venereal Control Division of State Health Department; conducted venereal disease control conferences on West Coast for U.S. Public Health Service (1922). Developed a program of public health work in flooded Ark. areas, including malarial control, with funds from the federal government and the Rockefeller Foundation (1923-24). Chosen by Rockefeller Foundation, because of accomplishments with Foundation grants, to be one of two state health officers to represent the United States at the Copenhagen International Health Conference (1924). Established a Child Health Division in State Health Department to administer benefits under the Sheppard-Towner program (1920s). REFERENCES: Auxiliary to Sebastian County Medical Society, *Physicians and Medicine: Crawford and Sebastian Counties* (1977), 304-6; Dallas T. Herndon, *Centennial History of Arkansas* 2 (1922) 1025.

D. Konold

GARRISON, FIELDING HUDSON (November 5, 1870, Washington, D.C.-April 18, 1935, Baltimore, Md.). *Medical historian; Bibliographer; Librarian*. Son of John Rowzee II, comptroller, and Jennie (Davis) Garrison. Married Clara Augusta Brown, 1910; three daughters. EDUCATION: 1886, Washington Central High School; 1890, A.B., Johns Hopkins University; 1893, M.D., Georgetown University. CAREER: At Army Medical Library: 1891-99, clerk; 1899-1912, assistant librarian; and 1912-17, principal assistant librarian; in Officers Reserve

Corps: 1917-18, major; 1918-20, lieutenant colonel; and 1920-30, colonel, Medical Corps; 1930-35, librarian, William H. Welch Medical Library, Johns Hopkins University. CONTRIBUTIONS: After developing intensive bibliographical and historical expertise in compiling the *Index-Catalogue of the Library of the Surgeon General's Office* and editing *Index Medicus*, wrote the first comprehensive American treatise on the history of medicine. Prepared plans and collected material for the history of the U.S. Medical Department in World War I. Performed detailed, invaluable reference services in the Army Medical Library. Wrote countless articles and reviews instructing and encouraging medico-historical activity in the United States.

WRITINGS: *Introduction to the History of Medicine* (1913; 4th ed., 1929); *John Shaw Billings, a Memoir* (1915); *Notes on the History of Military Medicine* (1922); *The Principles of Anatomic Illustration Before Vesalius* (1926); *Contributions to the History of Medicine from the Bulletin of the New York Academy of Medicine, 1925-1935* (1966). Writings listed in Claudius Frank Mayer, "The Literary Activity of Fielding H. Garrison, M.D., with an Annotated Bibliography of His Publications Related to Medicine," *Bull. Inst. Hist. Med.* 5 (1937): 378-403. REFERENCES: *BHM* (1964-69), 101; (1970-74), 70; (1975-79), 50; *DAB*, Supplement 1: 334-35; "Fielding H. Garrison Memorial Number," *Bull. Inst. Hist. Med.* 5 (1937): 299-403; Solomon R. Kagan, *Fielding H. Garrison, a Biography* (1948); Miller, *BHM*, p. 40; *NCAB*, 26: 51.

G. Miller

GARVIN, CHARLES HERBERT (October 27, 1890, Jacksonville, Fla.-July 17, 1968, Cleveland, Ohio). *Urology*. Son of Charles Edward, mailman, and Theresa (De Courcey) Garvin. Married Rosalind West, 1920; two children. EDUCATION: Howard University: 1911, A.B., and 1915, M.D.; 1915-16, internship, Freedmen's Hospital, Washington, D.C. CAREER: 1916, visiting assistant surgeon, Freedmen's Hospital; 1916-17; 1919-68, private practice, Cleveland; 1917-19, Army Medical Corps (served 11 months in France); 1920-56, staff urologist, Lakeside Hospital, Cleveland; 1920-56, urology faculty member, Western Reserve University Medical School. CONTRIBUTIONS: First black to receive commission in army in World War I (1917, first lieutenant in Medical Corps); first black to study at Army Medical School in Washington, D.C. At a time when Cleveland's black physicians and surgeons could get no hospital privileges or appointments and had to do surgery in homes, obtained first appointment of a black to a Cleveland hospital, Lakeside Hospital (1920), after impressing Dr. George W. Crile (q.v.) and his associates with his surgical knowledge. After he and his family moved into a new house in a "white" section of Cleveland (1927), it was twice bombed. The Garvins remained in that house for 40 years. Served the black community of Cleveland from his downtown office. Involved in black business and community affairs, as well as NAACP (one of earliest life members). Compiled an "Index Medicus of Negro Authors, 1924-34" and wrote 17 clinical papers in urology and 7 on the Negro in medicine. Contributing editor (1943-49) and member, Editorial Board, (1950-68) of the *Journal of the National Medical Association (JNMA)*. Contributed at least one item to every issue of *JNMA* from 1950 until his death. Served as alumni trustee and then as regular member of Howard's Board of Trustees (1931-64). WRITINGS: Twenty-six publications, including "Chronic Prostatitis," *Ohio State Med. J.* 24 (1928): 618-23; "The Negro Physicians and Hospitals of Cleveland," *JNMA* 22 (1930): 711-44; "Index Medicus of Negro Authors," *ibid.*, 27 (1935): 146-53; 28 (1936): 91; "Immunity to Disease Among Dark Skinned Peoples," *Opportunity* (Aug. 1926). Writings listed in *JNMA* 61 (1969): 89. REFERENCES: W. Montague Cobb, "Charles Herbert Garvin, 1889-1968," *JNMA* 61 (1969): 85-89; Charles H. Garvin, "Desmoid Tumor: A Tumor That Shaped a Career," *JNMA* 56 (1964): 209-10; "Men of the Month," *The Crisis* 19 (1920): 334; *NCAB*, 55: 8-9; *WWICA* 7 (1950): 204. His private papers are at Western Reserve Historical Society, Cleveland, Ohio.

T. Savitt

GARY, THOMAS PORTER (April 10, 1835, Cokesbury, Abbeville District, S.C.-June 10, 1891, Ocala, Fla.). *Physician; Surgeon; Public Health.* Son of Thomas R., physician, and Mary (Porter) Gary. Married Tommie Ann Howell; two children. EDUCATION: Public school, Cokesbury; studied medicine under preceptorate of his brother, Dr. Frank Gary, S.C.; 1855-56, student, Jefferson Medical College, Philadelphia, Pa.; 1857, M.D., Medical College of South Carolina, Charleston, S.C. CAREER: 1858-62, practice, Brooksville, Fla. (Feb.-Jul. 1859, partner of Dr. John P. Wall [q.v.]); 1862, volunteered for Confederate Army service; commissioned surgeon, 7th Florida Infantry Regiment; field service with Gen. Braxton Bragg's Army, Tenn. campaigns; 1865-67, practice, Brooksville; 1867-91, practice, Ocala; eight times mayor of Ocala. CONTRIBUTIONS: Having studied at Jefferson under Joseph Pancoast (q.v.), became a distinguished surgeon, considered to be the foremost in central Fla. Paramount interest was public health. As mayor of Ocala, established the city Board of Health. Later organized the South Florida Board of Health. Elected to membership in Florida Medical Association (1887), two days later becoming chairman, Committee on Medicine. Provided strong support for establishing the Florida State Board of Health, having co-authored the bill that the state legislature passed (1889). President, Florida Medical Association (1889); reelected for second term. Incumbent at time of his death.

WRITINGS: "The Selection of Medicines," *Proc., Fla. Med. Assoc.* (1890): 51-58; "Malarial Haematuria" (Paper read, annual meeting, Florida Medical Association, 1889), *ibid.* (1889), p. 25. REFERENCES: *Banner* (Ocala), June 12, 1891; *New Capitol* (Ocala), June 10, 1891; *Proc., Fla. Med. Assoc.* (1887-92), especially report of Necrology Committee, 1892; Bradford T. Williams, "Dr. Thomas P. Gary, Florida's Frontier Physician, 1835-91," *J. Fla. Med. Assoc.* 65 (Aug.1978): 644-47; *Boston Med. and Surg. J.* 124 (1891): 618; Personal Papers preserved in Medical History Collection, J. Hillis Miller Health Center Library, University of Florida, Gainesville, Fla.

E. A. Hammond

GASSER, HERBERT SPENCER (July 5, 1888, Platteville, Wis.-May 11, 1963, New York, N.Y.). *Physiologist; Neurophysiology.* Son of Herman, physician, and Jane Elizabeth (Griswold) Gasser. Never married. EDUCATION: University of Wisconsin: 1910, A.B.; and 1911, A.M.; 1915, M.D., Johns Hopkins Medical School. CAREER: Pharmacology and physiology faculties: 1911-16, University of Wisconsin; and 1916-31, Washington University; 1918, pharmacologist, Chemical Warfare Service; 1931-35, physiology faculty, Cornell University Medical College; 1935-53, director, Rockefeller Institute for Medical Research. CONTRIBUTIONS: Built an electronic amplifier attached to a string galvanometer for use in electrophysiology (1921); instrument revealed the value of electronic amplification in studying the transmission of nerve impulses through muscles; its full research potential was realized during the following years when Gasser and his mentor, Joseph Erlanger (q.v.), developed the cathode-ray oscillograph. Two men made many important discoveries together for which they were awarded the 1944 Nobel Prize in medicine and physiology. Showed that impulse-conduction velocity varies with the thickness of the fiber, being more rapid for thicker fibers. Demonstrated the existence of three main types of nerve fibers: myelinated sensory and motor nerve fibers, myelinated autonomic nerve fibers, and nonmyelinated fibers. Elucidated the essential differences between sensory and motor nerves and demonstrated the mechanism of pain and reflex action. Other subjects that attracted Gasser's attention included the functions of the various afferent fibers, the morphology of unmyelinated nerve fibers (research on which was done with the aid of an electron microscope), and the excitability of nerve fibers in relation to after-potentials.

WRITINGS: "Physiological Action Currents in the Phrenic Nerve. An Application of the Thermionic Vacuum Tube to Nerve Physiology," *Am. J. of Physiol.* 57 (1921): 1-26 (with H. S. Newcomer); *Electrical Signs of Nervous Activity* (1937, with J. Erlanger). A bibliography is in *BMFRS.* Two other bibliographies are cited in *DSB.* REFERENCES: *BHM* (1964-69), 102; *BMFRS* 10 (1964): 75-82; *DAB*, Supp. 7: 279-81; *DSB*, 5: 290-91; *McGraw-Hill Modern Men of Sci.* 1 (1966): 186-87; *NCAB*, 61: 243; *Who Was Who in Am.*, 4: 348.

S. Galishoff

GATES, FREDERICK TAYLOR (July 2, 1853, Maine, N.Y.-February 6, 1929, Phoenix, Ariz.). *Baptist clergyman; Business and philanthropic executive.* Son of Granville, Baptist minister, and Sarah Jane (Bowers) Gates. Married Lucia F. Perkins, 1882; Emma Lucile Cahoon, 1886, seven children. EDUCATION: University of Rochester: 1877, A.B.; and 1879, A.M.; 1880, graduated from Rochester Theological Seminary. CAREER: 1880-88, pastor, Central Church, Minneapolis, Minn.; 1888-93, corresponding secretary, American Baptist Education Society; 1893-1912, business and benevolent representative of John D. Rockefeller; 1901-29, president, Board of Trustees, Rockefeller Institute for Medical Research; 1905-12, chairman, General Education Board; 1907-17, director, Rockefeller Foundation. CONTRIBUTIONS: Planned and organized Rockefeller's philanthropies and thereby played a major role in the promotion of medical education and research in the first half of the twentieth century. Asked by

Rockefeller to help him put his vast wealth to good use; decided that in light of the inability of physicians to cure most illnesses, encouragement of medical science should take priority; led to the establishment of the Rockefeller Institute for Medical Research (1901). Combatted the commercialization of medical education and the consequent lowering of medical standards by getting the General Education Board to make large grants to the better schools on the condition that they use the money to upgrade their institutions; money was instrumental in enabling medical schools to make the reforms proposed in the Flexner Report of 1910. Developed the principles and policies that led to the establishment of the Rockefeller Foundation.

WRITINGS: "The Memoirs of Frederick T. Gates," with an Introduction by Allan Nevins, *Am. Heritage*, n.s., 6, no. 3 (Apr. 1955): 65-86. REFERENCES: George Washington Corner, *A History of the Rockefeller Institute, 1901-1953* (1964); *DAB*, 7: 182-83; Raymond B. Fosdick, *Adventures in Giving: The Story of the General Education Board* . . .(1962); *NCAB*, 23: 250-51; *Who Was Who in Am.*, 1: 444.

S. Galishoff

GATHINGS, JOSEPH GOUVERNEUR (July 11, 1898, Richmond, Tex.-June 28, 1965, Washington, D.C.). *Physician; Dermatology; Syphilology*. Married Elizabeth Parr, 1924; one child. EDUCATION: c.1924, A.B.(?), Howard University; 1924-25, Meharry Medical College; 1925-28, M.D., Howard University; 1928-29, internship, Freedmen's Hospital, Washington, D.C.; 1941-43, Rosenwald Fellow in Dermatology and Syphilology, New York Skin and Cancer Hospital. CAREER: 1929-41, private practice, general medicine, Houston, Tex.; private practice, dermatology and syphilology: 1944-46, Houston; and 1946-65, Washington, D.C.; 1944-46, clinical assistant, dermatology and syphilology, Baylor University Medical Center; 1944-46, in charge of venereal disease clinics for Houston Health Department; 1946-65, clinical faculty, dermatology and syphilology, Howard University Medical College. CONTRIBUTIONS: In addition to practice and teaching in dermatology and syphilology, was deeply involved in NMA activities; board member (1941-49; chair, 1947-49), first vice-president (1949-50), president (1951-52). Involved in many activities of black medical societies in Houston and Washington, D.C., and as a guest lecturer and clinician at black medical societies and meetings around the country. Supported and fostered growth of NMA and its *Journal*. REFERENCES: W. Montague Cobb, "Joseph Gouverneur Gathings, M.D., 1898-1965," *JNMA* 57 (1965): 427-28.

T. Savitt

GAY, FREDERICK PARKER (July 22, 1874, Boston, Mass.-July 14, 1939, New Hartford, Conn.). *Physician; Pathology; Microbiology; Immunology*. Son of George Frederick, businessman, and Louisa Maria (Parker) Gay. Married Catherine Mills Jones, 1904; four children. EDUCATION: 1897, A.B., Harvard University; 1899, assistant, Johns Hopkins Medical Commission to the Philippines; 1901, M.D., Johns Hopkins University; 1901-3, fellow, Rockefeller Institute for Medical Research; and assistant demonstrator in pathology, University of Pennsylvania; 1903-6, studied under Jules Bordet, Pasteur Institute, Brussels. CAREER: 1906-7, bacteriological staff, Danvers (Mass.) State Hospital for the Insane; 1907-10, pathology faculty, Harvard Medical School; at University of California, Berkeley: 1910-21, pathology faculty; and 1921-23, bacteriology faculty; 1918-19, Medical Corps, U.S. Army; assigned to the Yale Army Laboratory School; at National Research Council: 1917-24, member, medical section; 1922-23, chairman, and 1922-26, chairman, Medical Fellowship Board; 1926-27, exchange professor, Belgian universities; *post* 1929, bacteriology faculty, College of Physicians and Surgeons (Columbia). CONTRIBUTIONS: Made numerous and diverse contributions in the emerging fields of bacteriology and immunology. Under the influence of Jules Bordet, studied serum reactions accompanying infection and immunity, particularly conglutination and the complement fixation reaction (1905-10); undertook prolonged studies of tissue immunity and the possibility of inducing antibody formation by the use of antigens. As a bacteriologist, investigated the carrier state in typhoid fever (1913-19), the pathogenesis and chemotherapy of hemolytic streptococcus infections (1919-39), and viral diseases, especially the herpetic and encephalitic (1929-39). Published the first English translation (1909) of the classic *Studies in Immunology* by Bordet and his collaborators. Published *Agents of Disease and Host Resistance* (1935), the best work on that subject in its time.

WRITINGS: "The Value of the Conglutination Reaction as a Means of Diagnosis of Acute Bacterial Infections," *Proc., Soc. Exp. Biol. Med.* 7 (1910, with William P. Lucas): 21-24; *Typhoid Fever* (1918); "The Functions of the Tissues in Immunity," *Trans., Assoc. of Am. Physicians* 41 (1926): 262-67; "The Herpes Encephalitis Problem, II.," *J. of Infectious Diseases* 53 (1933): 287-303; *The Open Mind: Elmer Ernest Southard, 1876-1920* (1937). A bibliography is in *BMNAS*. REFERENCES: *BMNAS* 28 (1954): 99-116; *DAB*, Supplement 2: 224-26; *DSB*, 5: 316-17; *NCAB*, B: 268; *N.Y. Times*, July 15, 1929.

S. Galishoff

GEDDINGS, ELI (1799, Newberry District, S.C.-October 9, 1878, Charleston, S.C.). *Physician.* Married Mrs. (Wyatt) Grey, four children; Laura Postal. EDUCATION: 1818-20, studied medicine, Abbeville Academy, under Drs. Miller and Arnold; 1820, graduated from the Medical College of South Carolina and received license from the "Examining Board," Medical Society of South Carolina. CAREER: 1820, practice, St. George's Parish, Colleton, S.C.; 1821, practice, Abbeville, with Dr. E. S. Davis; winter of 1821-22, practiced medicine, Calhoun settlement, Abbeville District; 1825, voluntarily discharged duties of demonstrator, Medical College of South Carolina; 1826, visited the hospitals of Paris and London; 1827, returned to Charleston to practice and resumed position as demonstrator of anatomy until he opened the Charleston Academy of Medicine, a successful private school; 1833, edited *Baltimore Medical and Surgical Journal*; 1831-37, chairman of anatomy and physiology, University of Maryland;

1837, returned to Charleston to accept the new chair of pathological anatomy and medical jurisprudence, Medical College, until he was elected to the chair of surgery; 1847-50, filled Dr. Samuel Henry Dickson's (q.v.) position as professor of the practice of medicine, resuming the chair of surgery upon Dr. Dickson's return; gave lectures in his private library and conducted a course at the Alms House Hospital in the new-to-Charleston practice of auscultation; 1858, resigned his professorship but upon Dr. P. C. Gaillard's unexpected death, filled Gaillard's position as professor of practice, Medical College; the Civil War destroyed Dr. Geddings's livelihood, as well as his prized library, forcing him to return to practice; served on an Army Medical Board of the Confederacy; 1871, elected emeritus professor of the institute and practice of medicine; accepted a newly created chair of clinical medicine, which he held until 1873; after retirement, continued to give occasional lectures and consultations.

WRITINGS: Contributed many papers to the *Am. J. of Med. Sci.* While chairman of the committee on medical education, American Medical Association, wrote the first report of recommendations for improving educational facilities (1870). REFERENCES: *Appleton's CAB* 2 (1900); "Biographical Sketch of Eli Geddings, M.D.," *Charleston Med. J. and Rev.* 12 (1857); Eli Geddings, *Introductory Lecture of the Medical College of the State of S.C.* (1838); *In Memoriam, Eli Geddings. . .* (1878); Kelly and Burrage (1920), 431; *News and Courier*, Centennial (1903); *S.C. Gazette and Columbia Advertiser*, September 27, 1828; Joseph I. Waring, *History of Medicine in South Carolina, 1825-1900* (1967), 235-38.

J. P. Dolan

GERHARD, WILLIAM WOOD (July 23, 1809, Philadelphia, Pa.-April 28, 1872, Philadelphia). *Physician.* Son of William and Sarah (Wood) Gerhard. Married the daughter of Major William A. Dobbyn, 1850; three children. EDUCATION: 1826, A.B., Dickinson College; apprenticed to Dr. Joseph Parrish (q.v.), Philadelphia; 1828-31, resident pupil, Philadelphia Almhouse infirmary; 1830, M.D., University of Pennsylvania; 1831-33, postgraduate study, principally in Paris under Pierre Louis, but also in Great Britain. CAREER: 1834-35, resident physician, Pennsylvania Hospital; 1835-45, attending physician, Philadelphia Hospital; 1838-45, assistant professor (clinical medicine), University of Pennsylvania; 1838-42, editor, *Medical Examiner* (Philadelphia); 1845-68, visiting physician, Pennsylvania Hospital. CONTRIBUTIONS: Greatest contribution to medical science was distinction (1836) between typhoid and typhus fevers. Also reported important clinical-pathological observations on cholera (1832), smallpox and rubella (1833), and pneumonia and meningitis (1834) based on his Paris experience at L'Hopital des Enfants Malades. Nevertheless, such contributions pale beside role in clinical teaching at Philadelphia. Clinical lectures were well attended. Introduced many students to the new methods of clinical-pathological-anatomical correlation as practiced in Paris. Achieved great fame in physical diagnosis and his monograph *Diseases of the Chest* (1842) was particularly influential. While editor, *Medical Examiner*, regularly published his clinical lectures in that journal and collected and appended them (1842) to his edition of Robert Graves' *Clinical Lectures*. A founder and first president (1838), Pathological Society of Philadelphia, which was patterned on the Paris experience of the Societé Médicale d'Observation, of which Gerhard was also a founding member. Suffered a mysterious illness (1843) that left his health permanently impaired, and although he continued to practice and did some limited teaching, original research stopped, and Pathological Society ceased meeting until 1857 when it was reorganized.

WRITINGS: "On the Typhus Fever Which Occurred at Philadelphia in the Spring and Summer of 1836. . . ," *Am. J. of Med. Sci.* 19 (1837): 289-322; 20: 289-322; "Clinical Lectures," in Robert Graves, *A System of Clinical Medicine, with Notes and a Series of Lectures of W. W. Gerhard*, 2nd Am. ed. (1842), 479-557; *Lectures on the Diagnosis, Pathology, and Treatment of the Diseases of the Chest* (1842). Gerhard's early papers are listed by Joseph Garland. REFERENCES: *DAB*, 4, pt. 1: 218-19; Joseph Garland, "William Wood Gerhard (1809-72)," *New England J. of Med.* 273 (1965): 280; W. S. Middleton, "William Wood Gerhard," *Annals of Med. Hist.* 6 (1934): 1-18; *NCAB*, 23: 340; William Osler, "The Influence of Louis on American Medicine," in W. Osler, *An Alabama Student and Other Essays* (1908), 189-210; F. B. Rogers, "William Wood Gerhard: Pioneer in Nosography," in J. Dickinson, ed., *Early Dickinsoniana: The Boyd Lee Spahr Lectures in Americana, 1957-61* (1961), 237-51; Thomas Stewardson, "William Wood Gerhard," *Trans., Coll. of Physicians of Phila.* 4 (1874): 473-81.

D. C. Smith

GERRISH, FREDERIC HENRY (March 21, 1845, Portland, Maine-September 8, 1920, Portland). *Surgeon*. Son of Oliver, jeweler, and Sarah (Little) Gerrish. Married Emily Manning Swan, 1879; no children. EDUCATION: 1866, A.B., Bowdoin College; 1869, A.M. and M.D., Bowdoin Medical School. CAREER: 1873-75, lecturer on therapeutics and materia medica, medical faculty, University of Michigan; 1873-82, at Bowdoin Medical School: professor of therapeutics; 1882-1904, professor of anatomy; 1904-11, professor of surgery; and 1911-15, lecturer on medical ethics and emeritus professor of surgery; director and consulting surgeon, Maine General Hospital. CONTRIBUTIONS: One of the first surgeons to adopt and apply the Lister system of antiseptic surgery. A leader in the movement to establish a Public Health Service in Maine. President of several state and national professional associations and wrote and presented many papers.

WRITINGS: "Cases Treated by the Lister Method" (Presented before the Portland Clinical Society, September 1880); Championiere's *Antiseptic Surgery* (1881, translator and editor); "The Best Equipment for Medical Study" (Presented before the American Academy of Medicine, October 1886); "Best Order of Topics in a Two-Year Course of Anatomy in a Medical School," *Sci.* (Mar. 1895); "A Criticism of the Report of the Carnegie Foundation on Medical Education" (Presented to the Medical Club of Portland, November 10, 1910). A prolific writer who had many articles published in the *Transactions of the Maine Medical Association.* REFERENCES: *DAB*, 4, pt. 1: 221-22; *J. of the Maine Med. Assoc.* 11, no. 8 (1921): 263-64; Maine Historical Society Collection #85, Records of the Portland School for Medical Instruction, 1871-1904; Maine Historical Society

Collection #513, Maine Physicians compiled by James Spalding; Maine Historical So-
ciety, Portland Obituary Scrapbook, Vol 3, 133; *NCAB*, 12: 233; Walter Tobie, "Three
Outstanding Individualists" (Presented as the annual oration of the Portland Medical
Club, December 1, 1936).

B. Lister

GESELL, ARNOLD LUCIUS   (June 21, 1880, Alma, Wisconsin-May 29,
1961, New Haven, Connecticut). *Physician; Pediatrics; Mental health; Special
education.* Son of Gerhard, photographer. and Christine (Giesen) Gesell, schoolteacher. Married Beatrice Chandler, 1909; two children. EDUCATION: Graduated
c. 1896 from Stevens Point (Wis.) Normal School; 1915, M.D., Yale University;
1903, B.Ph. (education), University of Wisconsin; 1906, Ph.D. (psychology),
Clark University. CAREER: 1899-1909, teacher, Stevens Point High School, Chip-
pewa Falls (Wis.) High School, state normal schools in Platteville, Wis., and
Los Angeles, Calif.; 1909-15, assistant professor of education, Yale; 1911-15
(summers), instructor of teachers of defective children, New York University;
1911-48, director, Yale Clinic for Child Development; 1915-48, professor of
child hygiene, Yale Medical School; 1915-19, child psychologist, Connecticut
State Board of Education; 1928-48, attending pediatrician, New Haven Hospital;
1950-58, research consultant, Gesell Institute of Child Development. CONTRI-
BUTIONS: Through the use of psychological testing innovations and one-way
window observation and photography, pioneered understanding of child development. Ascertained standards of and deviations from normal mental and physical growth of children. Developed concepts, tests, and child-rearing systems
which influenced the direction of childhood education thinking. Established child
development as a legitimate aspect of pediatrics, child psychiatry, and child
neurology.

WRITINGS: Numerous books and articles. *The First Five Years of Life* (1940); *Devel-
opmental Diagnosis* (1941); *Infant and Child in the Culture of Today* (1943); *The Child
From Five to Ten* (1946). Writings listed in Miles (see below). REFERENCES: *DAB*,
Supplement 7: 283-85; *DSB*, 5: 377-78; Walter R. Miles, "Arnold Lucius Gesell,"
BMNAS, 37 (1964): 55-96; *NCAB*, 49: 119-20.

T. L. Savitt

GIBBON, JOHN HEYSHAM, JR.   (September 29, 1903, Philadelphia, Pa.-
February 5, 1973, Philadelphia). *Physician; Cardiology.* Son of John Heysham,
physician, and Marjorie (Young) Gibbon. Married Mary Hopkinson, 1931; four
children. EDUCATION: 1923, A.B., Princeton University; 1927, M.D., Jefferson
Medical College (Philadelphia); 1927-29, intern, Pennsylvania Hospital. CAREER:
1930-31, 1933-34, fellow in surgery, Harvard Medical School; 1936-42, fellow
in surgical research, University of Pennsylvania; 1943-45, Medical Corps, U.S.
Army; 1945-67, surgery faculty, Jefferson Medical College; 1950-73, consulting
surgeon, Pennsylvania Hospital; consultant, numerous governmental, educational, and service organizations; president: American Surgical Association,

American Association of Thoracic Surgery, Society for Clinical Surgery, and Society for Vascular Surgery. CONTRIBUTIONS: Devised an extracorporeal heart-lung machine for use in vascular surgery (1953); machine consisted of an artificial lung with a pump of sufficient capacity to oxygenate the blood while the patient's heart was completely bypassed; paved the way for open-heart surgery including procedures for correction of congenital heart defects, repair of heart valves, coronary bypass, and heart transplant.

WRITINGS: "An Oxygenator with a Large Surface-Volume Ratio," *J. Lab. and Clin. Med.* 24 (1939): 1192-98; "Application of a Mechanical Heart and Lung Apparatus to Cardiac Surgery," *Minnesota Med.* 37 (1954): 171-80, 185. REFERENCES: James Bordley and A. McGehee Harvey, *Two Centuries of Am. Med.* (1976), 508-9; *N.Y. Times*, February 6, 1973; *Who Was Who in Am.*, 5: 268.

S. Galishoff

GIBBONS, HENRY (September 20, 1808, Wilmington, Del.-November 4, 1884, Wilmington). *Physician.* Son of William, physician, and Rebecca (Donaldson) Gibbons. Married Martha Poole, 1833; four children. EDUCATION: 1829, M.D., University of Pennsylvania. CAREER: 1829-41, practice, Wilmington; 1841-50, practice, Philadelphia, Pa., and faculty member, College of Medicine, Philadelphia; 1850-84, practice, San Francisco, Calif.; 1862, professor of materia medica and therapeutics, the medical department, University of the Pacific; 1864, moved to the Toland Medical College as professor of materia medica; 1870, returned to the reorganized medical department, University of the Pacific, as professor of medicine and clinical medicine. CONTRIBUTIONS: An original member of both the State Board of Health (Calif.) (president, 1873-86) and the Board of Examiners. Represented Calif. at the International Medical Congress in Philadelphia (1876). Editor, *Pacific Medical and Surgical Journal*, 1865-84, and made it one of America's best medical journals. A founder of Female Medical College of Philadelphia; and California State Medical Society (president, 1857 and 1871). REFERENCES: Henry Harris, *California's Medical Story* (1932), 347-54; *NCAB*, 7: 287; *Who Was Who in Am.*, Hist. Vol.: 202.

Y. V. O'Neill

GIBSON, SAMUEL CARROLL (September 9, 1857, Steelville, Mo.-March 11, 1919, Reno, Nev.). *Physician; Public Health.* Son of Alexander, physician, and Haney C. (Halbert) Gibson. Married Mary E. Roycroft, 1882; four children. EDUCATION: Steelville Academy; Mo. School of Mines; 1879, M.D., Missouri Medical College (St. Louis, Mo.). CAREER: General practitioner: 1880-95, Alturlas, Calif.; and *post* 1895, Reno, Nev.; *post* 1900, chief surgeon, California, Nevada and Oregon Railroad. Active in local civic affairs. CONTRIBUTIONS:

Served Nev. as secretary (1896-99), and president (1899 to c.1914), State Board of Health, and as superintendent (1905-10), Nevada State Hospital. REFERENCE: *Who Was Who in Am.*, 4: 355.

J. Edwards

GIES, WILLIAM JOHN (February 21, 1872, Reisterstown, Md.-May 20, 1956, Lancaster, Pa.). *Biological chemist; Dentistry.* Son of John, Jr., and Ophelia Letitia (Ensminger) Gies. Married Mabel Loyetta Lark, 1899; four children. EDUCATION: Gettysburg College: 1893, B.S.; and 1896, M.S.; at Yale University: 1894, Ph.B.; and 1897, Ph.D.; 1899, studied at the University of Berne; 1901, 1902, studied at Marine Biological Laboratory, Woods Hole, Mass. CAREER: 1894-98, physiological chemistry faculty, Yale University; at Columbia University: 1898-1907, physiological chemistry faculty; 1907-37, biological chemistry faculty; and 1905-21, secretary, faculty of College of Physicians and Surgeons; 1904-22, physiological chemistry faculty, New York College of Pharmacy; 1909-28, physiological chemistry faculty, Teachers College (N.Y.); at New York Botanical Garden: 1902-21, consulting chemist; and 1911-28, member, Board of Scientific Directors; 1910-22, pathological chemistry staff, Bellevue Hospital; 1917-18, president, Annual Conference of Biological Chemists; 1916-17, chairman, Executive Committee, New York School of Dental Hygiene; 1917-21, secretary, administrative board, School of Dentistry, Columbia University; 1926-35, chairman, Dental Advisory Board, New York City Department of Health; 1921-31, in charge study of dental education for Carnegie Foundation; 1917-19, president, Society for Experimental Biology and Medicine; in International Association for Dental Research: 1939-40, president; and 1928-38, secretary; 1935-36, president, American Association of Dental Editors. CONTRIBUTIONS: In the twentieth century, led the movement to establish dentistry as a profession in the United States. Initiated the creation of Columbia University Dental School (1916). Organized the International Association of Dental Research and edited its organ *Journal of Dental Research* (1919-37). Conducted an intensive study (1920s) of American dental education, Carnegie Foundation for the Advancement of Teaching; report called attention to many weaknesses in dentistry and dental education and established an agenda for reform; led to the closing of proprietary dental schools and to the establishment of dentistry as another university branch of higher learning. Directed the negotiations that resulted in the merging of four separate dental education groups into one American Association of Dental Schools (1923). Authored textbooks in general chemistry, organic chemistry, and biological chemistry. At various times, edited *Proceedings of the Society for Experimental Biology and Medicine, Proceedings of the Society of Biological Chemists, Biochemical Bulletin, Chemical Abstracts, Journal of Dental Research*, and *Journal of the American College of Dentists*.

WRITINGS: *Biological Researches*, 8 vols. (1903-27); *Textbook of General Chemistry* (1904); *Textbook of Organic Chemistry* (1905); *Laboratory Work in Biological Chemistry* (1906); *Bulletin on Dental Education in the United States and Canada* (1926). REFER-

ENCES: N. Kobrin, "Builders of Modern Dentistry. William J. Gies—the Good Citizen," *Dental Outlook* 28 (1941): 315-18; Miller, *BHM*, p. 4l; Leuman M. Waugh, "Burkhart Memorial Scroll to William J. Gies. . .," *N.Y. Dental J.* 18 (1952): 330-36; *Who Was Who in Am.*, 3: 322.

S. Galishoff

GIFFORD, HAROLD (October 18, 1858, Milwaukee, Wis.-November 28, 1929, Omaha, Nebr.). *Physician; Ophthalmologist.* Son of Charles, horticulturist, and Mary Carolyn (Child) Gifford. Married Mary Louise Millard, December 30, 1890; four children, including Sanford R. (q.v.). EDUCATION: 1879, B.S., Cornell University; 1882, M.D., University of Michigan; postgraduate study, Erlangen and Heidelberg, Germany; Vienna, Austria; and Zurich, Switzerland. CAREER: At Omaha Medical College: 1890-98, lecturer in bacteriology; 1892-98, professor of clinical ophthalmology and otology; 1895-98, dean of the faculties; and 1898-1902, professor of ophthalmology and otology; at University of Nebraska College of Medicine: 1902-11, associate dean and professor of ophthalmology and otology; 1911-24, professor of ophthalmology and otology; 1919-25, chairman, Department of Ophthalmology; and 1925-29, professor emeritus of ophthalmology; 1897-1915, editor, *Ophthalmic Record*; 1907, president, Nebraska State Medical Society. CONTRIBUTIONS: Early research on sympathetic ophthalmia and drainage of the anterior chamber. First to note that organisms in normal conjunctival sac may become pathogenic when carried into the eye by trauma or operation. First to describe in English acute conjunctivitis caused by pneumococcus (1896). First English writer to describe involvement of the ocular conjunctiva with sporothrix. Described diagnostic eye symptoms in relation to exophthalmic goiter. Devised several modifications in ophthalmic surgery.

WRITINGS: "Sympathetic Ophthalmia," *Am. Encyclopedia of Ophthalmology* 16 (1913-21): 12369-417; "Congenital Defects of Abduction and Other Ocular Movements and Their Relation to Birth Injuries," *Am. J. of Ophthalmology* 9 (Jan. 1926): 3-22. Complete list of writings in University of Nebraska Medical Center Library of Medicine, Omaha. REFERENCES: *Arch. Ophthal.* 3, no. 2 (Feb. 1930): 217-22; archives, University of Nebraska Medical Center Library of Medicine, Omaha; *NCAB*, 22 (1932): 227; *Who Was Who in Am.*, 1: 452.

B. M. Hetzner

GIFFORD, SANFORD ROBINSON (January 8, 1892, Omaha, Nebr.-February 25, 1944, Chicago, Ill.). *Physician; Ophthalmology; Microbiology.* Son of Harold (q.v.), ophthalmic surgeon, and Mary Louise (Millard) Gifford. Married Mary Alice Carter, 1917; two children. EDUCATION: 1913, B.A., Cornell University; at University of Nebraska College of Medicine: 1918, M.D.; and 1924, M.A.; 1919, completed a two-year internship, Nebraska Lutheran Hospital; 1923-24, studied in the eye clinics and laboratories of Tubingen, Germany; and Vienna, Austria; and the Royal London Ophthalmic Hospital (Moorfields). CAREER: During World War I, in charge of the army's bacteriology laboratory in Base Hospital 49, Allery, France, and later in the army of occupation in Germany; 1919-29, practiced medicine with his father; and ophthalmology faculty, University of Nebraska College of Medicine; 1929-44, ophthalmology faculty, Northwestern University Medical School; ophthalmological staff: *post* 1930, Passavant Memorial; *post* 1941, Wesley; and *post* 1932, Cook County hospitals. CONTRIBUTIONS: Investigated ocular diseases produced by certain bacteria and fungi and did research in the biochemistry of the eye, particularly the crystalline lens. With James McDowell Patton, reported the probable etiologic agent of the hitherto unknown disease, agricultural conjunctivitis. Developed clinical and surgical procedures and studied ophthalmic problems associated with a general physical condition such as diabetes or vascular disease. Associate editor, *Archives of Ophthalmology* (*post* 1928); corresponding editor, *Klinische Monatsblätter für Augenheilbunde* (1928-40).

WRITINGS: "Agricultural Conjunctivitis," *Am. J. of Ophthalmology* 5 (Aug. 1922): 623-37 (with James M. Patton); "Iridencleisis with Water Tight Closure of the Conjunctiva," *Trans., Am. Acad. of Ophthal. & Otol.* (1927): 117-28; *A Handbook of Ocular Therapeutics* (1932); *A Textbook of Ophthalmology* (1938). REFERENCES: *DAB*, Supplement 3: 301-2; *NCAB*, 32: 457-58; *N. Y. Times*, February 26, 1944; *Who Was Who in Am.*, 2: 209-10.

S. Galishoff

GIHON, ALBERT LEARY (September 28, 1833, Philadelphia, Pa.-November 17, 1902, New York, N.Y.). *Physician; Naval medical officer.* Son of John Hancock, physician, and Mary J. Gihon. Married Clara M. Campbell, 1860; three children. EDUCATION: 1850, A.B., Central High School, Philadelphia; 1852, M.D., Philadelphia College of Medicine and Surgery; 1854, A.M., Princeton. CAREER: 1853-54, professor of chemistry and toxicology, Philadelphia College of Medicine and Surgery; 1855, entered navy as assistant surgeon; 1861, promoted to surgeon; served at sea on China station and in the Civil War on various ships as the surgeon; later stationed at the Bureau of Medicine and Surgery, commanded the hospital at the U.S. Naval Academy, and was fleet surgeon (1873) for the European Fleet; commanded naval hospitals, New York City and Washington, D.C.; president: American Academy of Medicine, American Public Health Association (APHA), and Association of Military Surgeons; 1895, became Commodore, retiring that year as senior medical officer of the navy after 40 years of active duty; in retirement, was the hospital director, Sailor's Harbor, on Staten Island, N.Y. CONTRIBUTIONS: Major contributions were in preventive medicine, public health, and vital statistics. Designed the hospital cot used by the navy of the period. Permanent navy medical delegate, American Public Health Association, and sponsored the project to build the Benjamin Rush (q.v.) statue erected in Washington. Contributed articles on naval medicine to various of the multivolume medical and surgical texts of the period and was well known as a lecturer at APHA, AMA, and other professional societies.

WRITINGS: *Practical Suggestions in Naval Hygiene* (1871). REFERENCES: *Boston Med. and Surg. J.* 145 (1901): 581; *Buffalo Med. J.* 41 (1901-2): 379-82; *DAB*, 4, pt. 1: 265-66; *JAMA* 37 (1901): 1403-4; *Med. Record* 70 (1901): 823; *NCAB*, 9: 154; R. P. Parsons, "History of the Medical Department of the United States Navy," in Francis R. Packard, *History of Medicine in the United States* 2 (1932): 659; Irving A. Watson, *Physicians and Surgeons of Am.* (1896).

R. J. T. Joy

GILES, ROSCOE CONKLING (May 6, 1890, Albany, N.Y.-February 19, 1970, Chicago, Ill.). *Surgeon*. Son of Francis Fenard, minister and attorney, and Laura (Caldwell) Giles. Married Frances Reeder; two children. EDUCATION: Cornell University: 1911, A.B.; and 1915, M.D.; 1915-17, intern, Provident Hospital, Chicago; 1930-31, postgraduate study in surgery, Vienna; 1933, postgraduate study in bone pathology and anatomy, University of Chicago. CAREER: 1917, passed examination for junior physician, Chicago Municipal Tuberculosis Sanitarium and Oak Park Infirmary, but was denied appointment on racial grounds; 1917, appointed a supervisor, Chicago Health Department; 1917-70, attending surgeon, Provident Hospital; honorary attending surgeon and then (1953) attending surgeon, Cook County Hospital; 1946-70, assistant professor of surgery, Chicago Medical School; 1942-45, Army Medical Corps, Chief of Medical Services, Hospital, Fort Huachuca, Ariz.; 1917-70, private surgical practice, Chicago. CONTRIBUTIONS: Served NMA and black medical profession as chair of NMA committee that succeeded in having the abbreviation "col." removed from the names of all black physicians listed in the AMA Directory (1938-40); president, NMA (1937); member, NMA Executive Board (1926-35). First black graduate, Cornell University Medical College (1915); first black diplomate, American Board of Surgery (1939); and first black attending surgeon, Cook County Hospital, Chicago. A key figure in NAACP campaign to open Bellevue Hospital in New York City to black interns (1915) and was involved in movements to open the military hospitals to black officers.

WRITINGS: Nine articles on surgery, including "A Report of Three Hundred and Forty-two Consecutive Cases of Appendicitis," *JNMA* 37 (1945): 177-80; "Anastomoses About the Terminal Ileum," *Am. J. of Surg.* 84 (1952): 473-75; "Chronic Duodenal Ileus," *ibid.*, 93 (1957): 824-28. Writings listed in *JNMA* 62 (1970): 256. REFERENCES: W. Montague Cobb, "Roscoe Conkling Giles," *JNMA* 62 (1970): 254-56.

T. Savitt

GILLETTE, ARTHUR JAY (October 28, 1864, Prairieville, Rice County, Minn.-March 24, 1921, St. Paul, Minn.). *Orthopedic surgeon*. Son of Albert J. and Ellen (Austin) Gilbert. Married Ellen Moore, 1890, one child; Katharine Kennedy, 1907, no children. EDUCATION: Hamline University (three years); 1883-85, Minnesota Hospital College; 1886, M.D., St. Paul Medical College; 1887, graduated from New York Polyclinic; postgraduate work, New York Polyclinic and New York Orthopedic Dispensary and Hospital; intern, St. Joseph's Hospital, St. Paul, as its first intern. CAREER: Medical practice, St. Paul;

post 1890, limited practice to orthopedics; at University of Minnesota: 1897, clinical professor of orthopedics; 1898, full professor; and 1913-15, head of the division. CONTRIBUTIONS: Among the first to operate for fracture of the neck of the femur (1898). Started orthopedic department (1897), Ancker Hospital (presently, the St. Paul-Ramsey Hospital). Worked to establish a state-supported hospital for poor crippled children (built in 1910-11). The Hospital for Crippled and Deformed Children was given Gillette's name (1925). It was the first state-supported orthopedic hospital for poor crippled children in the United States. President, Minnesota Academy of Medicine (1896).

WRITINGS: "Mechanical and Surgical Treatment of Fracture of the Neck of the Femur," *St. Paul Med. J.* (1898); "Advantages of a State Hospital for Indigent Crippled and Deformed Children. . . ," *Am. J. of Orthopedic Surgery* (1916). REFERENCES: Carl C. Chatterton, "Early Orthopedics in Minnesota," *Minnesota Med.* (1953); *NCAB*, 19: 227.

R. Rosenthal

GILLIAM, DAVID TOD (April 3, 1844, Hebron, Ohio-October 2, 1923, Columbus, Ohio). *Physician; Surgeon; Obstetrics and gynecology*. Son of William and Mary Elizabeth (Bryan) Gilliam. Married Lucinda Mintun, 1866; three children. EDUCATION: Bartlett's Commercial College; 1871, M.D., Medical College of Ohio, Cincinnati, Ohio. CAREER: 1861-63, Union Army; 1871-77, practice, Nelsonville, Ohio; 1879-1906, chair of general pathology, Columbus Medical College, and chairs of physiology and gynecology, Starling Medical College; faculty: 1907-14, Starling-Ohio Medical College; 1914-16, Ohio State University. CONTRIBUTIONS: Modified the Ferguson method of suspension of the uterus by shortening the round ligaments. Developed perforating forceps for use in operations, the Gilliam operating table, a new technique for cystocele operation and for cure of female urinary incontinence.

WRITINGS: *Pocket Book of Medicine* (1882); *Essentials of Pathology* (1883); "Abdominal Tumors and Conditions Simulating the Same, with Anomalous Features," *N.Y. Med. J.* 54 (1891); "The Vaginal Route for Operations on the Pelvic Viscera," *Am. Gyn. & Obst. J.* 7 (1895); *Textbook of Practical Gynecology for Practitioners and Students* (1903). REFERENCES: *DAB*, 7: 291; *NCAB*, 17: 60; *The Ohio State University College of Medicine: A Collection of Source Material Covering a Century of Progress, 1834-1934* 1 (1934); *Who Was Who in Am.*, 4: 358.

G. Jenkins

GILMAN, DANIEL COIT (July 6, 1831, Norwich, Conn.-October 13, 1908, Norwich, Conn.). *University president*. Son of William C., businessman, and Eliza (Coit) Gilman. Married Mary Ketcham, 1861, two children; Elizabeth Dwight Woolsey, 1877. EDUCATION: 1852, A.B., Yale University; 1852-55, studied in Cambridge, Mass., New Haven, Conn., and Berlin, Germany. CAREER: 1852-55, attaché, U.S. legation in St. Petersburg, Russia; 1855, commissioner to the French Exhibition; 1856-72, organizer of, librarian, and physical and political geography faculty, Sheffield Scientific School (Yale); 1872-75, president, University of California; 1875-1901, first president, Johns Hopkins

University; 1896-97, member, U.S. commission on boundary line between Venezuela and British Guiana; 1901-4, president, Carnegie Institution of Washington; trustee and board member of numerous educational and humanitarian organizations. CONTRIBUTIONS: Established the first modern university in the United States at Johns Hopkins and was instrumental in the founding of its hospital (1889) and medical school (1893). Patterned after German institutions, "The Hopkins" set a standard of excellence in medical education and served as a benchmark for medical school reformers. Notable features included what was then an unusually high entrance requirement—a baccalaureate degree or its equivalent, a four-year graded curriculum, clinical and laboratory instruction, and emphasis on research. Assembled a distinguished faculty, including William H. Welch (q.v.), William Osler (q.v.), William S. Halsted (q.v.), and Howard A. Kelly (q.v.), whose medical accomplishments, along with those of the bright, eager students they attracted, gave Hopkins an international reputation. Similar reforms effected in the other colleges of the university. With Charles W. Eliot (q.v.) and Andrew W. White, inaugurated a new era in American higher education by stressing graduate study, scholarship, and academic freedom.

WRITINGS: *Proposed Plan for a Complete Organization of the School of Science Connected with Yale College* (1856); *Launching of a University* (1906). REFERENCES: *DAB*, 7: 299-300; Abraham Flexner, *Daniel Coit Gilman, Creator of the American Type University* (1946); *NCAB*, 5: 170; *N.Y. Times*, October 14, 1908; *Who Was Who in Am.*, 1: 458.

S. Galishoff

GLASSER, OTTO (September 2, 1895, Saarbruecken, Germany-December 11, 1964, Cleveland, Ohio). *Biophysicist; Radiology.* Son of Alexander, businessman, and Lina (Gentsch) Glasser. Married Emmy von Ehrenberg, 1922; one child. EDUCATION: University of Heidelburg; 1919, Ph.D., University of Freiburg. CAREER: 1919-21, instructor, Radiological Institute of Freiburg; 1921-22, University of Frankfurt Medical School; 1922-23, biophysicist, Howard Kelly Hospital, Baltimore, Md.; 1923-25, Cleveland Clinic, Department of Biophysical Research; 1925-27, assistant professor of biophysics, New York Post Graduate Medical School; 1927-61, head, Department of Biophysics, Cleveland Clinic Foundation; 1937-60, professor of biophysics, F. E. Bunts Education Institute, Cleveland Clinic; 1950, curator, Roentgen Museum, Lennep, Germany. CONTRIBUTIONS: Internationally known for his work in biophysics and radiology. Inventor of the condenser dosimeter for the measurement of X-rays and radiation from radioactive substances (1932). As an early user of radioactive isotopes, was instrumental in standardizing them and providing a terminology. One of the first to measure radioactive fallout. Pioneered X-ray defraction of the kidney stone and the radioautograph of tissue sections. An early researcher in aviation medicine.

WRITINGS: Authored many books and articles, including "Roentgen-Ray Dosage," *Am. J. Roentgenol.* 10 (1923): 1-5; "Condenser Dosimeter and Its Use in Measuring Radiation Over Wide Range of Wave Lengths," *ibid.*, 20 (1928): 505 (with U. V.

Portmann and V. B. Seitz); *Science of Radiology* (1933, editor); *Medical Physics* (1944, 1950, 1960); *Physical Foundation of Radiology* (1944, 1952, 1961, collaborator); *Dr. W. C. Roentgen* (1945). REFERENCES: *Cleveland Clinic* 32 (Apr. 1965): 2; "Radium Therapy and Nuclear Medicine," *Am. J. Roentgenol.* 93 (Mar. 1965): 752-53; *Who Was Who in Am.*, 4: 361.

G. Jenkins

GODMAN, JOHN DAVIDSON (December 20, 1794, Annapolis, Md.-April 17, 1830, Germantown, Pa.). *Physician; Anatomy; Natural history.* Son of Samuel and Anna (Henderson) Godman. Married Angelica Kauffman Peale, 1821; at least three children. EDUCATION: 1811-12, printer's apprentice; 1815-18, studied medicine, first with William N. Luckey, Elizabethtown, Pa., and later with John B. Davidge (q.v.), Baltimore, Md.; 1818, M.D., University of Maryland. CAREER: c.1818, practiced medicine, New Holland, Pa., but soon moved to a small village near Baltimore in anticipation of obtaining an appointment at the University of Maryland; when position did not materialize, moved again to Philadelphia, where he lectured on anatomy and physiology; 1821-22, surgery faculty, Medical College of Ohio (Cincinnati, Ohio); 1823, assumed charge of Philadelphia School of Anatomy; 1826-27, anatomy faculty, Rutgers Medical College (New York City); 1828, went to West Indies to seek cure for his chest ailment; 1828-30, returned to Germantown, where he studied and wrote on natural history; is most famous for his work as a naturalist. CONTRIBUTIONS: A highly regarded anatomist. Published *Anatomical Investigations. . .*(1824), in which he described in minute detail the various fasciae of the human body. Edited *Western Quarterly Reporter of Medical, Surgical and Natural Science* (1822-23), the first trans-Allegheny medical journal. Helped edit (beginning in 1825) *Philadelphia Journal of the Medical and Physical Sciences* (later *American Journal of the Medical Sciences*). Translated Jacques Coster's *Manual of Surgical Operations* (1825). Edited Astley P. Cooper's *Treatises on Dislocations and on Fractures of the Joints* (1825) and John Bell and Charles Bell's *Anatomy and Physiology of the Human Body* (1827).

WRITINGS: *Anatomical Investigations Comprising Descriptions of the Various Fasciae of the Human Body* (1824); *Contributions to Physiological and Pathological Anatomy* (1825). REFERENCES: *BHM* (1974-79), 73; *DAB*, 7: 350; Clark A. Elliott, *Biog. Dict. of Am. Sci.* (1979), 104-5; Kelly and Burrage (1928), 474-76; Stephanie Morris, "John Davidson Godman (1794-1830): Physician and Naturalist," *Trans. and Studies of the Coll. of Physicians of Phila.* 41 (Apr. 1974): 295-303; *NCAB*, 7: 284.

S. Galishoff

GOLDBERGER, JOSEPH (July 16, 1874, Girált, Hungary-January 17, 1929, Washington, D.C.). *Physician; Epidemiology.* Son of Samuel, merchant, and Sarah (Gutman) Goldberger. Married Mary Humphreys Farrar, 1906; four children. EDUCATION: 1890-92, College of the City of New York; 1895, M.D.,

Bellevue Hospital Medical College; 1895-97, intern, Bellevue Hospital. CAREER: 1897-99, practiced medicine, Wilkes-Barre, Pa.; 1899-1929, U.S. Public Health Service: assigned to immigration and quarantine stations and to epidemiological investigations of yellow fever, typhus, and other diseases; 1899-1913, director, Hygienic Laboratory; *post* 1913, southern field investigations of pellagra. CONTRIBUTIONS: Best known for his work on pellagra. In field investigations of southern orphanages, insane asylums, and prison farms, demonstrated that the disease was caused by a nutritional deficiency resulting from an unbalanced diet and could be cured by the addition of fresh milk, meat, or yeast; led to a sharp decline in the incidence of pellagra, since dried yeast could be easily and inexpensively added to most diets and distributed to victims of the disease; named the curative nutritional element in the yeast the P-P factor; was later identified as niacin, a member of the vitamin B complex. With Edgar Sydenstricker (q.v.), conducted sophisticated epidemiological studies of the social, economic, and cultural factors that impinged upon the diet of selected noninstitutional populations in which there was a high incidence of pellagra. With J. F. Anderson, showed that measles is caused by a virus that can be recovered from the nasal secretions of its victims and is transmissible to monkeys (1911). With Anderson, demonstrated that both head and body lice can spread typhus and that "Brill's disease" and typhus are the same (1912).

WRITINGS: *The Nature of the Virus of Measles* (1911, with J. F. Anderson); *The Prevention of Pellagra, A Test of Diet Among Institutional Inmates* (1915, with C. H. Waring and D. C. Willetts); "A Further Study of Butter, Fresh Beef, and Yeast as Pellagra Preventatives, with Consideration of the Relation of Factor P-P of Pellagra (and Black Tongue of Dogs) to Vitamin B," *U.S. Public Health Reports* 41 (1926): 297-318 (with G. A. Wheeler, R. D. Lillie, and L. M. Rogers). Most important writings are in Milton Terris, ed., *Goldberger on Pellagra* (1964). REFERENCES: *BHM* (1964-69), 107; (1977), 14; *DAB*, 7: 363-64; *DSB*, 5: 451-53; Elizabeth Etheridge, *The Butterfly Caste; A Social History of Pellagra* (1972); Bess Furman, *A Profile of the United States Public Health Service, 1798-1948* (1973), 301-4, 362-63; Miller, *BHM*, p. 14; *NCAB*, 21: 83-84; *N.Y. Times*, January 18, 1929; *Who Was Who in Am.*, 1: 465.

S. Galishoff

GOLDMARK, JOSEPHINE CLARA (October 13, 1877, Brooklyn, N.Y.-December 15, 1950, White Plains, N.Y.). *Nursing; Reformer*. Daughter of Joseph, physician, and Regina (Wehle) Goldmark. Never married. EDUCATION: 1898, B.A., Bryn Mawr College; graduate work at Barnard College. CAREER: 1903, began to work with Florence Kelley (q.v.), National Consumer's League, as publications secretary and chair of the committee on legal defense of labor laws (legal research for her brother-in-law Louis Brandeis in the *Muller* v. *Oregon* case [1908] and for Felix Frankfurter); 1911-13, served on committee to investigate the Triangle Shirtwaist Company fire; 1919, completed survey of health and hospitals, Cleveland, Ohio; 1919, became secretary, Rockefeller Foundation committee for the study of nursing education; director, New York Visiting Nurses

Service. CONTRIBUTIONS: Worked with C.-E. A. Winslow (q.v.) on the Rockefeller Foundation survey of nursing and nursing education in America, and the
resulting Winslow-Goldmark report (1923) stressed higher standards of nursing
education, financially secure nursing schools, and procedures for evaluating and
accrediting schools of nursing, all of which developed after the report.
WRITINGS: *Fatigue and Efficiency* (1912); *Nursing and Nursing Education in the U.S.*
(1923). REFERENCES: *Notable Am. Women*, 2: 60-61; *N.Y. Times*, December 16, 1950.

M. Kaufman

GOLDSMITH, ALBAN GILPIN. See SMITH, ALBAN GILPIN

GOLDWATER, SIGISMUND SCHULTZ (February 7, 1873, New York,
N.Y.-October 22, 1942, New York). *Physician*; *Hospital administrator*. Son of
Henry, tobacconist and later pharmacist, and Mary (Tryoler) Goldwater. Married
Clara Aub, 1904; three children. EDUCATION: 1894-95, Columbia University;
1895-96, studied social problems, University of Leipzig; 1901, M.D., University
and Bellevue Hospital Medical College (New York University); 1901-3, intern,
Mount Sinai Hospital (N.Y.). CAREER: At Mount Sinai Hospital: 1903-16, superintendent; and 1917-29, director; 1914-15, commissioner of health, New York
City; 1924, medical counselor, Veterans' Bureau; 1939-40, commissioner, department of hospitals, New York City; president: 1940-42, Associated Hospital
Service (New York City "Blue Cross"); and 1908, American Hospital Association. CONTRIBUTIONS: A world-famous authority on hospital building and
administration. Made Mount Sinai a prototype of the well-rounded general hospital; added dentistry and social service departments and developed an extensive
outpatient service. As N.Y.'s commissioner of health, established the first municipal bureau of health education (1914-15). As head of the city's public hospitals, implemented a building and modernization program that made the N.Y.
hospital system one of the best anywhere (1934-39); rooted out politics and
brought all of the nonmedical staff under the civil service system; secured $7
million for the establishment of a center, Welfare Hospital (later Goldwater
Memorial Hospital), for the care and study of chronic diseases (1940). Consulted
in the planning and construction of nearly 200 hospitals in the United States and
abroad. Assisted in the reorganization of the British voluntary hospital system
(1927). With Associated Hospital Service of New York, sought to extend hospital
insurance to lower-income groups; with the aid of the city's medical, business,
and labor groups, established Community Medical Care, which made available
inexpensive medical treatment in hospital wards to the working class.
WRITINGS: *Fundamentals of Hospital Service* (1940-41); chapters and articles in
A. C. Bachmeyer and Gerhard Hartman, eds., *The Hospital and Modern Society* (1943).
Writings listed in American Hospital Association, comp., *Bibliography. . .of Sigismund
Schultz Goldwater, M.D.* (1944). REFERENCES: *DAB*, Supplement 3: 312-13; *NCAB*,

31: 411-12; Miller, *BHM*, p. 42; *N.Y. Times*, October 23, 1942; *Who Was Who in Am.*,
2: 214.

S. Galishoff

GOODFELLOW, GEORGE EMERY (December 23, 1855, Downieville,
Calif.-December 7, 1910, Los Angeles, Calif.). *Physician; Surgeon.* Son of
Milton J., mining engineer, and Amanda (Baskin) Goodfellow. Married Kath-
erine Colt, April 1876; one child. EDUCATION: University of California, Berkeley,
and the U.S. Naval Academy (expelled); 1876, M.D., Wooster University,
Cleveland, Ohio. CAREER: 1876-78, medical practice, Oakland, Calif.; contract
surgeon: 1878-79, U.S. Army, Fort Whipple, Ariz.; and 1879-80, Fort Lowell,
Ariz.; practice: 1880-91, Tombstone, Ariz.; and 1891-98, Tucson, Ariz.; 1898-
1900, civilian volunteer on the staff of Gen. William R. Shafter, U.S. Army,
Cuba; 1900-1907, practice, San Francisco, Calif.; 1907-8, chief surgeon, Arizona Eastern Railroad and Southern Pacific of Mexico. CONTRIBUTIONS: Expert
in treatment of gunshot wounds in abdomen. Performed first pure perineal prostatectomy ever done (September 29, 1891). Appointed first Ariz. quarantine and
health officer (June 1, 1893). REFERENCES: *Arizona Daily Star* (Tucson), December
8, 1910; "The History of Medicine in Arizona," *Arizona Med.* (Nov. 1956): 494-96;
John Hubner, "Just One 'Goodfellow' in Tombstone," *Arizona Highways* (Sept. 1976).

J. Goff

GOODPASTURE, ERNEST WILLIAM (October 17, 1886, Montgomery
County, Tenn.-September 20, 1960, Nashville, Tenn.). *Physician; Pathology;
Microbiology.* Son of Albert Virgil, lawyer, and Jennie Wilson (Dawson) Good-
pasture. Married Sarah Marsh Catlett, 1915, one child; Frances Katharine An-
derson, 1945. EDUCATION: 1907, A.B., Vanderbilt University; 1912, M.D.,
Johns Hopkins University; 1912-13, Rockefeller Fellow in Pathology, Johns
Hopkins; 1924-25, studied pathology, Vienna. CAREER: 1913-15, pathology faculty, Johns Hopkins University; 1915-18, pathology staff, Peter Bent Brigham
Hospital; 1918-21, pathology faculty, Harvard University; 1922, pathology and
bacteriology faculty, University of the Philippines; 1922-24, director, Singer
Memorial Research Laboratory (Pittsburgh, Pa.); at Vanderbilt University Medical School: 1924-55, pathology faculty; and 1945-50, dean; scientific director:
1938-40, 1942-44, International Health Division, Rockefeller Foundation; and
1955-59, Department of Pathology, Armed Forces Institute of Pathology; president: 1938-40, American Society for Experimental Pathology, and 1948-49,
American Association of Pathologists and Bacteriologists. CONTRIBUTIONS: Developed the technique of chick-embryo inoculation for viral growth and propagation. With Alice Woodruff, demonstrated that fowl pox virus could be cultivated
on the chorioallantoic membrane of the chick embryo (1931); next showed that
human viruses could be grown in the same way; provided inexpensive method
for viral research and made possible the commercial, mass production of vaccines
against viral diseases such as smallpox, yellow fever, and influenza. Did first

work on the progression of the herpes simplex virus along neural pathways to the central nervous system.

WRITINGS: "The Transmission of the Virus of Herpes Febrilis Along Nerves in Experimentally Infected Rabbits," *J. of Med. Research* 44, no. 2 (1923): 139-84 (with Oscar Teague); "The Susceptibility of the Chorio-allantoic Membrane of Chick Embryos to Infection with the Fowl-Pox Virus," *Am. J. of Path.* 7, (1931): 209-22; "Some Uses of the Chick Embryo for the Study of Infection and Immunity," *Am. J. of Hygiene* 28 (1937): 111-29. A bibliography is in *BMNAS*. REFERENCES: *BHM* (1975), 10; *BMNAS* 38 (1965): 111-44; Sir MacFarland Burnet, "The Influence of a Great Pathologist: A Tribute to Ernest Goodpasture," *Perspectives in Biol. Med.* 16 (Spring 1973): 333-47; Miller, *BHM*, p. 42; *N.Y. Times*, September 21, 1960; *Who Was Who in Am.*, 4: 366.

S. R. Breusch

GORGAS, WILLIAM CRAWFORD (October 3, 1845, Mobile, Ala.-July 4, 1920, London, England). *Physician; Sanitarian; Public health; Military medicine.* Son of Josiah, soldier, and Amelia (Gayle) Gorgas. Married Marie Cook Doughty, 1885; one child. EDUCATION: 1875, A.B., University of the South; 1879, M.D., Bellevue Hospital Medical College (New York University); 1879-80, intern, Bellevue Hospital. CAREER: 1880-1918, physician, Medical Corps, U.S. Army (rising in rank from first lieutenant to major-general in 1915): 1898-1902, chief sanitary officer, Havana; and *post* 1904, chief sanitary officer, Panama Canal Zone; 1919-20, director, yellow-fever control program, International Health Board, Rockefeller Foundation; 1909-10, president, American Medical Association. CONTRIBUTIONS: Directed programs of mosquito control, which greatly abated the ravages of yellow fever and malaria in the Caribbean. Following Walter Reed's (q.v.) discovery (1900) that the *aëdes aegypti* mosquito transmitted yellow fever, initiated a sanitary campaign to eliminate the breeding grounds of the vector, which rid Havana of yellow fever for the first time in 150 years. Undertook a similar program in the Panama Canal Zone, which eradicated yellow fever and brought malaria under control, enabling the United States to complete the building of the Panama Canal (1904-14). As surgeon-general of the army, mobilized the nation's medical personnel for World War I; organized one of the largest and most efficient medical corps in history; arranged for a complete medical examination of every soldier inducted into the army; and established a large network of hospitals in the United States and Europe to treat the sick and wounded.

WRITINGS: "A Short Account of the Results of Mosquito Work in Havana, Cuba," *J. of the Assoc. of Military Surgeons of the U.S.* (1903); "Sanitation of the Tropics with Special Reference to Malaria and Yellow Fever," *JAMA* 52 (1909): 1075-77; *Sanitation in Panama* (1915). REFERENCES: *BHM* (1964-69), 108; (1970-74), 75; (1975-79), 53; (1980), 17; *DAB*, 7: 430-32; M. C. Gorgas and B. J. Hendrick, *William Crawford Gorgas; His Life and His Work* (1924); Kelly and Burrage (1928): 481-82; Miller, *BHM*, p. 42; *NCAB*, 32: 4-6; *Who Was Who in Am.*, 1: 471.

S. Eichold

GORRIE, JOHN (c.October 3, 1803, Nevis Island, British West Indies-June 29, 1855, Apalachicola, Fla.). *Physician; Inventor.* Son of Captain Gorrie,

Scottish army officer in service of Spain, and a Spanish woman of cultivation, thought to have been a governess in the home of a Spanish nobleman. Married Caroline Frances (Myrick) Beeman, a widow, May 15, 1838; two children. EDUCATION: Schools of Charleston and Columbia, S.C.; 1827, M.D., College of Physicians and Surgeons, West District of N.Y., Fairfield. CAREER: General practice: 1827-31, Abbeville, S.C.; 1831-33, Jackson County, Fla., near present town of Sneads; and 1833-55, Apalachicola, Fla. CONTRIBUTIONS: Keen student of malarial diseases endemic to Fla. Was prompted to seek means of cooling rooms of fever patients as a therapeutic measure in tropical climates. Led him to experiment with machinery for condensing and expanding air. Preliminary success in producing artificial ice (1845). Perfected apparatus (1848) and patent granted by U.S. Patent Office (1851). Basic principles were those applied to refrigeration and air-conditioning today. Received no personal profit from the invention; the original machine is now in Smithsonian Institution.

WRITINGS: "Essay on Neuralgia," *N.Y. Med. & Phys. J.* (Sept. 1828): 325-43; "Fatal Case of Delerium Tremens," *ibid.* (Jul. 1829): 313-17; "On the Prevention of Malarial Diseases," 11 articles, using pseudonym Jenner, *Apalachicola Commercial Advertiser*, April 6-June 15, 1844; "An Inquiry, Analogous and Experimental, into the Different Electrical Conditions of Arterial and Venous Blood," *New Orleans Med. and Surg. J.* 10 (1853-54): 584-602, 738-757; "On the Nature of Malaria, and Prevention of its Morbid Agency," *ibid.* (1854-55): 611-34, 750-69; several articles on artificial production of ice. REFERENCES: Raymond B. Becker, *John Gorrie, M.D.* (1972); *DAB*, 7: 436-37; Alfred R. Henderson, "John Gorrie, M.D., 1803-1855," *JAMA* 185 (1963): 330-33; Edward Jelks, "John Gorrie, M.D.," *J. Fla. Med. Assoc.* 54 (Aug. 1967): 797-98; *NCAB*, 15: 345. Gorrie's statue stands in Statuary Hall, the Capitol, Washington, D.C.

E. A. Hammond

GRAHAM, EVARTS AMBROSE (March 19, 1883, Chicago, Ill.-March 4, 1957, St. Louis, Mo.). *Surgeon (thoracic).* Son of David W., surgeon, and Ida (Barnett) Graham. Married Helen Tredway (q.v., Helen Tredway Graham), 1916; two children. EDUCATION: 1904, A.B., Princeton University; 1907, M.D., Rush Medical College, Chicago; 1907-8, intern, Presbyterian Hospital, Chicago; 1907-9, university fellow in chemistry, University of Chicago. CAREER: 1910-14, assistant surgeon, Rush Medical College; 1915-18, private practice, Mason City, Ia.; 1918-19, captain to major, U.S. Army Medical Corps; 1919-51, Bixby Professor of Surgery and head, then (1951-57) professor emeritus, Department of Surgery, Washington University, St. Louis, Mo. CONTRIBUTIONS: Through his work with the Army's Empyema Commission, achieved a significant improvement in mortality rates by delaying operation until the acute phase of the lung infection had passed. With Warren H. Cole and Glover Copher, developed (early 1920s) cholecystography. Developed an excellent training program in chest diseases and surgery (late 1920s). Accomplished the first successful one-stage pneumonectomy (1933). Concentrated for the remainder of his career on the problem of bronchogenic carcinoma, culminating (1950s) in a series of articles with Ernst Wynder and A. B. Croninger on the carcinogenicity of cigarette tar and the links between smoking and cancer. Widely recognized for his leading role in the founding of the American Board of Surgery, of which he was the first chairman.

WRITINGS: "Pneumonectomy with the Cautery: A Safer Substitute for the Ordinary Lobectomy in Cases of Chronic Suppuration of the Lung," *JAMA* 81 (1923): 1010-12; "Roentgenologic Examination of the Gall Bladder: Preliminary Report of a New Method of Utilizing the Intravenous Injection of Tetrabromophenolphthalein," *ibid.*, 82 (1924): 613-14 (with Warren H. Cole); "Visualization of the Gall Bladder by The Sodium Salt of Tetrabromophenolphthalein," *ibid.*, 82 (1924): 1777-78 (with Warren H. Cole and Glover H. Copher); "Successful Removal of an Entire Lung for Carcinoma of the Bronchus," *ibid.*, 101 (1933): 1371-74; "Tobacco Smoking as a Possible Etiological Factor in Bronchogenic Carcinoma," *ibid.*, 143 (1950): 329-36 (with Ernst L. Wynder); "Experimental Production of Carcinoma with Cigarette Tar," *Cancer Research* 13 (1953): 855-64. Writings listed in *BMNAS*. REFERENCES: *BHM* (1964-69), 109; (1970-74), 75; (1975-79), 53; *BMNAS* 48 (1976): 221-50; *DAB*, Supplement 6: 245-47; Miller, *BHM*, p. 43; *NCAB*, 48: 644-45; *N.Y. Times*, March 5, 1957; Peter D. Olch, "Evarts A. Graham, the American College of Surgeons, and the American Board of Surgery," *J. Hist. Med.* 27 (1972): 247-61.

D. Sneddeker

GRAHAM, HELEN (TREDWAY) (July 21, 1890, Dubuque, Ia.-April 4, 1971, St. Louis, Mo.). *Pharmacologist.* Daughter of Harry E. and Marian (McConnell) Tredway. Married Evarts Ambrose Graham (q.v.), 1916; two children. EDUCATION: Bryn Mawr College: 1911, A.B. (first in her class); and 1912, M.A.; 1912-13, fellowship, University of Göttingen; 1915, Ph.D. (chemistry), University of Chicago. CAREER: 1918-19, assistant in pharmacology, Johns Hopkins Medical School; 1925-59, faculty in pharmacology, Washington University School of Medicine; 1959-71, professor emerita, pharmacology. CONTRIBUTIONS: Published more than 40 papers on both nerve physiology and histamines over her long and distinguished career. Despite family obligations and constraints on women in science, was a productive scientist who moved into a new field (histamine) at 60 and obtained a renewal of her NIH research grant at the age of 71. Listed in *American Men of Science* for over 50 years. Early work (some of it with Nobel Laureate Herbert Gasser [q.v.]) involved the physiology and pharmacology of peripheral nerve. Credited with the independent discovery of the histamine function of mast cells and blood basophils and the development of highly sensitive methods for measuring histamine in body fluid. A community leader, active in the promotion of interracial understanding, consumer and environmental protection, and education.

WRITINGS: "The End of Spike Potential of Nerve and Its Relation to the Beginning of Afterpotential," *Am. J. of Physiol.* 101 (1932): 316 (with Herbert S. Gasser); "Potentials Produced in the Spinal Cord by Stimulation of Dorsal Roots," *ibid.*, 103 (1933): 303 (with Herbert S. Gasser); "Rate of Conduction in Mamalian Nerve in Vivo," *ibid.*, 116 (1936): 63 (with Lorente de No); "After-potentials of Polarized Nerve," *ibid.*, 123 (1938): 79; "Distribution of Histamine Among Blood Elements," *Federation Proceedings* 11 (1952): 350 (with F. Wheelwright, H. Parish, O. Marks, and O. Lowry). REFERENCES:

Oliver H. Lowry, "Helen Tredway Graham," *The Pharmacologist* 13 (Fall, 1971): 2; *NCAB*, 56: 39.

M. *Hunt*

GRAHAM, SYLVESTER (July 5, 1794, West Suffield, Conn.-September 11, 1851, Northampton, Mass.). *Nutritionist.* Son of John, clergyman, and Ruth Graham. Married Sarah Earls, 1826. EDUCATION: 1823, entered Amherst College, left with no degree; 1826, ordained Presbyterian minister, Newark, N.J. CAREER: 1830-31, agent for the Pennsylvania State Society for the Suppression of the Use of Ardent Spirits; *post* 1831, delivered speeches on human physiology and diet; 1837, published lectures on the "science of human life;" 1837-40, American Physiological Society spread Graham's ideas; chapters in Boston, New York City, and Lynn, Mass., published the *Graham Journal*; May 1838, spirit behind American Health Convention, which resolved to condemn the use of medicines and advocated hygiene courses in schools; 1850, Mass. required teaching of physiology in public schools; 1850, retired from lecture tours. CONTRIBUTIONS: Leader of one of the first popular health movements in the United States. Conceived the notion that intemperance could be prevented and cured by a purely vegetable diet; stated that white bread brought on "atrophy and death." Name was given to bread made with unbolted flour. Paved the way for use of cereal foods and fruits as a cure for dyspepsia. Against eating meat, which he claimed excited vile tempers, sexual abuse, and loss of energy; lectured on the virtue of chastity. Founder of the Grahamites, who believed that all diseases had their source in the alimentary canal. Drugs could not touch the source of the diseases, and the best treatment lay in proper diet, fresh air, frequent bathing, sensible dress, temperance in food and drink, and sexual restraint. A strict regimen promised health and "longevity and prosperity in pursuit of life." Graham boarding houses and vegetarian tables at colleges were organized by his followers. Established Ladies Physiological Reform Societies throughout New England to work for emancipation from tight laced garments. In the twilight of his career, joined hydropathy advocates in support of water cures, turkish baths, and wet sheets. The graham cracker has been the most enduring product of the cult.

WRITINGS: *Lectures on the Science of Human Life* (1837), republished with biographical sketch (1858); *Lecture to Young Man of Chastity* (1839); "View of Beaumont's Experiments," *Graham J. of Health & Longevity*, 1 (1837): 262-64. REFERENCES: *DAB*, 4, pt. 1: 479-80; *NCAB*, 5: 516; S. Nissenbaum, *Sex, Diet, and Debility in Jacksonian America* (1980); Richard Harrison Skyrock, *Medicine in America, Historical Essays* (1966), ch. 5.

R. *Edwards*

GRASSICK, JAMES (June 29, 1850, Strathdon, Scotland-December 20, 1943, Grand Forks, N.Dak.). *Physician; Public health; Pulmonary medicine; History.* Son of Donald, farmer, and Helen (Edward) Grassick Grant. Married Christina

McDougall, 1889; two children. EDUCATION: 1882-83, read medicine with Dr.
John McDiarmid of Hensel, Ontario, Canada; 1885, M.D., Rush Medical College (Chicago, Ill.); 1888, M.D.C.M., University of Michigan; 1896, postgraduate study, University of Chicago. CAREER: 1885-88, 1889-1905, physician
and surgeon, Buxton, Dakota Territory, and N.Dak.; 1905-41, physician and
surgeon, Grand Forks, N.Dak.; 1909-13, superintendent of public health, N.Dak.;
1909-28, founder and first president, North Dakota Tuberculosis Association
(now the North Dakota Lung Association); 1909-13, member, Board of Directors, North Dakota State Tuberculosis Sanitarium; 1909-43, lecturer, School of
Medicine, University of North Dakota; 1913-27, editor, *The Pennant* (newsletter,
North Dakota Tuberculosis Association); 1916-32, university physician, University of North Dakota; 1923-24, president, North Dakota Medical Association;
1928, founder, Camp Grassick (near Dawson, N.Dak.); 1928-43, president emeritus, North Dakota Tuberculosis Association. CONTRIBUTIONS: Initiator and leader
of struggle against tuberculosis in N.Dak.; founded North Dakota Tuberculosis
Association (1909); member of citizens' board that planned and developed the
North Dakota State Tuberculosis Sanitarium, San Haven, N. Dak.; led statewide
educational movement to eliminate tuberculosis; led movement to create the
summer camp that bears his name as a rehabilitation site for tubercular children.
Efforts have been credited with a major part in the eradication of tuberculosis
from N.Dak. Compiled, wrote, and published a history of medicine in N.Dak.,
that is a basic source.

WRITINGS: "Pioneer Physicians of North Dakota," *Quarterly J. of the Univ. of North
Dakota* 13 (1923); *North Dakota Medicine: Sketches and Abstracts* (1926); "Joseph G.
Millspaugh: First President of the North Dakota Medical Association," *J.-Lancet* 51
(1931). Writings listed at the School of Medicine, University of North Dakota. REF-
ERENCES: *Compendium of History and Biography of North Dakota* (1900), 501-2; *Grand
Forks Herald*, December 21, 1943; James Grassick, *North Dakota Medicine: Sketches
and Abstracts* (1926).

L. Remele

GRAY, JOHN PURDUE (August 6, 1825, Center County, Pa.-November 29,
1886, Utica, N.Y.). *Physician; Alienist.* Son of Peter D., farmer and clergyman,
and Elizabeth (Purdue) Gray. Married Mary B. Wetmore, 1854; three children.
EDUCATION: Bellefonte (Pa.) Academy; 1846, A.M., Dickinson College; 1849,
M.D., University of Pennsylvania Medical School; 1849-51, resident physician,
Blockley Hospital. CAREER: At New York State Lunatic Asylum, Utica: 1851-
53, medical staff; and 1854-86, superintendent; 1853-54, superintendent, Michigan State Lunatic Asylum, Kalamazoo, Mich.; medical faculty: 1874-82, Bellevue Hospital Medical College; and 1876-82, Albany Medical College; 1854-82,
editor, *American Journal of Insanity*; 1885, president, Association of Medical
Superintendents of the American Institutions for the Insane. CONTRIBUTIONS:
Introduced modern management to the care of the insane and urged the improvement of the physical conditions and construction of asylums. Regarded the
insane as physically rather than mentally ill. Established postgraduate training

for alienists at Utica. Pioneered in the microscopic examination of the brain. An expert forensic witness in prominent court trials.

WRITINGS: *Heredity* (1884); *Insanity: Its Dependence on Physical Diseases* (1871); *Suicide* (1878); *Insanity: Some of Its Preventable Causes* (1880). REFERENCES: *DAB*, 4, pt. 1: 521-22; Kelly and Burrage (1928), 488-89; *NCAB*, 7: 273; Willis G. Tucker, "John Purdue Gray, M.D., LL.D.," *Report of the Committee on Necrology, University of the State of New York, Twenty-Sixth Convocation*, 23-26; *N.Y. Times*, November 30, 1886; R. J. Waldinger, "Sleep of Reason. . .," *J. Hist. Med.* 34 (1979): 163-79.

D. O. Powell

GREEN, HORACE (December 4, 1802, Chittendon, Vt.-November 29, 1866, Ossining, N.Y.). *Physician; Laryngologist.* Son of Deacon Zeeb, farmer and Revolutionary War veteran, and Sarah (Cowee) Green. Married Mary Sigourney Butler, 1829 (d.1833), no surviving children; Harriet Sheldon Douglas, 1841, 12 children (one source says 10), 8 of whom survived. EDUCATION: Self-educated, with little formal schooling; 1824, M.D., Castleton Medical College, Vt., after apprenticeship with two brothers and a brother-in-law in Vt.; 1830-31, attended lectures and dissections at the University of Pennsylvania; 1838, visited hospitals and medical schools in London and Paris during a visit of five months. CAREER: Private practice: 1824-29, 1831-35, 1839-40, Vt.; and 1835-38, 1840-60, New York City; 1839-40, professor of medicine and president, Castleton Medical College; 1842-60, member and president, Board of Trustees, president of the faculty, and professor of the theory and practice of medicine, New York Medical College. CONTRIBUTIONS: The first specialist in the United States to devote his practice exclusively to diseases of the throat. Excited an international controversy (beginning in 1846) by claiming the ability to explore and apply medication to the larynx by means of a probang, a curved instrument of whalebone ten inches long, tipped with a tiny sponge. Accused of plagiarism and fraud, defended himself in books, a journal he founded (*American Medical Journal*), and by demonstrating his technique on patients (1855) before a committee appointed by the New York Academy of Medicine. The outcome of these controversies was inconclusive. Had defenders and detractors in the United States, France, and Britain. His practice, which consisted mainly of the application of silver nitrate to the lining membrane and of surgery, was large and lucrative until his retirement as a result of invalidism from tuberculosis (1860).

WRITINGS: *A Treatise on Diseases of the Air Passages* (1846 and three subsequent editions); *On the Surgical Treatment of Polyps of Larynx and Oedema of the Glottis* (1852); *A Practical Treatise of Pulmonary Tuberculosis* (1864); numerous articles and speeches, *Autobiography*, MSS., 1865, New York Academy of Medicine, New York City. REFERENCES: *DAB*, 4, pt. 1: 547-48; Kelly and Burrage (1920), 490; William Snow Miller, "Horace Green and his Probang," *Johns Hopkins Hosp. Bull.* 30 (1919): 246-52; *NCAB*, 26: 91; Charles Snyder, "The Investigation of Horace Green," *Laryngoscope* 85 (1975): 2012-22. Letters from a patient, Julia Robertson Pierpont, 1850, written from Green's home, vividly describe his appearance, manner, methods of practice, and family setting (New York Academy of Medicine).

D. M. Fox

GREENBERG, MORRIS (June 6, 1890, Rumania-May 25, 1960, New York, N.Y.). *Physician; Pediatrician; Health officer.* Son of Harry and Henrietta (Spitzer) Greenberg. Married Clara Katz, 1924; two children. EDUCATION: 1911, A.B., City College of New York; 1917, M.D., College of Physicians and Surgeons, Columbia University; 1943, M.S., Columbia University. CAREER: Medical staff: 1926-43, New York Nursery and Child's Hospital; 1936-42, Gouverneur Hospital; 1937-42, Sydenham Hospital; and 1938-55, Beth David Hospital; 1920-60, clinic physician, chief epidemiologist (1941), director of Bureau of Preventable Diseases (1946), New York City Department of Public Health; medical faculty, Columbia University School of Public Health. CONTRIBUTIONS: A leader in the diagnosis and control of communicable diseases. Headed the task force that conducted mass inoculation with Salk vaccine for poliomyelitis and ordered that pregnant women be given priority after his research established they were more susceptible to polio. An authority on infant diarrhea.

WRITINGS: *Studies in Epidemiology: Selected Papers of Morris Greenberg* (1965); *Modern Concepts of Communicable Disease* (1953). REFERENCES: *JAMA* 173 (1960): 1373; *N.Y. State J. of Med.* 60 (1960): 2320; *N.Y. Times*, May 26, 1960; Berton Roueche, *Eleven Blue Men and Other Narratives of Medical Detection* (1953); *WWAPS*, p. 468.

D. O. Powell

GREENE, CLARENCE SUMNER (December 26, 1901, Washington, D.C.-October 9, 1957, Washington, D.C.). *Neurosurgeon.* Son of Samuel B. and Pharien (Gordon) Greene. Married Evelyn Gardner, 1945; two children. EDUCATION: c. 1920-c.1922, University of Pennsylvania; 1926, D.D.S., University of Pennsylvania Dental School; 1927-29, Harvard College; 1932, A.B., University of Pennsylvania; 1936, M.D., Howard University; 1936-37, intern, Cleveland City Hospital; 1937-39, resident, Douglass Hospital, Philadelphia, Pa.; 1939-42, resident, surgery, Freedmen's Hospital, Washington, D.C.; 1947-49, resident, neurosurgery, Montreal Neurological Institute of McGill University. CAREER: 1926-27, dental practice, Long Island, N.Y.; 1939-40, 1942-47, 1949-57, Howard University Medical School faculty member (1949-55, chief, Division of Neurosurgery; and 1955-57, chair, Department of Surgery). CONTRIBUTIONS: First professor of neurosurgery, Howard. Greatly improved status of neurosurgery at Freedmen's Hospital, making this kind of surgery routine work (1949-57); also improved quality of undergraduate and resident training in surgery at Howard Medical School (1955-57). First black diplomate of American Board of Neurosurgery (1953).

WRITINGS: "One Stage Suprapubic Prostatectomy as a Routine," *JNMA* 34 (1942): 188-91 (with E. Jones); "Cerebral Arteriography in the Diagnosis of Unilateral Exophthalmos," *ibid.*, 48 (1965): 10-16 (with J. B. Barber). Writings listed in *JNMA* 60

(1969): 254. REFERENCES: W. Montague Cobb, "Clarence Sumner Greene, A.B., D.D.S., M.D., 1901-1957," *JNMA* 60 (1968): 253-54; obituary, *ibid.*, 50 (1958): 139-40.

T. Savitt

GREENE, CORDELIA AGNES (July 5, 1831, Lyons, N.Y.-January 28, 1905, New York, N.Y.). *Physician.* Daughter of Jabez, physician, and Phila (Cooke) Greene. Never married; adopted six children. EDUCATION: 1854-55, student, Woman's Medical College, Philadelphia, Pa.; 1856, M.D., medical department, Western Reserve University. CAREER: 1856-59, assisted father at his "Water Cure" institution, Castile, N.Y.; 1859-65, practiced, Clifton Springs Sanitarium, N.Y.; 1865-1904, head, Castile Sanitarium. CONTRIBUTIONS: One of the earliest regular medical college female graduates, established one of the first sanitaria for the treatment of a variety of chronic diseases affecting women and children.

WRITINGS: *The Art of Keeping Well; or, Common Sense Hygiene for Adults and Children* (1906). REFERENCES: "Dr. Mary T. Greene Sanitarium: 100 Year Celebration," *Med. Woman's J.* 56 (Jun. 1949): 21-25; Elizabeth Putnam Gordon, *The Story of the Life and Work of Cordelia A. Greene, M.D.* (1925); "Obituary—Cordelia Agnes Greene, M.D.," *Woman's Med. J.* 15 (Apr. 1905): 80-81.

N. Gevitz

GREENWOOD, JOHN (May 17, 1760, Boston, Mass.-November 16, 1819, New York, N.Y.). *Dentist.* Son of Isaac, ivory-turner, mathematical instrument-maker, and dabbler in dentistry, and Mary (Pans) Greenwood. Married Elizabeth Weaver, 1788. EDUCATION: Apprenticed to uncle, Thales Greenwood, a cabinetmaker, in Portland, Me.; 1806, studied dentistry in France. CAREER: During early years of American Revolutionary War, served as a fife-major and as a scout; toward the end of the war, studied dental mechanics, possibly with money made from privateering; in 1784 or 1785 began to practice dentistry in New York City. CONTRIBUTIONS: A self-taught, mechanical genius, pioneered in American dentistry with regard to mechanics and instrumentation. Credited with inventing the foot-power drill, spiral springs which held the plates of artificial teeth in position, and the use of porcelain in the manufacture of false teeth. Treated George Washington, for whom he made several sets of false teeth. REFERENCES: *BHM* (1970-74), 76; (1975-79), 53; *DAB*, 7: 592; Miller, *BHM*, p. 43; *Who Was Who in Am.*, Hist. Vol.: 288.

S. Galishoff

GREGORY, SAMUEL (April 19, 1813, Guilford, Vt.-March 23, 1872, Boston, Mass.). *Medical educator; Advocate of the medical education of women.* Son of Stephen, farmer, and Hannah (Palmer) Gregory. Never married. EDUCATION: 1840, A.B., Yale University; 1845, A.M., Yale University. CAREER: 1840-45, itinerant teacher of English grammar; *post* 1844, wrote pamphlets on personal hygiene; *post* 1846, gave popular lectures throughout New England on health care and especially obstetrical practice; 1848-56, founder and secretary,

American Medical Education Society (incorporated 1850 as the Female Medical Education Society); 1848-72, founder, secretary, and chief administrative officer, Boston Female Medical School (reorganized 1856 as the New England Female Medical College). CONTRIBUTIONS: Attacked the practice of obstetrics by male physicians as indecent; advocated and gained popular support for the medical education of women. Founded and directed the first medical school for women in the United States. Belief in the immorality of male midwifery, not feminist commitments, animated his drive for the medical training of women as midwives, physicians, and nurses.

WRITINGS: *Facts and Important Information for Young Men on the Self-Indulgence of Sexual Appetite* (1841); *Man Midwifery Exposed and Corrected Together with Remarks on the Use and Abuse of Ether and Dr. Channing's "Cases of Inhalation of Ether in Labor"* (1848); *Letters to Ladies in Favor of Female Physicians for Their Own Sex* (1850); *Female Physicians* (1864). REFERENCES: *DAB*, 4, pt. 1: 604-5; "Historical Incidents. New England Female Medical College," 1847-1865, scrapbook kept by Gregory, Countway Library, Harvard Medical School, Boston; Frederick C. Waite, *History of the New England Female Medical College* (1950), esp. 11-16; Mary Roth Walsh, *"Doctors Wanted: No Women Need Apply"* (1977), 35-75.

J. H. Warner

GRIDLEY, SELAH (June 3, 1770, Farmington, Conn.-February 17, 1826, Exeter, N.H.). *Physician*. Son of Timothy, farmer, and Beulah (Langdon) Gridley; six children. EDUCATION: 1791, studied under a preceptor in Conn.; 1794, licensed by the censors of the Connecticut State Medical Society; probably never received M.D. CAREER: 1794, practiced, Conn.; 1795, moved to Castleton, Vt., where he became the leading physician in Rutland County; 1818, having more applicants for preceptorship than he could manage, founded the Castleton Medical Academy (later called the Vermont Academy of Medicine) with Theodore Woodward (q.v.) and John Cazier; 1818-22, president and professor of institutes and practice of medicine; 1820, became depressed; 1822, was divorced by his wife after which he went to live with his brother in Exeter, where he saw a few patients and died, probably of influenza (1826). CONTRIBUTIONS: President, First Medical Society of Vermont (1813). Chairman, organizing committee of the Vermont State Medical Society (1813), charter member, and president (1815-17).

WRITINGS: *A Dissertation on the Importance and Associability of the Human Stomach* (1816); *The Mills of the Muses*, a volume of poetry (1828). REFERENCES: F. C. Waite, *The First Medical College in Vermont* (1949), 37-44.

L. J. Wallman

GRIFFIN, JOHN STROTHER (1816, Va.-August 23, 1898, Los Angeles, Calif.). *Surgeon*. Orphaned at the age of nine. Married Louisa Hayes, first female schoolteacher in Los Angeles, 1856; no children. EDUCATION: 1837, M.D., University of Pennsylvania. CAREER: Until 1840, practice in Louisville, Ky.; 1840-54, surgeon, U.S. Army; 1854, resigned commission in army and returned to Los Angeles to establish surgical practice; 1856, became superintendent of schools, Los Angeles; 1871, first president, Los Angeles County Medical Association. CONTRIBUTIONS: Sought new treatments; was not hesitant to discard old methods. Showed great concern for patients. A leader in civic and business affairs, Los Angeles.

WRITINGS: George W. Ames, Jr., "A Doctor Comes to California: Diary of John S. Griffin, Asst. Surgeon to Kearney's Dragoons," *California Hist. Soc. Q.* 21 (1942): 193-224; 333-57. REFERENCES: Ames, "A Doctor Comes to California;" D. L. Clarke, "Soldiers Under Stephen Watts Kearney," *ibid.*, 45 (1966): 133-48; Henry Harris, *California's Medical Story* (1932), 70.

Y. V. O'Neill

GRISCOM, JOHN HOSKINS (August 14, 1809, New York, N.Y.-April 28, 1874, New York). *Physician; Public health.* Son of John, chemist, and Abigail (Hoskins) Griscom. Married Henrietta Peale, 1835; eight children. EDUCATION: Collegiate School of Friends; New York High School; apprentice to John D. Godman (q.v.) and Valentine Mott (q.v.); 1827-29, Rutgers Medical College; 1832, M.D., University of Pennsylvania; 1832-33, resident physician, New York Hospital. CAREER: 1833-36, assistant physician and physician, New York Dispensary; 1836-74, private practice, N.Y.; 1836-38, professor of chemistry, New York College of Pharmacy; 1842, city inspector, N.Y.; 1843-c.1870, physician, New York Hospital; 1848-51, general agent and physician, New York State Commissioners of Emigration. CONTRIBUTIONS: A prime mover in social, political, and medical efforts to organize a systematic and ongoing public health program in midnineteenth-century New York City; urged improved vital statistics and comprehensive sanitary surveys to pinpoint community public health needs; advocated a scientifically based health department and suggested a model for such a body. Contributed important scientific studies of the ventilation of buildings and ships. Became a leader of orthodox medical reform in antebellum N.Y.; played significant roles in early development of the American Medical Association, New York Academy of Medicine, National Quarantine and Sanitary Conventions, New York Prison Association, and other medical and philanthropic organizations.

WRITINGS: *Animal Mechanism and Physiology* (1840 and later editions); *The Sanitary Condition of the Laboring Population of New York* (1845); *First Lessons in Human Physiology* (1846 and later editions); *The Uses and Abuses of Air* (1848-49 and later editions); *Anniversary Discourse Before the New York Academy of Medicine* (1855); *Sanitary Legislation, Past and Future* (1861). Writings listed in Kelly and Burrage (1928); *Appleton's CAB*; *Lamb's Biographical Dict. of the U.S.* REFERENCES: James H. Cassedy, "The Roots of American Sanitary Reform, 1843-47. Seven Letters from John H. Griscom to Lemuel Shattuck," *J. Hist. Med.* 30 (1975): 136-47; Samuel W. Francis, "John H. Griscom," *Med. & Surg. Reporter* 15 (1866): 118-22; Duncan R. Jamieson, "Towards a Cleaner New York. John H. Griscom and New York's Public Health, 1830-1870" (Ph.D. diss., Michigan State University, 1972); Charles E. Rosenberg and Carroll S.

Rosenberg, "Pietism and the Origins of the American Public Health Movement: A Note on John H. Griscom and Robert M. Hartley," *J. Hist. Med.* 23 (1968): 16-35.

J. H. Cassedy

GROSS, SAMUEL DAVID (July 8, 1805, near Easton, Pa.-May 6, 1884, Philadelphia, Pa.). *Physician; Educator; Author*; *Surgery*. Son of Philip, farmer, and Johanna (Brown) Gross. Married Louisa Weissell, 1828; survived by four children, including Samuel W. Gross (q.v.). EDUCATION: 1828, M.D., Jefferson Medical College (Philadelphia). CAREER: 1828-30, practiced medicine, Philadelphia; 1830-33, practiced medicine, Easton; 1833-35; anatomy faculty, Medical College of Ohio; 1835-40, pathological anatomy faculty, Cincinnati Medical College; surgery faculty: 1840-56, University of Louisville; 1850-51, University of the City of New York; and 1856-62, Jefferson Medical College. CONTRIBUTIONS: Through his teaching and writings, made American surgery as good as that found anywhere in the world. Translated several French and German texts, including Alphonse Tavernier's *Elements of Operative Surgery* (1829), the first treatise on that subject published in America. Wrote *Elements of Pathological Anatomy* (1839), the first systematic treatment of that subject to appear in English and long the standard reference in its field. Made numerous pioneering contributions to medical literature, including *A Practical Treatise on the Diseases and Injuries of the Urinary Bladder, the Prostate Gland, and the Urethra* (1851) and *A Practical Treatise on Foreign Bodies in the Air Passages* (1854). Most famous work was *System of Surgery, Pathological, Diagnostic, Therapeutic and Operative* (1859), considered by many to be the greatest surgical treatise of its time; went through six editions between 1859 and 1882 and was translated into several languages. A highly skilled surgeon, especially eminent for his operations for bladder stones, hernias, and intestinal obstructions. Originator of the modern method of suturing intestinal wounds and restoring damaged intestines by resection and of suturing divided nerves and tendons. A founder, American Medical Association and American Surgical Society. Edited *Louisville Medical Review* and *North American Medico-Chirurgical Review* (Philadelphia, 1857-61). Edited and contributed to *The Lives of Eminent American Physicians and Surgeons of the Nineteenth Century* (1861).

WRITINGS: *Treatise on the Anatomy, Physiology, and Diseases and Injuries of the Bones and Joints* (1830); *An Experimental and Critical Inquiry into the Nature and Treatment of Wounds of the Intestines* (1843); *A Manual of Military Surgery* (1861). REFERENCES: *BHM* (1964-69), 111; (1970-74), 77; (1975-79), 54; *DAB*, 8: 18-20; John Garraty, *Encyclopedia of Am. Biog.* (1974), 461; Kelly and Burrage (1928), 503-6; Miller, *BHM*, p. 44; *NCAB*, 8: 216-17; John H. Talbott, *Biographical Hist. of Med.* (1970), 412-15; *Who Was Who in Am.*, Hist. Vol.: 291.

S. Galishoff

GROSS, SAMUEL WEISSELL (February 4, 1837, Cincinnati, Ohio-April 16, 1889, Philadelphia, Pa.). *Physician*; *Surgery*; *Oncology*. Son of Samuel David

(q.v.) and Louisa (Weissell) Gross. Married Grace Linzee Revere, 1876. ED-
UCATION: Received early education at Shelby College (Ky.) and Louisville University; 1857, graduated from Jefferson Medical College. CAREER: 1857-61,
1865-89, practiced medicine, Philadelphia; 1861-65, surgeon, U.S. Army; surgical staff, Philadelphia and Jefferson Medical College hospitals; at Jefferson
Medical College: genito-urinary surgery faculty; and post 1882, principles of
surgery and clinical surgery faculty. CONTRIBUTIONS: One of the foremost surgeons of his times. As a result of his Civil War experience, espoused idea that
instead of relying on pressure alone to combat hemorrhaging, as was usually
done, veins should be ligated as arteries were. In his book A Practical Treatise
on Tumors of the Mammary Gland (1880), argued that breast tumors could be
operated on successfully if the disease had not metastasized. Made the first
comprehensive study of bone sarcoma and broadened and solidified the conception of giant-cell sarcoma (1879). With William S. Halsted (q.v.) and others,
developed the modern radical operation for cancer. One of the first persons in
Philadelpia to adopt antiseptic surgery.

WRITINGS: "Sarcoma of the Long Bones; Based upon a Study of One Hundred and
Sixty-Five Cases," Am. J. of Med. Sci., n.s., 78 (1879): 17-57, 338-77; A Practical
Treatise on Impotence, Sterility, and Allied Disorders of the Male Sexual Organs (1881).
REFERENCES: DAB, 8: 20-21; Kelly and Burrage (1928), 506; Who Was Who in Am.,
Hist. Vol.: 292.

S. Galishoff

GRUENING, EMIL (October 2, 1842, Hohensalza, Prussia [now Inowraclaw,
Poland])-May 30, 1914, New York, N.Y.). Physician; Ophthalmology; Otology.
Son of Moritz and Bertha (Thorner) Gruening. Married Rose Fridenberg, 1874;
Phebe Fridenberg, 1880; one child by first marriage and four by the second.
EDUCATION: Graduated from Thorn Gymnasium; 1862, immigrated to the United
States; 1864, began study at College of Physicians and Surgeons (Columbia),
M.D., 1867; 1867-70, postgraduate study in London, Paris, and Berlin. CAREER:
1862-64, taught the classics and foreign languages to students in private homes;
1864-65, served in the 7th New Jersey Volunteer Infantry; post 1870, practiced
medicine in New York City; 1870, appointed to the staff of the Ophthalmic and
Aural Institute, became personal assistant to Dr. Hermann Knapp (q.v.), chief
surgeon; ophthalmic surgeon: 1878-1912, New York Eye and Ear Infirmary;
1879-1904, Mt. Sinai Hospital; 1880-1904, German (Lenox Hill) Hospital; 1882-
95, ophthalmology faculty, New York Polyclinic; president, American Otological Society (1903), American Ophthalmological Society (1910). CONTRIBU-
TIONS: Pioneered in ophthalmology and otology, conducting original investigations
and inventing instruments for surgical use. One of the first to describe and to
operate successfully upon brain abscess of otitic origin. Called attention to the
danger of blindness from the consumption of wood alcohol. Most enduring
achievement was the development of the modern mastoid operation.

WRITINGS: Contributed the chapter on "Wounds and Injuries of the Eyeball and Its Appendages" in W. F. Norris and C. A. Oliver, eds., *System of Diseases of the Eye*, 3 (1898); "Two Cases of Otitic Brain Abscess; Operation; Recovery," *Mt. Sinai Hospital Reports*, 2 (1900); "Methyl Alcohol Amblyopia," *Arch. of Ophth.* 39: (Jul. 1910) 333-36. REFERENCES: *DAB*, 8: 32; Kelly and Burrage (1928), 506-7; *NCAB*, 19: 47.

S. Galishoff

GUNDERSEN, ADOLF (October 8, 1865, near Flisa, Norway-September 15, 1938, near Flisa). *Physician; Surgeon.* Son of Martin Gundersen Löfsgaard, civil servant, and Oliane Andersdatter Melby. Married Helga Sara Theresa Isaksaetre, September 18, 1893; eight children. EDUCATION: Studied medicine, University of Christiania (Oslo); 1882-89, interned, Bergen's Kuminale Sykhus (Community Hospital); 1890, M.D. "with commendation," University of Christiania; and resident surgeon, Rigshospitalet, Christiania; additional study: 1893, Berlin, Germany; and 1896, Vienna, Austria; and Berne, Switzerland. CAREER: 1891, to gain surgical experience and repay educational debts to a maternal uncle, immigrated to La Crosse, Wis., in Apr. and joined Dr. Christian Christensen as an assistant; 1892, became a partner and retained this position until the partnership dissolved in 1918; 1924, co-founded with three of his sons, the Gundersen Clinic, which became one of Wis.'s largest and most successful group practices; practiced, La Crosse, until shortly before his death, which occurred during a visit to Norway. CONTRIBUTIONS: Set new standards for surgical practice in western Wis. and reputedly performed the first appendectomy in the state (c. 1894). Established (1925) an exchange program that brought young Norwegian physicians to the Gundersen Clinic. One of the original preceptors for the University of Wisconsin Medical School. Delivered the opening address, Scandinavian Surgical Society meeting, Copenhagen (1905). Knighted by the king of Norway for his service to Norwegian physicians (1925). Member, University of Wisconsin Board of Regents (1925-31).

WRITINGS: "Appendicitis," *Norsk Magasin for Laegevidenskaben* (1898); "Spinal Anesthesia," *ibid.*, 90 (1929): 514-21. REFERENCES: *NCAB*, 30: 574; obituaries, *Norsk Magasin for Laegevidenskaben* 99 (1939): 1279-82; *Who Was Who in Am.*, 1: 495; *Wisconsin Med. J.* 37 (1938): 932-33.

H. B. Midelfort

GUNN, JOHN C. (June 22, 1800, Savannah, Ga.-October 22, 1863, Louisville, Ky.). *Physician; Author.* Son of Christopher, innkeeper and tavern operator, and Ann (Morinow) Gunn. The 1800 birthyear is inscribed on the tombstone in Cave Hill Cemetery, Louisville; other evidence indicates, however, that Gunn was born earlier, perhaps in 1795. Married Clarissa (maiden name unknown) before 1830; one child reached maturity. EDUCATION: Mercantile and Mathematical Academy, Savannah, Ga.; preceptorship under a Va. physician; no evidence that he ever attended medical lectures or received an M.D.; probably was largely self-taught. CAREER: 1816-27, left Savannah and traveled along East Coast to N.Y. and then settled in Va., where he did a preceptorship and practiced medicine, Montgomery and Botetourt counties; 1827-38, practiced medicine, East Tenn., mainly in Knoxville; 1830, published the first edition of his popular domestic medicine; thereafter, largely abandoned the practice of medicine and devoted himself to selling and revising his book; 1838-63, lived in Louisville. CONTRIBUTIONS: Author of one of the most popular of the nineteenth-century domestic medical works. Book sold so well that by 1839 Gunn could state, "the astonishing number of *one hundred thousand copies have been sold.*" The number of "editions" multiplied rapidly, the 234th edition published in New York City (1920). Gunn's diagnostic and therapeutic principles were not greatly different from those of regular practitioners of his day. Quoted extensively from the leading works of prominent European and American physicians. Gunn's book also became the basic textbook for the largely self-taught medical practitioners of the frontier.

WRITINGS: *Gunn's Domestic Medicine, or Poor Man's Friend, in the Hours of Affliction, Pain, and Sickness.* By 1857 the title had become *Gunn's New Domestic Physician: or Home Book of Health, a Complete Guide for Families.* . . . REFERENCES: Compiled from newspapers, census reports, city directories, court records, and other sources.

S. R. Bruesch

GUNN, MOSES (April 20, 1822, East Bloomfield, N.Y.-November 4, 1887, Ann Arbor, Mich.). *Surgeon; Medical education.* Son of Linus, farmer, and Esther (Bronson) Gunn. Married Jane Augusta Terry, 1848; four children. EDUCATION: East Bloomfield (N.Y.) Academy; studied medicine with Edson Carr, Canandaigua, N.Y.; 1846, M.D., Geneva (N.Y.) Medical College; 1849-50, studied in N.Y. and Pa. hospitals. CAREER: 1846-49, private lecturer in anatomy, Ann Arbor, Mich.; at University of Michigan medical department: 1849-54, founding professor of anatomy; 1854-67, professor of surgery; and 1858-59, dean; 1857-60, co-editor, *Peninsular and Independent Medical Journal;* 1861-62, surgeon, Fifth Michigan Infantry; 1867-87, chairman, Department of Surgery, Rush Medical College (Chicago, Ill.); 1885, president, American Surgical Association. CONTRIBUTIONS: Delivered the first anatomy lectures in Mich. A founder and leader of the early faculty, University of Michigan medical department. Major surgical contribution was to devise an improved procedure for reducing shoulder and hip dislocations, based on his anatomical observations of the role of untorn capsule portions in such dislocations.

WRITINGS: *Luxations of the Hip and Shoulder Joints, and the Agents Which Oppose Their Reduction* (1859). REFERENCES: C. B. Burr, *Medical History of Michigan* 1 (1930): 463-64; Jane Augusta Gunn, *Memorial Sketches of Dr. Moses Gunn, by His Wife* (1889); Martin Kaufman, *American Medical Education: The Formative Years* (1976), 105-6; Kelly and Burrage (1928), 510; *NCAB,* 12: 423; Wilfred B. Shaw, *The University of Michigan: An Encyclopedic Survey* (1951), pt. 5.

M. Pernick

GUTHRIE, SAMUEL (1782, Brimfield, Mass.-October 19, 1848, Sacketts Harbor, N.Y.). *Physician; chemist; Industrial chemistry.* Son of Samuel, physician, and Sarah Guthrie. Married Sybil Sexton, 1804; four children. EDUCA-TION: Studied medicine with father; 1810-11, College of Physicians and Surgeons (Columbia); 1815, University of Pennsylvania. CAREER: 1802-11, practiced medicine, Smyrna, N.Y.; 1811, moved to Sherburne, N.Y.; during War of 1812, examination surgeon; after war, resumed medical practice; *post* 1817, moved to Sacketts Harbor, where he engaged in farming, medicine, and industrial chemistry; best known to contemporaries for his manufacture of the first successful priming powder and the punch lock that exploded it. CONTRIBUTIONS: Discovered chloroform while attempting to produce chloric ether by distilling chloride of lime with alcohol. Devised a method for the rapid conversion of potato starch to molasses.

WRITINGS: "New Mode of Preparing a Spiritous Solution of Chloric Ether," *Am. J. of Sci.* 21 (1832): 64-65; "On Pure Chloric Ether," *ibid.*, 21 (1832): 105-6. Most important writings reproduced in Jesse R. Pawling, *Dr. Samuel Guthrie: Discoverer of Chloroform, Manufacturer of Percussion Pellets, Industrial Chemist* (1947). REFERENCES: *DAB*, 8: 62; Clark Elliott, *Biographical Dict. of Am. Sci.* (1979), 111-12; Kelly and Burrage (1928), 511-12; *NCAB* 11: 406; *Who Was Who in Am.*, Hist. Vol.: 293.

S. Galishoff

H

HAGGARD, WILLIAM DAVID, JR. (September 28, 1872, Nashville, Tenn.-January 28, 1940, Palm Beach, Fla.). *Surgeon.* Son of William David, surgeon, and Jane (Douglass) Haggard. Married Mary Laura Champe, 1899, no children; Lucile Holman, 1926, two children. EDUCATION: 1893, M.D., University of Tennessee, Nashville. CAREER: 1893-1925, surgeon, St. Thomas Hospital, Nashville; at University of Tennessee, Nashville: 1896-1900, assistant professor of gynecology; and 1900-1911, professor of gynecology and abdominal surgery; 1911-38, professor of clinical surgery, Vanderbilt; in American Medical Association: 1912-21, Council on Medical Education, 1916-17, chairman, Surgical Section; and 1925-26, president; at American College of Surgeons: 1913-20, regent, and 1933-34, president; in Southern Surgical Association: 1903-16, secretary; and 1917, president; 1914-15, president, Tennessee Medical Association; 1918-19, surgeon, Evacuation Hospital #1, Toul, France. CONTRIBUTIONS: Surgeon and scientist, an investigator on clinical subjects, especially the abdominal and pelvic region of the body. Originated the concept of the periodic health examination. Wrote, "Prevention runs a thread of gold through the fabric of medicine" (1924). Provided outstanding leadership in medicine, including the presidency of AMA and American College of Surgeons. Excelled in undergraduate teaching of medical students, and such activity gave him great pleasure.

WRITINGS: More than 150 papers, beginning in 1908; *The Romance of Medicine and Other Addresses* (1927); *Surgery, Queen of the Arts and Other Papers and Addresses* (1935). REFERENCES: Morris Fishbein, *A History of the American Medical Association, 1847 to 1947* (1947), 766-68; *J. Tenn. Med. Assoc.* 33 (1940): 68-70, 84-85; *NCAB*, 33: 87; obituary notice, *JAMA* 114 (1941): 428; *Who Was Who in Am.*, 1: 500.

S. R. Bruesch

HAIGHT, CAMERON (September 2, 1901, San Francisco, Calif.-September 25, 1970, Ann Arbor, Mich.). *Surgeon; Thoracic surgery.* Son of Louis Montrose, physician, and Minnie (Schuler) Haight. Married Isabel Hubbard, 1936;

two children. EDUCATION: 1923, A.B., University of California; 1926, M.D., Harvard University; 1926-28, surgical intern, Peter Bent Brigham Hospital; 1928-31, assistant resident surgeon, New Haven Hospital. CAREER: 1931-70, surgical faculty, University of Michigan, including 1950-70, professor of surgery; 1952-54, chairman, American Board of Thoracic Surgery; 1956-57, president, American Association of Thoracic Surgeons. CONTRIBUTIONS: First American, second in the world, to remove an entire lung successfully (1932). First to repair congenital tracheal-esophageal fistula, by primary anastomosis (1941). Pioneered transnasal tracheo-bronchial aspiration (1940). A founder of the thoracic surgery board (1949).

WRITINGS: "Total Removal of Left Lung for Bronchiectasis," *Surg. Gyn. & Obst.* 58 (1934): 768-80; "Congenital Atresia of the Esophagus with Tracheoesophageal Fistula," *ibid.*, 76 (1943): 672-88 (with H. A. Towsley). Writings listed in Lyman A. Brewer III, *Cameron Haight: Personal Recollections* (1977). REFERENCES: *Am. Men of Med.* (1961), 277; Lyman A. Brewer III, *Cameron Haight: Personal Recollections* (1977); *Michigan Med.* 69 (1970): 1039; *Who Was Who in Am.*, 5: 297.

M. Pernick

HALE, JOHN HENRY (June 5, 1878 [or 1879, 1882, or 1885], Estill Springs, Tenn.-March 27, 1944, Nashville, Tenn.). *Surgeon; Medical educator.* Son of Aaron and Emma (Gray) Hale. Married Millie E. Gibson (d. 1930), c. 1904, three children; Carrie Jordan, no children. EDUCATION: 1903, A.B., Walden University (Nashville); 1905, M.D., Meharry Medical College; postgraduate courses, Mayo Clinic (Rochester, Minn.) and Crile Clinic (Cleveland, Ohio). CAREER: 1905-44, private practice, Nashville; 1905-44, member, Meharry Medical College faculty, and staff of George W. Hubbard Hospital, beginning as instructor in histology (1905-11), becoming chief of hospital surgical staff (1923), professor of surgery (1931), and chairman of surgery department (1938). CONTRIBUTIONS: Strong figure in development of Meharry Medical College in a transitional period as founder George Whipple Hubbard (q.v.), and his generation of faculty passed on (1910s-20s). Co-founded Millie E. Hale Hospital (1916) and served as its surgeon-in-chief (1916-38). Medical advisor and head, Student Health Service, Tennessee Agricultural and Industrial State College, for 33 years. President, NMA (1935). Involved in local charitable and civic work for betterment of blacks. REFERENCES: W. Montague Cobb, "[John Henry Hale, M.D.]," *JNMA* 46 (1954): 79-80; obituary, *ibid.*, 36 (1944): 130-31; *WWAPS* 1 (1938): 486; *WWCR* 1 (1915): 127.

T. Savitt

HALL, GEORGE CLEVELAND (February 22, 1864, Ypsilanti, Mich.-June 17, 1930, Chicago, Ill.). *Surgeon.* Son of John Ward and Romelia (also given as Emiline or Ameline) (Buck) Hall. Married Theodosia Brewer, 1894; two children. EDUCATION: 1886, A.B., Lincoln University, Pennsylvania; 1888, M.D., Bennett Medical College. CAREER: 1888-1930, practiced medicine and surgery,

Chicago; 1894-1930, on staff, Provident Hospital, Chicago, in gynecology and surgery. CONTRIBUTIONS: Leading black physician in Chicago (1900-1930) and prominent surgeon and leader of Provident Hospital staff. Had frequent disagreements with Dr. Daniel Hale Williams (q.v.), the established, nationally reputed black Chicago surgeon who had founded Provident Hospital (1891). Williams tried to destroy Hall's reputation, but Hall continued giving clinics throughout the country, teaching other black surgeons his ideas and techniques, and treating patients at Provident. As a member, Board of Trustees (1900-1930); chairman, Medical Advisory Board (1910-26); and chief of staff (1926-30), Provident Hospital, played a major role in the hospital's development and operation. Was deeply involved in humanitarian and fund-raising activities for the improvement of Chicago's blacks throughout his career. Founded Cook County Physicians' Association of Chicago. Organized and directed first postgraduate course, Provident Hospital (1918), beginning a program that became (1933) a national center for postgraduate training of black physicians.

WRITINGS: "Negro Hospitals," *Southern Workman* 39 (1910): 551. REFERENCES: John A. Kenney, *The Negro in Medicine* (1912): 20-21; John W. Lawlah, "George Cleveland Hall, 1864-1930, A Profile," *JNMA* 46 (1954): 207-10; "Some Chicagoans of Note," *The Crisis* 10 (1915): 241; *WWCR* 1 (1915): 128.

T. Savitt

HALL, G[RANVILLE] STANLEY (February 1, 1844, Ashfield, Mass.-April 24, 1924, Worcester, Mass.). *Psychologist*; *Philosopher*. Son of Granville Bascom, farmer, and Abigail (Beals) Hall. Married Cornelia Fisher, 1879 (d. 1890), two children; Florence E. Smith, 1899. EDUCATION: 1862-63, Williston Academy; 1867, A.B., Williams College; 1867-69, Union Theological Seminary; 1869-71, 1878-80, studied in Germany; 1878, Ph.D., Harvard University. CAREER: Taught: 1872-76, Antioch College; 1876-78, 1880-81, Harvard College; and 1882-88, Johns Hopkins University; 1888, accepted presidency, Clark University; remained there until retirement (1920). CONTRIBUTIONS: One of the major figures in the rise of psychology in the late nineteenth and early twentieth centuries. Established the *American Journal of Psychology* (1887). Founded American Psychological Association (1891) and served as its first president. A leader in the child study movement (1880s and 1890s), which served subsequently as the foundation for the progressive education movement. From Hall's work emerged a number of specialized fields, including child development, educational psychology, and psychological testing. Founding president, Clark University, which in its early days was a graduate university emphasizing scientific research and scholarship. Taught psychology and helped to train a generation of psychologists who in the early twentieth century transformed their discipline. A prolific writer of books and articles, played a key role in developing an awareness of the importance of childhood, adolescence, and sex, all of which he placed at the center of genetic or developmental psychology; integrated concepts of the life cycle from infancy to senescence and incorporated into his framework Freud's psychoanalytic theories. Organized the famous Clark Conference of 1909 that brought Freud to America for the first and only time and helped to stimulate discussions about psychoanalysis.

WRITINGS: *Adolescence*, 2 vols. (1904); *Youth, Its Education, Regimen and Hygiene* (1906); *Founders of Modern Psychology* (1912); *Jesus the Christ in the Light of Psychology*, 2 vols. (1917); *Morale* (1920); *Senescence* (1922); *Life and Confessions of a Psychologist* (1923). Writings listed in Louis N. Wilson, ed., "Bibliography of the Published Writings of G. Stanley Hall, 1866-1924," in "Granville Stanley Hall. In Memoriam," *Clark Univ. Library Publications* 7 (May 1925): 109-35, and Dorothy Ross, *G. Stanley Hall: The Psychologist as Prophet* (1972), 439-50. REFERENCES: *BHM* (1964-69), 115; (1970-74), 79; (1975-79), 56; *DAB*, 4, pt. 2: 127-30; Miller, *BHM*, p. 45; *NCAB*, 39: 469-70; Dorothy Ross, *G. Stanley Hall* (1972).

G. Grob

HALL, JAMES LOWELL (December 30, 1892, Waxahachie, Tex.-June 10, 1965, Chicago, Ill.). *Physician; Allergist.* Son of James Porter, schoolteacher and principal, and Josie (Briggs) Hall. Married Allie Mary Hughes, 1916; two children. EDUCATION: 1911, A.B., Prairie View College; 1923, B.S., University of Chicago; 1925, M.D., Rush Medical College; 1925-26, intern, Homer G. Phillips Hospital, St. Louis; postgraduate study: 1930-32, Allegemeine Krankenhaus, Vienna; and 1932, Billings Hospital of University of Chicago. CAREER: 1911-16, schoolteacher; 1926-41, general medical practice, Chicago; 1932-40, director of medical research laboratory, University of Chicago; 1936-41, director of clinics, Provident Hospital, Chicago; at Howard University Medical School: 1941-47, professor; and 1941-44, chairman, Department of Medicine; at Freedmen's Hospital, Washington, D.C.: 1941-44, medical director; and 1944-47, superintendent; 1947-65, private practice and hospital affiliations, Chicago. CONTRIBUTIONS: In addition to service to Provident and Freedmen's hospitals, where he also established allergy clinics, did research in allergic diseases, histamines, and vitamin deficiency diseases. Was among the first black physicians to obtain certification from American Board of Internal Medicine. Involved in antidiscrimination legislation for Chicago and Ill. hospitals. Worked 15 years with Selective Service Board of Ill. and with Illinois National Guard.

WRITINGS: "Effect of Histamine on Alkali Reserves and on Blood Sugar in Man," *Arch. of Int. Med.* 49 (1932): 799-807; "Major Allergic Diseases and Their Treatment," *JNMA* 34 (1942): 225-29; "Vitamin B-Complex Deficiencies," *ibid.*, 34 (1942): 91-98. REFERENCES: John W. Lawlah, "James Lowell Hall, Sr., M.D., 1892-1965," *JNMA* 58 (1966): 82-83; *NCAB*, 53: 137.

T. Savitt

HALL, JOSIAH NEWHALL (October 11, 1859, North Chelsea, Mass.-December 17, 1939, Denver, Colo.). *Physician.* Son of Stephen and Evalina (Newhall) Hall. Married Carrie Ayres, 1885; two children. EDUCATION: 1878, B.S., Massachusetts Agricultural College; 1882, M.D., Harvard University; 1882-83, house physician, Boston City Hospital. CAREER: 1883-92, practice, Sterling, Colo.; 1888-89, mayor, Sterling; 1891, president, Colorado State Board of Medical Examiners; 1892, moved to Denver; 1893-97, professor of materia medica, therapeutics, and clinical medicine, University of Colorado; 1897-1910, professor of medicine, Gross Medical College (later Denver & Gross); president: 1895, Denver Medical Society; 1900, Colorado Medical Society; 1903-4, Colorado State Board of Health; 1916, American Therapeutic Society; 1917-18, major, M.C., U.S. Army; chief of medical service, base hospital, Camp Logan, Tex. CONTRIBUTIONS: Widely known and respected as an able diagnostician. Medical interests were broad, with some special emphasis on gunshot wounds, about which he provided a section in Peterson and Haines's *Legal Medicine and Toxicology*. His *Borderline Diseases* (2 vols., 1915) is a comprehensive manual of medical diagnosis but not notably "with especial reference to its surgical bearings," as title and subtitle would suggest. His *Tales of Pioneer Practice* (1937) is interesting but undocumented.

WRITINGS: Some 140 of his papers are listed in *Medical Coloradoana* (1922). REFERENCES: Nolie Mumey, Preface, "An Ideal Physician," in J. N. Hall, *Reminiscences of Past Presidents of the Colorado State Medical Society* (1932), 7-9; *NCAB*, A: 206; *Who Was Who in Am.*, 1: 506.

F. B. Rogers

HALL, WILLIAM WHITTY (October 15, 1810, Paris, Ky.-May 10, 1876, New York, N.Y.). *Physician; Popular medicine.* Son of Stephen and Mary (Wooley) Hall. Married to Hannah Mattock, and then to Magdalen Matilda Robertson. EDUCATION: 1830, graduated from Centre College; 1836, M.D., Transylvania University; 1836, ordained in the Presbyterian ministry. CAREER: Did missionary work in Texas, 1837, but gradually abandoned preaching for medicine; practiced medicine in New Orleans and Cincinnati until 1851; practiced in New York City thereafter. CONTRIBUTIONS: Pioneer editor of popular health magazines and wrote extensively on hygiene and related subjects for laymen. 1854, began publication of *Hall's Journal of Health* and in 1875 began a new periodical, *Hall's Medical Adviser*. Wrote several works advising the general public on how to stay healthy, including *Health and Disease as Affected by Constipation and Health by Good Living* (1870), and *How to Live Long* (1875). Also wrote several books for physicians on ailments of the throat and lungs as well as two works in which he claimed to have found a cure for consumption.

WRITINGS: *Consumption a Curable Disease, Illustrated in the Treatment of 150 Cases* (1845); *Observations on the Curability of Consumption by a New, Safe and Painless Method, Illustrated in Selections of 350 Cases* (1847); *Bronchitis, Chronic Laryngitis, Clergyman's Sore Throat* (1848, 5 ed., with S. W. Hall); *The Nature, Cause, Symptoms and Cure of Diseases of the Throat and Lungs* (1850). REFERENCES:

DAB, 8: 147-48; Kelly and Burrage, (1928), 515; *NCAB*, 11: 437; *Who Was Who in Am.*, Hist. Vol.: 297.

S. Galishoff

HALSTED, WILLIAM STEWART (September 23, 1852, New York, N.Y.-September 7, 1922, Baltimore, Md.). *Surgeon.* Son of William Mills, businessman, and Mary Louisa (Haines) Halsted. Married Caroline Hampton, 1890; no children. EDUCATION: 1874, A.B., Yale University; 1877, M.D., College of Physicians and Surgeons of New York City; 1876-77, intern, Bellevue Hospital, New York City; 1877-78, house physician, New York Hospital; 1878-80, studied in Vienna, Austria, and Leipzig and Würzburg, Germany. CAREER: 1880-88, combined private practice in New York City with serving for varying periods as attending physician and attending surgeon, Charity Hospital, Blackwell's Island Hospital, Emigrants Hospital, Roosevelt Hospital, Bellevue Hospital, and Presbyterian Hospital; 1889-1922, professor of surgery and surgeon-in-chief, Johns Hopkins Medical School and Hospital. CONTRIBUTIONS: World-famous surgeon, clinical teacher, and member of Johns Hopkins "Big Four" who left an indelible impress upon an entire generation of American surgeons. Combined experimental work in physiology and pathology with innovative surgical techniques; originated procedure of "blood refusion" for carbonic oxide poisoning; pioneered the use of cocaine for local anesthesia and laid the foundations for neuroregional anesthesia; introduced a host of new surgical techniques and procedures for dealing with cancers, hernias, goitres, and aneurysms; early proponent of aseptic surgery; emphasized need for careful exacting procedures in operating room. Over and above skill and originality in surgery, made significant physiological and clinical studies of cancer, thyroid and parathyroids, blood vessels, and other subjects. Many contributions to surgery won him honorary memberships in leading scientific and medical societies throughout the world.

WRITINGS: Best known work is "The Training of the Surgeon," *Am. Med.* 7 (1904): 66-77. During his career, published 169 articles in various medical journals. In 1924 virtually all of them were collected and published under the editorship of Walter C. Burket, *Surgical Papers of William Stewart Halsted*, 2 vols. (1924). REFERENCES: A. J. Beckhard and W. D. Crane, *Cancer, Cocaine and Courage: The Story of Dr. William Halsted* (1960); *BHM* (1964-69), 116; (1970-74), 79; (1975-79), 56; (1980), 18; S. J. Crowe, *Halsted of Johns Hopkins* (1957); *DAB*, 8: 164-65; *DSB*, 6: 77-78; *JAMA* 79 (1922): 984; Kelly and Burrage (1928), 516-17; W. G. MacCallum, *William Stewart Halsted, Surgeon* (1930); Rudolph Matas (q.v.), "In Memoriam—William Stewart Halsted," *Johns Hopkins Hosp. Bull.* 36 (1925): 2-27; Miller, *BHM*, pp. 45-46; *NCAB*, 20: 209-10.

J. Duffy

HAMILTON, ALICE (February 27, 1869, New York, N.Y.-September 22, 1970, Hadlyme, Conn.). *Physician; Industrial medicine.* Daughter of Montgomery, wholesale grocer, and Gertrude (Pond) Hamilton. Never married. EDUCATION: 1893, M.D., University of Michigan; 1894-95, intern, Women's and

Children's Hospital (Minneapolis, Minn.) and Women's Hospital (Roxbury, Mass.); studied at: 1895-96, universities of Leipzig and Munich; 1896-97, Johns Hopkins; 1898-1900, University of Chicago; and 1903, Pasteur Institute. CAREER: 1897-1919, resident, Hull House, active in settlement work; 1897-1902, pathology faculty, Women's Medical College of Northwestern University; 1902-10, bacteriologist, McCormick Memorial Institute for Infectious Diseases; 1910, medical investigator, Illinois Occupational Disease Commission; 1910-21, investigator of industrial poisons, U.S. Department of Labor; 1919-35, industrial medicine faculty, Harvard Medical School; 1924-30, member, health committee, League of Nations; 1937-38, 1940, medical consultant, U.S. Department of Labor. CONTRIBUTIONS: Awakened interest in the hazards of industrial employment and was the nation's leading industrial toxicologist. Directed the investigations of the Illinois Occupational Disease Commission, which led that state to enact its first workmen's compensation law (1910). Made similar studies for the national government, which induced other states to make investigations of their own and resulted in the adoption of preventive measures in factories. Investigated industrial toxicology in many dangerous industries, including lead, mining, munitions, painting, printing, and rayon. Helped start the *Journal of Industrial Hygiene* and played an active role in its direction for many years.

WRITINGS: *Industrial Poisons in the United States* (1925); *Industrial Toxicology* (1935); *Exploring the Dangerous Trades; An Autobiography* (1943). Main writings listed in W. R. Slaight, "Alice Hamilton: First Lady of Industrial Medicine" (Ph.D. diss., Case Western Reserve University, 1974). REFERENCES: *BHM* (1964-69), 116; (1970-74), 79; (1976), 15; *Current Biog.* (1946), 234-36; May R. Mayers, "Alice Hamilton," *J. Occupational Med.* 14 (Feb. 1972): 102-4; Miller, *BHM*, p. 46; *NCAB*, G: 107-8; *Who Was Who in Am.*, 5: 301.

S. Galishoff

HAMILTON, JOHN BROWN (December 1, 1847, Jersey County, Ill.-December 24, 1898, Elgin, Ill.). *Surgeon; Medical administrator*. Son of Benjamin Brown, clergyman, and Martha Hamilton. Married Mary L. Frost, 1871; two children. EDUCATION: 1869, M.D., Rush Medical College (Chicago, Ill.). CAREER: 1869-74, practiced medicine, Kane, Ill.; 1874-76, surgeon, U.S. Army; in U.S. Marine Hospital Service: 1876-79, 1891-96, surgeon; and 1879-91, surgeon-general; 1883-91, surgery faculty, Georgetown University; 1883-c. 1891, surgical staff, Providence Hospital; 1892-98, surgery faculty, Rush Medical College; 1892-98, surgical staff, various Chicago medical institutions; 1896-97, superintendent, Illinois Northern (Elgin) Hospital for the Insane. CONTRIBUTIONS: Raised the status of the U.S. Marine Hospital Service while he plotted to destroy the short-lived National Board of Health (1879-83). Induced Congress to place the Marine Hospital Service on an equal footing with the medical corps of the army and navy. Established the National Laboratory of Hygiene, a bacteriological laboratory devoted to research on communicable diseases, (later to become the National Institutes of Health) within the Marine Hospital Service (1887). Re-

garded the fledgling National Board of Health as a rival to the Marine Hospital
Service and with the help of states rights advocates succeeded in getting Congress
to end the board's quarantine powers, thereby destroying it. Introduced modern
procedures for herniotomy in Chicago. Edited the *Journal of the American
Medical Association* (1893-98). American editor of *Moulin's Surgery* (1893).

WRITINGS: "On the Radical Cure of Inguinal Hernia: a Review of the Existing Status
of the Operation with Remarks on Its Past History," *JAMA* 7 (1886): 256-62. A nearly
complete list of Hamilton's writings is in *Index Catalogue*. REFERENCES: Bess Furman,
A Profile of the United States Public Health Service, 1798-1948 (1973), 151-98; Kelly
and Burrage (1928), 520; *NCAB*, 23: 245-46; Wilson Smillie, *Public Health, Its Promise
for the Future* (1973), 151-98.

S. Galishoff

HAMMOND, WILLIAM ALEXANDER (August 28, 1828, Annapolis, Md.-
January 5, 1900, Washington, D.C.). *Physician; Army medical officer.* Son of
John W., physician, and Sarah (Pinckney) Hammond. Married Helen Nisbet,
1849, two children; Esther Chapin, 1888. EDUCATION: Private tutors; St. Johns
College; 1848, M.D., Medical College of the City of New York; 1849, internship, Pennsylvania Hospital. CAREER: Private practice, Maine; 1849, entered
active duty, U.S. Army Medical Corps, as assistant surgeon; served in N. Mex.
in Indian campaigns, in Fla. and at West Point, and at Fort Riley in the Sioux
campaign; 1860, resigned; appointed professor of anatomy and physiology, University of Maryland Medical School; 1861, re-entered army as first lieutenant;
1862, appointed brigadier general and surgeon-general; 1864, disagreements with
Secretary of War Edwin Stanton led to dismissal by court-martial (reversed by
act of Congress on basis of perjury and lack of evidence in 1878); 1866-88,
practice of neurology, New York City; lecturer, nervous and mental diseases:
1866, College of Physicians and Surgeons; and 1867-74, Bellevue Hospital
Medical College; 1874-88, professor, University of City of New York; 1880, a
founder and professor, Post-Graduate Medical School of New York; 1888-1900,
practice, Washington, D.C.; 1889, founded Washington Sanitarium. CONTRI-
BUTIONS: An early physiological scientist, while in army (1849-60), published
with S. W. Mitchell (q.v.) and won research gold medal of AMA for work on
curare and in nutrition. Became Surgeon General with support of U. S. Sanitary
Commission. Reformed medical supply, organization, and staffing during his
17 months as Surgeon General. Strong supporter of Jonathan Letterman (q.v.).
Founded Army Medical Museum (1862) and started work on *Medical and Surgical History*. A leading founder and developer of neurology as a specialty in
this country; his *Treatise* (1871) was the first American textbook in the field. A
prolific writer, including novels and a play as well as textbooks, monographs,
and more than 300 journal articles. His *Treatise* went through eight editions.
First to describe athetosis (1871) or "Hammond's Disease." Founded and/or
edited four journals. Member of many professional societies and president (1883),
American Neurological Association. Made early contributions to work in aphasia,

insomnia, and forensic medicine. A contentious personality, was involved in controversy throughout his career on psychiatry, psychology, hypnotism, animal extract therapy, spiritualism, and women's rights. May be fairly credited with early leadership in clinical research in neurology in America.

WRITINGS: *Physiological Memoirs* (1863); *Military Medical and Surgical Essays* (1864, editor); *Sleep and Its Derangements* (1869); *Treatise on Diseases of the Nervous System* (1871); *Sexual Impotence in the Male and Female* (1887). Writings listed in the *Index Catalogue* and *Index Medicus*. REFERENCES: American Neurological Association, *Semicentennial Anniversary Volume* (1924); BHM (1964-69), 116; (1970-74), 79-80; (1975-79), 56; (1980), 18; Bonnie E. Blustein, "A New York Medical Man: William A. Hammond" (Ph.D. diss., University of Pennsylvania, 1979); *DAB*, 4, pt. 2: 210-11; Jack D. Key, *William Alexander Hammond* (1979); Miller, *BHM*, p. 47; *NCAB*, 26: 468; James M. Phalen, "Chiefs of the Medical Department," *Army Med. Bull.*, no. 52 (Apr. 1940); Joel M. Wileutz, *William Alexander Hammond: Surgeon General* (1964).

R. J. T. Joy

HANDY, JOHN CHARLES (October 20, 1844, Newark, N.J.-September 25, 1891, Tucson, Ariz.). *Physician; Public health*. Married Mary Page; four children. Shot and killed by wife's attorney in divorce action. EDUCATION: Public schools of Calif., where family moved when he was nine years old; 1864, M.D., Cooper Medical College, San Francisco, Calif. CAREER: 1865-66, contract surgeon, U.S. Army, Calif.; 1869-71, at forts Apache, Thomas, and Grant, Ariz.; 1871-91, private practice, Tucson; in later years, chief surgeon for Southern Pacific Railroad. CONTRIBUTIONS: City and county physician and city health officer. Member, County Board of Supervisors. Campaigned to promote better sanitation and for licensing of physicians. A founder, University of Arizona. REFERENCES: *Arizona Star* (Tucson), October 2, 1932; *Arizona Weekly Citizen* (Tucson), September 26, 1891; "The History of Medicine in Arizona," *Arizona Med.* (Dec. 1956); Frances E. Quebbeman, *Medicine in Territorial Arizona* (1966).

J. Goff

HARALSON, HUGH HARDIN (March 10, 1854, Wetumpka, Ala.-November 18, 1939, Vicksburg, Miss.). *Physician; Editor*. Son of Isaac C. and Jane (Hardin) Haralson. Married Belle Lack, 1878; Jane Stein Coats; seven children. EDUCATION: Cooper Institute, Lauderdale County, Miss.; 1883, M.D., Tulane University Medical School. CAREER: 1877, entered drug business and began study of medicine in Harperville, Miss.; 1883, medical practice, Harperville; 1891-96, practiced medicine, Forest, Miss.; 1891-96, health officer, Scott County; 1895-96, president, Mississippi State Medical Association; moved practice to: 1896, Biloxi, Miss.; and 1898, Vicksburg; 1892-1904, member: Mississippi State Board of Health; staff of visiting physicians, Vicksburg Charity Hospital; and Board of Directors, visiting physician and surgeon, Vicksburg Infirmary. CONTRIBUTIONS: Editor and proprietor, *Mississippi Medical Monthly*, which appeared in Meridian, Miss. (1891). Began publication of the *Medical Record of Mississippi* (1897). Each publication indicated that it was the official organ of the Mississippi State Medical Association. Recognized as one of the most able physicians and surgeons of Miss.

WRITINGS: Numerous articles in his own publications. REFERENCES: Dunbar Rowland, ed., *Mississippi: Comprising Sketches of Counties, Events, Institutions, and Persons Arranged in Cyclopedic Form* (1907): 3: 317-18; James G. Thompson, *History of the Mississippi State Medical Association* (1949), p. 76.

M. S. Legan

HARE, LYLE (November 26, 1885, Cedar Rapids, Nebr.-October 31, 1975, Spearfish, S. Dak.). *Physician; General practice.* Son of Joseph, farmer and newspaper publisher, and Louisa (McFee) Hare. Married Edna Stone, 1911 (d. 1918), one child; Hazel Buckman, 1925, three children. EDUCATION: 1907, State Normal School, Spearfish; 1909, University of South Dakota School of Medicine; 1911, M.D., University of Illinois College of Physicians and Surgeons of Chicago; University Hospital of Illinois, one year. CAREER: Taught physiology and hygiene, State Normal School, Spearfish; practiced medicine, Spearfish; physician, Homestake Mining Company; 1917-18, U.S. Army Medical Corps, stationed in Vichy, France; 1920-24, mayor, Spearfish. CONTRIBUTIONS: Leading physician in western S. Dak. First graduate, University of South Dakota's two-year medical program. Received many honors and awards for distinguished service. REFERENCES: Helen Jane Hare, "First Graduate—USD School of Medicine, Lyle Hare, M.D. Family Practitioner," *South Dakota J. of Med.* 34, no. 5 (May 1981): 70-71; Doane Robinson, *History of South Dakota* 1 (1904): 416-17.

D. W. Boilard and P. W. Brennen

HARGIS, ROBERT BELL SMITH (June 7, 1818, Hillsboro, N.C.-Nov. 30, 1893, Pensacola, Fla.). *Physician; General practice.* Son of Thomas N. L. Hargis. Married Modeste Sierra, November 23, 1854; seven children. EDUCATION: Student, University of North Carolina; read medicine for three years under Dr. T. J. Jordan, Fayetteville, N.C.; 1841, M.D., Medical College of Louisiana, New Orleans, La. (now Tulane University Medical School). CAREER: Practice: 1841-51, Mobile and Mt. Pleasant, Ala., interrupted by periods of poor health; and 1851-61, Pensacola; surgeon: 1861-65, Confederate States of America, 17th Alabama Infantry Regiment, field and hospital service; and 1865-93, Pensacola; 1851-54, health officer, Pensacola; 1854-61, surgeon, U.S. Marine Hospital; 1856, established private infirmary near Marine Hospital, in partnership with Dr. John Whiting; 1882, president, Florida Medical Association; appointed to National Board of Public Health; 1885, Fla.'s delegate to Gulf States Quarantine Convention, New Orleans. CONTRIBUTIONS: Fla.'s most prolific writer on medical subjects. Careful observations on the various fevers common to the area established him as a foremost authority on the care of fever victims, especially those suffering from yellow fever. Held tenaciously to the theory that yellow fever was imported into Fla., in support of which he wrote a lengthy article and an 80-page monograph, "The Ship Origin of Yellow Fever." Although he wrote on "Malaria and the Relation of Micro-Organisms to Disease" (1884), did not fully comprehend the implications of the work of Sir Patrick Manson, C. J. Finlay, and others on insect vectors.

WRITINGS: "Communicability of Yellow Fever," *New Orleans Med. News and Hosp. Gazette* (1859); "Muriated Tincture of Iron—A Specific of Erysipelas," *Am. Med. Bi-Weekly* (1860); "The Genius of Medicine," *New Orleans Med. and Surg. J.* (1882); important paper read before the American Public Health Association, "History and Origin of Yellow Fever, Its Cause, Communicability and Prevention" (1879). REFERENCES: *Daily News* (Pensacola), December 1, 1893; R. P. Rerick, *Memoirs of Florida*, 1 (1902): 561-62; *Proc., Fla. Med. Assoc.* (1878-84); Kelly and Burrage (1920), 491; Elizabeth Dwyer Vickers and F. Norman Vickers, M.D., "Notations on Pensacola's Medical History," *J. Fla. Med. Assoc.* (Jan. 1974): 83-105.

E. A. Hammond

HARGRAVE, FRANK SETTLE (August 27, 1874, Lexington, N.C.- March 11, 1942, Orange, N.J.). *Physician; Pulmonary medicine.* Son of Henry M. and Laura Hargrave. Married Bessie E. Parker, 1907. EDUCATION: B.S., Shaw University; 1901, M.D., Leonard Medical College (N.C.). CAREER: Private practice: 1901-3, Winston-Salem, N.C.; 1903-24, Wilson, N.C.; and 1924-42, Orange. CONTRIBUTIONS: Founder (1913) and medical director, Wilson Tuberculosis Hospital (1913-23), which later became Mercy Hospital (Wilson). Served NMA as president (1915), member of Executive Committee, and chair, Committee on Medical Education and Hospitals. Active in New Jersey Tuberculosis League and in local and state medical societies. Served New Jersey and Orange as assemblyman nine times (beginning in 1929) and as activist in economic, educational, and social problems. Author of a bill creating Migrant Welfare Commission, on which he served by governor's appointment. REFERENCES: "Dr. Frank S. Hargrave, An Assemblyman," *JNMA* 21 (1929): 165-66; obituary, *ibid.*, 34 (Jul. 1942): 174; "Our New President," *ibid.*, 6 (1914): 238-39; *WWICA* 5 (1938-40): 230.

T. Savitt

HARISON, BEVERLY DRAKE (May 8, 1855, Canton, N.Y.-December 6, 1924, Battle Creek, Mich.). *Physician; Medical legislation.* Son of Minturn and Susan (Drake) Harison. Married Josephine Lister, 1889; one child. EDUCATION: Bishops College School (Lennoxville, Quebec, Canada) and Trinity College, Toronto, Ontario, Canada; studied medicine with James Thorburn; University of Toronto: 1882, M.B.; and 1901, M.D. CAREER: 1882-85, general practice with Charles H. Bonnell, Toronto; 1885-88, surgeon, Ontario lumber company; 1888-1906, medical practice, Sault Ste. Marie, Mich.; 1896, founder, Upper Michigan Medical Society; president, State Hospital, Newberry, Mich.; 1899-1924, founding secretary, Michigan State Board of Registration in Medicine; 1905, president, Michigan State Medical Society; 1906-24, medico-legal practice, Detroit, Mich.; 1912, founding secretary, American Confederation of Reciprocating State Medical Boards; 1917-18, captain, Army Medical Corps. CONTRIBUTIONS: "Father of medical license legislation" in Mich. Wrote the legislation creating the State Board of Registration in Medicine. Nationally, pioneered the reciprocal recognition of licenses by states with similar license requirements.

WRITINGS: "Medical Reciprocity, or Interstate Exchange of Licensures," *Med. Record* (N.Y.) 62 (1902): 522-26. REFERENCES: C. M. Burton, *City of Detroit* 4 (1922): 354-58; *Detroit Evening News: Men of Progress* (1900), 397; *JAMA* 83 (1924): 1940; Kelly and Burrage (1928), 527; A. N. Marquis, *Book of Detroiters* (1908), 209-10; Michigan State Med. Soc., *J.* 24 (1925): 73; *Who Was Who in Am.*, 1: 519-20.

M. Pernick

HARKINS, HENRY NELSON (July 13, 1905, Missoula, Mont.-August 12, 1967, Seattle, Wash.). *Physician; Surgery.* Son of William Draper, educator, and Anna Louise (Hatheway) Harkins. Married Jean Hamilton Trester, 1937; four children. EDUCATION: University of Chicago: 1925, B.S.; 1926, M.S.; and 1928, Ph.D.; 1930, M.D., Rush Medical College; 1930-31, intern, Presbyterian Hospital; 1931, postgraduate work, University of Edinburgh, and National Hospital, London; 1931-38, residency in surgery, University of Chicago Hospital; 1938-39, Guggenheim Memorial Fellow in Surgery: University of Edinburgh; University of Ghent, Belgium; University of Frankfurt-am-Main, Germany; and University of Uppsala, Sweden. CAREER: 1939-43, surgical staff, Henry Ford Hospital, Detroit, Mich.; surgery faculty: 1943, Wayne University College of Medicine; and 1943-47, Johns Hopkins Medical School; and surgical staff, Johns Hopkins Hospital; 1943-45, secretary, subcommittee on shock, Office of Science, Research and Development, National Research Council; 1947-64, surgery faculty and first department chairman, University of Washington; surgical staff, King County Hospital; and, later, University of Washington Hospital; 1960-65, member, hematological study section; 1951-67, consultant, Veterans Administration hospitals, Seattle and Spokane, Wash.; guest lecturer and visiting professor at many American and foreign universities. CONTRIBUTIONS: Aided the development of surgery through his research, teaching, and editing. Made numerous experimental studies of gastric physiology and related subjects and developed new methods for the surgical treatment of peptic ulcer and hernia. Established and developed an excellent Department of Surgery, University of Washington. Author and co-editor of several surgical textbooks, including *The Treatment of Burns* (1942), *Surgery: Principles and Practice* (1957, with others), and *Surgery of the Stomach and Duodenum* (1962, with Lloyd M. Nyhus). Managing editor, *Johns Hopkins Hospital Bulletin* (1944-47); editor-in-chief, *Quarterly Review of Surgery* (later *Review of Surgery*) (1943 until his death); and served on the editorial boards of *Annals of Surgery* and *Western Journal of Surgery* (later *Pacific Medicine and Surgery*) (beginning in 1948).

WRITINGS: "The Present Status of Blood Examination in the Diagnosis of Surgical Infections, with a Study of Twenty-Seven Indices of Infection Reported in the Literature," *Surg. Gyn. & Obst.* 59 (Jul. 1934): 48-61; "A Cooper's Ligament Herniotomy," *Surgical Clinics of North Am.* 23 (Oct. 1943): 1279-97 (with S. A. Swenson); "The Billroth I

Gastric Resection: Experimental Studies and Clinical Observation on 291 Cases," *Trans., Am. Surg. Assoc.* 72 (1954): 145-64 (with Horace G. Moore, Jr., et al.); *Hernia* (1964, editor, with Lloyd M. Nyhus). REFERENCES: K. Alvin Merendino, "Henry Nelson Harkins," *Trans., Am. Surg. Assoc.* 85 (1967): 412-16; *NCAB*, 54: 185-86; Mark M. Ravitch, *A Century of Surgery*, 2 vols. (1981); *Who Was Who in Am.*, 4: 406.

S. Galishoff

HARPER, CORNELIUS ALLEN (February 20, 1864, Hazel Green, Wis.- June 26, 1951, Madison, Wis.). *Physician; Public health.* Son of Moses Allen, farmer, and Hester (Lewis) Harper. Married Elizabeth L. Bowman, 1901; two children. EDUCATION: 1889, B.S., University of Wisconsin; 1893, M.D., Columbian (later George Washington) University, Washington, D.C.; 1893-94, postgraduate work, Howard University, Washington, D.C. CAREER: 1884-85, taught rural schools, Wis.; 1889-90, high school principal, Cassville, Wis., schools; *post* 1894, practiced medicine, Madison; 1901, appointed member, Wisconsin State Board of Health; 1904-43, secretary, Wisconsin State Board of Health, and state health officer; 1943-48, specialist advisor, Wisconsin State Board of Health; 1903, member, Wisconsin Tuberculosis Commission, to select a site and erect the first State Tuberculosis Sanatorium in Wis.; 1908-9, president, State and Provincial Health Officers of North America; 1911, served in State Assembly representing Madison; 1930-31, president, Wisconsin State Medical Society; director, Wisconsin Anti-Tuberculosis Association, and fellow, American Public Health Association. CONTRIBUTIONS: Instrumental in transferring vital statistics from the Wis. secretary of state's office to the Board of Health and in the passage of a uniform vital statistic law, which he called "the bookkeeping of public health." One of the first in the state to use diphtheria antitoxin, a strong advocate of the prevention and eradication of diphtheria and typhoid fever and a key figure in Wis.'s war on tuberculosis. Led physicians, the public, and the legislature in a rapidly expanding disease-prevention program; was instrumental in establishing nurses registration laws; licensing plumbers, barbers, and restaurants; creating the bureaus of Sanitary Engineering and Maternal and Child Health.

WRITINGS: Wrote for and edited the State Board of Health Reports. Author of pamphlets on various diseases and health procedures. "History of the Wisconsin State Board of Health," MS., Archives, Wisconsin State Historical Society, Madison. REFERENCES: Cornelius A. Harper Papers, Archives, State of Wisconsin Historical Society Library, Madison; *Coronet*, 25 (Apr. 1949); 106-12; The State Historical Society of Wisconsin, *Dict. of Wisconsin Biog.* (1960), 158-59; *JAMA*, 147 (1951): 334; *N. Y. Times*, June 28, 1951; *Thirty Second Report of the State Board of Health of Wisconsin*, July 1, 1926-June 30, 1928 (1928), 560; Ellis Baker Usher, *Wisconsin: Its Story and Biography, 1848-1913* (1914) 5: 1333-34; *Who's Important in Med.* 5, 1st ed. (1945), 1022; *Who's Who in Am.* 25 (1948): 1044; *Who's Who in Am. Med.* (1925), 643; *WWAPS*, pp. 504-5.

M. Van H. Jones

HARRIS, CHAPIN AARON (May 6, 1806, Pompey, N.Y.-September 29, 1860, Baltimore, Md.). *Dentist; Educator.* Son of John and Elizabeth (Brundage)

Harris. Married Lucinda Heath Hawley, January 11, 1826; nine children. ED-UCATION: N.Y. public schools; 1824-26, studied medicine under his brother John, Madison, Ohio, after which he obtained license to practice medicine from the Board of Medical Censors of Ohio; 1833, following John's lead, studied dentistry and was licensed by the Medical and Surgical Faculty of Maryland; M.A., University of Maryland; 1838, M.D., Washington Medical College, Baltimore; 1854, D.D.S., Philadelphia Dental College; one historian has written, however, that Harris "purchased college degrees from a diploma mill in Illinois," thus casting doubt on the legitimacy of some of his scholastic distinctions. CAREER: 1827-28, private medical practice, Greenfield, Ohio; 1828, began dental practice, Greenfield; 1831-39, dental practice, Baltimore, Richmond, Va., and other southern cities; 1833, shared dental practice with his uncle James H. Harris, Baltimore; summers of 1833, and 1834, practiced dentistry with F. B. Chewning, Richmond; 1835, established himself permanently in Baltimore; 1839-60, editor, *American Journal of Dental Science*; 1839-60, independent dental practice, Baltimore; 1840-41, dean, Baltimore College of Dental Surgery; 1844, succeeded Horace H. Hayden (q.v.), as president, Baltimore College of Dental Surgery and American Society of Dental Surgeons; 1852, became member, AMA; president: 1856, American Dental Association; and 1856-57, American Dental Convention; on faculty, Baltimore College of Dental Surgery: professor of the principles and practice of dental science; chair, principles and practice of dental surgery; professor of practical dentistry and dental pathology; and professor of operative dentistry and dental prosthesis; first corresponding secretary, American Society of Dental Surgeons; member, Medical and Chirurgical Faculty of Maryland and Western Academy of Natural Sciences. CONTRIBUTIONS: With the help of some N.Y. dentists, founded (1839) the *American Journal of Dental Science* (first dental periodical in the world). With Hayden, established (1840) the Baltimore College of Dental Surgery (the first dental college in the world) after he failed to convince the University of Maryland to open a dental department. Again with Hayden, organized (1840) the American Society of Dental Surgeons (the first national dental association). Organizer, the American Dental Convention (1855).

WRITINGS: *The Dental Art, A Practical Treatise on Dental Surgery* (1839), appeared thereafter as *Principles and Practice of Dental Surgery*, 13 eds. (through 1896); *Dictionary of Dental Science, Biography and Medical Terminology* (1849), thereafter, *A Dictionary of Medical Terminology, Dental Surgery and the Collateral Sciences*, 6 eds. (through 1896), with every ed. after the third being revised and enlarged by F. J. S. Gorgas. Revised and enlarged Joseph Fox's *Diseases of the Human Teeth* . . . , 3rd Eng. ed., lst Am. ed. (1846). Writings listed in *DAB*, 8: 305-6; *Index Catalogue*, 1st series, 4: 854; 2nd series, 6: 759-60; 3rd series, 6: 445; and 4th series, 7: 87. REFERENCES: George H. Callcott, *History of the University of Maryland* (1982), 83-91; "A Chapter in Early Dental History," *Ohio Archaeological and Hist. Q.* 35 (Apr. 1926): 389-97, 400-401; *DAB*, 8: 305-6; *Index Catalogue*, 2nd series, 6: 760; 4th series, 7: 87; Kelly and Burrage (1928), 531-32; *NCAB*, 22: 432-33; J. R. Quinan, *Medical Annals of Baltimore* . . . (1884), 110-11.

C. Donegan

HARRIS, ELISHA (March 5, 1824, Westminster, Vt.-January 31, 1884, Albany, N.Y.). *Physician; Statistician; Public health reformer.* Son of John, farmer, and Eunice (Foster) Harris. Married Eliza Andrews (d. 1867); no children. EDUCATION: Attended and taught in rural schools, Vt.; 1849, M.D., College of Physicians and Surgeons, N.Y., following apprenticeship to Dr. S. B. Woolworth. CAREER: 1849-55, 1870-73, private practice, New York City; 1855-60, superintendent and physician-in-chief, Quarantine Hospital, Staten Island, N.Y.; 1858, active in series of National Quarantine Conventions; 1859, in charge of New York Floating Hospital; 1860-61, co-editor, *The Medical Times* (N.Y.); 1861-65, organizer, member, and corresponding secretary, U.S. Sanitary Commission; at New York City Metropolitan Board of Health: 1866-70, registrar of records; and 1873-76, registrar of vital statistics; 1880-84, secretary and superintendent of vital statistics, New York State Board of Health; an organizer and officer of many associations, notably the American Public Health Association (1877, president) and the Prison Association of New York. CONTRIBUTIONS: A pioneer in adapting European, particularly English, techniques of statistical investigation and sanitation to American cities. According to John Duffy, "possibly the outstanding health reformer of his day." For a generation, was an active participant in political, administrative, and scientific activities to apply the results of statistical and laboratory investigation to public administration. The causes he promoted included effective quarantine, accuracy in sanitary surveys and reporting of vital statistics, improved drainage and water supply, medical inspection of schoolchildren, vaccination, central organization of military hospitals and their coordination with sanitary work, and prison reform based on a concept of crime as a morbid condition caused by the environment. A synthesizer rather than an innovator, advocated measures to prevent miasmas as well as destroy germs, balanced the influence of heredity and environment in the causation of illness and social problems, participated in the politics of public health but deplored government by patronage, supported vaccination but reported on its ineffectiveness, and worked to develop public agencies and professional associations but always served in subordinate positions in their leadership. An international figure, winning a prize in Paris (1867) for the design of a railway ambulance and corresponding with William Farr and other notable figures in British statistical and sanitary affairs.

WRITINGS: A prolific author of reports, most of which are published as public documents or the proceedings of professional associations; subjects include quarantine hospitals, infectious diseases, ventilation and sanitation, the collection of vital statistics, the work of the U.S. Sanitary Commission, crime, and drunkenness. A useful list is in the *Author Catalogue* of the New York Academy of Medicine; also *Index Catalogue* 5 (1884): 854-55. REFERENCES: *DAB* 8 (1958): 307-8; John Duffy, *A History of Public Health in New York City*, 2 vols. (1968, 1974); Kelly and Burrage (1928), 532-33; *NCAB*, 9: 352.

D. M. Fox

HARRIS, SEALE (March 13, 1870, Cedartown, Ga.-March 16, 1957, Birmingham, Ala.). *Physician; Internal medicine.* Son of Charles Hooks, physician, and Margaret Ann (Monk) Harris. Married Stella Baskins Rainer, 1897; two children. EDUCATION: 1891-92, student, University of Georgia; 1894, M.D., University of Virginia; 1900, postgraduate courses, New York Polyclinic; 1904, studied at Post-Graduate Medical School, Chicago, Ill.; 1906, postgraduate work, Johns Hopkins, University of Vienna, and other European clinics. CAREER: Medical practice: 1894-1906, Union Springs, Ala.; 1907-15, Mobile, Ala.; *post* 1915, Birmingham; 1905, surgeon, Central of Georgia Railway Surgeon's Association; 1906-13, professor of medicine, Medical College of Alabama, Mobile; 1907-13, physician-in-chief, Mobile City Hospital; 1911-21, editor and owner, *Southern Medical Journal*; 1917, major, Medical Reserve Corps, U.S. Army; 1918-19, editor, *War Medicine*; during World War I, secretary, Research Committee, American Red Cross, in France; and completed medical and nutritional study in Europe following the war; president: 1919, American Medical Editors Association; 1921, Southern Medical Association; 1938, Medical Association of the State of Alabama; and American Medical Association. CONTRIBUTIONS: Established Chunnenuggee Sanitarium, Union Springs, Ala. (1904). Discovered hyperinsulinism and its cure (1923). Wrote several important historical works.

WRITINGS: "Tuberculosis in the Negro," *Alabama Med. J.* 15 (1902-3): 53-71; "The Nation's Greatest Need: A National Department of Health," *Am. J. of Public Health* 10 (1920): 633-36; "Insulin and Diet in the Treatment of Diabetes," *International Clinics*, 2nd series, 33 (1923): 6-20; "Hyperinsulinism and Dysinsulinism," *JAMA* 83 (1924): 729-33; *Clinical Pellagra* (1941); *Banting's Miracle: The Story of the Discovery of Insulin* (1946); *Women's Surgeon: Life of J. Marion Sims* (1950). REFERENCES: *JAMA*, 163 (1957): 1376-77; *NCAB*, A: 314; *N. Y. Times*, March 17, 1957; W. Owen, *History of Alabama* (1978); *Southern Med. J.* 50 (1957): 828-30; *Who's Who in Ala.* (1939-40); *Who Was Who in Am.*, 3: 374.

                                                                                    S. Eichold

HARRIS, WILLIAM HENRY (June 15, 1867, Augusta, Ga.-November 12, 1934, Athens, Ga.). *Physician*. Son of Nathan, farmer, and Harriet (Alexander) Harris. Married Jane Caroline Badger, 1895; five children. EDUCATION: A.B., Clark University; 1893, M.D., Meharry Medical College; 1906, postgraduate course in medicine, New York School of Clinical Medicine (Bellevue Hospital) and Massachusetts General Hospital, Boston, Mass. CAREER: 1893-1934, private practice, Athens. CONTRIBUTIONS: Co-founded Georgia State Medical Association (1893) and served in various capacities. Served Athens's black community with medical care for almost 40 years. Founded in Athens a black burial and fraternal insurance society, Improved Order of Samaritans (1897) and served as grand secretary (1897-1934). Involved in local, state, and national Republican party, religious affairs, black community concerns, and the Morris Brown College Board of Trustees and Finance Committee. REFERENCES: Henry S. Robinson, "William Henry Harris, M.D., 1867-1934," *JNMA* 62 (1970): 474-77.

                                                                                    T. Savitt

HARRISON, JOHN POLLARD (June 5, 1796, Louisville, Ky.-September 2, 1849, Cincinnati, Ohio). *Physician; Teacher*. Son of Maj. John, veteran of

Revolutionary War, and Mary Ann (Johnson) Harrison. Married Mary T. Warner, 1820; six children. EDUCATION: Began the study of medicine, possibly as early as 1814, under Dr. John Croghan of Louisville; 1817, attended lectures, University of Pennsylvania; 1819, M.D., University of Pennsylvania; private pupil of Dr. Nathaniel Chapman (q.v.) and William Dewee (q.v.) while attending lectures at the University of Pennsylvania. CAREER: 1819, began practice of medicine, Louisville, 1827, announced 32 clinical lectures as a course for medical students with an opportunity for dissection on a recent subject and for them to visit clinical cases in the Louisville Marine (City) Hospital; 1833, one of the incorporators listed on the first charter for the Louisville Medical Institute; 1835-46, professor of materia medica, Cincinnati College medical department; at Medical College of Ohio: 1841-46, professor of materia medica; and 1847-49, professor of theory and practice; September 1849, died of cholera during the epidemic. CONTRIBUTIONS: Medical staff of first hospital (Louisville Marine Hospital) in Louisville in which he taught his students. Gave the first formal medical lectures of record in Louisville, Marine (City) Hospital, beginning March 27, 1827. Writings on medical education were thorough and progressive. Associate editor (1847-49), *Western Lancet* (Cincinnati). Active in the Medical Convention of Ohio and president (1843). Elected a vice-president, American Medical Association (1849).

WRITINGS: *Essays and Lectures on Medical Subjects* (1835); "Address on Medical Education," *Proc., Med. Convention of Ohio* (1841); *The Elements of Materia Medica and Therapeutics*, 2 vols. (1844-1845). Writings listed in the *Index Catalogue*. REFERENCES: *Boston Med. and Surg. J.* 41 (1849): 415-17; O. Juettner, *Daniel Drake and His Followers* (1909).

E. H. Conner

HARRISON, ROSS GRANVILLE (January 13, 1870, Germantown, Pa.-September 30, 1959, New Haven, Conn.). *Biologist; Experimental embryology.* Son of Samuel, mechanical engineer, and Catherine Barrington (Diggs) Harrison. Married Ida Lange, 1896; five children. EDUCATION: Johns Hopkins University: 1889, A.B.; and 1894, Ph.D.; 1899, M.D., University of Bonn, Germany. CAREER: 1894-95, morphology faculty, Bryn Mawr College; 1896-1907, anatomy faculty, Johns Hopkins Medical School; 1908-38, anatomy, biology, and zoology faculties, Yale University; 1938-46, chairman, National Research Council. CONTRIBUTIONS: Made fundamental discoveries in neurology and developed a technique for cultivating cells in an artificial medium (hanging-drop culture method). Proved that nerve fibers are outgrowths of cells located in the central nervous system (1907); work settled a long-standing dispute over the formation of nerve fibers and furnished evidence that the cell is the building block of multicellular organisms; did work by taking cells from the central nervous system and placing them in hanging drops of clotted frog lymph, which he then placed under a microscope; left further development of tissue culture techniques to others; became one of the most important tools of biological and medical research, especially in oncology, virology, and genetics. Turned his attention thereafter to the study of embryonic development. Did major studies of polarity and asymmetry in embryonic organs and the control of organ growth. Worked earlier on the development of fish fins (1893-95), embryonic grafting in amphibian larvae (1903), and the histogenesis of the peripheral nervous system (1901). Helped found and edited the *Journal of Experimental Zoology* (from its beginning in 1903 until 1946).

WRITINGS: "Observations on the Living Developing Nerve Fiber," *Anat. Record* 1 (1907): 116-18, and *Proc., Soc. for Experimental Biol. & Med.* 4 (1907): 140-43; "The Outgrowth of the Nerve Fiber as a Mode of Protoplasmic Movement," *J. of Experimental Zool.* 9 (1910): 787-846; "The Cultivation of Tissues in Extraneous Media as a Method of Morphogenetic Study," *Anat. Record* 6 (1912): 181-93. Writings are listed in *BMNAS*. REFERENCES: *BHM* (1964-69), 117; (1975), 11; *BMFRS* 7 (1961): 111-26; *BMNAS* 35 (1961): 132-62; *DAB*, Supp. 6: 281-83; *DSB*, 6: 131-35; Miller, *BHM*, p. 47; J. Oppenheimer, "Ross Harrison's Contributions to Experimental Embryology," *Bull. Hist. Med.* 40 (1966): 525-43; *Who Was Who in Am.*, 3: 375.

                                                                                   S. Galishoff

HARTMAN, SAMUEL BRUBAKER (April 1, 1830, near Harrisburg, Pa.-January 30, 1918, Columbus, Ohio). *Physician; Patent medicine manufacturer.* Son of Christian, farmer, and Anna (Brubaker) Hartman. Married Sallie Ann Martzell, 1860; two children. EDUCATION: 1850s, Farmers College, Cincinnati, Ohio, and Western Reserve Medical College, Cleveland, Ohio; 1857, M.D., Jefferson Medical College, Philadelphia, Pa. CAREER: Began as rural carpenter and later itinerant Bible salesman; 1855-56, practiced medicine while studying, Vandalia and Tippecanoe City, Ohio; 1857-69, practiced, Millersville, Pa.; 1869-88, said to have operated as an itinerant "bonesetter"; 1888 until death, practiced, Columbus, Ohio; 1870s, began to make Peruna, patent medicine that achieved worldwide fame and sales; 1890s, manufacture on large scale began; 1890, opened sanitarium in Columbus and subsequently opened large hotel in conjunction with it; 1890s, Peruna Medicine Co. formed; produced Peruna and Manalin, a laxative, and Lacupia; reinvested profits widely in real estate around Columbus; after his death, Peruna Medicine Company was sold to a Chicago firm. CONTRIBUTIONS: At its height, Peruna was said to be "the most widely known trade name in the United States." The firm specialized in testimonials and advertised in newspapers all over the country. It spent $5,000 a day on newspaper spots and to distribute the 36 million booklets, almanacs, and pamphlets it printed each year. The most famous advertising stunt was to procure endorsements from 50 members of Congress (1903, 1904). Claimed that all diseases were forms of catarrh, which Peruna was said to cure. In fact, Peruna was as much as 30 percent alcohol, and addiction to it was not unknown. Office of Indian Affairs forbade its sale on reservations (1905), and the Commissioner of Internal Revenue made it subject to the federal excise tax on liquor sales. Changed the Peruna formula, adding powerful laxatives, and developed Ka-Tar-

No, a "new" medicine he made with the old Peruna recipe. Estate was valued at several million dollars, mostly in land and buildings.

WRITINGS: "Health and Beauty," "The Ills of Life," "The Real Truth About Peruna," and other advertising materials. REFERENCES: Samuel Hopkins Adams, "The Great American Fraud, II—Peruna and the 'Bracers,' " Collier's Weekly 36 (Oct. 28, 1905): 17-19; Robert Gunning, "The Hypocrite's Highball," Am. Mercury 55 (Dec. 1942): 722-29; Stewart H. Holbrook, "Dr. Hartman's Peruna," Ohio State Med. J. 56 (1960): 918-20, 1078-80; Henry W. Holcombe, "Peruna Medicine Company," in George B. Griffenhagen, comp., Patent Medicine Tax Stamps (1969), 396-98; NCAB, 13: 409.

E. Shoemaker

HARTMANN, ALEXIS FRANK (October 30, 1890, St. Louis, Mo.-September 6, 1964, St. Louis). Pediatrician. Son of Henry C., physician, and Bertha (Griesedick) Hartmann. Married Gertrude Krachmann, 1922; two children. EDUCATION: At Washington University: 1919, B.S.; 1921, M.S.; and 1921, M.D.; 1922-24, internship, St. Louis Children's Hospital; residency, St. Louis Children's Hospital. CAREER: At Washington University School of Medicine: 1924-1964, faculty in pediatrics; and 1936-64, chairman; physician-in-chief, St. Louis Children's Hospital. CONTRIBUTIONS: A student of W. McKim Marriott (q.v.), his predecessor as chairman of pediatrics. Principal contributions were in the understanding of pediatric biochemistry and metabolism. Obtained B.S., M.S., and M.D. within three years and worked in the laboratory of Dr. Philip Shaffer (q.v.). Their collaboration resulted in a technique known as the Shaffer-Hartmann method for determining sugar in the blood (1921). Always interested in the clinical applications of biochemistry, participated in early use of insulin for the treatment of diabetes at St. Louis Children's Hospital (1922). Among the early pediatricians who understood the importance of the biochemical approach to children's diseases. Did pioneering studies on the use of sodium lactate for the treatment of metabolic acidosis and was among the first to note important biochemical changes in the dehydration of infants and children. Published papers on neonatal hypoglycemia, hyperinsulinism, juvenile diabetes, galactosemia, and glycogen storage disease, maintaining a lifelong interest in carbohydrate metabolism and its disorders. Developed Lactate-Ringer's solution (1932), an important contribution to the development of parenteral fluid therapy. Described with his research associates (1962) the first known inborn error of lactic acid metabolism. Throughout his clinical career as a pediatrician, never lost interest in basic research as a means to approaching the treatment of children's diseases. According to his colleague, Dr. Gilbert Forbes, it was at his instigation that Carl and Gerty Cori (q.v.) undertook their famous studies of glycogen storage diseases in children.

WRITINGS: "The Iodometric Determinations of Copper and Its Use in Sugar Analysis," J. Biol. Chem. 45 (1921): 349 (with Philip A. Shaffer [q.v.]); "New Aspects of Acidosis," JAMA 91 (1928): 1675 (with McKim Marriott); "Studies in the Metabolism of Sodium r-Lactate," I, II, III, J. Clin. Invest. 11 (1932): 327, 337, 345 (with Milton Senn); "Subtotal Resection of the Pancreas for Hypoglycemia," Surg. Gyn. & Obst. 59

(1934): 474 (with Evarts Graham [q.v.]); "Lactate Metabolism: Studies of a Child with a Serious Congenital Deviation from the Normal," *J. Pediat.* 61 (1962): 165 (with H. Wohltmann, M. Purkerson, and M. Wesley). REFERENCES: Carl F. Cori, "Alexis F. Hartmann" (Memorial Address), *Med. Bull., St. Louis Children's Hosp.* (Spring 1966); Gilbert B. Forbes, "Alexis F. Hartmann: An Appreciation," *J. Pediat.* 64 (1964): 793-95; Park J. White, "Alexis F. Hartmann, Sr.," *ibid.*, 783-92; *Who Was Who in Am.*, 4: 414.

M. Hunt

HATCHER, ROBERT ANTHONY (February 6, 1868, New Madrid, Mo.-April 1, 1944, Flushing, N.Y.). *Pharmacologist.* Son of Richard Hardaway, lawyer, and Harriet Hinton (Marr) Hatcher. Married May Quinn Burton, 1904; one child. EDUCATION: 1889, Ph.G., Philadelphia College of Pharmacy; 1898, M.D., Tulane University. CAREER: 1890s, pharmacist in New Orleans, first in the employ of I. L. Lyons and Company and then for a short time in business for himself in the firm of Godbold and Hatcher; 1899-1904, materia medica faculty, Cleveland School of Pharmacy; pharmacology faculty: 1900-1904, Western Reserve University; and 1904-35, Cornell University Medical College; 1910-35, member, Committee of Revision, U.S. Pharmacopeia; 1934, president, American Society for Pharmacology and Experimental Therapeutics; inaugurated the teaching of pharmacology at Harvard University and University of Chicago. CONTRIBUTIONS: A founder of experimental pharmacology in the United States. Approach to investigating the diverse behavior of drugs in humans—absorption, distribution, elimination, bioassay—developed into the present discipline of clinical pharmacology. Investigated strychnine, morphine, the cinchona alkaloids, and local anesthetics. Best known for his work on digitalis; helped define the Hatcher-Brody cat unit of digitalis that made possible safe, rational, and effective use of the drug in heart disease. Analyzed the physiology and pharmacology of emesis (vomiting).

WRITINGS: *A Textbook of Materia Medica* (1904, with Torald H. Sollmann [q.v.]); *The Pharmacopeia and the Physician* (1906); *The Pharmacology of Useful Drugs* (1915, with Martin I. Wilbert); "Standardization of Digitalis—a Preliminary Report," *J. of the Am. Pharmacy Assoc.* 8 (Nov. 1919): 913-14. REFERENCES: *DAB*, Supplement 4: 342-43; Harry Gold, "Robert Anthony Hatcher (1868-1944)," *J. of Clinical Pharmacology* 11 (Jul.-Aug. 1971): 245-48; *NCAB*, 33: 289-90; *N.Y. Times*, April 2, 1944; *Who Was Who in Am.*, 2: 241.

S. Galishoff

HAYDEN, HORACE H. (no middle name) (October 13, 1769, Windsor, Conn.-January 26, 1844, Baltimore, Md.). *Dentist.* Son of Thomas, architect and builder, and Abigail (Parsons) Hayden. Married Marie Antoinette Robinson, 1805; six children. EDUCATION: Apprentice to John Greenwood, New York, N.Y., c. 1792-1800, and read dentistry on his own. CAREER: c. 1784-1790s, mechanic, Windsor, Conn.; 1800-1844, general dental practice, Baltimore area; 1840-44, professor at Baltimore College of Dental Surgery, the first dental school in the United States. CONTRIBUTIONS: Founded, with Chapin A. Harris (q.v.), the independent Baltimore College of Dental Surgery (1840) after University of Maryland trustees denied them affiliation. First president and first professor of the principles of dental science, then professor of dental physiology and pathology (1840-44). An early advocate (1817) of a national professional organization for dentists. A founder (1840) and first president (1840-44) of the American Society of Dental Surgeons. Recognized as father of professional dentistry in America.

WRITINGS: Published articles on dental physiology and pathology in early medical journals which were reprinted in 1840s in the new *American Journal of Dental Science*. REFERENCES: *Appleton's CAB*, 3: 131-32; Asbell, M.B., "Horace H. Hayden (1769-1844): Father of Professional Dentistry," *N.Y. J. Dentistry* 39 (1969): 226-29; *DAB*, 8: 440-42; Kelly and Burrage (1928), 544; *NCAB*, 13:525.

T. L. Savitt

HAYS, ISAAC (July 5, 1796, Philadelphia Pa.-April 12, 1879, Philadelphia). *Physician; Ophthalmologist; Editor.* Son of Samuel, wealthy merchant, and Richae (Gratz) Hays. Married Sarah Minis, 1834; four children. EDUCATION: Taught by Rev. Samuel B. Wylie; 1816, A.B., University of Pennsylvania; 1817, became medical student of Nathaniel Chapman (q.v.); 1820, M.D., University of Pennsylvania. CAREER: 1822, appointed to the staff, Pennsylvania Infirmary for Diseases of the Eye and Ear; 1827, became editor, *Philadelphia Journal of Medical and Physical Sciences*; changed the name to *American Journal of the Medical Sciences*; edited it until 1879; 1834-54, appointed surgeon to the Wills Eye Hospital, Philadelphia; 1843, publisher, *Medical News*; 1874, began publishing *Monthly Abstract of Medical Science*. CONTRIBUTIONS: As ophthalmologist, one of the first to detect astigmatism and to study color blindness; invented a special knife for cataract operations. Primary importance as a medical editor, exposing quackery and medical delusions, promoting professionalism. Active in the development of the AMA, serving as treasurer of the conventions (1847-52) and chairing the committee to create state and county medical societies (1853). Became chairman, Pennsylvania State Medical Society committee that drafted the organization's constitution. Founder and first president, Ophthalmological Society of Philadelphia.

WRITINGS: Edited and enlarged Sir William Lawrence's *Treatise on the Diseases of the Eye* (1843). REFERENCES: *BHM* (1975-79), 58; *DAB*, 4, pt. 2: 462-63; Kelly and Burrage (1920); *NCAB*, 11: 256; Alfred Stillé, "Memoir of Isaac Hays," *Trans., Coll. of Physicians*, 3rd series, 5 (1881): 27-60.

D. I. Lansing

HAYWOOD, EDMUND BURKE (January 15, 1825, Raleigh, N.C.-January 18, 1894, Raleigh). *Physician; Surgeon.* Son of John, planter and state treasurer, and Eliza Eagles (Williams) Haywood. Married Lucy A. Williams, 1850; seven children. EDUCATION: Raleigh Male Academy; apprentice to Fabius J. Haywood (his brother), Raleigh; *post* 1843, University of North Carolina; 1849, M.D.,

University of Pennsylvania. CAREER: 1850-61, 1865-94, private general practice, Raleigh; 1861-65, various medical positions, N.C. and Confederate armies, including commander of Pettigrew Hospital, Raleigh (1862-65). CONTRIBUTIONS: Considered eminent by N.C. contemporaries and historians for his long career of distinguished public service in medicine, including vice-president (1866) and president (1868), state medical society; chair of surgery, State Board of Medical Examiners (1866-72); co-organizer (1870), secretary (1872), and president (1874, 93), Raleigh Academy of Medicine; member (1866-89) and president (1875-89), Board of Directors, North Carolina Insane Asylum, Raleigh; chairman (1889-91) and member (1891-94), State Board of Public Charities; president, Board of Health, Wake County; physician, at time of his death, Peace Institute, and Deaf, Dumb, and Blind Institute, Raleigh. Represented the state government and the state and local medical societies at various national and international meetings. As president, asylum board, influenced legislature (1875) to reject establishment of asylum for blacks in an old building in Wilmington, N.C., and to build new asylums in Goldsboro, N.C. (for blacks), and later, in Morganton, N.C. (for whites). Established the right of N.C. physicians to receive compensation for serving as expert witnesses in court cases (1872). Performed numerous surgical procedures, some for the first time in N.C. Considered preeminent in his field in the state.

WRITINGS: Several case reports published in state journal and medical society transactions. Writings listed in *Cyclopedia of . . . the Carolinas*, 2 (1892): 234-35. REFERENCES: S. A. Ashe, ed., *Biographical History of North Carolina*, 6 (1907): 289-95; *Cyclopedia of Eminent and Representative Men of the Carolinas in the 19th Century*, 2 (1892): 230-36; Kelly and Burrage (1920), 510; *NCAB*, 9: 324-25; *North Carolina: The Old North State and the New*, 3 (1941): 7-10.

T. Savitt

HAZEN, ALLEN (August 28, 1869, Hartford, Vt.-July 26, 1930, Miles City, Mont.). *Hydraulic and sanitary engineer*. Son of Charles Dana, farmer, and Abbie Maria (Coleman) Hazen. Married Elizabeth McConway, 1903; seven children. EDUCATION: c. 1885, B.S., New Hampshire College of Agriculture and the Mechanic Arts; 1887-88, studied sanitary chemistry, Massachusetts Institute of Technology. CAREER: 1888-93, director, State Board of Health Experiment Station, Lawrence, Mass.; 1893, in charge of sewage disposal, Chicago Exposition; 1894-1930, private consulting practice, Boston, Mass., and New York City. CONTRIBUTIONS: Played a prominent role in hydraulic engineering and sanitary science in the late nineteenth and early twentieth centuries. As first director, Lawrence Experiment Station, guided the work of an interdisciplinary team of engineers, biologists, and chemists, which became internationally famous for its research on sewage and water purification. An authority on the properties of sands, gravels, and other materials and their suitability for use in water and sewage purification. Designed the Albany (N.Y.) water purification plant, the nation's first slow sand filter plant with continuous filtration (1900). Retained

as a consulting engineer on water supply by many cities and states throughout
the nation. Expanded his interests in later years into the fields of hydrology,
appraisal and rate making, design of large dams, and distribution pipes. With
Gardner S. Williams, developed the widely used Williams and Hazen pipe-flow
formula (1905). Pioneered in the development of probability concepts in hy-
drological studies, which he explored in his last book, *Flood Flows* (1930).

WRITINGS: *The Filtration of Public Water-Supplies* (1895); *Hydraulic Tables* (1905);
Clean Water and How to Get it (1907); *Meter Rates for Water Works* (1917). REFER-
ENCES: *DAB*, Supplement 1: 389-90; *NCAB*, 28: 342; *Who Was Who in Am.*, 1: 541-
42.

S. Galishoff

HEALY, HENRY HERBERT (December 30, 1869, Drayton, Ontario, Canada-September 2, 1935, Grand Forks, N.Dak.). *Physician; Public Health.* Son
of Henry Wilkinson, farmer, and Lucy (Dales) Healy. Married Mary Maude
Wallace, 1893; four children. EDUCATION: 1891, A.B., University of Minnesota;
1892, M.D., Rush Medical College (Chicago, Ill.). CAREER: Physician and
surgeon: 1892-1901, Michigan, N. Dak.; and 1901-35, Grand Forks; 1901-7,
superintendent of public health, N. Dak.; 1903-4, founder and secretary, Grand
Forks District Medical Association; 1910-11, president, North Dakota Medical
Association; 1912-14, superintendent of health, Grand Forks County, N. Dak.;
1918-19, captain, Medical Corps, American Expeditionary Forces. CONTRIBU-
TIONS: First N. Dak. superintendent of public health to advocate establishment
of a state tuberculosis sanitarium and public care for victims of this disease.
Established (1912) first county-level visiting nurse program for rural schools, an
idea that quickly spread throughout the nation. REFERENCES: *Grand Forks Herald*,
September 3, 1935, pp. 1-2; James Grassick, *North Dakota Medicine: Sketches and
Abstracts* (1926), 110-13.

L. Remele

HEALY, WILLIAM (January 20, 1869, Buckinghamshire County, England-
March 15, 1963, Clearwater, Fla.). *Physician; Psychiatry; Child psychology.*
Son of William and Charlotte (Hearne) Healy, farmers. Married Mary Sylvia
Tenney, 1901, one child; Augusta Bronner, 1932. EDUCATION: 1893-99, Harvard
College and Harvard Medical School, B.A., 1899; 1900, M.D., Rush Medical
College; 1906-7, postgraduate work in neurology, Vienna, Berlin, and London.
CAREER: 1883-93, employed by Fifth National Bank of Chicago; 1900, medical
staff, Women's Division of the Mendota State Hospital, Wis.; *post* 1901, prac-
ticed medicine, Chicago, Ill., specializing first in gynecology and after 1907 in
neurology; early 1900s, first instructor in gynecology for two years, Northwestern
University, and then member of neurology faculty for three years, Chicago
Polyclinic; 1909-17, director, Juvenile Psychopathic Institute of Chicago; 1917-
49, founder and director, Judge Baker Foundation, Boston, Mass. (later Judge
Baker Guidance Center); president, American Psychopathological Association;

made significant studies of juvenile delinquency and criminal behavior and was a leader in the movement to establish child guidance clinics. CONTRIBUTIONS: Helped introduce psychoanalysis in America in his book *The Structure and Meaning of Psychoanalysis* (1930, with Augusta Bronner and A. M. Bowers). A pioneer in the field of mental testing. *Manual of Individual Mental Tests and Testing* (1929, with Augusta Bronner et al.) was widely used (1920s, 1930s). A founder and first president, American Orthopsychiatric Association. Helped organize the child mental health movement in the United States.

WRITINGS: *The Individual Delinquent* (1915); "Pictorial Completion Test. II.," *J. of Applied Psychology* 5 (1921-22): 225-39. Author of 14 books and numerous articles. REFERENCES: George E. Gardner, "William Healy (1869-1963)," *J. of the Am. Acad. of Child Psychiatry*, 11 (Jan. 1972): 1-29; Sheldon Glueck, "Remarks in Honor of William Healy, M.D.," *Mental Hygiene* 48 (1964): 318-22; H. Meltzer, "Contributions to the History of Psychology: VI. Dr. William Healy—1869 to 1963—the Man in His Times," *Psychological Reports* 20 (Jun. 1967): 1028-30; *Who's Important in Medicine* (1952), 457.

S. Galishoff

HEATH, LILLIAN (December 29, 1865, Burnett Junction, Wis.-August 5, 1962, Rawlins, Wyo.). *Physician.* Daughter of William Albert, railroader, and Calleta (Hunter) Heath. Married Lou Nelson, 1898; no children. EDUCATION: University of Colorado, Boulder, Colo.; and College of Physicians and Surgeons, Keokuk, Ia.; 1893, M.D.; studied under Drs. F. B. Forsey and J. C. Hughes (q.v.) for three months in obstetrics. CAREER: 1893-1909, practice, Rawlins; before her schooling in medicine, was a nurse for Dr. Thomas Maghee (q.v.). CONTRIBUTIONS: First woman physician in Wyo. Assisted Dr. Thomas Maghee at the first "plastic surgery" facial reconstruction in Wyo. REFERENCES: *Denver Post, Empire Magazine*, August 28, 1955; *Rawlins Daily Times*, August 15, 1955.

A. Palmieri

HEERMAN, LEWIS (August 3, 1779, Cassel, Germany-May 21 or 25, 1833, New Orleans, La.). *Surgeon; Naval medical officer.* Son of Johann Heerman, farmer. Married Eliza Potts, 1821; five children. EDUCATION: Probably received M.D. in Germany; 1806-8, postgraduate work, European and British hospitals; 1827, M.D., Geneva Medical College. CAREER: Before 1802, immigrated to United States; 1802, joined navy as surgeon's mate; 1803-5, served in Barbary Coast Wars under Preble and Decatur; 1804, famous for heroism at burning of USS *Philadelphia*; promoted to surgeon; served two years, Norfolk Navy Yard; 1810-26, founded and commanded U.S. Naval Hospital, New Orleans, La.; sick leave, New Haven, Conn.; 1829, lectured on surgery, Yale Medical School; 1830, fleet surgeon, Mediterranean Fleet; developed first insignia of senior medical rank. CONTRIBUTIONS: Early proponent of permanent U.S. Navy hospitals. Developed example of operation and command of one of first naval hospitals. Widely known in South as consultant in infectious diseases. Contributed to

Benjamin Silliman's (q.v.) work during joint geological field trips. Willed his large 250-volume medical library to Yale—a nucleus of present collection. Example of heroism at Tripoli (1804) established precedent of American naval surgeons volunteering for medical support in dangerous missions.

WRITINGS: *Directions for the Medicine Chest* (1811). Writings listed in Robert B. Austin, *Early American Imprints*, no. 897 (1961). REFERENCES: R. P. Parsons, "History of the Medical Department of the United States Navy," in Francis R. Packard, *History of Medicine in the United States* 2 (1932): 659-734; F. L. Pleadwell and W. M. Kerr, "Lewis Heerman, Surgeon in the United States Navy," *Annals of Med. Hist.* 5 (1923): 113-45.

R. J. T. Joy

HEG, ELMER ELLSWORTH (February 23, 1861, Waupun, Wis.-September 25, 1922, Stanwood, Wash.). *Physician; Surgeon; Pulmonary medicine.* Son of Hans C., editor and historian, and Cornelia Einong (Jacobson) Heg. Married May Thornton, 1890 (d. 1911), two children; Mrs. Evelyn Robbins Sampson, 1918, no children. EDUCATION: 1880, A.B., Beloit College; 1887, M.D., Bellevue Hospital Medical College. CAREER: *Post* 1888, private practice, Yakima, Wash., and Seattle, Wash.; surgeon: 1896-98, Washington National Guard; and 1898-1900, Spanish-American War; 1909-11, Wash. State commissioner of health; 1909-15, medical director, Pulmonary Hospital of Seattle. CONTRIBUTIONS: Highly respected specialist in pulmonary medicine and surgery in Wash. Deeply involved in Wash. State public health matters as member, State Board of Health (1897-98, 1902-16), serving as secretary (1897-98, 1903-11) and president (1912, 1916). Became interested in public health affairs in Yakima while residing there; served on Seattle Board of Health (1900-1902) and as state commissioner of health (1909-11). Chosen U.S. delegate to 14th International Congress on Hygiene (Berlin, 1907). Secretary, AMA's section on hygiene and sanitary science (1905-7) and Washington State Medical Society (1891-92). President, King County Medical Society (1904-5). REFERENCES: *NCAB*, 20: 72; *Who Was Who in Am.*, 4: 425.

T. Savitt

HEKTOEN, LUDVIG (July 2, 1863, Westby, Wis.-July 5, 1951, Chicago, Ill.). *Pathologist; Editor.* Son of Peter P., farmer and teacher, and Olave (Thorsgaard) Hektoen. Married Ellen Strandh, 1891; two children. EDUCATION: 1883, B.A., Luther College, Decorah, Ia.; 1887, M.D., College of Physicians and Surgeons, Chicago; 1887-89, intern, Cook County Hospital. CAREER: 1889-1903, pathologist, Cook County Hospital; 1890-94, coroner's physician, Chicago; pathology faculty: 1891-94, College of Physicians and Surgeons; and 1895-1933, Rush Medical College; 1901-32, pathology and bacteriology faculties, University of Chicago; 1902-39, director, McCormick Institute for Infectious Diseases. CONTRIBUTIONS: Proved that measles could be transmitted between humans (1905). Produced cirrhosis of the liver experimentally (1900-1901). Showed that X-rays could suppress antibody response (1915). First to suggest that selection of a blood donor who belongs to the same group as the recipient will eliminate many dangers of blood transfusion; probably the first in the United States to make blood cultures from living patients. Greatly improved the medical section of the coroner's office in Chicago. A founder, McCormick Institute for Infectious Diseases (1902), renamed the Ludvig Hektoen Institute for Medical Research of Cook County (1943), and of the Chicago Tumor Institute (1938). Chairman, National Research Council (1936-38). Founder and editor, *Archives of Pathology* (1926-49). First editor, *Journal of Infectious Diseases* (1904-41). A founder, Institute of Medicine of Chicago (1915).

WRITINGS: "Experimental Bacillary Cirrhosis of the Liver," *J. Path. Bact.* 7 (1901): 214-20; "Experimental Measles," *J. Infect. Dis.* 2 (1905): 238-55; "The Influence of the X-ray on the Production of Antibodies," *J. Infect. Dis.* 17 (1915): 415-22; "Precipitin-Production in Allergic Rabbits," *J. Infect. Dis.* 21 (1917): 279-86. Writings listed in *BMNAS*, 28: 181-97; *Arch. Path.* 26: 20-31. REFERENCES: *Arch. Path.* 26 (1938): 1-31; *Arch. Path.* 52 (1951): 390-94; *BMNAS* 28 (1954): 163-97; *DSB*, 6: 232-33; *NCAB*, 18: 146-47; *Proc., Inst. Med. Chicago* 19 (1952-53): 3-11 (includes *JAMA* obit.).

W. K. Beatty

HELMUTH, WILLIAM TOD (October 30, 1833, Philadelphia, Pa.-May 15, 1902). *Surgeon; Homeopath.* Son of John Henry and Jeanette (Tod) Helmuth. Married Fannie Ida Pritchard, 1859; two children. EDUCATION: St. Timothy's College, Baltimore, Md.; studied medicine with his uncle, Dr. William S. Helmuth, Homeopathic Medical College of Pennsylvania; 1853, M.D., Homeopathic Medical College of Pennsylvania; 1868, surgical studies, Europe. CAREER: At Homeopathic Medical College of Pennsylvania: 1854-55, dispensary physician and prosector of anatomy; and 1856 (at age 22), became professor of anatomy; 1858, moved to St. Louis, Mo.; 1858-70, professor of anatomy, Homeopathic Medical College of Missouri and surgeon to Good Samaritan Hospital; 1870-1902, at New York Homeopathic Medical College: 1870-1902, professor of surgery; and 1893-1902, dean. CONTRIBUTIONS: Leading homeopathic surgeon in America (from 1860s to death in 1902). A founder, Homeopathic Medical College of Missouri. President, American Institute of Homeopathy (1867). Prolific author of works on homeopathic surgery.

WRITINGS: *Surgery and Its Adaption to Homeopathic Practice* (1855); *A Treatise on Diphtheria* (1862); *A System of Surgery* (1873); and numerous others. Also edited the *Western Homeopathic Observer* (1863-71) and co-edited the *North American Journal of Homeopathy* (1862-69) as well as other journals. REFERENCES: T. L. Bradford, *Hist. of the Homeopathic Medical College of Pennsylvania* (1898); *DAB*, 8: 516-17; *NCAB*, 12: 471; *N.Y. Times*, May 16, 1902.

M. Kaufman

HEMMETER, JOHN CONRAD (April 25, 1864, Baltimore, Md.-February 25, 1931, Baltimore). *Physician; Physiology; Gastroenterology.* Son of John, railroad employee, and Mathilde (Ziegler) Hemmeter. Married Helene Emilie

Hilgenberg, 1893; no children. EDUCATION: 1882, A.B., Baltimore City College; 1884, M.D., University of Maryland; 1890, Ph.D., Johns Hopkins University; *post* 1890, studied physiology in Berlin and pathology of the digestive system in Vienna. CAREER: 1884-88, medical staff, Bayview Hospital (Baltimore); *post* 1888, practiced medicine, Baltimore; 1903-22, physiology and clinical medicine faculties, University of Maryland; associate editor, *Archives for Digestive Diseases* (Berlin); composer for orchestra, voice, and piano. CONTRIBUTIONS: Won international acclaim for clinical and experimental investigations of gastrointestinal diseases. One of the first persons to use X-rays for studying the stomach (1896). Devised a method of intubating the duodenum that made possible direct observation and examination of that organ (1896). Did important work on the physiology of digestion and early diagnosis of stomach cancer. Wrote on medical history toward the end of his life.

WRITINGS: *Diseases of the Stomach* (1897); *Diseases of the Intestines* (1901-2); *Manual of Practical Physiology* (1912); *Master Minds in Medicine: A History of Evolution of Ideas in Medicine* (1927). REFERENCES: *DAB*, 8: 519; *NCAB*, 30: 230-31; *Who Was Who in Am.*, 1: 548.

S. Galishoff

HENCH, PHILIP SHOWALTER (February 28, 1896, Pittsburgh, Pa.- March 30, 1965, Ocho Rios, Jamaica). *Physician; Rheumatoid arthritis*. Son of Jacob Bixler, classics scholar and preparatory schoolteacher, and Clara John (Showalter) Hench. Married Mary Genevieve Kahler, 1927; four children. EDUCATION: 1916, A.B., Lafayette College; 1920, M.D., University of Pittsburgh; 1920-21, intern, St. Francis Hospital (Pittsburgh); 1921-23, fellow in medicine, Mayo Foundation (Rochester, Minn.); 1928-29, postgraduate study, Germany; 1931, M.S., University of Minnesota. CAREER: 1923-57, medical staff, Mayo Clinic; 1928-57, medicine faculty, Mayo Graduate School of Medicine, University of Minnesota; 1942-46, director, Army rheumatism center, Army and Navy General Hospital. CONTRIBUTIONS: Noticed that jaundice, pregnancy, and starvation diets reduced the pain and swelling in arthritic joints (1929); reasoned that since the blood of such patients was high in steroids, arthritis could be treated with the steroid hormones of the adrenal cortex; enlisted the aid of Edward C. Kendall (q.v.), who crystallized six steroids, which he designated compounds A to F; administered compound E, cortisone (1948), to 14 bedridden arthritic patients whom he subsequently filmed running and jumping; for this work, was awarded the 1950 Nobel Prize in medicine or physiology with Kendall and Tadeus Reichstein of Switzerland. A founder, American Rheumatism Association, chief editor of its annual *Rheumatism Reviews* (1932-48), and associate editor, *Annals of Rheumatic Disease* (London).

WRITINGS: "The Effect of a Hormone of the Adrenal Cortex. . . and of Pituitary Adrenocorticotropic Hormone on Rheumatoid Arthritis; Preliminary Report," *Annals of the Rheumatic Diseases* 8 (1949): 99-104 (with E. C. Kendall, C. H. Slocumb, and H. F. Polley). Authored about 200 papers, chapters in books, and other writings. REFER-

ENCES: *BHM* (1964-69), 122; *Current Biog.* (1950), 230-31; Miller, *BHM*, p. 48; *DAB*, Supp. 7: 340-41; *McGraw-Hill Modern Men of Sci.* 1: 217-18; *Nature* 206 (1965): 1195-96; *N.Y. Times*, April 1, 1965; *Who Was Who in Am.*, 4: 428.

S. Galishoff

HENDERSON, LAWRENCE JOSEPH (June 3, 1878, Lynn, Mass.-February 10, 1942, Boston, Mass.). *Biochemist; Physiologist.* Son of Joseph, businessman, and Mary Reed (Bosworth) Henderson. Married Edith Lawrence Thayer, 1916; one child. EDUCATION: Harvard University: 1898, A.B.; and 1902, Ph.D.; 1902-4, studied biochemistry with Franz Hofmeister, Strasbourg, France. CAREER: 1904-42, biochemistry faculty, Harvard University; 1921, Harvard University exchange professor, Harvard to University of Paris; 1928, Silliman Lecturer, Yale University, and Leyden Lecturer, University of Berlin; 1931, Mills Lecturer, University of California; exerted considerable influence as a sociologist, natural philosopher, and historian of science. CONTRIBUTIONS: Described quantitatively the physiological mechanism regulating the acid-base equilibrium in the body. Recognized that a mixture of carbonic acid and biocarbonates is particularly effective in stabilizing the hydrogen ion concentration of blood and many other physiological fluids. Argued that the properties of the elements of carbon, hydrogen, and oxygen uniquely favored the evolution of complex life forms; expounded and elaborated on this idea in his books *The Fitness of the Environment* (1913) and *The Order of Nature* (1917). Believed that every one of the variables involved in the respiratory changes of blood must be a mathematical function of all the others. With the help of P. M. D'Ocagne, devised a simplified way of visualizing the relations between several variables and of computing the data, which found wide use in biology; summarized his findings in a great work, *Blood: A Study in General Physiology* (1928). Was responsible for many improvements at Harvard University: founded the Department of Physical Chemistry in the medical school (1920) but left its direction to a younger colleague, Edwin J. Cohen; with financial assistance from the Rockefeller Foundation, established the Fatigue Laboratory (1927) to study the chemical changes that produce fatigue and the environmental factors that trigger them; organized Harvard's Society of Fellows (1932), which each year awards stipends to promising young scholars to enable them to pursue investigations of their own choosing for a period of three years or more.

WRITINGS: "Concerning the Relationship Between the Strength of Acids and Their Capacity to Preserve Neutrality," *Am. J. of Physiol.* 21 (1908): 173-79; "The Theory of Neutrality Regulation in the Animal Organism," *ibid.*, pp. 427-48; "On the Intensity of Urinary Acidity in Normal and Pathological Conditions," *J. Biol. Chem.* 13 (Jan. 1913): 393-405 (with W. W. Palmer); *Pareto's General Sociology: A Physiologist's Interpretation* (1935); "The Practice of Medicine as Applied Sociology." *Trans., Assoc. of Am. Physicians* 51 (1936): 8-22. A bibliography is in *BMNAS* 23 (1943): 52-58, and in J. Parascandola, "Lawrence J. Henderson and the Concept of Organized Systems" (Ph.D. diss., University of Wisconsin, 1968), 233-38. REFERENCES: *BHM* (1965-69),

122; (1970-74), 82-83; *DAB*, Supplement 3: 349-52; *DSB*, 6: 260-62; *Who Was Who in Am.*, 1: 549.

S. Galishoff

HENDERSON, YANDELL (April 23, 1873, Louisville, Ky.-February 18, 1944, La Jolla, Calif.). *Physiologist*; *Toxicologist*. Son of Isham, engineer, lawyer, and newspaper publisher, and Sally Nielsen (Yandell) Henderson. Married Mary Gardner Colby, 1903; two children. EDUCATION: Yale University: 1895, B.A.; and 1898, Ph.D. (physiological chemistry); 1898-1900, studied under Albrecht Kossel in Marburg, Germany, and Carl Voit in Munich, Germany. CAREER: During Spanish-American War, ensign, U.S. Navy; at Yale University: 1900-1921, physiology faculty; and 1921-38, professor of applied physiology (with no teaching duties); 1913-25, consulting physiologist, U.S. Bureau of Mines; during World War I: chief of physiological section, U.S. war gas investigation conducted by the Bureau of Mines; chairman, Medical Research Board, Aviation Section, Signal Corps, U.S. Army. CONTRIBUTIONS: An authority on the physiology of respiration and circulation and on the pharmacology and toxicology of gases. Pointed out the role of severe pain in stimulating overventilation and argued that the decrease in carbon dioxide that accompanies excessive pulmonary ventilation is the cause of shock. Introduced the technique of administering a mixture of carbon dioxide and oxygen, instead of only oxygen, after anesthesia as a means of eliminating the anesthetic and preventing postoperative illness. With Howard Wilcox Haggard, invented the Henderson-Haggard inhalator for use in resuscitation (1922); was widely used in the treatment of carbon monoxide poisoning, surgical shock, asphyxia of newborn babies, and similar conditions; became a standard piece of equipment for rescue squads and is credited with having saved numerous lives. With Haggard, determined ventilation standards for the Holland Tunnel under the Hudson River, which were adopted in tunnels throughout the world.
WRITINGS: "Acapnia and Shock.I. Carbon Dioxide as a Factor in the Regulation of the Heart Rate," *Am. J. of Physiol.* 21 (Feb. 1, 1908): 126-56; 23 (Feb. 1, 1909): 345-73; 24 (Apr. 1, 1909): 66-85; "Carbon Monoxide Poisoning," *JAMA* 67 (Aug. 19, 1916): 580-83; "A Lecture On Respiration in Anaesthesia: Control by Carbon Dioxide," *British Med. J.* 2 (1925): 1170-75; *Noxious Gases and the Principles of Respiration Influencing Their Action* (1927, with Howard W. Haggard). A bibliography is in his *Adventures in Respiration* (1938). REFERENCES: *DAB*, Supplement 3: 352-54; *DSB*, 6: 264-65; *NCAB*, 36: 25-26; *N.Y. Times*, February 20, 1944; *Who Was Who in Am.*, 2: 242-43.

S. Galishoff

HENRY, MORRIS HENRY (July 26, 1835, London, England-May 19, 1895, New York, N.Y.). *Physician*; *Dermatology*; *Venereal diseases*; *Surgery*. Son of Henry A., Orientalist, educator, and Esther (Henry) Henry. Married Elizabeth Rutherford Hastings, 1872; Mrs. Harrison Everett Maynard, 1880. EDUCATION: Polytechnic schools at Brussels and art courses at the Government School, Somerset House, London; 1852, immigrated to the United States; 1860, M.D.,

University of Vermont; 1860-61, studied medicine in Europe. CAREER: 1857, prosector and assistant to the chair in surgery, New York Medical College; 1861-63, assistant surgeon, U.S. Navy; *post* 1864, practiced medicine in New York City; 1864, surgeon, Northern Dispensary; 1869, surgeon, New York Dispensary; 1873-80, surgeon-in-chief, New York State Emigrant Hospital; 1872-1884, chief police surgeon of New York City. CONTRIBUTIONS: Helped arouse the interest of American physicians in dermatology and venereal diseases. Founded (1870) and edited for five years the *American Journal of Syphilography and Dermatology*, the first American periodical on these subjects. 1871, published an American edition of W.T. Fox, *Skin Diseases: Their Description, Pathology, Diagnosis, and Treatment*, which was adopted for use in the medical departments of the American armed services and became the standard textbook in its field. Was equally renowned as a surgeon. Invented numerous surgical instruments, notably forceps and scissors for various purposes. Won fame in the United States and abroad for his operation for varicocele by the removal of the redundant scrotum. REFERENCES: *DAB*, 8: 553-54; Kelly and Burrage (1928), 554-55; *NCAB*, 2: 485-86; *Who Was Who in Am.*, Hist. Vol.: 317.

S. Galishoff

HERING, CONSTANTINE (January 1, 1800, Oschatz, Saxony, Germany-July 30, 1880, Philadelphia, Pa.). *Homeopathic physician; Educator.* Son of Christian Gottlieb Karl, musician and educator, and Christiane Fredericke (Kreutzberg) Hering. Married Charlotte Kemper, 1829; Marianne Hussman; Theresa Bucheim, 1845; two sons. EDUCATION: Classical school of Zittau; 1820, surgical academy of Dresden, Germany; 1820-24, University of Leipzig; 1826, M.D., University of Wurzburg. CAREER: 1826, math and science teacher, Blochmann Institute (Dresden, Germany); zoological research, Surinam, and medical practice, Paramaribo, South America; 1833-80, medical practice, Philadelphia; 1835-42, organizer and principal teacher, first homeopathic school in the world, the North American Academy of the Homeopathic Healing Arts (Allentown, Pa.); 1844, presiding officer, first convention of the American Institute of Homeopathy; at Homeopathic Medical College of Pennsylvania: 1848, a founder; and 1864-67, professor of the institutes of homeopathy and the practice of medicine; 1867, founder Hahnemann Medical College of Philadelphia, serving as dean and professor (1867-71). CONTRIBUTIONS: German physician who brought homeopathy to America (1833) and worked to establish medical institutions (homeopathic), including Hahnemann Medical College of Philadelphia. Originally was commissioned to write a pamphlet against homeopathy but became a convert when he became more familiar with the theories of Samuel Hahnemann, founder of homeopathic medicine. An editor, *North American Homeopathic Journal* (1851-53); *Homeopathic News* (1854-56), and *American Homeopathic Materia Medica* (1867-71).

WRITINGS: *Antisporic Remedies in Their Relation to Leprosy* (1831); *The Homeopathist, or Domestic Physician* (1835-38); *Materia Medica* (1873); *Analytical Therapeu-*

tics (1875); *Guiding Symptoms*, 10 vols. (1878-91); died after the first three were published. REFERENCES: *DAB*, 4, pt. 2: 575-76; Arthur Eastman, *Life and Reminiscences*; Kelly and Burrage (1920); *NCAB*, 3: 477.

D. I. Lansing

HERRICK, JAMES BRYAN (August 11, 1861, Oak Park, Ill.-March 7, 1954, Chicago, Ill.). *Physician; Cardiology.* Son of Origen White, banker, and Dora Ellen (Kettlestrings) Herrick. Married Zellah P. Davies, 1889; two children. EDUCATION: 1882, A.B., University of Michigan; 1888, M.D., Rush Medical College (Chicago); 1888-89, intern, Cook County Hospital (Chicago). CAREER: 1882-86, high school teacher, Oak Park and Peoria, Ill.; at Presbyterian Hospital (Chicago): 1890-1924, internal medicine staff; 1903-7, vice-president, medical board; 1908-13, president; 1890-1910, medical staff, Cook County Hospital; 1890-1927, medical staff, Central Free Dispensary (Chicago); 1890-1927, internal medicine faculty, Rush Medical College. CONTRIBUTIONS: First physician to describe and diagnose coronary thrombosis in a living person (1912). Formulated a clear, clinical picture of the disease based on many years of bedside and postmortem examinations. Pointed out that often conditions diagnosed as angina pectoris, acute indigestion, or ptomaine poisoning were actually cases of coronary occlusion; stated that coronary thrombosis occurred frequently, could be diagnosed at the bedside, and was not invariably fatal as was then believed. Through his writings, obtained widespread medical recognition of coronary vascular disease and stimulated clinical and experimental study of heart ailments. Introduced the string galvanometer, the predecessor of the electrocardiograph, in Chicago. Provided the first description of sickle cell anemia (1910).

WRITINGS: *A Handbook of Medical Diagnosis* (1895); "Peculiar Elongated and Sickle-Shaped Red Blood Corpuscles in a Case of Severe Anemia," *Arch. of Int. Med.* 6 (1910): 517-21; "Clinical Features of Sudden Obstruction of the Coronary Arteries," *JAMA* 59 (1912): 2015-20; *A Short History of Cardiology* (1942). Writings through October 1935 are listed in William Henry Holmes, *James Bryan Herrick: An Appreciation* (1935). REFERENCES: *BHM* (1975-79), 60; (1980), 19-20; James Herrick, *Memoirs of 80 Years* (1949); *JAMA* 154 (Jan.-Apr. 1954): 1016; Miller, *BHM.*, p. 49; *NCAB*, 42: 595-96; *N.Y. Times*, March 9, 1954; John H. Talbott, *Biog. Hist. Med.* (1970), 1158-60; *Who Was Who in Am.*, 3: 394.

S. Galishoff

HERSEY, EZEKIEL (September 21, 1709, Hingham, Mass.-December 9, 1770). *Physician.* EDUCATION: 1728, graduated from Harvard College; studied medicine with Lawrence Dal'Honde, Boston, Mass. CAREER: Practiced medicine, Hingham. CONTRIBUTIONS: A prominent colonial physician whose practice extended into Plymouth, Norfolk, and Barnstable counties, Mass. With his wife and brother, Dr. Abner Hersey, endowed the Hersey Professorship of Anatomy and Surgery and the Hersey Professorship of the Theory and Practice of Physic, Harvard University. REFERENCES: Kelly and Burrage (1928), 560.

S. Galishoff

HERTER, CHRISTIAN ARCHIBALD (September 3, 1865, Glenville, Conn.-December 5, 1910, New York, N.Y.). *Physician; Biochemistry; Pathology*. Son of Christian, artist and interior decorator, and Mary (Miles) Herter. Married Susan Dows, 1886; five children. EDUCATION: 1885, M.D., College of Physicians and Surgeons (Columbia); 1886, studied at Johns Hopkins and in Europe. CAREER: 1886-c.1896, practiced medicine, N.Y.; 1894-1904, visiting physician, New York City Hospital; 1898-1903, pathological chemistry faculty, University and Bellevue Hospital Medical College (New York University); 1903-10, pharmacology and therapeutics faculty, College of Physicians and Surgeons; *post* 1901, member, Board of Directors, and treasurer, Rockefeller Institute for Medical Research; 1907, member, Board of Scientific Referees (established by President Theodore Roosevelt to act as advisers to the Department of Agriculture in the enforcement of the Pure Food and Drug Act of 1906); 1908-10, medical staff, Hospital of the Rockefeller Institute. CONTRIBUTIONS: Through his research, editorial labors, and involvement with the Rockefeller Institute for Medical Research, played a prominent role in the advancement of scientific medicine in the United States. Organized one of the nation's first medical research laboratories in his home, which became an important center of scientific investigation. Did earliest work on diseases of the nervous system and published a textbook on the subject in 1892. Turned next to pathological chemistry; studied metabolic disorders and the formation of gallstones and glycosuria, which he reported in his well-known book *Lectures on Chemical Pathology in Its Relation to Practical Medicine* (1902). Examined the chemistry and bacteriology of digestion; investigated the pathology caused by toxins secreted by intestinal bacteria and described a condition of infantilism in children under ten arising from chronic intestinal infection ("celiac disease" or "Herter's infantilism"). Was instrumental in the founding of the Rockefeller Institute and its establishment of an associated teaching and research hospital. Co-founded (1905) and edited the *Journal of Biological Chemistry* and participated in the organization of the American Society of Biological Chemists (1908). With his wife, Mary, endowed lectureships, Johns Hopkins Medical School and Bellevue Hospital Medical College.

WRITINGS: *The Diagnosis of Diseases of the Nervous System* (1892); *The Common Bacterial Infections of the Digestive Tract and the Intoxication Arising from Them* (1907); *On Infantilism Arising from Chronic Intestinal Infection* (1908). REFERENCES: *DAB*, 8: 597-98; Robert M. Hawthorne, Jr., "Christian Archibald Herter, MD (1865-1910)," *Perspectives in Biol. Med.*, 18 (Autumn 1974): 24-39; Kelly and Burrage (1928): 560-61; *Who Was Who in Am.*, 1: 556.

S. Galishoff

HERTZLER, ARTHUR EMANUEL (July 25, 1870, West Point, Ia.-September 12, 1946, Halstead, Kans.). *Surgeon; Surgical pathologist*. Son of Daniel, a farmer, and Hannah (Krehbiel) Hertzler. Married Myrtle Arnold, 1894, three daughters, divorced; Edith Sarrasin, 1909, divorced; Dr. Irene Koeneke, 1935. EDUCATION: 1890, A.B., Southwestern (Kans.); 1894, M.D., Northwestern University; 1896, B.S., Southwestern; 1897, M.A., Illinois Wesleyan; studied in Berlin with Wilhelm Waldeyer and Hans Virchow. CAREER: 1902-7, professor of histology and pathology, University Medical College of Kansas City (Kans.); 1907-46, surgical faculty, University of Kansas School of Medicine, becoming full professor in 1919. CONTRIBUTIONS: Attained worldwide popular acclaim (1938) with publication of the autobiographical *Horse and Buggy Doctor*, which sold more than 200,000 copies the first year and eventually was translated into some 17 languages. Divided career between teaching in Kansas City and developing a clinic-hospital in Halstead. The latter was occupied (1902) and expanded repeatedly to become a multispecialty clinic along Mayo lines; hospital was transferred to the Sisters of Saint Joseph (1933). Ranked among the most accomplished surgical pathologists of his time. In part this resulted from religious adherence to the advice of mentor Christian Fenger (q.v.), who urged his students to beat a path between operating room and laboratory. From the outset, saved every surgical specimen he excised and amassed a collection of 150,000 slides. Authored some 150 scientific articles and 25 books, including the first English work on local anesthesia.

WRITINGS: *Surgical Operations with Local Anesthesia* (1912); *A Treatise on Tumors* (1912); *The Peritoneum* (1919); *Clinical Surgery by Case Histories* (1921); *Diseases of the Thyroid Gland* (1922); *Minor Surgery* (with V. E. Chesky, 1927); *Surgical Pathology of Various Organs Systems*, 10 vols. (1930-38). REFERENCES: Edith Coe, *Hertzler Heritage* (1975); Edward Hashinger, *Arthur E. Hertzler: The Kansas Horse and Buggy Doctor* (1961), contains bibliography; Jerrad Hertzler, "Arthur E. Hertzler: The Kansas Horse and Buggy Doctor," *J. Kans. Med. Soc.* 63 (1962): 424-33; *NCAB*, C: 189; 16: 144.

R. Hudson

HESS, ALFRED FABIAN (October 19, 1875, New York, N.Y.-December 5, 1933, New York). *Physician*; *Pediatrics*; *Public health*. Son of Selmar, art publisher, and Josephine (Solomon) Hess. Married Sarah Strauss, 1904; three children. EDUCATION: 1897, A.B., Harvard University; 1901, M.D., College of Physicians and Surgeons (Columbia); for two and one-half years, intern, Mt. Sinai Hospital, New York City; for two additional years, studied in Prague, Vienna, and Berlin. CAREER: Upon return to the United States, on the staff, Rockefeller Institute for Medical Research, for a short period and then began the practice of medicine, New York City; 1915-31, clinical pediatrics faculty, New York University and Bellevue Hospital School of Medicine; medical staff, Hebrew Infant Asylum, Willard Parker Hospital, Harlem Hospital. CONTRIBUTIONS: One of the foremost pediatric investigators of his time, best known for clinical and experimental studies of scurvy and ricketts. Popularized the use of pasteurized milk formulas for infants supplemented with suitable antiscorbutic substances, such as fresh orange juice. Demonstrated that bleeding in scurvy is due to leakage from the capillaries rather than abnormal blood composition. Discovered that antirachitic properties could be imparted to certain foodstuffs, notably milk, by exposing them to ultraviolet rays. Discoveries revolutionized infant feeding practices. Urged upon Adolf Windaus the studies that resulted in the identification of the sterol ergosterol as provitamin D. His books *Scurvy, Past and Present* (1920) and *Rickets, Including Osteomalacia and Tetany* (1929) are medical classics. Was active in the movement to improve New York City's market milk supply and urged the pasteurization of cream for butter manufacture to prevent the spread of tuberculosis. Instrumental in the establishment of a tuberculosis preventorium for children in Farmingdale, N.J., the first such institution, of which he was medical director and, at the time of his death, president. First to advocate splenectomy for purpura. Also made important studies of hemophilia, gastrointestinal disorders, and infectious diseases of childhood.

WRITINGS: "German Measles (Rubella): An Experimental Study," *Arch. of Int. Med.* 13 (1914): 913-16; "Infantile Scurvy: The Blood, the Blood Vessels, and the Diet," *Am. J. of Diseases of Children* 8 (Dec. 1914): 385-405 (with Mildred Fish); "A Consideration of the Reduction of Blood Platelets in Purpura," *Proc., Soc. for Experimental Biol. & Med.* 14 (1917): 96-97; "Prophylactic Therapy for Rickets in a Negro Community," *JAMA* 69 (1917): 1583-86 (with L. J. Unger); "A Tuberculosis Preventorium for Infants," *Am. Rev. of Tuberculosis* 1 (1917-18): 669-73. A bibliography is in *Collected Writings: Alfred Fabian Hess* (1936). REFERENCES: *DAB*, Supplement 1: 397-98; Miller, *BHM*, p. 49; *NCAB*, 32: 357-58; *N.Y. Times*, December 7, 1933; George Rosen, "The Case of the Consumptive Conductor, or Public Health on a Streetcar: A Centennial Tribute to Alfred F. Hess, M.D.," *Am. J. of Public Health* 65 (Sept. 1975): 977-78.

                                                                                    S. Galishoff

HEWITT, CHARLES NATHANIEL (June 3, 1835, Vergennes, Vt.-July 7, 1910, Summit, N.J.). *Public health.* Son of Henry, physician, and Althea F. Hewitt. Married Helen Robinson Hawley, 1869. EDUCATION: At Hobart College: 1856, B.A.; and 1859, A.M.; 1857, M.D., Albany Medical College. CAREER: 1857-61, practice, Geneva, N.Y.; 1861-65, surgeon, 50th New York Regiment, and surgeon-in-chief, engineer brigade, Army of the Potomac; 1866, settled in Redwing, Minn.; 1873, became professor of public health, University of Minnesota; 1872-97, executive secretary, Minnesota State Board of Health. CONTRIBUTIONS: Responsible for the creation of the Minnesota State Board of Health (1872) and was its director for its first 25 years. Founder, *Public Health in Minnesota* (1885-94). Founded and directed the Minnesota Vaccine Station (1889), supplying free vaccine to all medical personnel in the state. Studied abroad with Pasteur (1889). When he returned, brought a Koch sterilizer and the equipment to set up the first bacteriological laboratory west of the Allegheny Mountains concerned with human infection. President, Minnesota State Medical Association

(1881-82). REFERENCES: Philip D. Jordan, *The People's Health, A History of Public Health in Minnesota to 1944* (1953); *NCAB*, 13: 57; *Who Was Who in Am.*, 1: 557.

R. Rosenthal

HILL, FREDERICK THAYER (June 14, 1889, Waterville, Maine-April 22, 1969, Waterville). *Physician*; *Otolaryngology*. Son of James F., physician, and Angie (Foster) Hill. Married Ruby Winchester Choate, 1924; four children. EDUCATION: Preparatory work, Coburn Classical Institute; 1910, A.B., Colby College; 1914, M.D., Harvard Medical School, where he was a pupil of Harris Peyton Mosher, professor of otolaryngology; residency as aural house surgeon, Massachusetts Eye and Ear Infirmary. CAREER: During World War I, became a 1st lieutenant, Army Medical Corps; after a year, returned briefly to the Massachusetts Eye and Ear Infirmary as a staff member; 1919, returned to Waterville to begin practice; founder and medical director, Thayer Hospital, for 13 years and became director of Development and Future Planning (1964). CONTRIBUTIONS: Established and participated in the teaching programs for interns and nurses at Thayer. Received a number of honors. Respected and dedicated ENT practitioner. Made medical care accessible to citizens of Maine.

WRITINGS: *J. of the Maine Med. Assoc.*: "Otological Cases of Interest to the General Practitioner," 14 (Mar. 1924): 165-70; "What Is Wrong with the Tonsil Operation," 17 (Jan. 1926): 1-16; "Treatment of Deafness," 23 (Jun. 1933): 126-29; "The Problem of Financing Hospital Care for Indigent and Geriatric Patients," 51 (Oct. 1960): 353-54; "Functions of Area-Wide Planning as Seen in the Local Hospital," 54 (Jun. 1963): 120-22. REFERENCES: *J. of the Maine Med. Assoc.* 52 (Jun. 1961): 225-26; 60 (Jun. 1969): 149; *NCAB*: J: 98; *Portland Press Herald*, April 23, 1969; *Who Was Who in Am.*, 5: 334.

B. Lister

HILL, LUTHER LEONIDAS (January 22, 1862, Montgomery, Ala.-April 4, 1946, Montgomery). *Physician; Surgeon*. Son of Luther Leonidas and Laura Sarah (Croom) Hill. Married Lillie Lyons, 1888; five children. EDUCATION: 1878, Howard College, Marion, Ala.; 1880-81, M.D., University of the City of New York (later New York University); 1882, postgraduate studies under Dr. Samuel Gross (q.v.), Jefferson Medical College; 1882, M.D., Jefferson Medical College; 1883, study at Wyeth's New York Polyclinic Medical School and Hospital; 1883-84, studied surgery under Sir Joseph Lister, King's College Hospital, London. CAREER: 1884, began medical and surgical practice, Montgomery; 1888, appointed surgeon of the Second Regiment of Alabama State Troops with rank of captain; 1893, appointed Montgomery County physician to the Poor House; 1893, president, Montgomery County Board of Health; 1896-99, 1902-4, member, Board of Examining Surgeons (president, 1899); 1897, president, Medical Association of the State of Alabama; 1897-1932, visiting surgeon, Laura Hill Hospital, Montgomery (named after his mother; owned and operated by him and his brother Dr. Robert Hill); 1911, appointed surgeon-general with the rank of colonel, Alabama National Guard; 1915, surgeon, Mobile and Ohio Railroad;

1932, retired from practice. CONTRIBUTIONS: Performed the first successful operation in the United States of suture of the heart (for a stab wound penetrating the left ventricular cavity).

WRITINGS: "Wounds of the Heart," in *Reference Handbook of the Med. Sciences*, 2nd, 3rd, and 4th eds. (1886, 1893, 1895); "Elephantiasis," *Med. News* (Philadelphia) 64 (1894): 712-15; "Wounds of the Heart with a Report of Seventeen Cases of Heart Suture," *Med. Record* 58 (1900): 921-24. REFERENCES: E. B. Carmichael, "L. L. Hill," *Southern Surgeon* 14 (1948): 659-69; *NCAB*, 36: 455; *Who's Who in Ala.* (1939-40).

S. Eichold

HILLEBRAND, WILHELM (November 13, 1821, Nieheim, Westphalia, Germany-July 13, 1886, Heidelberg, Germany). *Physician*. Son of Judge Franz Joseph and Louise Pauling (Koening) Hillebrand. Married Anna Post, November 16, 1852; two sons. EDUCATION: Early education in Nieheim; studied in Goettingen, Heidelberg, and Berlin, Germany, and received medical degree in Berlin. CAREER: Practiced in Paderborn, Germany, and Manila, Philippines; 1850, arrived in Hawaii; 1852-58, practiced with Dr. Wesley Newcomb; 1859-71, physician at Queen's Hospital, Honolulu, Hawaii; 1863, member, Board of Health; 1868, physician, Insane Asylum; 1871, left Hawaii for the last time; 1872-86, traveled in Europe and settled in Heidelberg, where he continued work on *Flora of the Hawaiian Islands*. CONTRIBUTIONS: One of signers of the charter of incorporation, Hawaiian Medical Society (1856), and served as its first vice-president. As commissioner of immigration, arranged for the emigration of workers from Portugal to Hawaii (1877). Investigated methods for control of leprosy at request of Board of Health. While on a world tour (1865-66), collected plants and animals that he believed would make a valuable addition to those species already in the Islands. Carefully preserved and studied native plants of Hawaii wherever he went. Foster Gardens, Honolulu, Hillebrand's former home, has a collection of exotic trees and flowers he planted; lovely native begonia is named Hillebrandia in his honor.

WRITINGS: *Flora of the Hawaiian Islands* (1888, published posthumously); "On Leprosy," *Indian Medical Gazette*, 1 (1866): 131-33; *Ueber Form und Ursache des schrägverengten Beckens* (1849). REFERENCES: *Honolulu Advertiser*, November 8, 1951.

J. Breinich

HINSON, EUGENE THEODORE (November 20, 1873, Philadelphia, Pa.-June 7, 1960, Philadelphia). *Gynecologist*. Son of Theodore C. and Mary E. (Cooper) Hinson. Married Marie E. Hopewell, 1902; no children. EDUCATION: 1892, graduated from Institute for Colored Youth, Philadelphia; 1898, M.D., University of Pennsylvania; denied internship, University of Pennsylvania, because of race, despite fact that these positions were awarded to top 15 graduates in the class (he ranked 12th). CAREER: 1892-94, schoolteacher, Harford County, Md. (1892-93), and Philadelphia (1893-94); 1898-1905, staff, Frederick Douglass Memorial Hospital, Philadelphia; 1907-55, staff, Mercy Hospital, Philadelphia (chief of Gynecological Service, 1907-55); 1898-1955, private practice, Philadelphia. CONTRIBUTIONS: A founder of Mercy Hospital, the second oldest black hospital in Philadelphia (1907). Member of board, Douglass Hospital (until 1905), and Mercy Hospital (1907-55). Highly respected physician of Philadelphia; involved in black community improvement through NAACP and other organizations for many years. Co-founder, with Dr. Henry M. Minton (q.v.), of Sigma Pi Phi (Boule), first Negro American Greek letter fraternity. REFERENCES: W. Montague Cobb, "Eugene Theodore Hinson, M.D. 1873-," *JNMA* 48 (1956): 213; Russell F. Minton, "Eugene Theodore Hinson," *JNMA* 52 (1960): 454-55; *WWICA* 7 (1950): 263.

T. Savitt

HINTON, WILLIAM AUGUSTUS (December 15, 1883, Chicago, Ill.-August 7, 1959, Canton, Mass.). *Physician; Syphilology.* Son of Augustus and Maria Hinton, farmers and former slaves. Married Ada Hawes, 1909; two children. EDUCATION: 1905, B.S., Harvard College; 1912, M.D., Harvard Medical School. CAREER: 1912-15, voluntary assistant, Pathological Laboratory, Massachusetts General Hospital; 1915, appointed director, Laboratory Department, Boston Dispensary; and chief, Wassermann Laboratory, Massachusetts Department of Public Health; 1923-59, medicine faculty (bacteriology, immunology, preventive medicine, and hygiene), Harvard Medical School; 1949, at the age of 66, promoted to professor, making Hinton the first black professor in the history of Harvard Medical School; lecturer, Simmons College, Harvard School of Public Health, and Tufts College; 1935, appointed consultant on venereal disease, U.S. Public Health Service. CONTRIBUTIONS: Developed the Hinton flocculation test for the diagnosis of syphilis; with Dr. John A. V. Davies, Children's Hospital, developed the Davies-Hinton test for the detection of syphilis in the nervous system through the analysis of spinal fluid. Helped establish at the Boston Dispensary, one of the first training schools for medical technicians in the United States. As director, Wassermann Laboratory, contributed to the establishment of more than 100 new diagnostic laboratories for the detection of venereal disease.

WRITINGS: *Syphilis and Its Treatment* (1936); "Glycerol-Cholesterol Precipitation Reaction in Syphilis," *Boston Med. and Surg. J.* 196 (1927): 993-96; "Hinton and Davies-Hinton Tests for Syphilis," *Ven. Dis. Inform.*, Supplement 9 (1939): 172-82 (with J.A.V. Davies). Writings listed in Harvard Medical School Archives, Cambridge, Mass.; and Barbara Anne Nabrit, "A Question of Merit: A Study of William Augustus Hinton" (Senior honors thesis, Harvard University, 1972), app. 4. REFERENCES: Dr. Albert Coons et al., "William Augustus Hinton," *Harvard Univ. Gazette* (Jul. 16, 1960): 243-44; *JNMA* 49 (1957): 427-28; Nabrit, "A Question of Merit."

M. H. Warner

HIRSCHFELDER, ARTHUR DOUGLASS (September 29, 1879, San Francisco, Calif.-October 11, 1942, Minneapolis, Minn.). *Physician; Cardiology;*

Pharmacology. Son of James Oakland, physician, and Clara (Honigsberg) Hirschfelder. Married Mary R. Straus, 1905; two children. EDUCATION: 1897, B.S., University of California; 1898-99, studied at Pasteur Institute, Paris, and University of Heidelberg; Johns Hopkins: 1903, M.D.; and 1903-4, intern; 1904-5, resident and assistant in medicine, Cooper Medical College (San Francisco). CAREER: 1905-13, medicine faculty, Johns Hopkins Medical School; 1913-42, pharmacology faculty, University of Minnesota; 1918, pharmacologist, War Department, U.S. government. CONTRIBUTIONS: Appointed director, physiological laboratory, Johns Hopkins medical clinic (1905), one of three full-time clinical research divisions established that year at Johns Hopkins—the first of such facilities in the United States. Made some of the first measurements of blood pressure in man using the wide cuff. Did important research in variations in the form of the venous pulse and cardiac arrhythmias. Investigated the physiological mechanisms by which maladies in distant organs cause cardiac disturbances. Wrote *Diseases of the Heart and Aorta* (1910), the first comprehensive American monograph on cardiology; work brought together all that was then known about cardiovascular diseases in a manner that instructed both the scientific researcher and the practicing physician. With Merrill C. Hart, synthesized saligenin, a local anesthetic with low toxicity. During World War I, synthesized several brominated and chlorinated cresols whose louse-killing vapors were effective for much longer periods than the ordinary cresol and naphthol then in use.

WRITINGS: "Diuretics in Cardiac Disease: A General Review," *JAMA* 61 (1913): 340; *Textbook of Pharmacology; An Investigation of the Louse Problem* (1918, with William Moore); "Applications of Saligenin and Other Aromatic Alcohols and Their Derivatives to the Problems of Therapeutics," *Trans. Assoc. of Am. Physicians* 36 (1921): 387. Most important writings are in *Johns Hopkins Med. J.* REFERENCES: A. McGehee Harvey, "Arthur D. Hirschfelder—Johns Hopkins's First Full-Time Cardiologist," *Johns Hopkins Med. J.* 143 (Oct. 1978): 129-39; *JAMA* 120 (Sept.-Dec. 1942): 638; *Who Was Who in Am*, 2: 255.

S. Galishoff

HITCHCOCK, EDWARD (May 23, 1828, Amherst, Mass.-February 15, 1911, Amherst). *Physician; Hygiene; Physical education.* Son of Edward, geologist and president, Amherst College, and Orra (White) Hitchcock. Married Mary Lewis Judson, 1853; three children. EDUCATION: 1849, A.B., Amherst College; 1853, M.D., Harvard Medical School; 1860-61, studied comparative anatomy under the British naturalist Sir Richard Owen (1804-92), London. CAREER: 1854-60, taught chemistry and natural history, Williston Seminary, Easthampton, Mass.; 1861-1911, chair of hygiene and physical education, Amherst College; 1869-1910, trustee, Mt. Holyoke College; 1879-89, member, Massachusetts State Board of Health, Lunacy and Charity; 1885-87, first president, American Association for the Advancement of Physical Education; 1897, founder, Society of the Directors of Physical Education in Colleges; at Amherst College: 1898, acting president; and 1898-1910, dean of faculty. CONTRIBUTIONS: Influential advocate of physical education for college students. The purpose of physical education, according to Hitchcock, was not to produce athletes or prodigies but to establish and preserve health. In addition to directing physical exercises, position at Amherst included instruction in hygiene, visiting sick students, and in general supervising student health. To demonstrate the beneficial effect of regular exercise (the department at Amherst was "experimental" and badly needed justification), kept detailed anthropometric statistics of his students, based on a battery of physical tests and measurements. The pattern established at Amherst was widely emulated at other American colleges. Pursued other bio-statistical studies and included the eugenicist Francis Galton (1822-1911) among his correspondents.

WRITINGS: *Elementary Anatomy and Physiology* (1852, with his father, Edward Hitch-cock; rev. eds., 1861, 1871); *A Report of Twenty Years Experience in the Department of Physical Education in Amherst College* (1881); *The Need of Anthropometry* (1887). Writings listed in *Am. Phys. Ed. Rev.* 11 (1906): 121-30. REFERENCES: *DAB*, 5, pt. 1: 71-72; Kelly and Burrage (1920), 532; Kenneth D. Miller, "Edward Hitchcock," *J. Health & Phys. Ed. Rev.* 31 (1960): 35, 132; idem, "Stearns, Hitchcock, and Amherst College," *J. Health, Phys. Ed. Rev.* 28 (1957): 29-30; *NCAB*, 13: 95; P. C. Phillips, "Edward Hitchcock," *Am. Phys. Ed. Rev.* 16 (1911): 217-28.

M. H. Warner

HITCHCOCK, HOMER OWEN (January 28, 1827, Westminster, Vt.-December 7, 1888, Kalamazoo, Mich.). *Surgeon; Public health.* Son of David and Hannah (Owen) Hitchcock. Married Fidelia Wellman, 1856, three children; Kate B. Wilcox, 1875, one child. EDUCATION: Kimball Union Academy (N.H.); at Dartmouth College: 1851, A.B.; and 1854, A.M.; studied medicine with his brother Alfred Owen Hitchcock; Dartmouth Medical College; 1855, M.D., College of Physicians and Surgeons (N.Y.); 1855-56, house surgeon, Bellevue Hospital. CAREER: 1852-53, principal, Orford Academy (N.H.); 1856-88, surgical practice, Kalamazoo; 1872, president, Michigan State Medical Society; 1873-78, founder and first president, Michigan State Board of Health; trustee, Olivet College. CONTRIBUTIONS: Led the Mich. medical profession in efforts to create one of the nation's pioneer state health boards; as first president of the board, devoted attention to public school conditions, alcohol abuse, and eugenics.

WRITINGS: *The Entailments of Alcohol* (1874); "The Laws of Heredity and Their Relation to Public Health," *Annual Reports Michigan State Board of Health* 5 (1878). Writings listed in *Index Catalogue*, 2nd series, 7: 182. REFERENCES: C. B. Burr, *Medical History of Michigan* 2 (1930): 113-14; Kelly and Burrage (1928), 571-72; Theodore R. MacClure, *The State Board of Health and a Quarter Century of Public-Health Work in Michigan* (1897), 11; *Representative Men of Michigan: American Biographical History of Eminent and Self-Made Men*, district 4 (1878), 33.

M. Pernick

HOCKER, WILLIAM ARTHUR (February 7, 1848, Lincoln County, Ky.-April 30, 1919, Omaha, Neb.). *Physician; Surgeon; Asylum superintendent.* Son of Tilman, agriculturalist, and Sarah W. (Morrison) Hocker. Married Alice Reynolds, June 16, 1873; seven children. EDUCATION: M.D., 1868, Bellevue Hospital Medical College; intern, Bellevue Hospital. CAREER: Practice: 1870-75, Harrisonville, Mo.; and 1875-99, Evanston, Wyo.; 1898-1917, physician and surgeon, Union Pacific Railroad, Kemmerer, Wyo., and practice. CONTRIBUTIONS: First superintendent, Wyoming State Hospital (then known as the State Insane Asylum). Had been a member of the legislature when the enabling legislation authorizing the hospital had been passed and was primarily instrumental in its passage. Personally attended to the relocation of the state insane wards from Jacksonville, Ill., to Evanston. REFERENCES: *History of Wyoming* 1 (1918): 260; *Kemmerer Republican* (1917-19); Woods Hocker Manly, *The Doctor's Wyoming Children: A Family Memoir* (1953); *Progressive Men in the State of Wyoming* (1903), 102-3.

A. Palmieri

HODGE, HUGH LENOX (June 27, 1796, Philadelphia, Pa.-February 26, 1873, Philadelphia). *Physician; Obstetrics and gynecology.* Son of Hugh, physician, and Maria (Blanchard) Hodge. Married Margaret E. Aspinwall, 1828; seven children. EDUCATION: 1814, A.B., Nassau Hall, Princeton; 1814, apprentice to Casper Wistar (q.v.), Philadelphia; 1818, M.D., University of Pennsylvania; 1818-20, ship's surgeon. CAREER: *Post* 1820, practiced surgery, Philadelphia; *post* 1821, taught anatomy at Dr. Horner's private school; *post* 1823, taught at Dr. Chapman's Summer School (the Medical Institute), Philadelphia; 1835-63, professor of obstetrics and diseases of women and children, University of Pennsylvania. CONTRIBUTIONS: Highly regarded teacher of obstetrics and gynecology. An accurate observer of great experience, clarified concepts of the mechanism of labor, anticipated Credé method of placental expulsion. Championed proper indications for use of obstetrical forceps. Invented pessary of particular value for uterine retroversion. Opposed accouchement forcé in eclampsia and the concept of the contagiousness of puerperal sepsis. Inveighed against criminal abortion.

WRITINGS: *On the Non-contagious Character of Puerperal Fever: An Introductory Lecture* (1852); *On Diseases Peculiar to Women, Including Displacements of the Uterus* (1860); *The Principles and Practice of Obstetrics* (1864); *Foeticide, or Criminal Abortion. . .* (1869). REFERENCES: *DAB*, 5, pt. 1: 99-100; William Goodell, *Biographical Memoir of Hugh L. Hodge, M.D., LL.D.*(1874); *NCAB*, 10: 244-45; R.A.F. Penrose, *A Discourse Commemorative of the Life and Character of Hugh L. Hodge, M.D., LL.D., . . .* (1873); Herbert Thoms, "Hugh Lenox Hodge," *Am. J. Obstet. Gynecol.* 33 (1937): 886-93; John Whitridge Williams, "Hugh Lenox Hodge (1796-1873)," in "A Sketch of the History of Obstetrics in the United States up to 1860," *Am. Gynecol.* 3 (1903).

L. D. Longo

HODGEN, JOHN THOMPSON (January 19, 1826, Hodgenville, Ky.-April 28, 1882, St. Louis, Mo.). *Surgeon.* Son of Jacob and Frances (Brown) Hodgen. Married Elizabeth Delphine Mudd, March 28, 1854; four children. EDUCATION:

Collegiate course, Bethany College, Bethany, Va.; 1848, M.D., Missouri Medical College (medical department, University of Missouri), St. Louis; 1848-49, assistant resident physician, St. Louis City Hospital. CAREER: 1849-53, demonstrator of anatomy, Missouri Medical College; at St. Louis Medical College, St. Louis: 1854-58, professor of anatomy; 1858-64, professor of anatomy and physiology; 1864-75, professor of physiology and anatomy; and 1875-82, professor of surgical anatomy and dean. CONTRIBUTIONS: A widely known surgeon in the western United States, was originally the protege of Joseph Nash McDowell (q.v.), Missouri Medical College. During the Civil War, transferred allegiance to the rival St. Louis Medical College because of his adherence to the Union cause. Member, first permanent Board of Health, St. Louis (1867-71), and first president. Helped organize the Association of American Medical Colleges (1876), although the St. Louis Medical College decided not to join it. During tenure as dean, a third year of medical instruction was introduced by the St. Louis Medical College, an option selected by an overwhelming majority of its students. Best remembered for the invention of the Hodgen splint, a wire suspension device for thigh fractures.

WRITINGS: "Treatment of Oblique and Compound Fractures of the Leg." *St. Louis Med. & Surg. J.*, n.s. 8 (1871); "On Fractures," *ibid.*, n.s. 7 (1870). Listed in the *Index Catalogue* 6 (1885): 273. REFERENCES: *DAB*, 5, pt. 1: 100; Kelly and Burrage (1920), 536; Harvey Hodgen Mudd, "Dr. Abram Litton and Dr. John T. Hodgen" (pamphlet, Missouri Historical Society, 1895); *NCAB*, 8: 214; "A Sketch of the Life of the late John T. Hodgen, M.D., LL.D. of St. Louis," *Med. Mirror*, (St. Louis), January 1890.

D. Sneddeker

HOERR, NORMAND LOUIS (May 3, 1902, Peoria, Ill.-December 14, 1958, Cleveland, Ohio). *Histologist; Neuroanatomist.* Son of Christian J. and Lydia (Dallinger) Hoerr. Married Virginia Collier Gale, 1927. EDUCATION: 1923, B.A., Johns Hopkins University; University of Chicago: 1929, Ph.D. (anatomy); and 1931, M.D. CAREER: 1923-24, chemist, DuPont Company; anatomy faculty: 1925-39, Chicago University; and 1939-58, Western Reserve University. CONTRIBUTIONS: With Robert Russell Bensley, inaugurated the modern era of organelle chemistry (1934), when they separated mitochondria from the liver cell; led biochemists to realize the value of localizing specific enzymes and biochemical functions within morphologic constituents of the cell; cell fractionation procedure employed in study is still in use today. Helped establish the field of cytochemistry by organizing a symposium entitled "Frontiers in Cytochemistry" and by editing the proceedings (published in 1943). With George William Bartelmez, elucidated the structure of the synapse. Associate editor, *Gray's Anatomy* (1942) and *Anatomical Record* (1948-58), and co-editor, *New Gould Medical Dictionary* (1949, 1956).

WRITINGS: "The Vestibular Club Endings in *Ameiurus*. Further Evidence on the Morphology of the Synapse," *J. of Comparative Neurology* (1933): 401-28 (with G. W. Bartelmez); "The Preparation and Properties of Mitochondria from Guinea Pig Liver,"

Anatomical Record (1934): 251-66, 449-55 (with R. R. Bensley). His major scientific writings are cited in *DAB*. REFERENCES: *DAB*, Supplement 6: 295-96; *Who Was Who in Am.*, 4: 450.

S. Galishoff

HOFFMAN, FREDERICK LUDWIG (May 2, 1865, Varel, Germany-February 23, 1946, San Diego, Calif.). *Statistician; Public health.* Son of Augustus Franciscus, lawyer, and Antoinette (von Laar) Hoffman. Married Ella George Hay, 1891; six children. EDUCATION: Largely self-taught. CAREER: 1884, immigrated to the United States; 1884-86, odd jobs in the West and South; 1887-90, agent, Metropolitan Life Insurance Company; 1890-94, agent and then superintendent, Newport News office, Life Insurance Company of Virginia; 1894-1934, statistician, Prudential Insurance Company; 1922-27, research staff, Babson Institute (Wellesley Hills, Mass.); 1934-38, consultant, Biochemical Research Foundation of the Franklin Institute. CONTRIBUTIONS: Made extensive statistical studies of the diseases and mortality rates of blacks, which were published in *Arena* (April 1892) and later in an expanded form in *Race Traits and Tendencies of the American Negro* (1896); concluded that the high mortality rates of blacks, nearly double that of whites, had been brought about by emancipation and the loss of white supervision, which formerly, he maintained, had enabled the race to overcome its "inferior constitution and vitality;" findings were used to justify disenfranchisement and higher insurance premiums for blacks. Made statistical analyses of many of the health hazards of man, several of which were used by health reformers seeking remedial legislation; examination of "The Mortality from Consumption in the Dusty Trades," United States Bureau of Labor, *Bulletin No. 79* (1908), was especially significant and influenced both the antituberculosis campaign and labor legislation. Aided the American life insurance industry in its early fight against national health insurance (1916-22). Was instrumental in the founding (1913) of the American Society for the Control of Cancer (later, American Cancer Society) and was active in its educational work. Instituted and directed the extensive San Francisco, Calif., cancer survey of the 1920s. Improved the reporting of vital statistics and enhanced the status of health statisticians.

WRITINGS: *Facts and Fallacies of Compulsory Health Insurance* (1919); *9th and Final San Francisco Cancer Report* (1934). Writings are described in *DAB* and *NCAB*. REFERENCES: *DAB*, Supplement 4: 384-85; John S. Haller, Jr., "Race, Mortality, and Life Insurance," *J. Hist. Med.* 25 (1970): 247-61; *NCAB*, 34: 66; *N.Y Times*, February 25, 1946; *Who Was Who in Am.*, 2: 257.

S. Galishoff

HOLMES, CHRISTIAN RASMUS (October 18, 1857, Engom, Denmark-January 9, 1920, New York, N.Y.). *Physician; Medical educator; Ophthalmology; Otolaryngology.* Son of C. R., employee of the railroad, and Karen (Mickelson) Holmes. Married Bette Fleishmann, 1892. EDUCATION: 1883, M.D.,

Miami (Ohio) School of Medicine; 1883-86, intern and resident, Cincinnati Hospital. CAREER: 1886, junior post, Cincinnati Hospital; 1886-1914, entered practice with Joseph Aub and gained a national reputation for his work in ophthalmology and otolaryngology; 1888-99, ophthalmologist and otologist, Cincinnati Hospital; 1890-1904, professor of otology, Miami Medical College; *post* 1904, professor of ophthalmology, Laura Medical College and Presbyterian Hospital; medical director, Cincinnati General Hospital; and advisory commissioner, new Cincinnati General Hospital; professor of otology, College of Medicine, Cincinnati University; 1914-20, dean, medical department, Cincinnati University; 1917, Base Hospital, Camp Sherman, Chillicothe, Ohio, head of ear, nose, and throat department. CONTRIBUTIONS: Prominent ophthalmologist and otologist. Modernized Cincinnati General Hospital and merged the Medical College of Ohio and Miami Medical College (1909) into a leading medical educational center. President: American Academy of Ophthalmology and Oto-Laryngology, American Ophthalmology Society, American Laryngology, Rhinology and Otological Society, and American Otological Society.

WRITINGS: "Extirpation of the Lacrymal Sac and Gland," *Arch. Ophthal.* 28 (1899); "Hypertrophy of the Turbinated Bodies and Their Relations to Inflammation of the Middle Ear," *N.Y. Med. J.* 72 (1900): 529; "Laryngology and Otology," *JAMA* 35 (1900): 199; "Report of Five Interesting Cases of Lateral Sinus Thrombosis," *Laryngoscope* 30 (1919): 1-13 (with Henry M Goodyear). REFERENCES: M. H. Fischer, *Christian R. Holmes. . .* (1937); *NCAB*, 18: 361; R. Sattler, "Incidents from the Life of Christian R. Holmes: His Early Student and Professional Experiences," *Univ. Cincinnati Med. Bull.* 1 (1920): 63-67; Cecil Striker, *Medical Portraits* (1963), 130-34; *Who Was Who in Am.*, 1: 581.

G. Jenkins

HOLMES, OLIVER WENDELL (August 29, 1809, Cambridge, Mass.-October 7, 1894, Cambridge). *Physician; Poet and essayist; Anatomy.* Son of Abiel, minister, and Sarah (Wendell) Holmes. Married Amelia Lee Jackson, 1840; three children. EDUCATION: Phillips Academy, Andover, Mass.; 1829, A.B., Harvard College, Cambridge; 1829-30, Harvard Law School; 1830, studied with Dr. James Jackson (q.v.), Boston, Mass.; studied in Paris and Edinburgh; 1836, M.D., Harvard Medical School. CAREER: 1836, began practice, Boston; 1838-40, professor of anatomy, Dartmouth College; at Harvard Medical School: 1847-71, Parkman Professor of Anatomy and Physiology; 1871-82, Parkman Professor of Anatomy; and 1847-53, dean. CONTRIBUTIONS: Combined evidence from the literature with logical arguments to establish the contagiousness of puerperal sepsis. Writings, which antedated Semmelweiss, were attacked by most physicians and were not accepted for many years. Popular lecturer on anatomy. Considered a precursor of Freud. Highly esteemed poet, wit, and author of numerous essays and books.

WRITINGS: *Boylston Prize Dissertations for the Years 1836 and 1837* (1838); "The Contagiousness of Puerperal Fever," *New Eng. Q. J. of Med. & Surg.* 1 (1842-43): 503-30; *Homeopathy and Its Kindred Delusions. . .* (1842); *Puerperal Fever as a Private Pestilence* (1855); *Currents and Counter-Currents in Medical Science* (1860); *Medical*

Essays, 1842-1882 (1883). REFERENCES: Charles J. Cullingworth, *Oliver Wendell Holmes and the Contagiousness of Puerperal Fever* (1906); T. F. Currier and E. M. Tilton, eds., *A Bibliography of Oliver Wendell Holmes...* (1953); *DAB*, 9: 169-76; G. B. Ives, *A Bibliography of Oliver Wendell Holmes* (1907); William Sloane Kennedy, *Oliver Wendell Holmes: Poet, Litterateur, Scientist* (1883); J. H. Mason, Jr., "The Medical Life of Oliver Wendell Holmes," *Johns Hopkins Hosp. Bull.* 18 (1907): 45-51; John T. Morse, *Life and Letters of Oliver Wendell Holmes*, 2 vols.(1896); *NCAB*, 2: 336; Clarence P. Oberndorf, *The Psychiatric Novels of Oliver Wendell Holmes* (1943); E. M. Tilton, *Amiable Autocrat* (1947).

L. D. Longo

HOLT, ERASTUS EUGENE (June 1, 1849, Peru, Maine-October 2, 1931, Portland, Maine). *Physician; Ophthalmology; Otology.* Son of Erastus, carpenter and farmer, and Lucinda (Packard) Holt. Married Mary Brooks Dyer, 1876; six children. EDUCATION: Public school education, Peru and Canton, Maine; brief training in business and then attended Hebron Academy and Westbrook and Gorham Seminaries; taught school, Canton and Cape Elizabeth, and served for a time as principal, City Reform School, Boston, Mass., to earn money for medical school; 1874, M.D., Maine Medical School; 1875, M.D., College of Physicians and Surgeons of Columbia University; interned, Maine General Hospital, Portland; attended additional medical lectures, Dartmouth Medical School; 1881, went to Europe to observe techniques in English, Irish, and continental hospitals. CAREER: 1876, entered practice, Portland; 1886, founded the Maine Eye and Ear Infirmary and served it to his death; the first house doctor of the Maine General Hospital; for two years, demonstrator in anatomy, Maine Medical School; for two years; attending physician, Portland Dispensary; 1917, appointed Governor Carl Milliken's medical advisor and head of an advisory board of 300 physicians who examined draftees for World War I. CONTRIBUTIONS: Member and frequent officer of numerous local, state, and national professional associations. First eye and ear specialist chosen president, Maine Medical Association (1916). A founder, New England Ophthalmological Society (1886) and the Maine Academy of Medicine and Science and its journal (1894). Founder and first president, Portland Medical Club (1876). A bill he prepared to prevent blindness, especially in infants, was enacted into law (1891) by the state legislature as was one requiring practitioners in Maine to be examined and registered (1896), which he had prepared with others.

WRITINGS: "Does Cocaine Hydrochlorate While Relieving the Pain in Acute Otitis Media Prolong the Congestion?" (Read before the American Otological Society, 1885); "Physical Economics," *J. of Med. and Sci.* 10 (Sept. 1904): 329-40. An incredibly prolific writer, the following represents a sample of his contributions to the *Trans., Maine Med. Assoc.*; a more complete listing is in Richard Herndon, *Men of Progress* (1897): "Diseases of the Lachrymal Apparatus" (1882): 484-98; "Diseases of the Mastoid" (1883): 59-68; "Angiosclerosis of the Retinal Vessels" (1925): 22-24. REFERENCES: *Biographical Review, Cumberland County, Maine* (1880), 62-63; Henry Chase, *Repre-*

sentative Men of Maine (1893), 127; Herndon, *Men of Progress*, pp. 599-601; *J. of the Maine Med. Assoc.* 22 (1931): 211-14; Maine Historical Society Portland Obituary Scrapbook, 8: 95; *Who Was Who in Am.*, 1: 582.

B. Lister

HOLT, LUTHER EMMETT (March 4, 1855, Webster, N.Y.-January 14, 1924, Peking, China). *Physician; Pediatrics.* Son of Horace, farmer, and Sabrah Amelia (Curtice) Holt. Married Linda F. Mairs, 1886; five children. EDUCATION: University of Rochester: 1875, A.B.; and 1878, A.M.; 1880, M.D., College of Physicians and Surgeons (Columbia); 1880-81, intern, Bellevue Hospital. CA-REER: *Post* 1881, practiced medicine, New York City; early 1880s, medical staffs, Northwestern Dispensary, New York Infant Asylum, and New York Foundling Hospital; *post* 1888, medical director, Babies Hospital of New York City; 1890-1901, diseases of children faculty, New York Polyclinic Hospital and Medical School; 1901-21, diseases of children faculty, College of Physicians and Surgeons; 1901-24, member, Board of Directors, and secretary, Rockefeller Institute for Medical Research. CONTRIBUTIONS: Through his books, organizational work, and influence as a teacher, helped establish pediatrics as a specialty and effected a significant improvement in the health of infants. Did important clinical research at Babies Hospital of New York City, which became world famous under his direction; made it the first children's hospital in the United States providing more than orthopedic and surgical care. Wrote *The Care and Feeding of Infants* (1894), which went through 75 printings. Authored *The Diseases of Infancy and Childhood* (1896), one of the first textbooks of pediatrics, which went through 12 editions and was the definitive English-language work in its field for many years. Set a standard of meticulous professionalism that became a part of the education of his many students. A founder and president, American Pediatric Society and the Child Health Association. A founder and an original editor, *Archives of Pediatrics* and *American Journal of Diseases of Children*. A leader in the fight for clean milk and the reduction of infant mortality.

WRITINGS: "Two New Factors in Blood Coagulation—Heparin and Pro-Antithrombin," *Am. J. of Physiol.* 47 (1918-19): 328-41 (with William H. Howell [q.v.]). REFERENCES: *DAB*, 9: 183-84; Kelly and Burrage (1928), 586-87; Miller, *BHM*, p. 52; *NCAB*, 20: 46; Edwards A. Park and Howard H. Mason, "Luther Emmett Holt (1855-1924)," in Borden S. Veeder, ed., *Pediatrics Profiles* (1957), 33-60; *Who Was Who in Am.*, 1: 583.

S. Galishoff

HOLT, WINIFRED (November 17, 1870, New York City-June 14, 1945, Pittsfield, Mass.). *Artist and sculptor; Social worker; Special education.* Daughter of Henry, publisher, and Mary Florence (West) Holt. Married Rufus Graves Mather, 1922; no children. EDUCATION: Attended the Brearly School, New York City; 1897, studied at the Art Students' League. CAREER: 1903, after having seen a group of blind boys enjoying a concert became an advocate of the blind;

1903, established a bureau providing theater and concert tickets to the blind in New York City; 1904, studied at the Royal Normal College and Academy of Music for the Blind, founded by Sir Francis Campbell who was blind; 1905, with her sister Edith, organized the New York Assoc. for the Blind; 1913, founded "The Lighthouse," a social settlement for the blind funded by the Russell Sage Foundation; during World War I, organized Lighthouses in France and consulted on the rehabilitation of soldiers blinded during the war; 1919, established the Italian Lighthouse at Rome; 1934, settled at Williamstown, Mass., and supervised expansion of the American lighthouses.

WRITINGS: *The Light Which Cannot Fail* (1922). REFERENCES: Edith Holt Bloodgood and Rufus Graves Mather, eds., *First Lady of the Lighthouse* (1952); *DAB*, Supp. 3: 364-65; *Notable Am. Women*, 2: 209-10; *Who Was Who in Am.*, 2: 259-60.

M. Kaufman

HOLTON, HENRY DWIGHT (July 24, 1838, Rockingham, Vt.-February 12, 1917, Brattleboro, Vt.). *Physician; Public health specialist.* Son of Elihu Dwight and Nancy (Grout) Holton. Married Ellen Hoit, 1862; two children. EDUCATION: Vermont Academy, Saxtons River; studied under J. H. Warren, Boston, Mass., and Valentine Mott (q.v.), N. Y.; 1860, M.D., University of New York. CAREER: 1860, physician, Williamsburg, N.Y., Dispensary; 1861-67, practice, Putney, Vt.; 1867-1917, practice of medicine, Brattleboro, Vt.; 1873-86, professor, materia medica and general pathology, University of Vermont; 1896-1916, member, Vermont Board of Health; 1900-1912, secretary and executive officer, State Board of Health. CONTRIBUTIONS: Lobbied to create the Vermont State Board of Health, which was authorized in 1886. In 1898 the State Laboratory was established largely through his efforts. Modernized the health department's division of vital statistics, kept careful records of outbreaks of infectious diseases, worked toward improvements in sanitation. First president, Austine Institute for the Deaf, Brattleboro, Vt. President, Vermont State Medical Society (1873). Vice-president, AMA (1900). Helped organize the Pan American Medical Congress (1893) of which he was chairman, Executive Committee.

WRITINGS: "Problems in Sanitation" (presidential address, American Public Health Association), *Phila. Med. J.* (Apr. 25, 1902); "Tuberculosis: Its Transmission and Prevention" (presidential address, American Congress of Tuberculosis); *Am. Med.* 4 (1902): 298-311. REFERENCES: *Brattleboro Reformer*, February 12, 1917; *Who Was Who in Am.*, 1: 583.

L. J. Wallman

HOLYOKE, EDWARD AUGUSTUS (August 1, 1728, Marblehead, Mass.-March 31, 1829, Salem, Mass.). *Physician.* Son of Edward, Marblehead pastor and president of Harvard College (1737-69), and Margaret (Appleton) Holyoke. Married Judith Pickman, 1755, who died in childbirth; Mary Vail, 1759, 12 children. EDUCATION: 1746, A.M., Harvard College; 1747-49, studied medicine with Dr. Thomas Berry, leading practitioner of Ipswich, Mass., and surrounding area; 1783, M.D. (hon.—first), Harvard University. CAREER: 1747-1829, leading practitioner of Salem, and indeed the entire North Shore, for four-fifths of a century; 1782-84, 1786-87, first president, Massachusetts Medical Society; president, Essex Medical Society; 1814-20, highly active in a wide range of community affairs as a founder and president, American Academy of Arts and Sciences; first president: 1810-29, Salem Atheneum; and 1821-29, Essex Historical Society; president, Institution for Savings and the Salem Dispensary; a justice of the peace and member, Salem Stamp Act Committee; pillar of the Salem Club. CONTRIBUTIONS: Best known as a leading force in the early years of the Massachusetts Medical Society, being an incorporator and its first president (although he attended only the inaugural meeting during his first term) and reporting to it interesting cases and meteorological observations. Another dimension of Holyoke's strong influence on eighteenth-century Massachusetts medicine was his role as a leading medical preceptor, training 35 physicians, including Nathaniel W. Appleton and James Jackson (q.v.). One of the earlier Bay State physicians to integrate normal deliveries into his practice, but seldom did surgery. Known as the "Honest Doctor," was representative of the best in the native, apprenticeship trained, public-spirited tradition of eighteenth-century New England medicine. Enthusiastic student of science, made observations on the transits of Mercury and Venus and presented a 28-foot telescope to Harvard.

WRITINGS: "An Account of the Weather and of the Epidemics, at Salem, in the County of Essex, for the Year 1786," *Med. Communications of the Mass. Med. Soc.* 1 (1790): 17-40; "A Letter. . .Respecting the Introduction of the Mercurial Practice in the Vicinity of Boston," *Med. Repository* 1 (1798): 500-503; *Memoir of Edward Augustus Holyoke, M.D., LL.D.* (1829); "Meteorological Journal from the Year 1786 to the Year 1829 Inclusive," Am. Acad. of Arts and Sci., *Memoirs,* n.s., 1 (1833): 107-216. REFERENCES: *DAB,* 5, pt. 1: 185-86; J. B. Felt, *Annals of Salem* (1827); "The Holyoke Family," in C. F. Dow, *The Holyoke Diaries, 1709-1856* (1911); *NCAB,* 7: 488; C. K. Shipton, "Edward Augustus Holyoke," *New England Life in the Eighteenth Century: Representative Biographies from Sibley's Harvard Graduates* (1963), 546-51; Richard Wiswell, "Dr. Edward Augustus Holyoke," *Essex Institute Historical Collections* 66 (1930): 441-63.

P. Cash

HOOD, WILLIAM HENRY (January 6, 1862, Adrian, Mich.-November 29, 1942, Reno, Nev.). *Physician; Public health.* Son of Andrew Jackson and Mary Sophia Hood, farmers. Married Eunice Standerwick Hobbs, December 23, 1891, four children; Susan Cloran Seager, June 25, 1933. EDUCATION: Rush Medical College; 1883, B.S., Adrian College; 1886, M.D., University of Michigan. CAREER: 1886-1942, practice, Nev.; 1905-26, president, Nevada State Board of Health. CONTRIBUTIONS: Leading pioneering physician in Nev. President: State Board of Health (1905-26); Board of Medical Examiners of Nevada (1904); and Pacific Association of Railway Surgeons (1929-30). Active in Nev. banking and financial circles, serving as an officer of Pershing County Bank (1911-31) and director of the First National Bank of Reno.

J. Edwards

HOOKER, WORTHINGTON (March 2, 1806, Springfield, Mass.-November 6, 1867, New Haven, Conn.). *Physician; General practice.* Son of John, judge, and Sarah (Dwight) Hooker. Married Mary Ingersoll, 1830, four children; Henrietta Edwards, 1855, two children. EDUCATION: 1825, A.B., Yale University; 1829, M.D., Harvard Medical School. CAREER: 1829-52, general practice, Norwich, Conn.; 1852-67, faculty, Yale Medical School. CONTRIBUTIONS: Especially active in reform movements involving medical education and medical ethics. Published only monograph on subject of medical ethics to be written by an American physician in the nineteenth century (1849). Chaired several committees of the AMA and was elected a vice-president (1864). Contributed to reform in general education by writing primary and secondary school texts in the natural sciences, some of which were still in print 20 years after his death.

WRITINGS: *Physician and Patient; or, A Practical View of the Mutual Duties, Relations and Interests of the Medical Profession and the Community* (1849); "Rational Therapeutics," *Publ. Mass. Med. Soc.* 1 (1856-60): 151-218. REFERENCES: Chester R. Burns, "Worthington Hooker (1806-1867): Physician, Teacher, Reformer," *Yale Med.* 2 (1967): 17-18; *DAB*, 5, pt. 1: 201-2; *NCAB*, 13: 552.

C. Burns

HOOPER, PHILO OLIVER (October 11, 1833, Little Rock, Ark.-July 29, 1902, Sayre, Okla.). *Physician.* Son of Alanson and Magdaline (Perry) Hooper. Married Georgia Carroll, 1860; five children. EDUCATION: 1852-55, apprentice to Dr. Lorenzo Gibson, Sr.; 1856, M.D., Jefferson Medical College. CAREER: 1857-61, 1865-87, private practice, Little Rock, Ark.; 1861-65, Confederate States of America Army Medical Corps; 1879-87, medical faculty and dean, medical department, Arkansas Industrial University; 1886-93, 1897-1902, superintendent, Arkansas State Lunatic Asylum. CONTRIBUTIONS: Championed the movement for medical organization in Ark. (1870s) and rallied educated physicians to close ranks against quacks and irregulars. Helped organize and served as first president, Arkansas State Medical Association (1870-71). President, Little Rock and Pulaski County Medical Society (1872-73). Helped organize Little Rock College of Physicians and Surgeons (1873) and State Medical Society of Arkansas (1875), when the State Medical Association fell victim to ethical disputes. Participation in the organization and administration of the medical department, Arkansas Industrial University, emphasized the importance of a regular medical education. Largely instrumental in the founding of the Arkansas State Lunatic Asylum (1882), in its successful early administration, and in the development of public sentiment favorable to its continuation. Elected vice-president, AMA (1882) and presided over the 1883 meeting. REFERENCES: Arkansas Medical Society, *An Anthology of Arkansas Medicine* (1975), 26, 30; W. David

Baird, *Medical Education in Arkansas* (1979), 25-26; *Goodspeed Biographical and Historical Memoirs of Central Arkansas* (1978), 462-63; Nolie Mumey, *University of Arkansas School of Medicine* (1975), 65-66; *NCAB*, 7: 452; *Who Was Who in Am.* 1: 585; Kelly and Burrage (1920), 552.

D. Konold

HOPKINS, LEMUEL (June 19, 1750, Naugatuck, Conn.-April 14, 1801, Hartford, Conn.). *Physician; Satirist; Poet.* Son of Stephen, farmer, and Dorothy (Talmadge) Hopkins. EDUCATION: Classical education under his father; studied medicine under Dr. Jared Potter of Wallingford, Conn., and Dr. Seth Bird of Litchfield, Conn. CAREER: 1776, began practice, Litchfield, but served briefly as a volunteer in the Revolutionary Army; 1784-1801, physician, Hartford. CONTRIBUTIONS: One of the most eminent practitioners in early Conn. Extensively employed in consultation and had a great reputation in chronic diseases. A founder of the Connecticut Medical Society. Well known as a man of letters because of his association with the little coterie of literary men known as the "Hartford Wits."

WRITINGS: Wrote two treatises about "consumption" and "colds" supposedly revealing "a knowledge far ahead of that time and prove Hopkins to be a rival with Rush for honors in treating the great white plague." Wrote several poems, including "The Hypocrite's Hope," "The Cancer Quack," and "Ethan Allen." REFERENCES: *DAB*, 9:215; Kelly and Burrage (1928); James Thatcher, *American Medical Biography* (1828; rep., 1967).

J. Ifkovic

HORINE, EMMET FIELD (August 3, 1885, Brooks, Bullitt County, Ky.-February 1, 1964, Brooks, Ky.). *Cardiologist; Medical historian.* Son of George H., physician, and Elizabeth (Barrell) Horine. Married Helen B. Ruthenburg, June 30, 1914; four children. EDUCATION: Preliminary education in public schools, Americus, Ga.; 1901-3, Emory College (now Emory University), Atlanta, Ga.; 1903-7, Kentucky School of Medicine (now University of Louisville); 1907-9, internship and residency, St. Anthony's Hospital, Louisville; 1922, National Heart Hospital, London; and studied briefly (July) in Sir Thomas Lewis's Laboratory, University College, London; 1922-23, Pathologische Institut, Allgemeines Krankenhaus, Vienna. CAREER: 1909-17, general practice of medicine and anesthesiology, Louisville; 1918-19, captain M.C., U.S. Army, and chief, Cardiovascular Service, Camp Hancock, Augusta, Ga.; 1923-46, private practice of cardiology, Louisville; 1935-63, historian, Kentucky State Medical Association; president, Medico-Chirurgical Society, Louisville, and Ohio Valley Medical Association; 1908, instructor in medicine, University of Louisville medical department; at University of Louisville School of Medicine: 1933, associate clinical professor of medicine; 1949, clinical professor of medicine and chief of section on medical history; 1950, professor of medicine and chief of section on medical history; and 1955, professor emeritus of medicine. CONTRIBUTIONS: During 46 years of association with the University of Louisville School of

Medicine, taught numerous students in the lecture room and in the clinics. Major contributions to the advance of medicine were in his specialty of cardiology. First cardiologist in Jefferson County (1922). A meticulous scholar; publications were recognized for their unimpeachable references to facts. Known best for his publications in cardiology and medical history.

WRITINGS: "An Epitome of Ancient Pulse Lore," *Bull. Hist. Med.* 10 (1943): 209-49; "Early Medicine in Kentucky and the Mississippi Valley: A Tribute to Daniel Drake, M.D.," *J. Hist. Med. & Allied Sci.* 3 (1948): 263-78; *Biographical Sketch and Guide to the Writings of Charles Caldwell, M.D. (1772-1853)* (1960); *Daniel Drake, M.D. (1785-1852): Pioneer Physician of the Midwest* (1961). Bibliography prepared by E. H. Conner for presentation at Convocation Honoring E. F. Horine, M.D., University of Louisville School of Medicine, May 1961. REFERENCES: [E. H. Conner], "Emmet Field Horine, 1885-1964," *J. Ky. State Med. Assoc.* 62 (1964): 216; D. Ruthenburg, "Destiny Fulfilled," *The Courier-Journal Magazine*, September 11, 1960; L. S. Thompson, *American Book Collector*, 14 (1964).

E. H. Conner

HORNER, WILLIAM EDMONDS (June 3, 1793, Warrenton, Va.-March 13, 1853, Philadelphia, Pa.). *Physician; Anatomy.* Son of William and Mary (Edmonds) Horner. Married Elizabeth Welsh, 1832; ten children. EDUCATION: Academy of Rev. Charles O'Neill (Va.); 1809-12, apprentice to John Spence, physician of Dumfries, Va.; 1811-12, University of Pennsylvania, M.D., 1814. CAREER: 1813-15, surgeon's mate, hospital department, U.S. Army (during War of 1812); 1815, practice, Warrenton; 1815-19, practice, Philadelphia; and prosector of anatomy, University of Pennsylvania; at University of Pennsylvania: 1819-31, adjunct professor of anatomy; and 1831-53, professor of anatomy and dean; member, medical and surgical staff, St. John's Hospital. CONTRIBUTIONS: As dean of the medical school, University of Pennsylvania, maintained very high standards, and in response to the AMA recommendations for all colleges simultaneously to raise standards of all American medical schools, Pennsylvania was only one of a handful of schools that tried to comply. Wrote the first American work on pathology (1829). Helped develop the anatomical collection of the University of Pennsylvania, building upon the material bequeathed by Caspar Wistar (q.v.). Bequeathed personal anatomical collection to the university, enlarging what became the Wistar-Horner Museum.

WRITINGS: *Lessons in Practical Anatomy* (1823); *Treatise on Special and General Anatomy* (1826); *A Treatise on Pathological Anatomy* (1829). REFERENCES: *DAB*, 9: 233-34; Samuel D. Gross, *Lives of Eminent Am. Physicians and Surgeons* (1861); Kelly and Burrage (1920); W. S. Middleton, article in *Annals of Med. Hist.* (1923); *NCAB*, 6: 383.

M. Kaufman

HORNEY, KAREN (DANIELSEN) (September 16 1885, Blankenese [near Hamburg], Germany-December 4, 1952, New York, N.Y.). *Physician; Psychoanalysis.* Daughter of Berndt Henrik Wackels and Clotilde Marie (Van Ronzelen) Danielsen. Married Oscar Horney, 1909 (separated, 1929; divorced, 1937); three children. EDUCATION: Hamburg Realgymnasium for girls and universities of Freiburg-am-Breisgau, Göttingen, and Berlin; 1911, M.D., University of Berlin; 1911-13, internship, Berlin Urban Hospital; 1913-15, residencies in neurology (with Hermann Oppenheim) and psychiatry (with Karl Bonhoeffer), Berlin Charity Hospital; 1914-15, psychoanalyzed by Karl Abraham; 1921, psychoanalyzed by Hans Sachs. CAREER: 1915-19, neurologist, Berlin hospitals; 1919-32, Berlin Psychoanalytic Clinic and Institute (at first, lecturer; later, training and supervising analyst); 1932-34, assistant director, Chicago Institute for Psychoanalysis; 1934-41, instructor and training analyst, New York Psychoanalytic Institute; *post* 1934, lectured at the New School for Social Research; 1941-52, dean and training analyst, American Institute for Psychoanalysis, N.Y. CONTRIBUTIONS: After "disqualification" as training analyst (because of challenges to Freud's theory) by New York Psychoanalytic Institute (1941), established (with Eric Fromm, Clara Thompson, and others) Association for the Advancement of Psychoanalysis, which supported American Institute for Psychoanalysis and *American Journal of Psychoanalysis* (which she edited). Emphasized sociocultural factors (as opposed to instinctive and biological factors) as determinants of personality and causes of neuroses. Disagreed with (and challenged) portions of Freudian theory that were interpreted to support ideas of inferiority of women (for example, concept of penis envy); developed a psychoanalytic psychology of women.

WRITINGS: Many early articles are collected in Harold Kelman, ed., *Feminine Psychology* (1966). Major books include *The Neurotic Personality of Our Time* (1937); *New Ways in Psychoanalysis* (1939); *Self-Analysis* (1942); *Our Inner Conflicts* (1945). REFERENCES: *Current Biog.* (1941), 409-10; *DAB*, Supplement 5: 315-18; Harold Kelman, *Helping People; Karen Horney's Psychoanalytic Approach* (1971); Joseph M. Natterson, "Karen Horney, 1885-1952: The Cultural Approach," *Psychoanalytic Pioneers*, ed. Franz Alexander (1966), 450-56; *Notable Am. Women*, 4: 351-54; *NUC Pre-1956 Imprints*, 255: 189-90; *N.Y. Times*, December 5, 1952, p. 27; Jack L. Rubins, *Karen Horney: Gentle Rebel of Psychoanalysis* (1978). A complete bibliography is in Frederick A. Weiss, "Karen Horney: A Bibliography," *Am. J. of Psychoanalysis* (1954).

M. M. Sokal

HORSFALL, FRANK LAPPIN, JR. (December 14, 1906, Seattle, Wash.-February 19, 1971, New York, N. Y.). *Physician; Microbiology.* Son of Frank, physician, and Jessie Laura (Ludden) Horsfall. Married Norma E. Campagnari, 1937; three children. EDUCATION: 1927, B.A., Washington University; 1932, M.D., C.M., McGill University; 1932-33, volunteer assistant in bacteriology, Harvard Medical School, and house officer, Peter Bent Brigham Hospital (Boston); 1933-34, resident physician, Royal Victoria Hospital (Montreal), and, during part of 1934, resident surgeon, Montreal General Hospital; 1938, studied at the Institute of Physical Chemistry, Uppsala, Sweden. CAREER: At Rockefeller Institute for Medical Research: 1934-37, 1941-60, researcher; and 1937-41, staff member, International Health Division, Rockefeller Foundation; 1942-46, Medical Corps, U.S. Navy Reserve; at Memorial Sloan-Kettering Institute for Cancer Research, N.Y.: 1949-53, member, Board of Scientific Consultants; and 1960-71, president, director, and member, Board of Trustees; 1960-71, medicine faculty, Cornell University Medical College; 1965-71, director, microbiology faculty, Sloan-Kettering Division, Graduate School of Medical Sciences, Cornell University; and director of research, Memorial Hospital for Cancer and Allied Diseases; advisor and consultant to numerous private agencies and government boards; president: 1956-57, Harvey Society; 1967-68, American Association of Immunologists; 1968-71, Association of American Cancer Institutes; and 1969-71, Practitioners' Society. CONTRIBUTIONS: Introduced antipneumococcus rabbit serum as a therapeutic agent in lobar pneumonia. Made important studies of pneumonia and influenza; helped explain the changes found in influenza virus from epidemic to epidemic. Directed the world's largest medical center for cancer research, where he investigated possible viral links to cancer (1960-71). Co-edited and wrote extensively for the third edition of the widely used *Viral and Rickettsial Infections of Man* (1959). Helped edit *Journal of Immunology* (1950-62), *Virology* (1954-60), *Journal of Experimental Medicine* (1958-60), and *American Journal of Public Health* (1958-60).

WRITINGS: "Formaldehyde Hypersensitiveness. An Experimental Study," *J. of Immunology* 27 (1934): 569-81; "Anti-pneumococcus Rabbit Serum as a Therapeutic Agent in Lobar Pneumonia," *JAMA* 108 (1937): 1483-90 (with K. Goodner, C. M. MacLeod [q.v.], and A. H. Harris II); "The Diverse Etiology of Epidemic Influenza," *U.S. Public Health Reports* 56 (1941): 1777-88 (with E. H. Lennette, E. R. Richard, and G. K. Hirst). A bibliography is in *BMNAS*. REFERENCES: *BMNAS* 50 (1979): 233-67; *Current Biog.* (1961), 208-9; *N.Y. Times*, February 20, 1971; *Who Was Who in Am.*, 5: 348.

S. Galishoff

HOSACK, DAVID (August 31, 1769, New York, N.Y.-December 22, 1835, New York). *Physician; Botanist*. Son of Alexander, merchant, and Jane (Arden) Hosack. Married Catherine Warner, 1791, one child; Mary Eddy, 1797, nine children; Mrs. Magdalena Coster, 1825. EDUCATION: Academy of Rev. Dr. Alexander McWhorter, Newark, N.J.; Academy of Dr. Peter Wilson, Hackensack, N.J.; 1786-88, Columbia College; May-Autumn 1788, private pupil of Dr. Richard Bayley (q.v.), New York City; 1788-89, B.A., College of New Jersey (Princeton); 1789-90, medical studies with Dr. Nicholas Romayne (q.v.) New York City; 1790-91, M.D., University of Pennsylvania; 1792-93, medical lectures, University of Edinburgh; 1793-94, St. Bartholomew's Hospital, London, under Sir James Earle; studied botany under William Curtis; befriended by Sir James Edward Smith who gave him duplicate specimens from the Linnaean Herbarium. CAREER: Private practice, 1791-92, Alexandria, Va.; and 1794-1825, New York City; partnership with Dr. Samuel Bard (q.v.) for some years; at Columbia College: 1795, professor of botany; and 1796-1811, professor of botany and materia medica; at College of Physicians and Surgeons, New York City: 1807-11, professor of botany and materia medica and lecturer on surgery and midwifery; and 1811-26, professor of theory and practice of physic and clinical medicine; 1826-27, professor of physic and clinical medicine, Rutgers Medical College, New York City; 1827-30, professor of physic and clinical medicine, Rutgers Medical Faculty of Geneva College, N.Y., New York City; 1830, retired as professor with dissolution of Rutgers Medical Faculty. CONTRIBUTIONS: Outstanding teacher. Internationally known botanist who founded Elgin Botanic Garden to cultivate native and imported plants, especially those with medicinal properties. Authority on yellow fever, favored botanical treatment, opposing bleeding with the scalpel and purging with calomel. A leading citizen of New York City, was a founder of the College of Physicians and Surgeons and Rutgers Medical College as well as a staunch supporter of the New York Public Library, Columbia College, New York Hospital, New York Horticultural Society, and New York Historical Society. Took an active part in civic movements for the benefit of the poor and was instrumental in the founding of Bellevue Hospital and in providing vaccination for the poor of New York City soon after the discovery by Jenner.

WRITINGS: *Essays on Various Subjects of Medical Science*, 3 vols. (1824); *Lectures on the Theory and Practice of Physic* (1838). Writings listed in *Memoirs of the Am. Philosophical Soc.* 62 (1964): 212-40; N.Y. Acad. of Med., *Author Catalog* 18 (1969): 675-82. REFERENCES: *DAB*, 5, pt.1: 234-40; Alexander Eddy Hosack, "David Hosack, 1769-1835," in S. D. Gross, *Lives of Eminent Am. Physicians & Surgeons of the Nineteenth Century* (1861), 289-337; Miller, *BHM*, p. 52; *NCAB*, 9: 354; Christine Chapman Robbins, "David Hosack, Citizen of New York," *Memoirs of the Am. Philosophical Soc.* 62 (1964): 1-246; idem, "David Hosack's Herbarium and Its Linnaean Specimens," *Proc. of the Am. Philosophical Soc.* 104 (1960): 293-313.

R. Batt

HOWARD, WILLIAM FORREST (July 26, 1868, Portsmouth, Ohio-October 19, 1948, Idaho). *Physician; Surgeon.* Son of Nelson, farmer, and Frances Ellen (Folin) Howard. Married Minnie Frances Hayden, 1894; four children. EDUCATION: 1894, A.B. and B.S., Central Normal College, Kans.; 1896-97, Kansas University; 1897-99, Kansas University Medical College, M.D., 1899; postgraduate study, New York City, Vienna, and Rochester, Minn., and at Johns Hopkins. CAREER: 1902, settled in Pocatello, Idaho, where he practiced for 43 years. CONTRIBUTIONS: A leading Idaho physician, who published over 20 articles in journals and was elected president, Idaho State Medical Association (1912). Elected fellow, American College of Surgeons (1913), serving on its Board of Governors (1920-39). President, the Tri-State Medical Association (1915) and Northwest Medical Association. President, Idaho Reclamation Association (1923-30). REFERENCES: H. T. French, *History of Idaho* 3 (1914): 1259.

A. A. Hart

HOWARD, WILLIAM TRAVIS (January 12, 1821, Cumberland County, Va.-July 31, 1907, Narragansett Pier, R.I.). *Physician; Gynecology.* Son of William

Alleyne, architect, and Rebecca Elizabeth Travis (Anderson) Howard. Married
Lucy M. Davis Fitts, Annis L. Waddell, Rebecca N. Williams. EDUCATION:
Graduated from Hampden-Sidney College; 1844, M.D., Jefferson Medical College; 1843, resident, Baltimore City Almshouse. CAREER: 1844-66, practiced
medicine and surgery, Warren County, N.C.; *post* 1866, practiced medicine and
surgery, Baltimore; at University of Maryland: 1866-67, physiology faculty; and
1867-97, diseases of women and children faculty; 1884, president, American
Gynecological Society; for many years, visiting surgeon, Hospital for the Women
of Maryland; consulting physician and surgeon, Johns Hopkins Hospital; and
consulting physician, Hebrew Hospital. CONTRIBUTIONS: Occupied the first chair
of diseases of women and children in the United States. First American to use
Tarnier's forceps successfully, later simplifying the instrument and popularizing
its use. Devised many gynecological instruments, including the bivalve, or Howard, speculum. A founder, American Gynecological Society.

WRITINGS: "Three Fatal Cases of Rupture of the Uterus, with Laparotomy," *Trans.,
Am. Gyn. Soc.* 5 (1880): 145-63; "Two Rare Cases in Abdominal Surgery," *ibid.*, 10
(1885): 39-73. Writings are found mainly in *Trans., Am. Gyn. Soc.* and *Trans., Med.
and Chirurgical Faculty of Md..* REFERENCES: *DAB*, Supplement 1: 436-37; Kelly and
Burrage (1928), 607-8; *NCAB*, 12: 316; *N.Y. Times*, August 1, 1907.

S. Galishoff

HOWE, LUCIEN (September 18, 1848, Standish, Maine-December 27, 1928,
Belmont, Mass.). *Physician; Ophthalmology.* Son of Marshall Spring, army
officer, and Anne (Cleland) Howe. Married Elizabeth M. Howe, 1893; no children. EDUCATION: Bowdoin College: 1870, A.B.; and 1873, A.M.; 1871, M.D.,
Long Island Hospital Medical College (Brooklyn); 1872, M.D., Bellevue Hospital Medical College; c.1872-c.1875, studied in Europe. CAREER: 1876-1926,
founder and member, ophthalmology staff, Buffalo Eye and Ear Infirmary; 1876-
1909, ophthalmology faculty, University of Buffalo; *post* 1885, ophthalmology
staff, Buffalo General Hospital; 1926-28, director, Howe Laboratory of Ophthalmology, Harvard University. CONTRIBUTIONS: Secured passage of the nation's first law for the prevention of ophthalmia neonatorum by requiring the
use of prophylactic drops of silver nitrate solution in the eyes of newborn babies
(N.Y. State, 1890); similar legislation soon passed in nearly every other state;
nearly eliminated gonorrheal ophthalmia, formerly the leading cause of infant
blindness. Donated $250,000 to Harvard University (1926) to establish a research
laboratory bearing his name for the investigation of diseases of the eyes; matching
grant was provided by the General Education Board and the Harvard Corporation.

WRITINGS: *The Muscles of the Eyes* (1907-8); *Hereditary Eye Defects* (1927). Authored
more than 130 scientific papers. REFERENCES: *DAB*, 9: 293; *JAMA* 92, no. 2 (1929):
165; *NCAB*, 23: 218-19; *N.Y. Times*, December 29, 1928; *Who Was Who in Am.*, 1:
596.

S. Galishoff

HOWE, PERCY ROGERS (September 30, 1864, North Providence, R.I.-
February 28, 1950, Belmont, Mass.). *Dentist.* Son of James Albert, Baptist

minister and educator, and Elizabeth Rachel (Rogers) Howe. Married Rose Alma Hilton, 1891, two children; Ruth Loring White, 1943. EDUCATION: 1887, B.A., Bates College; 1890, D.D.S., Philadelphia Dental College. CAREER: Practiced dentistry: 1890, Auburn, Maine; 1890-93, Lewiston, Maine; and *post* 1898 (part time until 1903), Boston, Mass.; at Forsyth Dental Infirmary for Children, Boston: *post* 1915, chief of research; and *post* 1927, director; at Harvard Dental School: 1917-25, dental research faculty; and 1925-40, dental science faculty; 1925-40, pathology faculty, Harvard Medical School; 1929-30, president, American Dental Association. CONTRIBUTIONS: Pioneered in dental research and brought dentistry into the mainstream of medical science. Investigated the role of microorganisms in producing caries and particularly the etiology of pyorrhea. Introduced the ammoniated silver nitrate solution for the treatment of dental caries. Showed that diets deficient in vitamins C and A caused serious deterioration in the tooth and bone structure. Conversely, opposed the prevailing theory that diseased teeth could act as foci for bodily infection and the practice of wholesale extraction of teeth as a method of treating bodily illness. Played an important part in the conversion of the Harvard Dental School to the School of Dental Medicine, with a four-year graded curriculum equally divided between medical science and clinical dentistry.

WRITINGS: "Studies upon Dental Caries," *J. of the Nat. Dental Assoc.* 4 (1917): 997-1002 (with Helen H. Gillette); "The Treatment of Root Canals by a Silver Reduction Method," *ibid.*, 5 (1918): 1008-18; "Report on the Pathology and Aetiology of Pyorrhea Alveolaris," *International Dental Cong.* (Sixth) *Trans.* (1919): 115-19, also in *Dental Cosmos* 57 (1915): 307-13, *British Dental J.* 36 (1915): 464-71, *British J. of Dental Sci.* 59 (1916): 43-50, 77-81; "To What Degree Are Oral Pathological Conditions Responsible for Systemic Disease?" *Dental Cosmos* 61 (1919): 33-40; "Report on Studies of the Effect of Vitamin-Deficient Diet upon the Teeth," *Dental Soc. of the State of N.Y., Trans.* (1921), 136-42, also in *Dental Cosmos* 63 (1921): 1086-92. A bibliography is in Rollo Walter Brown, *Dr. Howe and the Forsyth Infirmary* (1952). REFERENCES: *BHM* (1964-69), 131; Brown, *Dr. Howe*; *DAB*, Supplement 4: 401-2; *N.Y. Times*, March 1, 1950; *Who Was Who in Am.*, 2: 602-3.

S. Galishoff

HOWE, SAMUEL GRIDLEY (November 10, 1801, Boston, Mass.-January 9, 1876, Boston). *Reformer*. Son of Joseph Neals, ship owner and manufacturer, and Patty (Gridley) Howe. Married Julia Ward, 1843; five children. EDUCATION: 1821, graduated, Brown University; 1824, M.D., Harvard University. CAREER: 1824-30, combat officer and surgeon, Greek war of independence from Turkey; 1831, studied methods of educating the blind in Europe; 1832-76, founder and director, New England Asylum for the Blind (later Perkins Institution and Massachusetts Asylum); 1844-45, co-editor, antislavery newspaper, *The Commonwealth*; Civil War, member, U.S. Sanitary Commission and American Freedmen's Inquiry Commission; 1865-74, chairman, Massachusetts Board of State Charities; 1866-67, organized Cretan War relief expedition; 1870-71, member, presidential commission to report on the annexation of Santo Domingo; active in numerous causes to create a more just society, including abolitionism, public education, and prison reform. CONTRIBUTIONS: Secured the establishment of the nation's first schools for the blind, deaf, and mentally retarded. Founder and director, Perkins Institution, where he developed instructional methods for the education of blind children. Invented a new form of raised type and led the way in the printing of books for the blind. Succeeded in teaching a blind deaf-mute child (Laura Dewey Bridgman) to communicate after all others had failed; had significant impact on the fields of psychology, education, and public charities. Was instrumental in the opening of a school for mentally retarded children in Boston (1848). Championed oral communication as opposed to signing for instruction of the deaf.   REFERENCES: *DAB*, 9: 296-97; John Garraty, *Encyclopedia of Am. Biog.* (1974), 544-45; Kelly and Burrage (1928), 608-9; Miller, *BHM*, p. 53; *NCAB*, 8: 372-73; H. Schwartz, *Samuel G. Howe* (1956); *Who Was Who in Am.*, Hist. Vol.: 332.

S. Galishoff

HOWELL, WILLIAM HENRY (February 20, 1860, Baltimore, Md.-February 6, 1945, Baltimore). *Physiologist; Cardiology; Hematology.* Son of George Henry, businessman, and Virginia Teresa (Magruder) Howell. Married Anne Janet Tucker, 1887; three children. EDUCATION: Johns Hopkins University: 1881, A.B.; and 1884, Ph.D. CAREER: 1884-89, biology and physiology faculties, Johns Hopkins University; 1889-92, physiology and histology faculty, University of Michigan; 1892-93, physiology faculty, Harvard University; at Johns Hopkins University: 1893-1931, physiology faculty; 1899-1911, dean, medical faculty; 1916-25, assistant director, School of Hygiene and Public Health; and 1926-31, director; 1932-33, chairman, National Research Council; 1905-9, president, American Physiological Society. CONTRIBUTIONS: The nation's most eminent physiologist in the early twentieth century. Did his first work on the circulatory system, nerve tissue, and blood components. Demonstrated the importance of inorganic salts in regulating heart beat. Described the degeneration of peripheral nerve fibers after severance of a nerve. Made most important contributions in studies of blood coagulation. Isolated thrombin (1910) and established its importance in blood clotting. With L. Emmett Holt, Jr. (q.v.), isolated a powerful anticoagulant found in large amounts in the liver, which he named "heparin"; was used in the treatment of clots, their prevention in transfusions, and vascular surgery. At the University of Michigan, taught what is believed to be the first laboratory course in physiology in an American medical school. Wrote *Textbook of Physiology for Medical Students and Physicians* (1905), which was widely adopted by American medical schools and went through 14 editions during his lifetime. Helped found the American Physiological Society and presided over the meeting of the first international congress of physiology held in the Americas (1929).

WRITINGS: "A Physiological, Histological, and Clinical Study of the Degeneration and Regeneration in Peripheral Nerve Fibers after Severance of Their Connection with the Nerve Centers," *J. of Physiol.* 13 (1892): 335-406 (with G. C. Huber); "An Analysis of the Influence of the Sodium, Potassium, and Calcium Salts of the Blood on the Automatic Contraction of the Heart Muscle," *Am. J. of Physiol.* 6 (1901): 181-206; "The Preparation and Properties of Thrombin together with Observations on Antithrombin and Prothrombin," *ibid.*, 26 (1910): 453-73; "Two New Factors in Blood Coagulation, Heparin and Proantithrombin," *ibid.*, 47 (1918): 328-41 (with L. E. Holt, Jr.); "The Production of Blood Platelets in the Lungs," *J. of Experimental Med.* 65 (1937): 177-203 (with D. D. Donahue). A bibliography is in *BMNAS* 26 (1951): 153-80. REFERENCES: *BHM* (1975-79), 64; *DAB*, Supplement 3: 369-71; *DSB*, 6: 525-27; Miller, *BHM*, p. 53; *NCAB*, F: 478-79; *Who Was Who in Am.*, 2: 266.

S. Galishoff

HOWLAND, JOHN (February 3, 1873, New York, N.Y.-June 20, 1926, London, England). *Physician; Pediatrics.* Son of Henry Elias, judge, and Sarah Louise (Miller) Howland. Married Susan M. Sanford, 1903; four children. ED-UCATION: 1894, A.B., Yale University; 1897, M.D., New York University Medical School; 1897-99, intern, Presbyterian Hospital (N.Y.); 1899, M.D., Cornell Medical College; 1899-1900, intern, New York Foundling Hospital; 1900-1901, studied in Berlin and Vienna; 1910-11, studied with Czerny in Strassburg, France. CAREER: c.1901-8, assistant to Luther Emmett Holt (q.v.); 1901-9, medical staff, various N.Y. hospitals; pediatrics faculty: 1910-11, Washington University Medical School; and 1912-26, Johns Hopkins Medical School; 1912-26, pediatrics staff, Johns Hopkins Hospital; 1912-26, director, Harriet Lane Home for Invalid Children. CONTRIBUTIONS: Inaugurated the modern era in American pediatrics during tenure as chairman, Johns Hopkins pediatrics department, the first full-time pediatrics department in the United States and the first equipped for laboratory study of infant and children's diseases; success of department aided the acceptance of full-time professorships in the clinical disciplines at other universities. Made important studies of chloroform poisoning of the liver (1909) and chemical and energy metabolism of sleeping children (1910-11). Did his most important work on infantile tetany, diarrheal acidosis, and rickets; showed that tetany could be treated with calcium chloride (1917) and, with Edward A. Park, demonstrated the effectiveness of cod liver oil in rickets (1921). Revealed the importance of calcium and phosphorus in the diet of children. Trained about 30 students who became heads of pediatrics departments in the United States and abroad. Collaborated with L. Emmett Holt (q.v.) on the seventh and eighth editions of his famous textbook *The Diseases of Infancy and Childhood.*

WRITINGS: "Acidosis Occurring with Diarrhea," *Am. J. of Diseases of Children* 11 (1916): 309-25 (with W. McK. Marriott); "Observations upon the Calcium Content of the Blood in Infantile Tetany and upon the Effect of Treatment by Calcium," *Quarterly J. of Med.* 11 (1918): 289-319 (with W. McK. Marriott); "The Radiographic Evidence of the Influence of Cod Liver Oil in Rickets," *Johns Hopkins Hosp. Bull.* 32 (1921): 341-44 (with E. A. Park). A bibliography is in *J. Hist. Med.* REFERENCES: *BHM* (1964-69), 131; *DAB*, 9: 312-13; Wilburt C. Davison, "John Howland: The Seventy-Fifth

Anniversary of His Birth," *J. Hist. Med.* 5 (1950): 197-205; idem, "Pediatric Profiles: John Howland (1873-1926)," *J. of Pediat.* 46 (1955): 473-86; A. McGehee Harvey, *Adventures in Medical Research* (1976), 195-215; Miller, *BHM*, p. 53; *NCAB*, 21: 392; *Who Was Who in Am.*, 1: 598.

S. Galishoff

HOYT, JOHN WESLEY (October 13, 1831, Worthington, Ohio-May 22, 1912, Washington, D.C.) *Physician; Chemist; Attorney; Educator.* Son of Jacob, farmer, and Judith (Hawley) Hoyt. Married Elizabeth Orpha Sampson, November 28, 1854; two children. EDUCATION: Ohio Wesleyan University: 1849, A.B.; and 1852, A.M.; 1852, studied at Cincinnati Law School and in the law office of Salmon P. Chase; Ohio Medical College; M.D., 1853, Eclectic Medical Institute, Cincinnati, Ohio. CAREER: 1853-57, professor of chemistry and medical jurisprudence, Eclectic Medical Institute; 1855-57, professor of chemistry and jurisprudence, Cincinnati College of Medicine; 1885-87, professor of chemistry, Antioch College, Yellow Springs, Ohio; 1857, moved to Madison, Wis.; 1857-67, editor and publisher, *Wisconsin Farmer and Northwestern Cultivator*; 1858-72, managing officer, Wisconsin State Agricultural Society; 1878-83, appointed by President Rutherford B. Hayes as governor, Wyo.; 1887-90, first president, University of Wyoming; 1890, elected to the Wyo. Constitutional Convention, where he helped prepare the documents for admission to the union; 1891, due to health, moved to Washington, D.C., where he organized the National University Committee of One Hundred, composed mostly of university presidents. CONTRIBUTIONS: Although a physician, is best known for his educational and political accomplishments. Organized Academies of Sciences, tried to reorganize George Washington University into a national university. An ardent conservationist and proponent of Yellowstone Park.

WRITINGS: *Toxicological Charts* (1856); Reports, Wisconsin State Agricultural Society, 1860-72; *Resources of Wisconsin* (1866); *University Progress* (1869); Reports of Wisconsin Academy of Sciences, Arts, and Letters, 1870-77; U.S. government report on education in Europe and America (1870); *Agricultural Resources of Wyoming* (1892); histories of the universities of Bologna, Paris, Oxford, and Cambridge during the Middle Ages. REFERENCES: F. B. Beard, *Wyoming from Territorial Days to the Present*, 1 (1933); *Biographical Sketch of the Life of John Wesley Hoyt*; *Casper Tribune Herald*, September 25, 1944; *Chronicles of the University of Wyoming* (1911); *DAB*, 5, pt. 1: 321-22; M. D. Harrison, "A National University and the National Interest" (Ph.D. diss., University of Kentucky, 1968); *History of Wyoming* 1 (1918); *Laramie Republican Boomerang*, June 27, 1929; *NCAB*, 13: 158; *N.Y. Times*, May 24, 1912; J. R. Schumacher, "Life, Educational Work and Contributions of John Wesley Hoyt" (Ph.D. diss., University of Wyoming, 1969); *Who Was Who in Am.*, Hist. Vol.: 599; *Wyoming State Tribune*, September 22, 1944.

A. Palmieri

HUBBARD, GEORGE WHIPPLE (August 11, 1841, North Charlestown, N.H.-August 24, 1924, Nashville, Tenn.). *Physician; Medical educator.* Son of J. B. and Annie Hubbard. Married Annie Lyons, 1869. EDUCATION: New Hampshire Methodist Conference Seminary and New London (N.H.) Scientific and Literary Institution; 1876, M.D., University of Nashville Medical Department; 1879, M.D., Vanderbilt University Medical Department. CAREER: 1864-66, teacher of black troops, U.S. Army of the Potomac and Army of the Cumberland; 1866-76, schoolteacher of blacks, Clinton, Kans.; Pittsburgh, Pa.; and Nashville; at Meharry Medical College: 1876-1916, dean; and 1916-21, president. CONTRIBUTIONS: Co-organized the medical department, Central Tennessee College (1876), which eventually became Meharry Medical College, one of two black medical colleges to survive the medical education reforms of the early twentieth century. Played a key role in educating more than half the black physicians in the United States during his lifetime. Obtained funding to keep the school operating from the Freedmen's Aid Society of the Methodist Episcopal Church, private donors, and the General Education Board. Without Hubbard, Meharry would have had a very difficult time surviving its first 50 years.

WRITINGS: Numerous articles about medical education of blacks primarily published in missionary journals. REFERENCES: Cyril A. Crichlow, "The Last of His Generation," *The Brown Book* (n.d.), 13-18; editorial, "Dr. George W. Hubbard Retires," *JNMA* 13 (1921): 30-31; J. Manuel Smith, "The Pioneering Influences of Dr. George W. Hubbard on Medical Education," *JNMA* 45 (1953): 427-29; *Who Was Who in Am.*, 4: 468.

T. Savitt

HUGHES, HENRY ADAMS (November 12, 1848, Mahoning County, Ohio-September 26, 1928, Phoenix, Ariz.). *Physician; Surgeon.* Son of Mordecai B., physician, and Ann (Adams) Hughes. Married Mary Inge, 1873; eight children. EDUCATION: 1875, M.D., Louisville Medical College; 1886, postgraduate work, Jefferson Medical College; also took courses at Johns Hopkins. CAREER: Left home at early age and at 14 was a cowboy in Tex.; practiced medicine, Grayson County, and later, Glen Rose, Tex.; 1886-1928, practiced medicine, Phoenix. CONTRIBUTIONS: Member, Texas Board of Medical Examiners. Helped to organize the Arizona Medical Society and was its second president. Member, Arizona Board of Medical Examiners. Superintendent, Arizona Territorial Asylum (1896). County health officer and candidate for Democratic nomination for governor (1911, withdrew; 1914, lost in primary election). Champion of prohibition cause. REFERENCES: *Arizona Republican* (Phoenix), September 27, 1928; certain information from descendents; James H. McClintock, *Arizona* (1916).

J. Goff

HUGHES, JOHN CLOKEY (April 1, 1821, Washington County, Pa.-August 10, 1881, Keokuk, Ia.). *Physician; Surgery.* EDUCATION: Studied medicine in Baltimore, Md., with Dr. Joseph Perkins; 1845, M.D., University of Maryland. CAREER: c.1845-50, medical practice, Mt. Vernon, Ohio; 1850-81, medical faculty, College of Physicians and Surgeons, Keokuk: 1851, professor of anatomy; 1852-81, professor of surgery; and 1853-81, dean of the faculty; 1852, chairman, AMA section on surgery; 1861-65, surgeon-general, Ia., and chairman, Board of Medical Examiners; 1856, 1866, president, Iowa State Medical Society; 1853-58, 1867-69, editor, *Iowa Medical Journal*; charter member, American Surgical Association. CONTRIBUTIONS: A distinguished surgeon and an important figure in early medical education in the Midwest as dean of a medical school that was "unsurpassed in the Upper Mississippi Valley Before the Civil War" except perhaps by Rush Medical College in Chicago. Influential in the development of a medical journal for the Iowa State Medical Society.

WRITINGS: Several papers detailing successful operations read before the Iowa State Medical Society and published in its transactions. REFERENCES: David S. Fairchild, *History of Medicine in Iowa* (1923), 224-26; Peter T. Harstad, "Health in the Upper Mississippi River Valley, 1820-1861" (Ph.D. diss., University of Wisconsin, 1963), esp. ch. 10, "Medical Education"; Charles H. Lothrop, *The Medical and Surgical Directory of the State of Iowa* (1876); *One Hundred Years of Iowa Medicine, 1850-1950* (1950), 115-16.

R. E. Rakel

HULLIHEN, SIMON P. (December 10, 1810, Milton, Pa.-March 27, 1857, Wheeling, W.Va.). *Oral surgeon*. Son of Thomas and Rebecca (Freeze) Hullihen. EDUCATION: 1832, M.D., Washington Medical College, Baltimore, Md. CAREER: Established practice, Wheeling, and announced intention to specialize in surgical treatment of the head and mouth. CONTRIBUTIONS: Criticized by physicians who opposed both specialization and dentistry for educated physicians. Acknowledged as the founder of oral surgery. Founded Wheeling Hospital, the first in what is now W.Va. Received honorary D.D.S. from Baltimore College of Dental Surgery (1843). Helped in the process by which dentistry was recognized as a separate profession on the same scientific principles as medicine.

WRITINGS: "Case of Elongation of the Under Jaw and Distortion of the Face and Neck, Caused by Burn, Successfully Treated," *Am. J. of Dental Sci.* 9 (1849): 157-65; valedictory address delivered before the graduating class of the Baltimore College of Dental Surgery, at the annual commencement for the session of 1849-50. REFERENCES: E. C. Armbrecht, "Hullihen, the Oral Surgeon," *International J. of Orthodontia and Oral Surg.*, 23 (1937): 377, 511, 598; *DAB*, 5 pt. 1: 364-65; Kelly and Burrage (1920): 575-76; Robert L. Murphy, "Father of Oral Surgery," *West Virginia University* (Spring 1976).

K. Nodyne and R. Murphy

HULSE, ISAAC (August 31, 1797, Coram, Suffolk County, Long Island, N.Y.-August 29, 1856, Pensacola, Fla.). *Naval surgeon*. Son of Caleb M. and Jerusha (Petty) Hulse. Married Amelia Rogers, 1821 (d. 1827), three children; Melania Innerarity, 1833, four children. EDUCATION: Local schools, Coram, N.Y.; Union Hall Academy, Jamaica, N.Y.; 1823, M.D., University of Maryland School of Medicine. CAREER: c.1818-19, teacher, Latin and Greek, Westchester County, N.Y.; c.1820-21, teacher, Baltimore, Md.; 1823, joined U.S. Navy, soon after receiving medical degree; assigned to U.S.S. *Congress* as medical officer; 1824, duty at Naval Hospital, Gosport, Va., assistant surgeon; 1825, promoted to surgeon; November 1826, became chief medical officer, Naval Hospital, Pensacola; 1837-40, fleet surgeon, West Indies Squadron; after leave of absence, returned to Naval Hospital, Pensacola, remaining there except for brief duty, Tampico and Vera Cruz, during Mexican War, until 1851, when for short time, was medical officer, U.S.S. *Saranac*; once more to Naval Hospital, Pensacola, to deal with yellow fever outbreak; 1856, died after a long and painful illness. CONTRIBUTIONS: Chief claim to fame was success in treatment of yellow fever. Mortality rate among patients lowest on record. Gained vast experience during epidemics at Pensacola and among seamen entering harbor from Caribbean ports. Wrote several newspaper items instructing public in prevention and treatment of disease. President, Board of Medical Officers, army and navy, Pensacola. Gave much attention to improvement of hospital care in military hospitals. Remembered for establishing a library for convalescents at Naval Hospital; numbered more than 2,000 volumes (1851).

WRITINGS: *Monograph on Yellow Fever* (1842); published original in *Maryland Med. and Surg. J.* 2 (1842): 391-406; *Dissertatio physiologico-medico inaugurales de medicamentorum operationibus* (1845). REFERENCES: Frederick Eberson, "Dr. Isaac Hulse, 1797-1856," *J. Fla. Med. Assoc.* 59, no. 8 (August 1972): 30-36; occasional brief items in Pensacola newspapers of period; Pensacola *Gazette*, September 2, 1856; Charles J. Werner, *Dr. Isaac Hulse* (1922).

E. A. Hammond

HUME, DAVID MILFORD (October 21, 1917, Muskegon, Mich.-May 19, 1973, Chatsworth, Calif.). *Physician; Surgery; Endocrinology.* Son of Wallace C., university professor, and Fay (Hill) Hume. Married Martha Emily Egloff, 1943; four children. EDUCATION: 1940, B.S., Harvard University; 1943, M.D., University of Chicago; 1943-51, intern and resident, Peter Bent Brigham Hospital (Boston, Mass.). CAREER: 1945-46, 1953-54, Medical Corps, U.S. Navy Reserve; 1951-56, surgery faculty and director, Laboratory for Surgical Research, Harvard Medical School; 1956-73, surgery faculty, Medical College of Virginia (later Virginia Commonwealth University); member: program project committee, National Heart Institute; and nephrology planning committee and surgery study section, National Institutes of Health; advisory board, Atomic Energy Commission; task force committee, National Kidney Foundation; and advisory group on renal transplants, Veterans Administration. CONTRIBUTIONS: Pioneered in kidney transplantation and in the modern evolution of pituitary endocrinology. Performed a series of cadaver kidney transplants (1950-51) in human subjects dying of renal failure; led to first successful twin transplantation, performed by his colleagues at Peter Bent Brigham Hospital. Studied the suprapituitary control of the secretion of adrenocorticotrophic hormone and developed the first quantitative bioassay for serum ACTH. Played a leading role in the development of Virginia

Commonwealth University and established there a large surgical research laboratory renown for its work in kidney transplantation.

WRITINGS: "Comparative Results of Cadaver and Related Donor Renal Homografts in Man, and Immunologic Implications of the Outcome of Second and Paired Transplants," *Annals of Surg.* 164 (1966): 352-97 (with others); *Principles of Surgery* (1969). REFERENCES: W. A. Altemeier, "David Milford Hume, 1917-1973," *Trans., Am. Surg. Assoc.* 92 (1974): 41-43; *NCAB*, 61: 80; *N.Y. Times*, May 21, 1973; Mark M. Ravitch, *A Century of Surgery*, 2 vols. (1981); *Who Was Who in Am.*, 6: 204.

S. Galishoff

HUME, EDGAR ERSKINE (December 26, 1889, Frankfort, Ky.-January 24, 1952, Washington, D.C.). *Physician*; *Military medicine*; *Public health*. Son of Enoch Edgar, physician, and Mary (South) Hume. Married Mary Swigert Hendrick, 1918; one child. EDUCATION: Centre College (Danville, Ky.): 1908, B.A.; 1909, M.A; 1913, M.D., Johns Hopkins University; 1914-15, voluntary assistant in neurology, Johns Hopkins University; 1917, graduated from Army Medical School (Washington); 1921, M.P.H., Harvard University-Massachusetts Institute of Technology School of Public Health; 1922, D.T.M., Harvard University; 1924, D.P.H., Johns Hopkins University School of Hygiene and Public Health. CAREER: 1915, medical director, American Relief Expedition to Italy after earthquake; 1917-51, officer (rising in rank from first lieutenant to major-general), Regular Army Medical Corps; 1918, commanding officer, Base Hospital No. 102, first with the Italian Army and then with the British Expeditionary Force; 1919-20, chief medical officer (director of typhus fever campaign) and American Red Cross Commissioner to Siberia; 1920-22, in charge of army's medical laboratory at Fort Banks, Mass.; at Army Medical Library: 1922-26, assistant librarian; and 1932-36, librarian; 1936-43, director, Medical Field Service School, Carlisle Barracks, Pa.; 1943-45, in African, Sicilian and Italian campaigns (1943, chief of public health, Sicily; 1943-45, chief, Allied Military Government, 5th Army, Italy); 1945-47, chief, military government, U.S. Zone of Austria; 1947-49, chief, Reorientation Branch, Civil Affairs Division; 1949-50, chief surgeon, Far East Command; 1950-51, director general of medical services, U.N. Commmand, Korea. CONTRIBUTIONS: One of the most decorated soldiers in American history, had a long, distinguished career in international medical relief and public health. Fought a typhus epidemic that ravaged Siberia after World War I and kept the disease under control in war-torn Naples (1943). Twice directed relief efforts in Italy, first after an earthquake killed over 30,000 persons (1915) and again as chief of the Allied government of the region occupied by the Fifth Army. A prolific writer on medical and military history. Helped edit *Military Surgeon* (1924-34).

WRITINGS: *Pettenkofer's Theory* (1929); *The Medical Work of the Knights Hospitallers* (1930); *The Medals of the United States Army Medical Department* (1942). REFERENCES: *Current Biog.* (1944), 315-19; *DAB*, Supplement 5: 335-36; Willard Rouse Jillson, "Major General Edgar Erskine Hume: A Biographical Sketch," *Kentucky Historical Soc. Register* 50 (1952): 95-110; Miller, *BHM*, p. 53; *Who Was Who in Am.*, 3: 428.

S. Galishoff

HUNT, EZRA MUNDY (January 4, 1830, Metuchen, N.J.-July 1, 1894, Metuchen, N.J.). *Physician; Public health.* Son of Holloway Whitfield, Presbyterian minister, and Henrietta Mundy. Married Emma L. Ayres, 1853; Emma Reeve, 1870, four children. EDUCATION: 1849, B.A., Princeton University; 1852, M.D., College of Physicians and Surgeons; 1876, studied sanitation and health administration in Europe. CAREER: *Post* 1852, practiced medicine, Metuchen; 1854, materia medica faculty, Vermont Medical College, Woodstock, Vt.; 1862, assistant surgeon, 29th New Jersey Infantry; 1863-65, in charge, Calvert Street Hospital, Baltimore, Md.; 1874, president (N.J.) State Health Commission; 1876-94, first hygiene instructor, Trenton State Normal School (now New Jersey State Teachers College at Trenton); 1877-94, secretary, New Jersey State Board of Health; president: 1864, New Jersey Medical Society; and 1882, American Public Health Association. CONTRIBUTIONS: One of the pioneers of American public health. Organized and guided the work of the New Jersey State Board of Health during its first 16 years (1877-94). Well known for his work and writings on epidemiology, vital statistics, rural health services, and personal and school hygiene. Foresaw and developed plans to meet the need of sanitary organization in rural areas.

WRITINGS: "The Need of Sanitary Organization in Villages and Rural Districts," *Am. Public Health Assoc. Reports, 1872-1873* (1875); "How to Study an Epidemic," *Am. Public Health Assoc. Reports, 1877-1878* (1880); "The Prevention of Epidemics," *British Med. J.* 1 (Mar. 14, 1885): 534; *Principles of Hygiene for the School and Home* (1886). Writings listed in *Index Medicus*, 1859-94. REFERENCES: Kelly and Burrage (1928), 618; *NCAB*, 12: 129; Fred B. Rogers,"Ezra Mundy Hunt: 1830-1894, Pioneer of Public Health," *J. of the Med. Soc. of New Jersey* 53, no. 11 (Nov. 1956): 554-58.

S. Galishoff

HUNT, HARRIOT KEZIA (November 9, 1805, Boston, Mass.-January 2, 1875, Boston). *Physician; Personal hygiene reformer.* Daughter of Joab, ship joiner and shipping merchant, and Kezia (Wentworth) Hunt. Never married. EDUCATION: Mrs. Carter's private school, Boston; 1833-35, studied medicine, Boston, with Dr. and Mrs. Richard Mott, irregular practitioners from England who stressed botanic remedies; 1853, M.D. (hon.), Female Medical College of Philadelphia. CAREER: 1827-33, founded and taught with her sister in a private school for girls; 1835-75, practiced medicine, Boston. CONTRIBUTIONS: First successful woman physician in the United States. First woman to press (unsuccessfully in 1847 and again in 1850) for admission to the Harvard Medical School. Believed that ignorance of physiological laws was the main cause of ill health. Her leading role in organizing the Charlestown (Mass.) Ladies' Physiological Society (1843) awakened her to the possibility of lecturing to women on physiology and hygiene, which she did throughout New England (although she attacked itinerent lecturers on physiology who were more interested in pecuniary gain than sanitary reform). A founder, New England Women's Club (1868), which supported women doctors. Advocate of women's rights, antislavery, temperance, education of women, and entrance of women into medicine.

WRITINGS: *Glances and Glimpses; Or, Fifty Years Social, Including Twenty Years Professional Life* (1856). REFERENCES: *DAB*, 5, pt. 1: 385-86; Hunt, *Glances and Glimpses*; Regina Markell Morantz, "The Perils of Feminist History," *J. Interdiscip. Hist.* 4 (1974): 649-60; *NCAB*, 9: 259; *Notable Am. Women* 2 (1971): 235-37; Mary Roth Walsh, *"Doctors Wanted: No Women Need Apply"* (1977), 20-34; Ann Douglas Wood, " 'The Fashionable Diseases': Women's Complaints and Their Treatment in Nineteenth-Century America," *J. Interdiscip. Hist.* 4 (1973): 25-52; Marie E. Zakrewska, "Harriot Kezia Hunt," *Woman's Med. J.* 10 (1900): 202-5.

J. H. Warner

HUNT, REID (April 20, 1870, Martinsville, Ohio-March 10, 1948, Belmont, Mass.). *Pharmacologist.* Son of Milton L., banker, and Sarah E. (Wright) Hunt. Married Mary Lillie Taylor, 1908; no children. EDUCATION: Johns Hopkins University: 1891, B.A.; and 1896, Ph.D. (physiology); 1896, M.D., College of Physicians and Surgeons (Baltimore, Md.); at various times between 1902 and 1904, studied under Paul Ehrlich at his Institute for Experimental Therapeutics, Frankfurt, Germany. CAREER: 1896-98, tutor in physiology, College of Physicians and Surgeons (Columbia); 1898-1904, pharmacology faculty, Johns Hopkins University; 1904-13, chief, Division of Pharmacology, Hygienic Laboratory, U.S. Public Health and Marine Hospital Service; 1913-36, pharmacology faculty, Harvard Medical School; at Council on Pharmacy and Chemistry, American Medical Association: 1906-27, member; and 1927-36, chairman; president: 1916-18, Society for Pharmacology and Experimental Therapeutics; and 1920-30, U.S. Pharmacopeial Convention. CONTRIBUTIONS: One of the pioneers of modern pharmacology in the United States. Studied the reflex decrease in blood pressure caused by stimulation of afferent nerves; provided basis for his subsequent major studies on vasodilator reactions. Became internationally famous for his discovery of the powerful biological activity of acetylcholine, especially in lowering blood pressure, and his elucidation of the relation between chemical structure and pharmacological action of choline derivatives upon the autonomic system. Investigated the physiology and pharmacology of the thyroid gland and showed the activity of thyroid preparations to be proportional to their iodine content, thereby providing a means for making them therapeutically reliable. Helped keep *The Pharmacopeia of the United States of America* abreast of modern developments. Played a leading role on the Council on Pharmacy and Chemistry of the American Medical Association in its efforts to promote high standards of purity and reliability for important drugs.

WRITINGS: "The Fall of Blood Pressure Resulting from the Stimulation of Afferent Nerves," *J. of Physiol.* 18 (1895): 381-410; "On the Physiological Action of Certain Cholin Derivatives and New Methods for Detecting Cholin," *British Med. J.* 2 (1906):

1788-91 (with René de M. Taveau); *Studies on Thyroid. I. The Relation of Iodine to the Physiological Activity of Thyroid Preparations. U.S. Hygienic Laboratory Bull.* 47 (1909, with A. Seidell); "Vasodilator Reactions," *Am. J. of Physiol.* 45 (1918): 197-267; "On Some Effects of Arsonium, Stibonium, Phosphonium and Sulfonium Compounds on the Autonomic Nervous System," *J. of Pharmacology and Experimental Therapeutics* 25 (1925): 315-55 (with R. R. Renshaw). A bibliography is in *BMNAS.* REFERENCES: *BMNAS,* 26 (1949): 25-37; *DAB,* Supplement 4: 410-12; *Who Was Who in Am.,* 2: 271.

S. Galishoff

HUNTER, JOHN FARRAR (February 19, 1860, Jackson, Miss.-October 5, 1918, Jackson). *Physician; Public health.* Son of Rev. John H. and Rosa M. (Farrar) Hunter. Married Perlie Prestidge, 1883; Mrs. Adine Poursine Kennington, 1915; one child. EDUCATION: Public and private schools of Jackson; began study of medicine under Dr. George K. Harrington, Jackson; attended medical lectures, Bellevue Hospital Medical College, N.Y.; 1882, A.B., M.D., Tulane University; 1888, postgraduate study, New York Polyclinic and Jefferson Medical College. CAREER: 1882, began practice of medicine, Jackson; at Mississippi State Board of Health: 1888-1908, member, and 1896-1908, secretary and executive officer; district surgeon, Illinois Central Railroad Company, and local surgeon, Gulf and Ship Island and Alabama and Vicksburg Railroads; medical director, Lamar Life Insurance Company, as well as examiner for other insurance companies; early 1900s, established a drug company in Jackson, and at time of death, was senior member of Hunter & McGee, druggists; 1900, formed professional partnership with Dr. Harris Allen Gant; 1909, opened an eight-bed hospital with Dr. Harley R. Shands, which eventually became the Mississippi Baptist Hospital, Jackson. CONTRIBUTIONS: As secretary and executive officer, Mississippi State Board of Health, took a leading part in stamping out the yellow fever epidemics (1897, 1898, 1899, and 1905). Played important role in establishment of the Mississippi Baptist Hospital, Jackson. REFERENCE: *NCAB,* 18: 189.

M. S. Legan

HUNTER, WILLIAM (1729 or 1730, Scotland-January 30, 1777, Newport, R.I.). *Physician.* Married Deborah Malbone, 1761; seven children. EDUCATION: Studied medicine under the elder Munro at Edinburgh, Scotland, and in Leyden, the Netherlands. CAREER: *Post* 1752, practiced medicine, Newport; during French and Indian War, surgeon, first to British forces and after 1758 to R.I. troops. CONTRIBUTIONS: Gave first systematic, advertised public lectures in anatomy and surgery in America (1754-56). First "male accoucheur" in the colonies. Contributed greatly to the reputation of Newport as a medical center in the colonial period. REFERENCES: Roland Hammond, "Doctor William Hunter," *R. I. Med. J.* 24

(Nov. 1941): 199-201; Kelly and Burrage (1928), 621; E. B. Krumbhaar, "Doctor William Hunter of Newport," *Annals of Surg.* (Jan. 1935): 506-28.

S. Galishoff

HUNTINGTON, GEORGE (April 9, 1851, Easthampton, N.Y.-March 3, 1916, Cairo, N.Y.). *Physician.* Son of George Lee, physician, and Mary (Hoogland) Huntington. Married Mary Elizabeth Hackard, 1874; six children. EDUCATION: 1868, began medical studies with his father; 1871, M.D., College of Physicians and Surgeons of New York (Columbia). CAREER: Practiced medicine: 1872-73, La Grangeville, N.Y.; 1901-3, Asheville, N.C.; and 1903-13, Hopewell Junction, N.Y.; early 1900s, health officer, East Fishkill, N.Y.; and visiting physician, Matteawan General Hospital, N.Y. CONTRIBUTIONS: Described a chronic degenerative hereditary chorea found in a small number of inbred families of old New England stock living on Long Island, now eponymally known as "Huntington's Chorea"; occurring in adult life and ending often in insanity and suicide, it had been earlier recognized by his grandfather and classified by his father, through whom he came into contact with the disease.

WRITINGS: "On Chorea," *Med. and Surg. Reporter of Phila.* 26 (Apr. 13, 1872): 317-21. REFERENCES: Kelly and Burrage (1928), 622; Charles S. Stevenson, "A Biography of George Huntington, M.D.," *Bull. Hist. Med.* 2 (1934): 53-76; John H. Talbott, *A Biographical Hist. of Med.* (1970) 850-52.

S. Galishoff

HURD, HENRY MILLS (May 3, 1843, Union City, Mich.-July 19, 1927, Ventnor, N.J.). *Physician; Psychiatry.* Son of Theodore C. and Eleanor Eunice (Hammond) Hurd. Married Mary Doolittle, 1874; two children. EDUCATION: 1858-60, Knox College; 1861-63, University of Michigan, B.A., 1863; 1863-66, Rush Medical College and University of Michigan, M.D., 1866. CAREER: 1860-61, schoolteacher; 1867-70, dispensary and general practice, Chicago, Ill., and New York, N.Y.; 1870-78, assistant physician, Michigan Asylum for the Insane, Kalamazoo, Mich.; 1878-89, medical superintendent, Eastern Michigan Asylum, Pontiac, Mich.; 1889-1911, (first) superintendent, Johns Hopkins Hospital; 1889-1906, professor of psychiatry, Johns Hopkins University. CONTRIBUTIONS: Editor, *Johns Hopkins Hospital Bulletin* and *Johns Hopkins Hospital Reports* (1890-1911). One of several editors, *American Journal of Insanity* (1897-1920). Editor, *Modern Hospital* (1913-20). Service to American Medico-Psychological Association (1892-97, secretary; and 1898-99, president; edited several volumes of its *Proceedings*). Developed standards for hospital care of the insane.

WRITINGS: *Suggestions to Hospital and Asylum Visitors* (1895, with John Shaw Billings [q.v.]); *The Institutional Care of the Insane in the United States and Canada*, 4 vols. (1916-17, editor). REFERENCES: *NCAB*, 12: 112; *NUC Pre-1956 Imprints*, 261: 362-63; *N.Y. Times*, July 20, 1927, p. 23; *Who Was Who in Am.*, 1: 611.

M. M. Sokal

HURD-MEAD, KATE CAMPBELL. See MEAD, KATE C. H.

HURTY, JOHN NEWELL (February 21, 1852, Lebanon, Ohio-March 27, 1925, Indianapolis, Ind.). *Physician; Pharmacist; Educator; Health officer.* Son of Josiah, teacher, and Ann (Walker) Hurty. Married Ethel Johnstone, 1877; two children. EDUCATION: 1870, graduated from Paris High School (Ill.); 1870-71, apprentice in pharmacy under Col. Eli Lilly; 1871-72, Philadelphia College of Pharmacy and Science; 1881, M.D. (hon.), Central College of Physicians and Surgeons; M.D., 1891, Medical College of Indiana. CAREER: 1872-73, worked as a pharmacist in Lilly's drug store, Paris, Ill.; 1873, foreman and chief chemist of the pharmaceutical company established by Lilly and Dr. John Johnstone (now Eli Lilly and Co.); 1879-96, opened his own prescription pharmacy and analytic laboratory; 1885-86, initiated the School of Pharmacy, Purdue University, and served as professor of pharmacy; 1881-1925, lecturer of hygiene and member, Board of Directors, Indiana Dental College (now Indiana University School of Dentistry); 1881-82, lecturer in pharmacy, Central College of Physicians and Surgeons; 1887-1905, lecturer in chemical philosophy and hygiene, Medical College of Indiana; 1905-7, professor of hygiene and state medicine, Purdue University department of medicine; 1909-25, professor of hygiene and sanitary science, Indiana University School of Medicine; 1896-1922, secretary, Indiana State Board of Health; 1923, representative, Ind. General Assembly. CONTRIBUTIONS: Service in establishing the Indiana State Board of Health as an effective force for the prevention and control of disease. Name is synonymous with "public health" in Ind. Authored the Ind. Pure Food and Drug Act of 1899. Wrote numerous articles for newspapers in promoting public health measures.

WRITINGS: Nine articles for various dental journals and a textbook on physiology and sanitation, *Life with Health* (1906); initiated *Bull. of the Indiana State Board of Health* and edited it (1897-1922). REFERENCES: *NCAB*, 23: 370; T. B. Rice, *The Hoosier Health Officer*, published in serial form, January 1939 to December 1946, in the *Bulletin*. Reprints were bound in book form and distributed to libraries through the nation; *Who Was Who in Am.*, 1: 612.

C. A. Bonsett

HUSON, FLORENCE (June 17, 1857, Ann Arbor, Mich.-August 12, 1915, Detroit, Mich.). *Physician; Surgery; Obstetrics.* Daughter of Capt. Frederick C., British Army, Ret., and farmer, and Mary L. (Bradley) Huson. Never married. EDUCATION: Ann Arbor public schools; studied surgery with Donald Maclean, Ann Arbor; 1885, M.D., University of Michigan; 1885, studied at Massachusetts General Hospital. CAREER: 1886-89, assistant to surgeon Donald Maclean, Ann Arbor; 1889-1915, surgical and obstetrical practice, Detroit; founder and first president: 1893, Woman's Hospital Free Dispensary, Detroit; and 1905, Blackwell Medical Society, Detroit; vice-president, Michigan State Medical Society; 1907, vice-chief of staff, Detroit Woman's Hospital; director, YWCA. CONTRIBUTIONS: Founding president, Detroit's first woman's medical society. First woman on the staff of Detroit's Woman's Hospital. Long active in charities for wayward girls. Patron of the arts. REFERENCES: *Detroit Saturday Night*, August 14, 1915; *Med. Woman's J*. 55 (Dec. 1948): 38; Michigan State Med. Soc., *J*. 30 (1931): 343; *NCAB*, 17: 277.

M. Pernick

HUTCHINSON, WOODS (January 3, 1862, Selby, England-April 26, 1930, Brookline, Mass.). *Physician; Writer*. Son of Charles and Elizabeth (Woods) Hutchinson. Married Cornelia Williams, 1893; one child. EDUCATION: 1880, A.B., Penn College (Iowa); 1884, M.D., University of Michigan. CAREER: 1884-96, medical practice in Des Moines, Iowa; 1891, professor of anatomy, State University of Iowa; 1896-99, professor of comparative pathology, University of Buffalo; 1899-1900, lecturer on comparative pathology, London Medical Graduates' College, on biology, University of London, extension department; 1900-1905, Oregon, practicing medicine; state health officer (1903-5); 1905, moved to New York City to devote his life to writing about medical subjects; during World War I served as an observer on the Western and Italian fronts; 1922-24, 1926-28, travel abroad; 1929, retired in Brookline, Mass. CONTRIBUTIONS: A well-known medical writer whose works were published in books, magazines, and newspapers throughout the country. Provided medical information to the layman, especially focussing on preventive medicine.

WRITINGS: Hundreds of articles in newspapers and popular magazines; *Instinct and Health* (1908); *Health and Common Sense* (1909); *We and Our Children*; *A Handbook of Health*; and *Exercise and Health* (all in 1911); *Common Diseases* (1913); *Community Hygiene* (1916). REFERENCES: *DAB*, 5, pt. 1: 443; *NCAB*, 21:376-77; *N. Y. Times*, April 27, 1930.

M. Kaufman

J

JACKSON, ALGERNON BRASHEAR (May 21, 1878, Princeton, Ind.-October 22, 1942, Washington, D.C.). *Physician.* Son of Charles A. and Sarah Luella (Brashear) Jackson. Married Elizabeth A. Newman, 1920; no children. EDUCATION: Three years at Indiana Normal University; 1901, M.D., Jefferson Medical College; postgraduate courses, University of Pennsylvania and Columbia University. CAREER: 1902-14, assistant surgeon, Philadelphia Polyclinic Hospital; at Mercy Hospital, Philadelphia, Pa.: 1907-21, surgeon-in-chief; and 1912-21, medical superintendent; 1921-34, professor and chairman, Department of Bacteriology, Preventive Medicine and Public Health, Howard University Medical College; 1921-42, private practice in gastroenterology (full-time, 1934-42), Washington, D.C. CONTRIBUTIONS: Described new treatment for acute rheumatism with injections of magnesium sulphate, which attracted wide attention (1911). A founder of Mercy Hospital, Philadelphia, Pa. (1907). Demonstrated concern for black health and black medical profession throughout his career, especially in his writings and speeches. During World War I, under special assignment from army surgeon-general's office, Jackson assisted in introducing measures to prevent venereal disease in army camps.

WRITINGS: *Evolution and Life* (1909); "The Treatment of Acute Articular Rheumatism by Injection of Magnesium Sulphate," *N.Y. Med. J.* (1911); 1223-25; *The Man Next Door* (1919); "Investigation of Negro Hospitals," *JAMA* 92 (1929): 1375-76. Writings listed in W. Montague Cobb, *The First Negro Medical Society* (1939), 108, and in sources below. REFERENCES: *NCAB*, 32: 299; *WWAPS* (1938): 597; *WWCR* 1 (1915): 149.

T. Savitt

JACKSON, CHARLES THOMAS (June 21, 1805, Plymouth, Mass.-August 28, 1880, Somerville, Mass.). *Chemist; Geologist; Mineralogical geology.* Son of Charles, merchant, and Lucy (Cotton) Jackson. Married Susan Bridge, 1834; survived by five children. EDUCATION: Studied medicine with James Jackson (q.v.) and Walter Channing (q.v.); 1829, M.D., Harvard Medical School; 1829-32, studied medicine and geology and mineralogy in Paris. CAREER: 1827, 1829, took mineralogical and geological tours of Nova Scotia; 1832-36, practiced medicine, Boston, Mass.; *post* 1836, established laboratory for teaching analytical chemistry, Boston; 1837-39, made geological survey of public lands of Maine and Mass. and was Maine state geologist; 1839-40, conducted geological survey of R.I. and was R.I. state geologist; 1839-44, conducted geological survey of N.H. and was N.H. state geologist; 1847, engaged by U.S. government to do mineral survey of the public lands in the Lake Superior region but resigned after two years because of conflict with other geologists employed in the project; returned to his laboratory and did work for various mining interests; 1873-80, committed to McLean Asylum for the insane; claimed to have invented guncotton, the electric telegraph, and ether anesthesia, all of which he had experimented with at one time or another; bitterly disputed the men credited with these inventions about the priority of their creations. CONTRIBUTIONS: Suggested to William T. G. Morton (q.v.) that ether, which he had discovered would render nerves insensible to pain, be used in tooth extractions. Later claimed to be the true discoverer of surgical anesthesia.

WRITINGS: *A Manual of Etherization: Concerning Directions for the Employment of Ether, Chloroform, and Other Anesthetic Agents by Inhalation in Surgical Operations. Comprising Also a Brief History of the Discovery of Anesthesia* (1861). An incomplete bibliography is in *Am. Geologist* 20 (1897): 87-110. REFERENCES: *BHM* (1964-69), 136; *DAB*, 9: 536-37; *DSB*, 7: 44-46; Elliott, *Biog. Dict. of Am. Sci.* (1979): 136; Kelly and Burrage (1928), 635-36; *NCAB*, 3: 97; *Who Was Who in Am.*, Hist. Vol.: 343.

S. Galishoff

JACKSON, CHEVALIER (November 4, 1865, Pittsburgh, Pa.-August 16, 1958, Philadelphia, Pa.). *Physician; Laryngology*. Son of William Stanford and Katharine Ann (Morange) Jackson. Married Alice Bennett White, 1899. EDUCATION: 1879-83, Western University (Pa.); 1886, M.D., Jefferson Medical College; studied laryngology in England. CAREER: *Post* 1886, practiced medicine, Philadelphia. CONTRIBUTIONS: Developed the method of removal of foreign bodies from the lungs and other air passages by insertion of tubes through the mouth; devised first an esophagus scope and later a bronchoscope for this purpose; replaced the more dangerous surgical methods of intervention used at this time; trained numerous students and physicians in these techniques in his bronchoscopic clinic in Philadelphia. Contributed to development of laryngeal surgery.

WRITINGS: *Tracheo-bronchoscopy, Esophagoscopy, and Gastroscopy* (1907); *Personal Endoscopy and Laryngeal Surgery* (1914); *Bronchoscopy, Esophagoscopy and Gastroscopy* (1934). REFERENCES: *BHM* (1964-69), 136; *DAB*, Supplement 6: 317-18; Miller, *BHM*, p. 54; Edward Podolsky, "Chevalier Jackson and the Blocked Passages," *Med. Record* 161 (1948): 535-38; *Who Was Who in Am.*, 3: 441.

S. Galishoff

JACKSON, EDWARD (March 30, 1856, West Goshen, Pa.-October 29, 1942, Denver, Colo.). *Ophthalmologist; Medical editor*. Son of Halliday and Emily

(Hoopes) Jackson. Married Jennie Price, 1878 (d. 1896), five children; Emily Churchman, 1898. EDUCATION: 1874, B.S., Union College, Schenectady, N.Y.; 1878, M.D., University of Pennsylvania. CAREER: 1878-84, general practice, West Chester, Pa.; following a postdiphtheritic paralysis involving ocular accommodation, began his lifelong study of ophthalmology; 1884-94, in Philadelphia, Pa., attached to Philadelphia Polyclinic and Wills Eye Hospital; 1894-96, after a stay in Denver, resettled there permanently in 1898; 1894-95, chairman, AMA section on ophthalmology; president: 1903, American Academy of Ophthalmology and Otolaryngology; and 1912, American Ophthalmological Society; 1905-21, professor of ophthalmology, University of Colorado; 1912, first to organize a postgraduate course in ophthalmology; president: 1918, Colorado Medical Society; and 1919, Denver Medical Society; 1914-19, chairman, American Board of Ophthalmology, from the time of its preliminary organization and served as a member of the board for another 11 years; founding editor: 1903, *Colorado Medicine*; 1904-17, *Ophthalmic Year Book*; and 1911-17, *Ophthalmic Literature* (bibliographical); 1918-28, editor, *American Journal of Ophthalmology*. CONTRIBUTIONS: Principal achievements were descriptions (1895) of skiascopy (retinoscopy), practical application of the principles of cross-cylinders to the measurement of astigmatic errors (1893-1907), and work as editor and educator.

WRITINGS: *Essentials of Diseases of the Eye. . .* (1890); *Skiascopy* (1895); *Manual of Diseases of the Eye* (1899). Wrote the section "Operations on the Extrinsic or Orbital Muscles," in Casey Wood, *System of Ophthalmic Operations* (1911). More than 500 of his articles (many of them editorials) are listed in Mabel Anderson's bibliography published in *Contributions to Ophthalmic Science Dedicated to Dr. Edward Jackson* (1926), 298-313. REFERENCES: Wm. H. Crisp, "Edward Jackson, Student and Teacher," *Am. J. of Ophthalmology* 26 (Jan. 1943): 1-12; *DAB*, Supplement 3: 377-78; Miller, *BHM*, p. 54; *NCAB*, 42: 439.

F. B. Rogers

JACKSON, HALL (November 11, 1739, Hampton, N.H.-September 28, 1797, Portsmouth, N.H.). *Surgeon*. Son of Clement, physician, and Sarah (Hall) Jackson. Married Mary (Dalling) Wentworth, 1765; three children. EDUCATION: Pupil of his father and his uncle Dr. Anthony Emery of Hampton, N.H.; 1762, spent one year in London hospitals; 1793, M.D. (hon.), Harvard. CAREER: 1763 until his death, practiced in Portsmouth; headed smallpox inoculation hospitals: 1764, Charlestown, Mass.; 1773, 1777, Marblehead, Mass.; and 1766, 1778, 1782, 1797, near Portsmouth; 1775, volunteer regimental surgeon at siege of Boston; 1776-77, chief surgeon, N.H. troops at Portsmouth; 1791, charter member, New Hampshire Medical Society. CONTRIBUTIONS: Famous among his contemporaries for his surgical skills, especially couching for cataract, amputations, and obstetrical care, as well as for inoculations. Remembered today chiefly because he introduced digitalis to American medical practice as a direct result of reading Withering's pioneering 1785 study of the drug's clinical efficacy. Honorary degree, election to honorary fellowship, Massachusetts Medical Society (1783), and correspondence reflect role as an opinion leader in late eighteenth-century New England.

WRITINGS: *Observations and Remarks on the Putrid Malignant Sore-Throat* (1786) was published anonymously; its reputation among his contemporaries is unknown today. REFERENCES: *DAB*, 5, pt. 1: 541; J. Worth Estes, *Hall Jackson and the Purple Foxglove: Medical Practice and Research in Revolutionary America, 1760-1820* (1979); *NCAB*, 16: 386.

J. W. Estes

JACKSON, JAMES (October 3, 1777, Newburyport, Mass.-August 27, 1867, Boston, Mass.). *Physician.* Son of Jonathan, banker and merchant, and Hannah (Tracy) Jackson. Father of James Jackson, Jr. (q.v.). Married Elizabeth Cabot, 1801, nine children; Sarah Cabot, c.1818. EDUCATION: Harvard University: 1796, A.B.; 1799, A.M.; 1802, M.B.; and 1809, M.D.; 1799, studied anatomy in London. CAREER: *Post* 1800, practiced medicine, Boston; *post* 1802, medical staff, Boston Dispensary; at Harvard University: 1810-12, clinical medicine faculty; and 1812-36, theory and practice of physic faculty; 1821-35, medical staff, Massachusetts General Hospital. CONTRIBUTIONS: First person in America to investigate vaccination in a scientific manner. Was instrumental in the founding of Massachusetts General Hospital. Gave an early description of peripheral alcoholic neuritis. *Letters to a Young Physician* (1855) embodied the highest ideals of medicine and quickly became a classic.

WRITINGS: "On a Peculiar Disease Resulting from the Use of Ardent Spirits," *New England J. of Med.* 2 (Oct. 1822): 351-53; *On the Theory and Practice of Physic* (1825); *Another Letter to a Young Physician* (1861). REFERENCES: *DAB*, 9: 547-48; Kelly and Burrage (1928), 638-40; *NCAB*, 5: 401; *Who Was Who in Am.*, Hist. Vol.: 344.

S. Galishoff

JACKSON, JAMES, JR. (January 1, 1810, Boston, Mass.-March 27, 1834, Boston). *Physician.* Son of James Jackson (q.v.) and Elizabeth (Cabot) Jackson. Never married.EDUCATION: 1828, graduated from Harvard University; c. 1828-31, studied medicine with his father and at Harvard Medical School; 1831-33, studied medicine in Paris; 1834, M.D., Harvard Medical School. CAREER: Died one month after receiving his medical degree. CONTRIBUTIONS: Called attention to the importance of the prolonged expiratory sound in the diagnosis of incipient pulmonary tuberculosis. Made astute observations about the clinical features and pathology of cholera during a Paris epidemic (early 1830s). Discovered that there was a familial tendency in emphysema. Played a leading role in the founding of the Société Médicale d'observation de Paris.

WRITINGS: *Notes on Sixty Cases of Cholera* (1834). Medical cases and extracts from letters were published by his father (1835) in a memoir of his son. REFERENCES: *BHM* (1964-69), 136; (1970-74), 92; Kelly and Burrage (1920), 602; Ronald J. Knudson,

"Familial Emphysema Discovered by James Jackson, Jr.," *New England J. of Med.* 300 (Jan.-Mar. 1979): 374.

S. Galishoff

JACKSON, JAMES CALEB (March 28, 1811, Manlius, N.Y.-July 11, 1895, Dansville, N.Y.). *Hydropath*. Son of James, physician, and Mary (Elderkin) Jackson. Married Lucretia Brewster, 1830; two children. EDUCATION: 1851, Central Medical College of New York (eclectic college in Syracuse). CAREER: 1834-37, lecturer and editor in temperance and abolitionist movements; 1847-58, managed water-cure institution, Skaneateles Lake, N.Y.; 1858-83, head of Our Home on the Hillside hydropathic resort (later Jackson Health Resort), Dansville, N.Y.; 1833-95, lecturer and writer on hygiene. CONTRIBUTIONS: Successful popularizer of hydropathy in America. Educated public in principles of hygiene and possibilities of preventive medicine (stressing dangers of alcohol, tobacco, and restrictive dress). Promoted "psychohygienic method," the recognition of the influence of mental and emotional factors on health. Pioneered in development of precooked breakfast cereals, inventing Granula (1863). Influenced health orientation of Seventh Day Adventist Church.

WRITINGS: *The Sexual Organism and Its Healthful Management* (1861); *American Womanhood: Its Peculiarities and Its Necessities* (1870); *How to Treat the Sick without Medicine* (1870); *The Debilities of Our Boys* (1872). REFERENCES: Gerald Carson, *Cornflake Crusade* (1957), 61-70; William Conklin, "The Jackson Health Resort. Pioneer in its Field" (unpublished ms.); *DAB*, 5, pt. 1: 547; *NCAB*, 3: 81; Ronald Numbers, *Prophetess of Health: A Study of Ellen G. White* (1976), 71-99.

J. Whorton

JACKSON, JAMES MADISON, JR. (March 10, 1866, White Sulphur Springs, Hamilton County, Fla.-April 2, 1924, Miami, Fla.). *Physician; General practice*. Son of James Madison, M.D., and Mary Glenn (Shands) Jackson. Married Ethel Barco, 1894; two daughters, one son died in infancy. EDUCATION: Public school, Bronson, Fla.; East Florida Seminary (Boys Preparatory), Gainesville, Fla.; 1884, A.B., Emory College, Oxford, Ga.; 1884-86, medical study under preceptorate of father; 1887, M.D., Bellevue Hospital Medical College, N.Y.; postgraduate courses, New York Polyclinic. CAREER: Practice: 1887-96, in partnership with father, Bronson, Fla.; and 1896-1924, Miami, Fla.; chief surgeon, Florida East Coast Railroad Hospital; 1905, president, Florida Medical Association. CONTRIBUTIONS: Constant champion of public health measures. Made earliest study of impact of Fla. phosphate mining in regard to its potential health hazards. As chairman, Ethics Committee, Florida Medical Association, instrumental in improving standards for medical licensing and practice. Periodically attended medical clinics and short courses in East and Middle West, practicing own precept, "one must, to be a successful physician, be always a student." Organized Miami Board of Health (1914). Was south Fla.'s preeminent physician. Served as administrator of two of Miami's earliest hospitals. Active in planning and building Miami's largest and most notable medical facility, James M. Jackson Memorial Hospital, a monument to his service.

WRITINGS: "Relation of Phosphate Mines to Health of Operatives and Surrounding Country," *Proc., Fla. Med. Assoc.* (1892), 119-23; presidential address (untitled), *ibid.* (1906). REFERENCES: *Herald* (Miami), April 2, 1924; *NCAB*, 28: 74; obituary, *News-Metropolis* (Miami), April 2, 1924; William M. Straight, M.D., "James M. Jackson, Jr., Miami's First Physician," *J. Fla. Med. Assoc.* 59 (Aug. 1972): 54-62.

E. A. Hammond

JACKSON, JOHN BARNARD SWETT (June 5, 1806, Boston, Mass.-January 6, 1879, Boston). *Physician; Pathological anatomy.* Son of Henry, sea captain, and Hannah (Swett) Jackson. Nephew of James Jackson (q.v.). Married Emily Jane Andrews, 1853; survived by two children. EDUCATION: Harvard University: 1825, B.A.; and 1829, M.D., 1829-31, studied medicine in Paris, London, and Edinburgh. CAREER: At Massachusetts General Hospital: 1827-28, apothecary; 1835-39, house physician and surgeon; and 1839-64, medical staff; at Harvard Medical School: 1847-79, pathological anatomy faculty and curator of Warren Anatomical Museum; and 1853-55, dean; curator for more than 40 years, museum of Boston Society for Medical Improvement. CONTRIBUTIONS: Made detailed studies of the gross morbid anatomy of diseased organs, and as curator of the museum of Boston Society for Medical Improvement and the Warren Museum, developed important collections of the same. Wrote *A Descriptive Catalogue of the Warren Anatomical Museum* (1870), which contained numerous medical case histories of the specimens described therein. Investigated the anatomy and diseases of lower animals.

WRITINGS: *Descriptive Catalogue of the Anatomical Museum of the Boston Society for Medical Improvement* (1847). REFERENCES: Clark A. Elliott, *Biog. Dict. of Am. Sci.* (1979), 136-37; Oliver W. Holmes (q.v.), memoir, *Proc., Am. Acad. of Arts and Sci.* 14 (1878-79): 344-52.

S. Galishoff

JACKSON, SAMUEL (March 22, 1787, Philadelphia, Pa.-April 4, 1872, Philadelphia). *Physician.* Son of David, pharmacist and medical practitioner, and Susan (Kemper) Jackson. Married "Miss Christie," daughter of a British army officer whom he met at Montreal, Quebec, Canada, in 1832; no children. EDUCATION: Apprenticed to James Hutchinson and after Hutchinson's death to Caspar Wistar (q.v.); attended the University of Pennsylvania as an arts student but did not earn a degree; 1808, M.D., University of Pennsylvania. CAREER: 1808-12, pharmacist; 1812-15, cavalry officer in Philadelphia volunteers; 1815-72, private practice, Philadelphia; 1820, president, Philadelphia Board of Health; 1821-27, professor, Philadelphia College of Pharmacy; 1822-45, physician and clinical lecturer, Philadelphia Almshouse Infirmary (after 1836 Philadelphia Hospital); 1827-35, assistant to Professor Nathaniel Chapman (q.v.); 1835-63, professor, Institutes of Medicine; 1863-72, professor emeritus, medical department,

University of Pennsylvania. CONTRIBUTIONS: Rendered important service toward improving the public health of Philadelphia in fighting the yellow-fever epidemic of 1820, which he regarded as caused by local accumulations of filth, and in investigating cholera (1832). Extremely important in the effort to establish the Philadelphia College of Pharmacy and to place the profession of pharmacist on a firm, scientific foundation. Greatest importance was role as a medical teacher who helped introduce new ideas into American medicine. As a clinical teacher at the almshouse infirmary, was instrumental in the introduction of mediate ausculation in Philadelphia. Text *Principles of Medicine* (1832), heavily dependent on the ideas of François Broussais, was the first general American medical textbook based on the new methods of clinical-pathological correlation. Personal influence was particularly important in the decision of many young Philadelphia physicians to visit Paris for postgraduate instruction.

WRITINGS: *The Principles of Medicine, Founded on the Structure and Functions of the Animal Organism* (1832). Incomplete lists of Jackson's many lectures and papers are in both *Index Catalogue* and Joseph Carson, *A Discourse Commemorative of the Life and Character of Samuel Jackson* (1872). REFERENCES: Carson, *Discourse*; Cato (pseud.), "Sketches of Eminent Living Physicians—no. XIV, Samuel Jackson, M.D., Prof. of Institutes in the University of Pennsylvania," *Boston Med. and Surg. J.* 41 (1849-50): 314-22; *DAB*, 5, pt. 1: 553; W. S. Middleton, "Samuel Jackson," *Annals of Med. Hist.* 7 (1935): 538-49; *NCAB*, 11: 169.

D. C. Smith

JACOBI, ABRAHAM (May 6, 1830, Hartum, Westphalia, Germany-July 10, 1919, Bolton Landing, N.Y.). *Physician; Pediatrics.* Son of poor Jewish parents. Married three times, last to Mary Corinna Putnam (Mary P. Jacobi [q.v.]), 1873; two children by second marriage. EDUCATION: 1847-49, studied at universities of Greifswald and Göttingen; 1851, M.D., University of Bonn; 1853, went to the United States to escape imprisonment for involvement in German revolutionary movement. CAREER: *Post* 1853, practiced medicine, N.Y.; diseases of children faculty: 1860-64, New York Medical College; 1865-70, University of the City of New York; and 1870-1902, College of Physicians and Surgeons (Columbia); medical staff, several New York City hospitals; president: 1891, 1906, American Pediatric Society; 1896, Association of American Physicians; 1896, American Climatological Society; 1912-13, American Medical Association; and several N.Y. medical associations. CONTRIBUTIONS: Considered the father of American pediatrics. Occupied the first American chair of pediatrics (1870) and pioneered bedside teaching in the field by establishing a pediatric clinic in New York Medical College, which he ran for nearly two years (1862-64). Made several important scientific contributions, notably his studies of infant hygiene, diphtheria, and dysentery; advocated the boiling of commercial milk in order to destroy its harmful bacteria and the use of intubation in laryngeal diphtheria. With Emil Noeggerath, founded (1862) and edited (1868-71) *American Journal of Obstetrics and Diseases of Women and Children.* Aided Nathan

Straus (q.v.) in the establishment of milk depots for the poor and the building of the first preventorium for tuberculosis in infants.

WRITINGS: *Infant Diet* (1872); *Treatise on Diphtheria* (1880); *Intestinal Diseases of Infancy and Childhood* (1887); *Therapeutics of Infancy and Childhood* (1896). Major writings are contained in William J. Robinson, ed., *Collectanea Jacobi* (1909). REFERENCES: *BHM* (1964-69), 137; (1970-74), 92; *DAB*, 9: 563-64; Jerome S. Leopold, "Abraham Jacobi (1830-1919)," in Borden S. Veeder, ed., *Pediatric Profiles* (1957), 13-19; Miller, *BHM*, p. 55; *NCAB*, 9: 345-46; R. Truax, *The Doctors Jacobi* (1952); *Who Was Who in Am.*, 1: 625.

S. Galishoff

JACOBI, MARY CORINNA (PUTNAM) (August 31, 1842, London, England-June 10, 1906, New York, N.Y.). *Physician.* Daughter of George Palmer, publisher, and Victorine (Haven) Putnam. Married Abraham Jacobi (q.v.), 1873; two children. EDUCATION: 1857-59, public high school, New York City; 1863, graduated New York College of Pharmacy; 1864, M.D., Woman's Medical College of Pennsylvania; 1864, brief internship, New England Hospital for Women and Children; 1871, M.D., École de Médecine, Paris. CAREER: At Woman's Medical College of the New York Infirmary: 1871-73, lecturer; and 1871-89, professor of materia medica and therapeutics; 1882-85, clinical lecturer, New York Post-Graduate Medical School; 1871-89, attending physician, New York Infirmary; 1873, established pediatric dispensary, Mt. Sinai Hospital; 1893, visiting physician, St. Mark's Hospital; in Association for the Advancement of the Medical Education of Women: 1872, founder; and 1874-1903, president; 1876, winner of Harvard Medical School's Boylston Prize for essay "The Question of Rest for Women during Menstruation"; among the first women members of numerous medical societies, including the New York Pathological Society, New York Neurological Society, Therapeutical Society of New York, and New York Academy of Medicine. CONTRIBUTIONS: Probably the most highly respected woman physician of her generation with more formal medical training than most men in her field. Author of more than 100 published papers in pathology, neurology, pediatrics, physiology, and medical education. Loyal supporter of the Woman's Medical College of the New York Infirmary and a firm believer in high standards. Untiring advocate of medical co-education. Pioneer among physicians concerned with the relationship between environment and health. Helped organize the Consumer's League (1890). Staunch feminist and supporter of women's suffrage. An inspiring role model to numerous younger women physicians and an effective spokeswoman for the cause of women physicians. Considerable achievements aided in dissipating public and professional skepticism about the capacity of women for medical practice.

WRITINGS: *The Question of Rest for Women* (1876); "Modern Female Invalidism," *Boston Med. and Surg. J.* 133 (1895): 174; "A Suggestion in Regard to Suggestive Therapeutics," *N. Y. Med. J.* 67 (1898): 485. Writings listed in Ruth Putnam, ed., *Life and Letters of Mary Putnam Jacobi* (1925). REFERENCES: *DAB*, 5, pt. 1: 564-65; Roy Lubove, "Mary Corinna Putnam Jacobi," *Notable Am. Women* 2 (1971): 263-65; *NCAB*,

8: 219; Putnam, *Life and Letters of Mary Putnam Jacobi*; *Mary Putnam Jacobi, M.D.,
A Pathfinder in Medicine* (1925); Rhoda Truax, *The Doctors Jacobi* (1952).

R. M. Morantz

JANEWAY, EDWARD GAMALIEL (August 31, 1841, New Brunswick,
N.J.-February 10, 1911, Summit, N.Y.). *Consulting physician; Clinical teacher.*
Son of George Jacob, Physician, and Matilda (Smith) Janeway. Married Frances
Strong Rogers, 1871; three children. EDUCATION: 1860, A.B., Rutgers Univer-
sity; 1864, M.D., College of Physicians and Surgeons (N.Y.); 1862-63, medical
cadet, army hospital, Newark, N.J.; 1864-66, house staff, Bellevue Hospital.
CAREER: 1866-1911, private practice, New York City; 1866-72, curator, Bellevue
Hospital; 1868-72, visiting physician and chief of staff (1871), Charity Hospital;
1872-92, visiting physician, Bellevue; 1875-81, commissioner of health, New
York City; at University of the City of New York: 1871-72, professor of pathological anatomy, medical department; and 1872-81, professor of pathological
anatomy and demonstrator of anatomy (1872-79); at Bellevue Hospital Medical
School: 1881-86, associate professor of medicine and professor of diseases of
the mind and the nervous system; and 1886-92, professor of the principles and
practice of medicine and clinical medicine; 1898-1905, professor of medicine
and dean, New York University-Bellevue Medical College; president: 1897-98,
New York Academy of Medicine; 1900, Association of American Physicians;
and 1910, National Association for the Study and Prevention of Tuberculosis;
officer of international congresses on tuberculosis. CONTRIBUTIONS: Widely regarded as one of the foremost diagnosticians and bedside teachers of his time.
Teaching at Bellevue Hospital helped to disseminate the ideas of Virchow,
Charcot, and Seguin in the United States. Although he preferred teaching and
consultation to writing and lecturing, was credited with the earliest description
of leukemia in the United States and with influential papers on tertiary syphilis
and the contagiousness of tuberculosis. A staunch Calvinist, disdained overt
medical politics and vigorously opposed corruption in hospital and public health
administration. Much in demand as a consultant and noted for treating neuras-
thenics with "positive terseness." Outstanding contribution to public health was
in the control of tuberculosis. Dr. Hermann Biggs (q.v.) sought his advice and
assistance in the early years of developing the pioneering New York City tuberculosis reporting program more frequently than that of "any other man in
New York." Became a statesman of tuberculosis control in his city and nation,
an active proponent of sanitoria; a forceful opponent of the social stigma attached
to victims of the disease.

WRITINGS: Fourteen of most significant articles and lectures are listed in the *Author
Catalogue*, New York Academy of Medicine. A representative essay on his beliefs about
the history and practice of medicine is "The Progress of Medicine," *Trans., N. Y. Acad.
of Med.* 12 (1895): 449-79. REFERENCES: James Bayard Clark, *Some Personal Recollections of Dr. Janeway* (1917); *DAB*, 5, pt. 1: 607-8; Kelly and Burrage (1928), 649-

52; S. Adolphus Knopf, "Dr. Edward G. Janeway," *N. Y. Med. J.* 95 (1912): 105-7; *NCAB*, 13: 499.

D. M. Fox

JARVIS, EDWARD (January 9, 1803, Concord, Mass.-October 31, 1884, Dorchester, Mass.). *Physician; Psychiatry; Public health.* Son of Francis, baker and farmer, and Millicent (Hosmer) Jarvis. Married Almira Hunt, 1834; no children. EDUCATION: 1826, A.B., Harvard College; 1830, M.D., Harvard Medical School. CAREER: Private practice: 1830-32, Northfield, Mass.; 1832-37, Concord; and 1837-42, Louisville, Ky.; 1842 until death, resided in Dorchester, where he accepted a small number of mentally ill patients into his home, a practice that afforded him the opportunity to conduct statistical researches in the fields of psychiatry and public health. CONTRIBUTIONS: Played a major role in the emergence of a statistically oriented medicine that combined science with morality and social activism. *Report on Insanity and Idiocy in Massachusetts* (1855) was one of the first demographic and epidemiological surveys in psychiatry. Also published extensively in the fields of psychiatry and public health in an effort to specify those conditions that accounted for morbidity and mortality. Had a key role in reorganizing the federal censuses (1842-71) and developing a statistical approach to the study of health and disease.

WRITINGS: "Insanity Among the Coloured Population of the Free States," *Am. J. of Med. Sci.* 7 (1844); "On the Comparative Liability of Males and Females to Insanity, and Their Comparative Curability and Mortality When Insane," *Am. J. of Insanity* 7 (1850); "On the Supposed Increase of Insanity," *ibid.*, 8 (1852); "Influence of Distance from and Nearness to an Insane Hospital on Its Use by the People," *Am. J. of Insanity* 22 (1866); "Mortality Statistics. . .Eighth Census," in *Statistics of the United States. . .Eighth Census* (1866). Writings listed in Gerald N. Grob, *Edward Jarvis and the Medical World of Nineteenth-Century America* (1978), 280-87. REFERENCES: *DAB*, 5, pt. 1: 621-22; Gerald N. Grob, *Edward Jarvis and the Medical World of Nineteenth-Century America* (1978); *NCAB*, 12: 116.

G. Grob

JARVIS, WILLIAM CHAPMAN (May 13, 1855, Fortress Monroe, Va.-July 30, 1895, Willet's Point, N.Y.). *Physician; Laryngology; Rhinology.* Son of Nathan Sturges, army physician, and Jane (Mamford) Jarvis. EDUCATION: 1875, M.D., University of Maryland; 1875-77, postgraduate study at Johns Hopkins University. CAREER: *Post* 1877, practiced medicine in New York City; worked as an assistant in Professor Franke H. Bosworth's (q.v.) Nose and Throat Service, Bellevue Hospital out-patient department; 1881-93, laryngology faculty, University of the City of New York (later New York University). CONTRIBUTIONS: Pioneered in laryngology and rhinology. 1881, introduced the Jarvis "snare" (cold wire écraseur) which revolutionized intranasal surgery. Was famous for his many innovations in the treatment of nasal and laryngeal diseases including the use of cocaine as a local anesthetic, the treatment of deviations of the nasal septum by electrically driven drills, and the illumination of the larynx by means of Edison's newly invented mignon lamp.

WRITINGS: "Cocaine in Intra-nasal Surgery," *New York Med. Rec.* 26 (1877): 655-56. REFERENCES: *DAB*, 9: 625; Kelly and Burrage (1928), 655-57; *Who Was Who in Am.*, Hist. Vol.: 346.

S. Galishoff

JAYNE, WALTER ADDISON (December 4, 1853, Orange, N.J.-August 29, 1929, Denver, Colo.). *Surgeon.* Son of Alfred Addison and Eleanor (Fordyce) Jayne. Never married. EDUCATION: 1875, M.D., Columbia University. CAREER: Practice: 1883-91, Georgetown, Colo.; and *post* 1891, Denver; 1897, president, Denver Medical Society; 1894-97, professor of gynecology and abdominal surgery, University of Colorado; 1897-1902, professor of gynecology, University of Denver; 1902-10, professor of gynecology and abdominal surgery, Denver & Gross College of Medicine; 1908-9, dean, Denver & Gross, led a movement to unite that school with the University of Colorado School of Medicine, a failed plan until following on the Flexner report (1910); 1912, president, Colorado Medical Society. CONTRIBUTIONS: Became president, Colorado Medical Library Association (1903), when it was in a moribund state, and in the same year, founded the Denver Academy of Medicine, which, in effect, served merely as a vehicle for transfer of the library holdings to the Denver Medical Society, a process that was completed in 1912, whereupon the academy ceased to exist. Nurtured, guided, and protected the society's library for the remainder of his life.

WRITINGS: "Medical Literature and Medical Libraries," *Bull. Med. Library Assoc.* 6 (1916): 1-12; *The Healing Gods of Ancient Civilization* (1925). REFERENCE: *Who Was Who in Am.*, 1: 630.

F. B. Rogers

JEAN, SALLY LUCAS (June 18, 1878, Towson, Md.-July 5, 1971, New York, N.Y.). *Health educator.* Daughter of George B. and Emilie Watkins (Selby) Jean. EDUCATION: 1896, graduated, Maryland State Normal School; 1898, graduated, Maryland Homeopathic Training School for Nurses. CAREER: 1898, nurse, U.S. Army hospitals; 1910-13, school nurse, health department, Baltimore, Md.; 1914-17, organizer and director, Social Health Service, Md.; 1917-18, organizer, Department of Health Service, Peoples' Institute, New York City; 1918-23, organizer and director, Child Health Association; 1923-24, executive secretary, Health Section, World Federation of Education Associations; *post* 1923, consultant in health education; 1934-35, supervisor, health education, U.S. Indian Service; 1937-40, president, Association of Women in Public Health; in Public Health Education Section of the American Public Health Association: 1939-41, secretary; and 1941-42, chairman. CONTRIBUTIONS: Responsible for the establishment of many ongoing health education programs in the schools of continental United States, Canal Zone, Virgin Islands, Philippines, Japan, and China.

WRITINGS: "Health Problems in Education," *Addresses & Proc., Nat. Ed. Assoc.* (1918): 443-46; "Health Education Work in Public Schools," *Addresses & Proc., Nat. Ed. Assoc.* (1920): 369-71; "Selling Health," *Am. Child Hyg. Assoc. Trans.* 11 (1920): 139-46; *Spending the Day in China, Japan and the Philippines* (1932, co-author). REFERENCES: Richard K. Means, *History of Health Education in the United States* (1962); *N. Y. Times,* July 7, 1971; Marguerite Vollmer, "Sally Lucas Jean, Health Education Pioneer," *Int'l J. Health Ed.* (1973); *Who Was Who in Am.,* 5: 370.

N. Gevitz

JELLIFFE, SMITH ELY (October 27, 1866, New York, N.Y.-September 25, 1945, Huletts Landing, N.Y.). *Physician; Medical editor; Neurology; Psychiatry.* Son of William Munson, teacher, and Susan Emma (Kitchell) Jelliffe. Married Helena Dewey Leeming, 1894, five children; Bee Dobson, 1917. EDUCATION: Brooklyn Polytechnic Institute: 1886, degree in civil engineering; and 1896, A.B.; at College of Physicians and Surgeons (Columbia): 1889, M.D.; 1899, Ph.D.; and 1900, A.M.; 1900-1901, intern, St. Mary's Hospital (Brooklyn); *post* 1890, studied in Europe at various times. CAREER: *Post* 1902, practiced medicine, Brooklyn; 1897-1907, pharmacognosy and materia medica faculty, New York College of Pharmacy; 1907-13, mental diseases faculty, Fordham University Medical School; 1911-17, diseases of the mind and nervous system faculty, Post Graduate Hospital and Medical School; president, various state and national neurological and psychiatric associations. CONTRIBUTIONS: Established psychosomatic medicine as a field of study and disseminated the latest European advances in psychoanalysis. Has been called the "father of psychosomatic medicine" for his studies of psychogenic factors in psoriasis, hypertension, and other bodily illnesses (1921-35). Exerted greatest influence by serving as a conduit for the ideas of others. Translated the works of leading European analysts, notably Paul C. Dubois's *Psychoneuroses* (1905). For more than 40 years (1902-45), was owner and managing editor, *Journal of Nervous and Mental Disorders,* oldest American neurological periodical. With William Alanson White (q.v.), edited a mongraph series under the sponsorship of the *Journal,* which provided an outlet for important but obscure or commercially unmarketable works on nervous and mental diseases (1907-45). With White, founded and edited *Psychoanalytic Review,* the first English-language journal devoted solely to psychoanalysis (1913-45). Edited *Medical News* (1900-1905) and co-edited its successor, *New York Medical Journal* (1905-9), one of the nation's outstanding medical periodicals. With White, wrote *Diseases of the Nervous System,* which went through seven editions (1915-48) and was widely adopted as a textbook in American and European schools.

WRITINGS: *Outlines of Pharmacognosy* (1904). The two best bibliographies are found in *Journal of Nervous and Mental Disorders* 106 (1947): 240-53, and in Alexander Grinstein, *The Index of Psychoanalytic Writings* 2 (1957): 970-90. REFERENCES: *BHM* (1970-74), 94; *DAB,* Supplement 3: 384-86; Miller, *BHM,* pp. 55-56; *NCAB,* 33: 360-61; *Who Was Who in Am.,* 2: 280.

S. Galishoff

JENKS, EDWARD WATROUS (March 31, 1833, Victor, N.Y.-March 19, 1903, on the train between Detroit, Mich., and Chicago, Ill.). *Surgeon; Ob-*

stetrics and gynecology; Medical education. Son of Nathan, storekeeper, and
Jane (Bushnell) Jenks. Married Julia Darling, 1859; Sarah R. Joy, 1867; two
children. EDUCATION: La Grange Collegiate Institute (Ind.); studied medicine
with James R. Wood (q.v.) and William Darling; attended University of New
York Medical College; 1855, M.D., Castleton Medical College (Vt.); 1864,
M.D., Bellevue Hospital (N.Y.). CAREER: 1855-63, surgical practice, Ontario,
Ind.; 1864, assistant surgeon, military hospitals, Detroit; 1866-69, founder and
editor, *Detroit Review of Medicine and Pharmacy;* 1868-80, founding president
and professor of obstetrics, Detroit Medical College; 1871, president, Detroit
Academy of Medicine; 1871-75, professor of surgical diseases of women, Bowdoin College (Maine); president: 1873, Michigan State Medical Society; and
1888, Detroit Gynecological Society; gynecologist: Harper, Woman's, St. Luke's,
and St. Mary's hospitals, Detroit; commissioner, Michigan State Board of Corrections and Charities. CONTRIBUTIONS: Founder and long-term president, Detroit
Medical College. Founding member and leader of many local professional
associations.

WRITINGS: "The Uses of Viburnum Prunifolium in Diseases of Women," *Trans., Am.
Gyn. Soc.* 1 (1876): 127; "The Practice of Gynecology in Ancient Times," *ibid.,* 6
(1882); *Disorders of Menstruation* (1888). Writings listed in *Index Catalogue,* 1st series,
7: 230; 2nd series, 8: 461-62; *Cyclopedia of Michigan* (1890). REFERENCES: *JAMA* 40
(1903): 862; Kelly and Burrage (1928), 660-61; *NCAB,* 4: 217; *Trans., Am. Gyn. Soc.*
28 (1903): 335-37; *Who Was Who in Am.,* 1: 632.

M. Pernick

JERMAIN, LOUIS FRANCIS (October 10, 1867, Meeme, Manitowoc
County, Wis.-July 24, 1935, Milwaukee, Wis.). *Physician; Internal medicine.*
Son of George, contractor, and Laura (Simon) Jermain. Married Rosa Barth,
1894; three children. EDUCATION: Oshkosh Normal School; 1894, M.D., Northwestern University; 1910, postgraduate study, Universities of Berlin and Vienna.
CAREER: 1894-1935, practitioner, Milwaukee; 1895-1905, professor of internal
medicine, Wisconsin College of Physicians and Surgeons; at Marquette University School of Medicine: 1905-30, professor of internal medicine; and 1913-
26, dean; 1908-10, assistant commissioner of health, Milwaukee. CONTRIBU-
TIONS: Prominent practitioner in Milwaukee and founder, Jermain Clinic. Played
a key role in creating (1913) the Marquette University School of Medicine from
the remains of the Wisconsin College of Physicians and Surgeons and the Milwaukee Medical College. Under his direction, new school won an "A" rating
from the AMA Council on Medical Education and a large endowment from the
Carnegie Foundation. When a fight between Marquette's Jesuit fathers and the
medical faculty over therapeutic abortions reduced the medical school to sham-
bles, stayed on to rebuild the school and return it to respectability. President,
Milwaukee Academy of Medicine (1912) and State Medical Society of Wisconsin
(1915).

WRITINGS: Contributed a chapter on diseases of the lungs to early editions of Frederick
Tice's *Practice of Medicine* as well as several articles to *Wisconsin Med. J.* REFERENCES:

William George Bruce, *History of Milwaukee City and County*, 3 vols. (1922), 2: 126-29; *Milwaukee Journal*, July 24, 1935; *Who Was Who in Am.*, 1: 634; *Wisconsin Med. J.* 34 (1935): 640-41.

W. J. Orr, Jr.

JERVEY, JAMES WILKINSON (October 19, 1874, Charleston, S.C.-November 1, 1945, Greenville, S.C.). *Physician; Ophthalmologist; Laryngologist.* Son of Eugene P. and Ella M. (Wilkinson) Jervey. Married Helen Doremus Smith, 1899, two children; Maude Earle Hammond, 1939, no children. EDUCATION: Charleston preparatory schools; University of South Carolina for two years; 1897, medical degree, Medical College of South Carolina; postgraduate studies, New York Eye Infirmary; 1908, 1913, European clinics. CAREER: 1898, began practice, Greenville; established Jervey Eye, Ear and Throat Hospital, where he was surgeon in charge; organizer, Greenville General Hospital; chief surgeon, Piedmont and North Railway Co. and North Railroad Co.; oculist, Southern Railway; fellow, American College of Surgeons; diplomate, American Board of Ophthalmic Examinations and American Board of Otolaryngology; member and president, American Laryngological, Rhinological, and Otological Society. CONTRIBUTIONS: Avid speaker, writer. Major contribution to medicine was in the area of his discoveries in the eye, ear, and throat genres.

WRITINGS: Edited *J. of the S. C. Med. Assoc.*, 1908-12; "Folliculosis or Trachoma Among School Children," *Kentucky Med. J.* (1922); "Mastoikitis hyperplastica serosa," *JAMA* (1922); "Practical Tonsil Hemostatics," *J. of the S. C. Med. Assoc.* (1923); "The Thesis on Etiology of Glaucoma, and a New Operation," *Southern Med. J.* (1924); "The Oculist, the Glasses, and the Emolument," *Southern Med. J.* (1926). REFERENCES: *Index Medicus*, 1922, 1923, 1924, 1927; *NCAB*, 36: 159; Joseph Ioor Waring, *History of Medicine in South Carolina, 1900-1970* (1971); *Who Was Who in Am.* 2 (1950).

J. P. Dolan

JOHNSON, A[RTHUR] HOLMES (October 18, 1894, Mapleton, Ia.-August 21, 1964, Kodiak, Alaska). *Physician; Thoracic surgeon.* Son of Eben S., Methodist bishop, and Sarah (Tillesley) Johnson. Married Fostina Bishop, 1925; one child. EDUCATION: 1918, B. A., Morningside College, Iowa; 1919, B. S., Univ. of Oregon; 1924, M.D., Northwestern University, Chicago; 1923-25, postgraduate study, Oxford University. CAREER: 1924-30, U.S. Army Medical Reserve Corps; 1928-29, general practice, St. Helens, Oregon; 1929-38, general practice and clinical instructor of surgery (1928-38), University of Oregon Medical School and teaching staff at Multnomah County Hospital; 1938-64, private practice, Kodiak, Alaska. CONTRIBUTIONS: Member, Alaska Medical Association (president, 1947) and Pan Pacific Surgical Association. Fellow: American College of Surgeons, American College of Chest Physicians (governor of Alaska), and American Society of Abdominal Surgeons. Chairman, Civil Defense, in hospital units during World War II. Many civic and community offices. With American Expeditionary Forces (1918-19).

WRITINGS: "Great Omentum and Omental Thrombosis," *Northwest Med.* 31 (1932):

285-90; "A General View of Tuberculosis in Alaska" *Dis. of Chest* 6 (1940) 266-69. REFERENCES: *Alaska Med.* 6; (1964) 78-79: *Who's Important in Med.* (1952), 522.

A.R.C. Helms

JOHNSON, JOHN BEAUREGARD (April 29, 1908, Bessemer, Ala.-December 16, 1972, Washington, D.C.). *Physician; Medical educator; Cardiologist.* Son of John B., postman, and Leona (Duff) Johnson. Married Audrey Amelia Ingram, 1964; two children. EDUCATION: 1931, A.B., Oberlin College; 1935, M.D., Western Reserve University; 1935-36, intern, Cleveland City Hospital; 1939-41, postgraduate study in internal medicine (General Education Board Fellowship), University of Rochester; 1948-49, fellow in cardiology (General Education Board Fellowship), Columbia University Division of Bellevue Hospital, N. Y. CAREER: 1936-72, at Howard University: 1936-37, laboratory assistant in physiology; 1937-38, assistant in medicine; 1938-41, instructor; 1941-44, director, clinical laboratories; 1944-49, acting chair, Department of Medicine; 1949-72, professor, Department of Medicine; and 1969-72, director, Division of Cardiology. CONTRIBUTIONS: A highly respected, long-time teacher at Howard Medical College. Groomed to take over as Department of Medicine chair at Howard after receiving advanced training at University of Rochester. Part of Dean Numa Adams's (q.v.) plan to bring blacks into positions of medical leadership at the Howard Medical College. One of two physicians appointed to staff of Georgetown University Hospital (1954) as part of plan to obtain equal opportunity for black physicians in the District of Columbia. Served the NMA as chair of its Council on Scientific Assembly (1954-63, 1966-72). Involved in many D.C. health agencies as an officer and active worker.

WRITINGS: Sixty-four publications, primarily in cardiology. "Effect of Oxalic Acid Given Intravenously on the Coagulation Time in Hemophilia," *Proc., Soc. for Experimental Biol. & Med.* 46 (1941): 496; "Observations on the Effect of Pyrogens in the Treatment of Patients with Hypertension," *JAMA* 43(1951): 300; "The T Wave of the Unipolar Precordial Electrocardiogram in Normal Adult Negro Subjects," *Am. Heart J.* 44 (1952): 494 (with Donald H. Keller); "Scimitar Syndrome: Anomalous Venous Drainage of the Right Lung into the Inferior Vena Cava with Malformation of Pulmonary Structure," *JNMA* 64 (1972): 297-301 (with Sughok K. Chun, Roscoe C. Young, and Edwin L. McCampbell). REFERENCES: W. Montague Cobb, "John Beauregard Johnson, M.D., D.Sc., F.A.C.P., 1908-1972," *JNMA* 65 (1973): 166-70; *Who Was Who in Am.*, 6: 214.

T. Savitt

JOHNSON, PETER A. (July 17, 1851, Pine Brook, N.J.-January 1, 1914, New York, N.Y.). *Physician; Surgeon.* Married Elizabeth Whittle, 1881; two children. EDUCATION: 1882, M.D., Long Island College Hospital; assistant to Drs. E. I. and Coroner Messemer in medical out-patient department, Mt. Sinai Hospital, N. Y., for seven years. CAREER: 1882-1914, private practice, at first with Dr. David K. McDonough, New York City; on staff, People's Dispensary,

N. Y., for four years during early practice. CONTRIBUTIONS: One of best-known physicians of his time in United States, serving both black and white patients of N. Y. area for 32 years. Served NMA as one of its charter members (1895); member, Executive Committee (1895-1914); and president (1908). A founder and surgeon-in-chief (1898-1903), McDonough Memorial Hospital, one of the first voluntary hospitals to open its doors to physicians, nurses, and patients regardless of race or nationality. Served in tuberculosis department, New York Board of Health and New York Milk Committee for prevention and care of infant diseases. Active in racial affairs as, for example, a founder, Urban League, and treasurer, Public Porters' Association. Also active in state and local politics. REFERENCES: "Dr. P. A. Johnson Dies on January 1," *JNMA* 6 (1914): 58; John A. Kenney, *The Negro in Medicine* (1912), 7-8; Herbert N. Morais, *Afro-American in Med.* 84 (1967): 87.

T. Savitt

JOHNSTON, GEORGE P. (March 6, 1863, Osborn, Greene County, Ohio-September 18,1956, Cheyenne, Wyo.). *Physician; Surgeon.* Son of Thomas P. and Elizabeth (Shellabarger) Johnston. Married Fanny Phelps; two sons. EDUCATION: 1888, Antioch College; 1891, M.D., Medical College of Ohio; 1896, M.S., Antioch College; 1912-13, interned at National Soldiers Home, Dayton, Ohio, and studied surgery, University of Vienna. CAREER: 1892, moved to Cheyenne and practiced there for more than 60 years; consulting physician, Union Pacific R.R. and Colorado and Southern Railroad; stopped practice due to failing eyesight. CONTRIBUTIONS: Holder of Wyo. Medical License #7, was one of three physicians responsible for the licensing act (for physicians) passed by the legislature (1899). Performed first appendectomy and first abdominal section in the state. Many of his surgical techniques were "firsts" for Wyo. Credited with bringing the first nurse (from Omaha, Nebr.) to the state. While a member of the City Council of Cheyenne (1900), noticed that the typhoid epidemic crippling the city centered around homes with private, contaminated wells. As a result, successfully lobbied for city and state sanitation laws. Brought the first water testing methods to Wyo., often assaying the water himself. Delivered more than 11,000 babies in 60 years of practice. Until death, represented Wyo. in the AMA House of Delegates, being the oldest member of that body. REFERENCES: *Casper Tribune Herald*, September 19, 1956; *Wyoming State Tribune* (Cheyenne), September 19, 1956.

A. Palmieri

JONES, JOHN (March 10, 1729, Jamaica, N.Y.-June 23, 1791, Philadelphia, Pa.). *Physician; Surgery; Obstetrics.* Son of Evan, physician, and Mary (Stephenson) Jones. EDUCATION: Studied medicine: 1747-50, Philadelphia, with Thomas Cadwalader (q.v.); and 1751, London with William Hunter and Percival Pott; Paris with Jean-Louis Petit and Henri-François LeDran; Edinburgh with Alexander Munro; and in Leyden, the Netherlands, with Boerhaave; 1751, M.D.,

University of Rheims. CAREER: c. 1751-58, 1765-76, practiced medicine, New York City; 1758-65, surgery, French and Indian War; *post* 1767, surgery and obstetrics faculty, medical department, King's College (N.Y.); 1771-75, medical staff, New York Hospital; 1777-81, surgeon, Tenth Massachusetts Regiment; 1781-91, practiced medicine, Philadelphia; 1781-91, medical staff, Pennsylvania Hospital; 1787, first vice-president, College of Physicians of Philadelphia. CONTRIBUTIONS: Leading surgeon and obstetrician in colonial N.Y. Said to have been the first American lithotomist. One of the first medical school teachers to offer a formal course of instruction in obstetrics. With Samuel Bard (q.v.) and others, founded and designed New York Hospital. Participated in the organization of the medical department of the Continental Army. Most famous for the publication of *Plain, Concise, Practical Remarks on the Treatment of Wounds and Fractures* (1775), first American textbook of surgery, which he wrote for physicians in the American Revolutionary Army; was largely adapted from the work of his teachers Pott and LeDran, to which he added (1776) his translation of Gerhard L. B. van Swieten's *Diseases Incident to Armies*. Helped establish both King's College and College of Physicians of Philadelphia.

WRITINGS: *Observations on Wounds* (1765); *Account of the Last Illness of Dr. B. Franklin* (1790); *A Case of Anthrax* (1794). REFERENCES: *BHM* (1964-69), 141; (1975-79), 69; Steven T. Charles, "John Jones. American Surgeon and Conservative Patriot," *Bull. Hist. Med.* 39 (1965): 435-49; *DAB*, 10: 181; Edgar Erskine Hume (q.v.), "Surgeon John Jones, U.S. Army. Father of American Surgery and Author of America's First Medical Book," *Bull. Hist. Med.*, 13 (1943); 10-32; Kelly and Burrage (1928), 675-76; Miller, *BHM*, p. 57; *NCAB*, 5: 149.

S. Galishoff

JONES, JOSEPH (September 6, 1833, Montevideo, Liberty County, Ga.- February 17, 1896, New Orleans, La.). *Physician; Research scientist; Teacher.* Son of Rev. Charles Colcock and Mary (Jones) Jones. Married Caroline Smelt Davis, October 26, 1859; Susan Rayner Polk, June 21, 1870; seven children. EDUCATION: Private tutoring; University of South Carolina; 1853, A.B., Princeton; 1856, M.D., University of Pennsylvania School of Medicine. CAREER: 1856-57, opened practice, Savannah, and named professor of chemistry, Savannah Medical College; 1858, professor of natural philosophy, botany, and natural theology, University of Georgia; 1858-61, professor of medical chemistry, Medical College of Georgia; 1861-62, service with the Liberty Independent Troop of Horse; 1862-65, surgeon, Confederate Army, with rank of major; 1866-68, professor of the institutes of medicine, University of Nashville; 1868-94, professor of chemistry and clinical medicine, medical department, University of Louisiana; 1870-94, visiting physician, Charity Hospital, New Orleans; president: 1880-84, Board of Health of Louisiana; and 1885-86, Louisiana Medical Society; 1889, surgeon-general, United Confederate Veterans. CONTRIBUTIONS: A prolific and tireless researcher who was particularly well known for his work in the nature, history, and pathology of fevers. Vitally concerned with educational reforms, medical history, public health, archaeology, diseases of the South.

Exhaustive note taking and research into the health and sanitary conditions of the Confederate armies were notable as was his investigation into the appalling conditions that prevailed in the Confederate prison camps, particularly at Andersonville. Much of the information he compiled was tellingly used in the federal government's suit against Henry Wirz. Work with hospital gangrene was carefully researched and the most thorough investigation of its kind to be done up to that time; was published by the U.S. Sanitary Commission after the war— as were his writings dealing with diseases among the prisoners at Andersonville. Has a substantial claim to have been the first to see the gangrene bacillus. Fight for effective quarantine restrictions in Louisiana was noteworthy; is considered to be one of the first to introduce the techniques of up-to-date medical bacteriology into the United States.

WRITINGS: Published extensively in most of the leading medical journals of the day, including the *Am. J. of Med. Sci., New Orleans Med. and Surg. J., Southern Med. and Surg. J.,* and *Nashville J. of Med. and Surg.* Publication that may be remembered longest, however, is his discursive but valuable *Medical and Surgical Memoirs*, 3 vols. (1876-90). REFERENCES: James O. Breeden, "Andersonville—A Southern Surgeon's Story," *Bull. Hist. Med.* 47 (1973): 317-43; idem, "Joseph Jones: Confederate Surgeon" (Ph.D. diss., Tulane University, 1967); idem, "Joseph Jones, a Major Source for Nineteenth Century Southern Medical History," *Bull. of the Tulane Univ. Med. Fac.* 26 (1967): 41-48; idem, *Joseph Jones, M.D., Scientist of the Old South* (1975); *DAB*, 10: 193; Kelly and Burrage (1920): 640-41; Joseph Krafka, "Joseph Jones, Surgeon," *J. of the Med. Assoc. of Ga.* 31 (1942): 353-63; Robert Manson Myers, *A Georgian at Princeton* (1976); *NCAB*, 10: 285; I. A. Watson, *Physicians and Surgeons of Am.* (1896), 593-97, contains a good listing of Jones's writing. Jones family papers are in the libraries of Tulane, Louisiana State University, University of Georgia, and Duke University.

P. Spalding

JONES, NOBLE WILEY (June 13, 1876, Wauseon, Ohio-February 7, 1975, Portland, Oreg.). *Physician; Internist; Medical educator.* Son of Philo Everett, physician, and Mary Eveline (Noble) Jones. Married Nellie S. Sturtevant, 1908; three children. EDUCATION: 1895, A.B., Stanford University; 1901, M.D., Rush Medical College; 1901-3, intern, Cook County Hospital; postgraduate study: 1906-7, Universities of Berlin and Vienna; 1913-14, hospitals of Vienna and London; and 1923-24, London. CAREER: Practice: 1903-5, Wilmot, S.Dak.; and 1908-44, Portland, Oreg.; 1913-47, medical faculty, University of Oregon; 1918, U.S. Army Medical Corps. CONTRIBUTIONS: Did first prostatectomy in S. Dak. One of first in Pacific Northwest to advocate multispecialty group practice. Opened such a practice in Portland with Robert C. Coffey (q.v.) and Thomas M. Jones (1913). Built Portland Convalescent Hospital (1910) and Portland Medical Hospital (1916). Established Portland Clinic (1921). Distinguished teacher of internal medicine. Brought first electro-cardiograph to Portland (1924). Moving force in development of library at the University of Oregon and library of the Multnomah County Medical Society. Endowed pathology research fellowship at University of Oregon Medical School (1919) and a visiting scholar lectureship

(1927). Helped to reinvigorate the Portland Academy of Medicine after 1913. First recognized specialist in internal medicine in Portland. Did clinical research in pernicious anemia, coronary heart disease, local infection as it related to rheumatic and arthritic conditions.

WRITINGS: "Secondary Pellagra Caused by Multiple Augentaffin Carcinoma of the Ileum and Jejunum," *Gastroenterology* 6 (1946): 443-48 (with R. G. D. McNeely); "Chronic Infection and Atherosclerosis; Some Additional Experimental Data," *Arch. Path.* 45 (1948): 271-77 (with A. L. Rogers). REFERENCES: Charles H. Carey, *History of Oregon* 3 (1922): 592-95; *Who's Important in Med.* (1952), 530.

G. Dodds

JORDAN, EDWIN OAKES (July 28, 1866, Thomaston, Maine-September 2, 1936, Lewiston, Maine). *Bacteriologist; Public health.* Son of Joshua Lane, ship captain and later banker, and Eliza (Bugbee) Jordan. Married Elsie Fay Pratt, 1893; three children. EDUCATION: 1888, S.B., Massachusetts Institute of Technology; 1892, Ph.D., Clark University. CAREER: 1888-90, chief assistant biologist, Massachusetts State Board of Health; 1889-90, biology faculty, Massachusetts Institute of Technology; at University of Chicago: 1892-95, anatomy faculty; 1895-1933, bacteriology faculty; and 1914-33, hygiene and bacteriology faculty; 1902-33, trustee, McCormick Memorial Institute for Infectious Diseases; 1920-33, associated with Rockefeller Foundation. CONTRIBUTIONS: Made diphtheria antitoxin available to Chicago's poor by establishing a serum division in the McCormick Institute for Infectious Diseases, which undertook the manufacture of the drug. Helped Chicago secure a clean and pasteurized milk supply. Demonstrated that the colon bacillus is a reliable indicator of fecal pollution of water supply. Provided evidence that Chicago's sanitary canal did not endanger the health of persons living downstream, indicating that the Illinois River, into which it drained, had the ability to purify itself of sewage contamination after a few miles of flow (1899-1903)—first proof that some streams undergo self-purification, a fact of great importance to developers of sanitary works. Wrote *Textbook of General Bacteriology* (1908) which went through numerous editions and was used all over the world. Made important discoveries concerning intestinal organisms and food-borne infections, which were incorporated in his classic work on *Food Poisoning* (1917). Compiled and arranged the literature on the baffling occurrence of *Epidemic Influenza* (1927). Joint editor, McCormick Institute's *Journal of Infectious Diseases* (1904-36), and editor, *Journal of Preventive Medicine* (1926-33). Trained more than 150 graduate students who went on to careers in commercial laboratories and universities.

WRITINGS: *The Newer Knowledge of Bacteriology and Immunology* (1928, editor with I. S. Falk). Writings are listed in *BMNAS*. REFERENCES: *BMNAS* 20 (1939): 197-228; *DAB*, Supplement 2: 352-54; *DSB*, 7: 170-71; *NCAB*, 42: 622; *Who Was Who in Am.*, 1: 652.

S. Galishoff

JUDD, GERRIT PARMELE (April 23, 1803, Paris, N.Y.-July 12, 1873, Honolulu, Hawaii). *Surgeon; Physician.* Son of Elnathan, physician, and Betsy

(Hastings) Judd. Married Laura Fish, September 20, 1827; nine children. ED-UCATION: Clinton Grammar School (N.Y.), which was supplemented by private tutoring in the classics by the Rev. Edwin W. Dwight; 1825, graduated, Medical College, Fairfield, N.Y. CAREER: 1828-42, service with the American Board of Missions, Honolulu; 1842-53, in service to King Kamehameha III; 1843, minister of foreign affairs; 1845, minister of the interior; 1846, minister of finance; sat in legislature: 1843-53, as a noble; and 1858, 1859, as a representative. CON-TRIBUTIONS: Entire life was devoted to the creation of a strong constitutional government for Hawaii. Was sent on a diplomatic mission (1849-50) to negotiate treaties with France, England, Belgium, and the United States guaranteeing the independence of the Hawaiian Islands. Established for the Hawaiian government an enviable financial reputation. Conceived the idea of independent ownership of the land by the Hawaiian people. A founder, Punahou School, Honolulu (1841) and one of first trustees. A signer of the charter of incorporation, Hawaii Medical Association. Master of the Hawaiian language, translated books about hygiene and the life of Abraham Lincoln and assisted in translations of the Bible.

WRITINGS: *Anatomia: he palapala ia e hoike ai i ke ano o ko ke kanaka kino* (1838). REFERENCES: *Builders of Hawaii* (1925), 135; *DAB*, 5, pt. 2: 229-30; *Dr. Judd; Hawaii's Friend* (1960, by Gerrit P. Judd IV); Kelly and Burrage (1920), 644-45; *Hawaii Gazette*, July 16, 1873; *Missionary Album: Sesquicentennial Edition, 1820-1970*; *NCAB*, 25: 193; *9 Doctors & God* (1954, by Francis John Halford, M.D.).

J. Breinich

JUST, ERNEST EVERETT (August 14, 1883, Charleston, S.C.-October 27, 1941, Washington, D.C.). *Biologist.* Son of Charles Frazier, wharf builder, and Mary (Matthews) Just. Married Ethel Highwarden, 1912; three children. EDU-CATION: 1907, A.B., Dartmouth College; 1916, Ph.D., University of Chicago. CAREER: 1907-41, Howard University faculty: 1907-9, English; 1909-41, zo-ology; and 1912-20, physiology; spent many summers doing research at Marine Biological Laboratory, Woods Hole, Mass.; worked for short periods throughout his career at research laboratories in Naples, Berlin, and other European cities; turned down an offer early in his career to join the Rockefeller Institute for Medical Research in order to remain at and support Howard University; later in his career, when Howard University failed to support him as a research professor, no other major university would offer him a post; although consulted frequently for selections to the National Academy of Sciences, was always passed over because of his race and school; in later life, grew embittered because of lack of opportunities for blacks in the United States and ceased encouraging younger students; because he received more acceptance in Europe, left the United States (early 1930s), returning only a few months before his death. CONTRIBUTIONS: Recognized as the premier black scientist up to his time. As the leading researcher in fertilization (early 1920s), wrote the chapter on that subject for Edmund V. Cowdry's *General Cytology*, a standard reference book (1924). First time a black scientist's work had appeared in such a book. Continued research in cell biology and fertilization, developing new techniques and concepts of cell differentiation and generation (summarized in *DAB*). Taught medical and graduate students at Howard.

WRITINGS: About 80 scientific papers and 2 books, *The Biology of the Cell Surface* (1939); *Basic Methods for Experiments on Eggs of Marine Animals* (1940). Writings listed in *JNMA* 49 (1957): 350-51. REFERENCES: W. Montague Cobb, "Edmund Vincent Cowdry, Ph.D., 1888-," *JNMA* 59 (1967): 150-51; idem, "Ernest Everett Just, 1883-1941," *JNMA* 49 (1957): 349-51; *ibid.*, 50 (1958): 138-39; *DAB*, Supplement 3: 402-3; Kenneth R. Manning, *Black Apollo of Science: The Life of Ernest Everett Just* (1983).

T. Savitt

K

KANE, JOHN KINTZING (Dec. 18, 1833, Philadelphia, Pa.- March 22, 1886, Summit, N.J.). *Surgeon; Public health.* Son of John Kintzing, judge, and Jane (Duval) Kane. Married Mabel Bayard, 1863; seven children. EDUCATION: c. 1852-55, apprentice to John Kearsley Mitchell (q.v.) and Dr. S. Weir Mitchell (q.v.), Philadelphia; 1855, M.D., Jefferson Medical College; 1857, studied at Ecole de Medicine (Paris). CAREER: 1856, sailed on polar expedition; 1856, on staff, Blockley (Philadelphia General) Hospital; 1857-61, private practice, Philadelphia; 1861-62, surgeon, U.S. Army; 1862-86, private practice, Wilmington, Del.; 1865-86, surgeon, Pennsylvania R.R. CONTRIBUTIONS: A significant force behind the campaign to make the vaccination of schoolchildren compulsory in Del. President, Medical Society of Delaware (1879).
REFERENCES: *DAB*, 5, pt. 2: 257-58; Meridith I. Samuels, *Med. Soc. of Del., 150th Annual Session* (1939), 68, 69; J. Thomas Scharf, *History of Delaware* 1 (1888): 495.
W. H. Williams

KEARSLEY, JOHN (June 4, 1684, Durham County, England-January 11, 1772, Philadelphia, Pa.). *Physician; Architect.* Son of John Kearsley, Anglican minister. Married Anne Magdalene (Fauconnier) Caillé, one child; Margaret Brand, 1748, no children. EDUCATION: Trained in England for the medical profession. CAREER: *Post* 1717, practiced medicine, Philadelphia; 1727-47, designed and built Christ Church, Philadelphia; member, several terms, Pennsylvania House of Assembly. CONTRIBUTIONS: One of the leading physicians of colonial Philadelphia. Medical preceptor of several of the most prominent colonial physicians, including John Redman (q.v.), Thomas Cadwalader (q.v.), William Shippen (q.v.), and Thomas Bond (q.v.). Wrote at least two medical treatises, one on yellow fever and one on smallpox, malaria, pneumonia, and various fevers "incidental to the Province." Founded and endowed Christ Church Hospital for the support of elderly, indigent women who attended the Episcopal Church.

WRITINGS: *Remarks on a Discourse on Preparing for the Small-pox* (1751); *The Case of Mr. Thomson* (1760). REFERENCES: *DAB*, 10: 274; Kelly and Burrage (1928), 685; Miller, *BHM*, p. 57; R. F. Stone, *Biog. of Eminent Am. Physicians and Surgeons* (1894), 262-63.

S. Galishoff

KEEFER, CHESTER SCOTT (May 3, 1897, Altoona, Pa.-February 3, 1972, Brookline, Mass.). *Physician; Medical administrator; Microbiology.* Son of John Henry and Gertrude (Scott) Keefer. Married Jean Balfour, 1928, one child; Dorothy Campbell, 1971. EDUCATION: Bucknell University: 1918, B.S.; and 1922, M.S.; 1922, M.D., Johns Hopkins Medical School; 1922-26, intern and resident, Johns Hopkins Hospital. CAREER: 1923-26, medicine faculty, Johns Hopkins Medical School; 1926-28, medical staff, Billings Hospital, University of Chicago Clinics; medicine faculty: 1928-30, Peiping Union Medical College, China; and 1930-40, Harvard Medical School; 1930-40, scientific staff, Thorndike Memorial Laboratories; 1930-40, medical staff, Boston City Hospital; at Boston University School of Medicine: 1940-64, medicine faculty; and 1955-59, dean; 1940-59, director, Evans Department of Clinical Research and Preventive Medicine, Boston University Hospital; 1940-59, medical staff, Massachusetts Memorial Hospital; 1959-60, director, Boston University-Massachusetts Memorial Hospitals Medical Center; at National Research Council: 1942-46, member, Executive Committee, Division of Medical Science; and 1944, medical administrative officer, Committee on Medical Research, National Office of Scientific Research and Development. CONTRIBUTIONS: One of the nation's leading clinical investigators of infectious diseases both before and during the antibiotic era. During World War II, was given the major responsibility for organizing medical research to combat infectious diseases in the armed services. Most notable accomplishment was direction of the clinical evaluation and distribution of penicillin that, together with the work of Newton Richards, resulted in the rapid development of penicillin from a laboratory curiosity to an important therapeutic agent.

WRITINGS: "The Absorption, Excretion and Toxicity of Penicillin Administered by Intrathecal Injection," *Am. J. of Med. Sci.*, 205 (1943): 342-50; *The Therapeutic Value of Penicillin, A Study of 10,000 Cases* (1948, with Donald G. Anderson); *The Therapeutic Value of Streptomycin, A Study of 3,000 Cases* (1948, with William L. Hewitt). REFERENCES: *Am. Philosophical Yearbook* (1972), pp. 202-204; *N.Y. Times,* February 4, 1972; *Trans., Am. Assoc. of Physicians,* 85 (1972): 24-26; *Who Was Who in Am.,* 5: 358.

S. Galishoff

KEEN, WILLIAM WILLIAMS, JR. (January 19, 1837, Philadelphia, Pa.-June 7, 1932, Philadelphia). *Surgeon.* Son of William Williams and Susan (Budd) Keen. Married Emma Corinna Borden, 1867; four children. EDUCATION: Graduate of Philadelphia's Central High School; 1859, M.A., Brown University; additional study, Brown University, in sciences; 1860-61, Jefferson Medical

College, M.D., 1862; postgraduate studies, Paris and Berlin. CAREER: 1861, service as assistant surgeon, Fifth Massachusetts Regiment; 1862, after graduation, commissioned acting assistant surgeon, U.S. Army; selected to assist S. Weir Mitchell (q.v.) at Turner's Lane Hospital, Philadelphia, special hospital for neurological casualties; 1866-75, taught pathological anatomy, Jefferson Medical College; 1866-75, taught surgical anatomy, his own Philadelphia School of Anatomy; 1876-89, taught artistic anatomy, Pennsylvania Academy of the Fine Arts; 1884, became professor of surgery, Women's Medical College of Pennsylvania; 1889, appointed professor of surgery, Jefferson Medical College. CONTRIBUTIONS: Brilliant innovative surgeon, gained worldwide recognition for a series of surgical procedures: drainage of the cerebral ventricles and successful removal of large brain tumors (meningiomas). With James White (q.v.), wrote the first American surgery text (1892) based on Listerian principles. That was superseded by *Keen's System of Surgery* (1906-21), which became the Bible of American surgeons in the first few decades of the twentieth century. President: American Medical Association, College of Physicians of Philadelphia, American Congress of Physicians and Surgeons, American Surgical Association, American Philosophical Society, and International Congress of Surgery. Effective spokesman for various causes, including the theory of evolution and importance of animal experimentation for the progress of biomedical research (the latter with Walter B. Cannon [q.v.]).

WRITINGS: *American Textbook of Surgery* (with James White, 1892); *Keen's System of Surgery* (1906-21). REFERENCES: *BHM* (1970-74), 97; (1975-79), 71; (1980), 23; *DAB*, Supplement 1: 459-60; D. Geist, with discussion by G. E. Erikson, "The Writings of William Williams Keen: A Selective Annotated Bibliography," *Trans. and Studies of the Coll. of Physicians of Phila.* 43 (1976): 337-71; Miller, *BHM*, p. 57; *NCAB*, 11: 367. See also his writings for the flavor of the man, the range of accomplishments, and the charm of his writings: *Addresses and Other Papers* (1905); *Medical Research and Human Welfare* (1917); *Papers and Addresses* (1923); *The Surgical Operations on President Cleveland in 1893* (1917).

G. E. Erikson

KELLEY, FLORENCE (September 12, 1859, Philadelphia, Pa.-February 17, 1932, Germantown, Pa.). *Industrial hygienist.* Daughter of William, legislator, and Caroline (Bonsall) Kelley. Married Lazare Wischnewtzky, physician, 1884, later divorced; three children. EDUCATION: 1882, B.Litt., Cornell University; 1894, LL.B., Northwestern University. CAREER: 1893-97, chief inspector of factories, Ill.; 1897-98, American editor, *Archiv for Soziale Gesetzgeburg*, Berlin; 1899-1932, general secretary, National Consumer's League; 1899-1924, resident, Henry Street Settlement, New York City; 1917-18, secretary, U.S. Board of Control of Labor Standards for Army Clothing; a Socialist, made the first English translation of Engel's *The Conditions of the Working Class in England in 1844*. CONTRIBUTIONS: Documented existence of unhealthy working conditions in factories and leader in national effort to secure remedial legislation. Also credited with helping to establish the U.S. Children's Bureau (1912).

WRITINGS: "Has Illinois the Best Laws in the Country for the Protection of Children," *Am. J. of Soc.* 10 (1905): 299-314; *Some Ethical Gains Through Legislation* (1905); "The Sex Problems in Industrial Hygiene," *Am. J. Pub. Hyg.* 6 (1910): 252-57; "Wanted: A New Standard Child Labor Bill," *Child Lab. Bull.* 6 (1917): 32-35. REFERENCES: *DAB*, Supplement 1: 462-63; Miller, *BHM*, p. 57; *NCAB*, 23: 111-12.

N. Gevitz

KELLOGG, JOHN HARVEY (February 26, 1852, Livingston County, Mich.-December 14, 1943, Battle Creek, Mich.). *Surgeon, Health reformer.* Son of John Preston, farmer, grocer, and broom manufacturer, and Ann Janette (Stanley) Kellogg, schoolteacher. Married Ella Ervilla Eaton, 1879; 42 foster children. EDUCATION: Michigan State Normal School; studied medicine, Russell Trall's Hygeio-Therapeutic College (Florence, N.J.) and medical department, University of Michigan; 1875, M.D., Bellevue Hospital College of Medicine; 1883, 1889, 1899, 1902, 1907, 1911, 1925, studied in Europe. CAREER: 1875, converted to the health reform ideas of Ellen G. White (q.v.), became editor of the Adventist *Health Reformer*, later *Good Health*; 1876, medical superintendent, Western Health Reform Institute, changed name to Battle Creek Sanitarium; 1879-91, 1911-17, member, Michigan State Board of Health; 1895, founder, American Medical Missionary College of Chicago; 1914, member, American College of Surgeons. CONTRIBUTIONS: Promoted "biologic living"—avoiding stimulants and condiments; eating fruits and grains; obtaining rest, exercise, sunlight, and bathing. Built Battle Creek Sanitarium into a world-renowned health center for the Seventh-Day Adventist Church; although in dispute (1907) was excommunicated. At the sanitarium food laboratory, created a number of new foods, including the first flaked cereals; cereals were developed and promoted by brother Will Keith, with whom he soon split over policy. Disputes with brother and Adventists both involved his refusal to subordinate hygienic concerns to either religion or marketing concerns.

WRITINGS: Works were voluminous. *Good Health* (1878-1943); *Plain Facts for Old and Young* (1881); *Rational Hydrotherapy* (1901); *The New Dietetics* (1921); *How to Have Good Health Through Biologic Living* (1932). Writings listed in Richard W. Schwarz, *John Harvey Kellogg, M.D.* (1970). REFERENCES: Gerald Carson, *Cornflake Crusade* (1957); *DAB*, Supplement 3: 409-11; Michigan State Med. Soc. *J.* 43 (1944): 162; *NCAB*, 35:122-24; Schwarz, *John Harvey Kellogg*; *Who Was Who in Am.*, 2: 293.

M. Pernick

KELLY, GEORGE LOMBARD (October 8, 1890, Augusta, Ga.-October 24, 1972, Augusta). *Physician; Educator; Scientist.* Son of Jefferson Davis and Carrie Winslow (Lockwood) Kelly. Married Adeline Mina Weatherly, March 21, 1913; Ina Belle (Todd) Hoffman, June 9, 1920; three children. EDUCATION: Academy of Richmond County; 1911, A.B., University of Georgia; Johns Hopkins University; at Medical College of Georgia: 1921, B.S. in medicine; and 1924, M.D. CAREER: At Medical College of Georgia: 1918-21, 1926-53, anatomy faculty; 1934, acting dean; and 1935-50, dean; 1944, secretary, Council on

Medical Services and Public Relations, AMA; 1950-53, first president, Medical College of Georgia. CONTRIBUTIONS: As dean, Medical College of Georgia (MCG), worked feverishly to restore the confidence of the public in MCG and to revive the esprit of the faculty. Succeeded in having the college's "A" rating restored and developed a program that would create a state board to administer all state hospitals and infirmaries. Developed a system of rotating internships in state-operated hospitals and led the movement that culminated in the construction of a state-owned, state-controlled referral hospital on MCG's campus. Work on this hospital was authorized in 1945; construction began in 1953; dedication of the Eugene Talmadge Memorial Hospital, in 1956. Instituted an ambitious and effective building program for MCG, added new departments, developed the successful course in Domiciliary Medicine. In short, was the father of the modern Medical College of Georgia.

WRITINGS: Worked with Dr. George Papanicolaou (q.v.), Cornell University, in 1926-27, and the two men published the first report of their findings in the *Am. J. of Anatomy* (1927); *Sex Manual for Those Married or About to Be* (1945); "Medical Education and Medical Care in Georgia—Past, Present, Proposed," *J. of the Med. Assoc. of Ga.* 36 (1947): 23-30. For the best listing of his publications, see *WWAPS* 641. REFERENCES: *Am. Men of Sci.*, 6th ed. (1937); 9th ed. (1955); Robert B. Greenblatt, "G. Lombard Kelly—A Man to Remember," *J. of the Med. Assoc. of Ga.* 59 (1970): 344-45; George Lombard Kelly and Irvine Phinizy, "Domiciliary Medicine in Fourth Year Medical Teaching," *JAMA* 9 (1928): 1895-97; *WWAPS* 641; *Who's Who in Am., 1954-55*, p. 1433. For a useful obituary, see *Augusta Chronicle*, October 25, 1972, sec. C., p. 1.

P. Spalding

KELLY, HOWARD ATWOOD (February 20, 1858, Camden, N.J.-January 12, 1943, Baltimore, Md.). *Surgeon; Biographer; Gynecology*. Son of Henry Kuhl, businessman, and Louise Warner (Hard) Kelly. Married Laetitia Bredow, 1889; nine children. EDUCATION: 1877, A.B., University of Pennsylvania; 1882, M.D., University of Pennsylvania Medical School; 1882-83, intern, Episcopal Hospital, Kensington, Pa. CAREER: 1883-88, private practice in association with Kensington Hospital for Women, Philadelphia, Pa.; 1888-89, associate professor and professor of obstetrics, University of Pennsylvania Medical School; 1889-1919, associate professor and professor of obstetrics and gynecology, Johns Hopkins Medical School; 1892-1940, physician-in-chief, Howard A. Kelly Hospital, Baltimore. CONTRIBUTIONS: Major figure in development of gynecological and abdominal surgery. Devised new techniques for the diagnosis and treatment of kidney and bladder diseases. Established field of gynecology as distinct from that of obstetrics. Founded Kensington Hospital for Women (1883). Authored or co-authored 10 textbooks and published some 575 medical works. Man of wide-ranging interests. Wrote on diverse topics such as snakes, botanical leaders, and medical biography.

WRITINGS: *The Vermiform Appendix and Its Diseases* (1905, with Elizabeth Hurdon); *Walter Reed and Yellow Fever* (1906); *Gynecology and Abdominal Surgery*, 2 vols. (1907-8, with Charles P. Noble); *Medical Gynecology* (1908); *Stereo-Clinic* (1908-15,

1919, editor); *Cyclopedia of American Medical Biography* (1912); *Diseases of the Kidney, Ureters, and Bladder* (1914, with F. R. Burnham); *Some American Medical Botanists* (1914); *American Medical Biographies* (1920, with Walter L. Burrage); *Dictionary of American Medical Biography* (1928, with Walter L. Burrage). REFERENCES: *BHM* (1964-69), 145; (1970-74), 98; (1975-79), 71; Curtis F. Burnham, "Howard A. Kelly," *Johns Hopkins Med. Bull.* 73 (1943): 1-22; Stephen T. Cullen, *Dr. Howard A. Kelly, Professor of Gynecology in the Johns Hopkins University* (1919); *DAB*, Supplement 3: 411-13; Audrey W. Davis, *Dr. Kelly of Hopkins, Surgeon, Scientist, Christian* (1959); *JAMA* 121 (1943): 277; Miller, *BHM*, p. 58; *NCAB*, 15: 210.

J. Duffy

KEMPSTER, WALTER (May 25, 1841, London, England-August 21, 1918, Milwaukee, Wis.). *Physician; Alienist.* Son of Christopher, botanist and horticulturist, and Charlotte (Treble) Kempster. Married Frances S. Fraser, 1892; J. L. J. Poessell, 1913, no children. EDUCATION: 1864, M. D., Long Island College Hospital. CAREER: After serving in the Civil War, became assistant superintendent, New York State Asylum for Idiots, Syracuse, N.Y.; 1867, assistant physician, New York State Lunatic Asylum, Utica, N.Y., where he served as assistant editor, *American Journal of Insanity*; 1873-84, superintendent, newly opened Northern Hospital for the Insane, Oshkosh, Wis.; 1884, established himself in Milwaukee; subsequently traveled to Russia (1891-92) and Western Europe (1892) as special medical commissioner for the U.S. government; 1894-98, reform administration in Milwaukee appointed Kempster city health commissioner; controversy over handling of an ensuing smallpox epidemic led to his dismissal but was reinstated and served the rest of his term; professor of mental diseases, Wisconsin College of Physicians and Surgeons. CONTRIBUTIONS: Worked with John P. Gray (q.v.) in developing the first U.S. laboratory to make systematic microscopic study of the human brain. Demonstrating through photomicrographs that the brains of insane people exhibited abnormal lesions, testified at numerous criminal trials. During the murder trial of President James A. Garfield's assassin, Charles Guiteau, declared the latter to be sane and responsible for his actions. Introduced carbolic acid as an internal treatment for some diseases, used chloral as a sleep-procuring agent, and pioneered in the use of hyoscyamine in the treatment of insanity. As superintendent at Oshkosh, boasted the lowest death rates among comparable U.S. institutions; his hospital became a showplace for its treatment of patients and its well-equipped laboratory.

WRITINGS: *Some Preventable Causes of Insanity* (1879); *The Causes of Emigration from Europe* (1892); *The International Dissemination of Cholera and Other Infectious Diseases with a Plan for Effectual Quarantine* (1893). REFERENCES: *Am. J. of Insanity* 75 (1918-19): 449-52; *DAB*, 5, pt. 2: 324-25; Kelly and Burrage (1920), 652-53; Judith Walzer Leavitt, *The Healthiest City: Milwaukee and the Politics of Health Reform* (1982); *NCAB*, 5: 21; F. M. Sperry, comp., *A Group of Distinguished Physicians and Surgeons of Milwaukee* (1904), 56-69; J. A. Watrous, *Memoirs of Milwaukee County* 2 (1909): 30-33.

J. W. Leavitt

KENDALL, EDWARD CALVIN (March 8, 1886, South Norwalk, Conn.- May 4, 1972, Princeton, N.J.). *Chemist; Biochemistry; Endocrinology.* Son of George Stanley, dentist, and Eva Frances (Abbott) Kendall. Married Rebecca Kennedy, 1915; four children. EDUCATION: Columbia University: 1908, B.S.; 1909, M.S.; and 1910, Ph.D. CAREER: 1910-11, research chemist, Parke, Davis and Company (Detroit, Mich.); biochemistry staff: 1911-13, St. Luke's Hospital (New York City); 1914-51, Mayo Clinic and biochemistry faculty, University of Minnesota; *post* 1951, chemistry faculty, Princeton University. CONTRIBU-TIONS: Made fundamental studies of the chemical nature, physiological activity, and synthesis of hormones. Identified and crystallized the active agent of the thyroid, which he called thyroxine (1916); was used to regulate growth and metabolism when there was a hormone deficiency. Isolated six hormones of the adrenal cortex, one of which, cortisone, was used with great success by colleague Philip S. Hench (q.v.) in the treatment of rheumatoid arthritis (1949); hormone was also used to reduce inflammation and hypersensitivity in a variety of other illnesses. With Hench and Tadeus Reichstein of Switzerland, was awarded the 1950 Nobel Prize in medicine and physiology "for their discoveries regarding the hormones of the adrenal cortex, their structure and biological effects."
WRITINGS: "Studies of the Active Constituent, in Crystalline Form, of the Thyroid," *Trans., Assoc. of Am. Physicians* 31 (1916): 134-45; *Thyroxine* (1929); "The Chemical Constitution and Physiologic Activity of Crystalline Products Separated from the Suparenal Cortex," *Trans., Assoc. of Am. Physicians* 42 (1937): 123; "The Effect of a Hormone of the Adrenal Cortex . . . and of Pituitary Adrenocorticotropic Hormone on Rheumatoid Arthritis: Preliminary Report," *Proc. Staff Meetings of the Mayo Clinic* 24 (1949): 181-97 (with Philip S. Hench, C. H. Slocumb, and H. F. Polley); *Cortisone* (1971). A bibliography is in *BMNAS*. REFERENCES: *BHM* (1977), 18; *BMNAS* 47 (1974): 249-90; *Current Biog.* (1950), 292-94; *DSB* 15, Supplement 1: 258-59; *N.Y. Times*, May 5, 1972.

S. Galishoff

KENNEY, JOHN ANDREW (June 11, 1874, Albemarle County, Va.-January 29, 1950, Montclair, N.J.). *Physician; Surgeon.* Son of John A. and Caroline Kenney. Married Alice Talbot, 1902 (d. 1912), no children; Frieda Frances Armstrong, 1913, four children. EDUCATION: 1897, A.B., Hampton Institute; 1901, M.D., Leonard Medical College; 1901-2, intern, Freedmen's Hospital, Washington, D.C. CAREER: 1902-24, served Tuskegee Institute as organizer of nurse training course, school physician, and medical director and chief surgeon, John A. Andrew Memorial Hospital; 1924, had to leave Tuskegee because of Ku Klux Klan threats of violence when he pursued black staffing of new Veteran's Administration hospital; 1924-39, private practice, Newark, N.J.; 1939-44, medical director, John A. Andrew Memorial Hospital. CONTRIBUTIONS: A leader in black medical profession and NMA for 46 years (1904-50): secretary (1904-12) and president (1912-13), NMA. A founder (1909), business manager (1909-16), and editor (1916-48), *JNMA*. An initiator of John A. Andrew Clinic, Tuskegee (1912), and a founder, Andrew Clinic Society (1918). Insisted on and received approval from President Warren Harding for black staff at new Veteran's Administration Hospital, Tuskegee (1923). Personal physician to Booker T. Washington (1902-15) and George Washington Carver (1902-24). Founded what became the Newark (N.J.) Community Hospital (1927).

WRITINGS: Numerous, including: "Health Problems of the Negroes," *JNMA* 3 (1911): 127-35; *The Negro in Medicine* (1912). Edited *JNMA* for 32 years. Some of his writngs listed in Herbert N. Morais, *History of the Afro-American in Medicine* (1967), 287, 292, 298, 305, 308. REFERENCES: W. Montague Cobb, "John Andrew Kenney, M.D., 1874-1950," *JNMA* 42 (1950): 175-77; *J. Negro Hist.* 35 (1950): 229-30; *Who Was Who in Am.*, 2: 295.

T. Savitt

KENNY, ELIZABETH (September 20, 1886, Warialda, Australia-November 30, 1952, Toowoomba, Australia). *Nurse; Physical therapy.* Daughter of Michael, farmer, and Mary (Moore) Kenny. Never married. EDUCATION: Largely self-taught. CAREER: 1911-40, private nursing, Australian bush; 1915-19, member, Australian Army Nursing Service (thereafter was called "Sister Kenny"); 1933, operated clinic, Townsville, Australia, for paralyzed patients; 1940, went to the United States; 1940-50, demonstrated method for treating infantile paralysis and established institute to train nurses and physiotherapists, Minneapolis, Minn.; 1950, returned to Australia. CONTRIBUTIONS: Devised a method of treating poliomyelitis using heat and movement. Treated first case (c.1911) by applying hot moist packs to the affected muscles and then manipulating and retraining them until they regained much of their use; was unaware that her method contradicted the standard treatment of prolonged immobilization in splints and casts. Gained popular support for physical therapy (1930s) but failed to win the backing of the Australian and British medical professions. Received opportunity from physicians at University of Minnesota and Minneapolis General Hospital to prove that paralyzed muscles could be reeducated (1940); soon demonstrated to the satisfaction of the American medical profession and the National Foundation for Infantile Paralysis that early treatment with her methods relieved pain and stiffness and lessened deformity; led to establishment of clinics using the "Kenny treatment." After World War I, invented a stretcher-on-wheels for moving emergency cases over rough terrain.

WRITINGS: *Treatment of Infantile Paralysis in the Acute Stage* (1941); *The Kenny Concept of Infantile Paralysis and Its Treatment* (1943, with John P. Pohl). A bibliography is in *Sister Kenny* . . . REFERENCES: Victor Cohn, *Sister Kenny, the Woman Who Challenged the Doctors* (1975); *Current Biog.*, (1942), 444-46; *DNB*, Supplement (1951-

60) 575-76; Miller, *BHM*, p. 58; *N.Y. Times*, November 30, 1952; *Who Was Who in Am.*, 3: 472.

S. Galishoff

KERR, JOHN GLASGOW (November 30, 1824, near Duncansville, Adams County, Ohio -August 10, 1901, Canton, China?). *Medical missionary.* Son of Joseph and Jane (Loughridge) Kerr, farmers. Married Abby L. Kingsbury, 1853 (d. 1855); Isabella Jane Moseley, 1858 (d. 1885); Martha Noyes, 1886. EDU-CATION: 1840-42, student, Denison University (Ohio); 1842, apprentice to Dr. Sharpe and Dr. Duke, Maysville, Ky.; student, medical department, Transylvania University; 1846-47, student, Jefferson Medical College, M.D., 1847. CAREER: 1847-53, practice, Ohio; 1854-1901, medical missionary, China; *post* 1855, director, hospital of the Medical Missionary Society, Canton, China. CONTRI-BUTIONS: One of the earliest medical missionaries sent by the Presbyterian Board of Foreign Missions. Founded the first hospital for the insane in China. He and assistants treated over 750,000 people, introducing Western medicine into China. Translated medical works into Cantonese. Trained over 200 Chinese in Western medicine.

WRITINGS: Translations of medical works into Cantonese. REFERENCES: *DAB*, 10: 357; D. MacGillivray, *A Century of Protestant Missions in China* (1907); *Who Was Who in Am.*, Hist. Vol.: 292.

M. Kaufman

KETCHUM, GEORGE AUGUSTUS (April 6, 1825, Augusta, Ga.-May 29, 1906, Mobile, Ala.). *Physician.* Son of Ralph and Christina Colden (Griffith) Ketchum. Married Susan Burton, 1848; one child. EDUCATION: Early education by private tutors; at 16, about to enter sophomore class at Princeton, but father's failure in business forced him to accept position of assistant teacher, Female Academy, Livingston, Ala.; studied medicine under Dr. Frank A. Ross, Mobile; resident medical student, City Hospital, for two years; 1844-45, course of lectures, Medical College of South Carolina, Charleston, S.C.; 1845, intern for four months, Blockley Almshouse, Philadelphia, Pa.; 1846, M.D., University of Pennsylvania. CAREER: *Post* 1846, practice, Mobile; president, Medical Association of the State of Alabama; 1848, physician, City Hospital, Mobile; at Medical College of Alabama: *post* 1859, professor of theory and practice of medicine; and later served as dean of faculty until death in 1906; 1861, surgeon, Fifth Alabama Infantry; 1861-65, surgeon of an organization formed for the defense of Mobile; 1871, president, Mobile Board of Health; reelected many times; 1874, president, Medical Association of the State of Alabama. CONTRI-BUTIONS: During yellow fever epidemics of 1847 and 1848, was first to administer large doses of quinine in early stages of disease; this became very general in the southern states. Helped organize the Medical Association of the State of Alabama (1847) and Medical College of Alabama (1859). One of four delegates sent from Mobile to the Secession Convention (1861). Helped reorganize the Medical

Association of the State of Alabama (1868). Responsible for securing abundant supply of pure water to Mobile.

WRITINGS: "Periodicity of Disease," "Report on the Diseases of Mobile," "The Sanitary Needs of the State," all published in the *Proc. Med. Assoc. of Ala.* REFERENCES: *Ala. J. Med. Sci.* 5 (1968): 511-14; D. Cannon, *J., Med. Assoc. of Ala.* (1936), 315, 349; *NCAB*, 8: 211; T. M. Owen, *History of Alabama*, 4 vols. (1978).

S. *Eichold*

KEYES, EDWARD LAWRENCE (August 28, 1843, Charleston, S.C.-January 24, 1924, New York, N.Y.). *Surgeon; Urology; Dermatology; Venereal Disease.* Son of Erasmus Darwin (soldier) and Caroline M. (Clarke) Keyes. Married Sarah Maria Loughborough, 1870; four children. EDUCATION: Apprentice to William H. Van Buren, New York, N.Y.; 1863, M.A., Yale College; 1866, M.D., University of the City of New York; 1866-67, studied dermatology, syphilis and male genito-urinary diseases at various Paris hospitals. CAREER: *Post* 1867, general, then urological, private practice, New York, N.Y.; *post* 1868, surgery faculty, Bellevue Hospital Medical College; *post* 1868, attending surgeon at Bellevue Hospital, first in Dispensary, then in Hospital; *post* 1885, surgeon, New York Skin and Cancer Hospital and St. Elizabeth's Hospital. CONTRIBUTIONS: As a pioneer in American dermatology and urology, taught the first course in dermatology in the U.S. in 1870 (Bellevue Medical College), trained a new generation of students in genito-urinary surgery, established the first ward in America for genito-urinary patients at Bellevue (1875), founded and served as first president of the American Association of Genito-Urinary Surgeons, and introduced the technique of administering continued small doses of mercury in treating syphilis (1877), a method which became standard for over 20 years. Textbooks and articles gained wide acceptance and usage.

WRITINGS: "The Effect of Small Doses of Mercury in Modifying the Number of Red Corpuscles in Syphilis," *Amer. J. Med. Sci.* (1876); *The Tonic Treatment of Syphilis* (1877); *Venereal Diseases* (1880); *A Practical Treatise on the Surgical Diseases of the Genito-Urinary Organs Including Syphilis* (1874); *Diseases of the Genito-Urinary Organs* (1910). REFERENCES: *DAB*, 10: 364; Kelly and Burrage (1928), 693-94; *NCAB*, 9: 343-44.

T. L. *Savitt*

KIEFER, GUY LINCOLN (April 25, 1867, Detroit, Mich.-May 8-9, 1930, Detroit). *Physician; Infectious diseases; Public health.* Son of Herman[n], physician, and Franciska (Kehle) Kiefer. Married Josephine Fannie Henion, 1893; two children. EDUCATION: Detroit High School; University of Michigan: 1887, A.B.; and 1891, M.D., A.M.; later studied in Berlin and Vienna. CAREER: 1893-95, medical practice, Detroit; 1895-1913, various municipal health positions, including 1901-13, Detroit health officer; 1926-30, Michigan state health commissioner; 1914, president, Michigan State Medical Society; 1911-30, chief of staff, Herman Kiefer Hospital, Detroit; professor and chairman of preventive medicine and contagious diseases, Detroit College of Medicine. CONTRIBUTIONS:

Shaped Detroit's public health policies in the formative era of modern medicine. Emphasized quarantine and personal hygiene over environmental approaches to preventive medicine. Sympathetic to the concerns of private practitioners. Responsible for school inspection law (1902), milk inspection, tuberculosis education, and other key legislation.

WRITINGS: "Value of Active Immunization Against Scarlet Fever," *JAMA* 91 (1928): 1885-88. REFERENCES: C. B. Burr, *Medical History of Michigan* 2 (1930): 878-80; *Detroit Free Press*, May 10, 1930; Michigan State Med. Soc., *J*. 29, Supplement (1930): 3-7, 459; *Who Was Who in Am.*, 1: 673.

M. Pernick

KING, JOHN (January 1, 1813, New York, N.Y.-June 19, 1893, North Bend, Ohio). *Eclectic physician; Pharmacology.* Son of Harman, New York custom house official, and Marguerite (La Porte) King. Married Charlotte M. Armington, 1833; Phebe (Rodman) Platt, 1853; eight children by first marriage. EDUCATION: 1838, graduated from Reformed Medical College of the City of New York. CAREER: 1838-45, taught at Reformed Medical College of the City of New York and later practiced medicine in New Bedford, Mass.; 1846-49, practiced medicine in Sharpsburg and Owingsville, Ky., and Cincinnati; 1848, secretary, first national convention of Reform Medical Practitioners, Cincinnati; 1849-51, materia medica faculty, Memphis Institute; *post* 1851, obstetrics faculty, Eclectic Medical Institute, Cincinnati; 1878, president, National Eclectic Medical Association. CONTRIBUTIONS: One of the founders of the Eclectic school of medicine. As a pharmacologist introduced several medicinal resins, including the oleo-resin of iris, the first and one of the most useful of the resin class of drugs. Discovered the active ingredient of many native plants. Most distinguished work was *The American Dispensatory* (1852) which went through eighteen editions during his lifetime; based on eclectic principles, it presented most of what was then known about the therapeutic value of American plants.

WRITINGS: *American Obstetrics* (1853); *Women: Their Diseases and Treatment* (1858); *The Microscopist's Companion* (1859); *The American Family Physician* (1860); *Chronic Diseases* (1866). REFERENCES: *DAB*, 10: 393-94; Kelly and Burrage (1928), 738-39; Miller, *BHM*, 59; *NCAB*, 15: 258-59; *Who Was Who in Am.*, Hist. Vol.: 364.

S. Galishoff

KINYOUN, JOSEPH JAMES (November 25, 1860, East Bend, N.C.-February 15, 1919, Washington D.C.). *Physician; Public health.* Son of John H. and Elizabeth (Conrad) Kinyoun. EDUCATION: 1882, M.D., Bellevue Hospital Medical College (New York University); 1896, Ph.D., Georgetown University; 1880s, 1890s, at various times studied bacteriology, Paris and Berlin, with Pasteur, Koch, Ehrlich, Roux, Behring, and Metchnikoff. CAREER: 1882-86, practiced medicine, United States; at Marine Hospital Service: 1886-1902, first director, Hygienic Laboratory, Staten Island, N.Y.; and 1899-1901, medical officer, U.S. Quarantine Station, San Francisco, Calif.; at George Washington

University: 1890-1892, hygienic and bacteriology faculty; and 1892-99, 1907-9, pathology and bacteriology faculty; 1903-7, director of biological laboratories, H. K. Mulford Co. Laboratories, Glenolden, Pa.; 1909-19, bacteriologist, health department, District of Columbia; 1909, president, Society of American Bacteriologists. CONTRIBUTIONS: Established one of the first bacteriological laboratories in the United States, Marine Hospital, Staten Island (1887). Facility was designated the "Hygienic Laboratory" (later National Institutes of Health) and Kinyoun named director. Marked the beginning of medical laboratory research in the U.S. government. Produced diphtheria antitoxin at the Hygienic Laboratory (1894), shortly after it became available in Europe, and helped standardize its preparation. Demonstrated the superiority of sulphur dioxide over other gases used in fumigation. Established the presence of bubonic plague in the Chinese quarters of San Francisco (1900), whereupon he quarantined the entire district. Was vilified by local merchants and politicians who demanded his dismissal. Existence of bubonic plague was then confirmed by an independent federal commission, but to appease local opposition, was transferred, which led him to resign from the Marine Hospital Service.

WRITINGS: *Observations on the Cholera Bacillus as a Means of Positive Diagnosis* (1887, with Samuel Treat Armstrong); *Ship Sanitation and Modern Treatment of Infected Vessels* (1892); *Dried Tetanus Antitoxin as a Dressing for Wounds* (1906). REFERENCES: Bess Furman, *A Profile of the United States Public Health Service, 1798-1948* (1973); *NCAB*, 23: 360-61; *Who Was Who in Am.*, 1: 681; Ralph Chester Williams, *The United States Public Health Service, 1798-1950* (1951).

S. Galishoff

KIRKBRIDE, THOMAS STORY (July 31, 1809, Morrisville, Pa.-December 16, 1883, Philadelphia, Pa.). *Physician; Asylum superintendent.* Son of John and Elizabeth (Story) Kirkbride. Married Ann West Jenks, 1839 (d. 1862); Eliza Butler, 1866. EDUCATION: Apprentice to Dr. Nicholas Belleville, Trenton, N.J.; 1832, M.D., University of Pennsylvania. CAREER: 1832, resident physician, Friends Asylum for the Insane, Frankford, Pa.; 1833-35, resident physician, Pennsylvania Hospital, Philadelphia; 1835-40, general practice, surgery, treating the mentally ill, Philadelphia; 1840-83, superintendent, Pennsylvania Hospital for the Insane. CONTRIBUTIONS: One of the "original 13" founding fathers, Association of Medical Superintendents of American Institutions for the Insane, and its president (1862-70). A vigorous advocate of moral treatment; identified the asylum as the key to curing the mentally ill, arguing that it provided a structured, disciplined milieu necessary for patient recovery. Main interest focused on the construction of mental institutions. What became known as the "Kirkbride plan" profoundly influenced the architectural style and planning of nineteenth-century American asylums. It consisted of a domed center structure with wings extending from each side in a step pattern.

WRITINGS: *On the Construction, Organization, and General Arrangement of Hospitals for the Insane* (1854). REFERENCES: L. V. Bell, *Treating the Mentally Ill from Colonial*

Times to the Present (1980), 22-24; *BHM*, (1975-79), 72; Earl D. Bond, *Dr. Kirkbride and His Mental Hospital* (1947); *DAB*, 10: 429-30; Miller, *BHM*, p. 59; *NCAB*, 6: 388; *One Hundred Years of American Psychiatry* (1944).

L. V. Bell

KIRKWOOD, JAMES PUGH (May 27, 1807, Edinburgh, Scotland-April 22, 1877, Brooklyn, N.Y.). *Civil engineer; Railroad and hydraulic engineering; Public health.* Married Mary Harper Adams; Sarah Elizabeth Richards; no children. EDUCATION: 1821-32, apprenticed to Granger & Miller, land surveyors and civil engineers, Scotland. CAREER: 1832-39, engineer, Norwich and Worcester, Boston and Providence, Stonington and Providence, and Long Island railroads; 1840-43, resident engineer, Western Railroad of Massachusetts; 1844-49, engineer, U.S. government and various railroad companies; 1850-55, chief engineer, Missouri Pacific Railroad; 1857-early 1860s, consultant and superintendent in charge of carrying out contracts, Brooklyn Waterworks; 1865-66, investigated and reported on the water supplies of Cincinnati, Ohio, and St. Louis, Mo.; 1867, studied European methods of water filtration; 1870s, consulting engineer, waterworks of St. Louis, Mo.; Pittsburgh, Pa.; Portland, Maine; New York, Brooklyn, Albany, Hudson, and Poughkeepsie, N.Y.; Salem, Lowell, Fall River, Lawrence, Lynn, and Boston, Mass.; and Hoboken, N.J.; 1875, investigated the pollution of rivers for the Massachusetts State Board of Health; 1867-68, president, American Society of Civil Engineers. CONTRIBUTIONS: First American authority on waterworks design and construction. Study of methods used by European cities to filter river water published in 1869, for more than two decades the only American textbook on that important subject. Consulting engineer for the waterworks of numerous northeastern cities. Designed the first successful slow sand filters in the United States at Poughkeepsie (1872). Helped introduce in America the technique of coating cast-iron water pipes with coal tar to prevent corrosion and was responsible for many of the improvements made in waterworks pumping machinery (1857-75). A founder, American Society of Civil Engineers.

WRITINGS: *Report* [to Brooklyn Waterworks] *in Relation to Proposals Made by Various Parties to Protect the Cast-Iron Pipes from Corrosion* (1858); *Report on the Filtration of River Waters, for the Supply of Cities, as Practiced in Europe, Made to the Board of Water Commissioners of the City of St. Louis* (1869); *Special Report on the Pollution of Rivers: An Examination of the Water-Basins of the Blackstone, Charles, Taunton, Neponset, and Chicopee Rivers; with General Observations on Water Supply and Sewerage* (1876). REFERENCES: Moses N. Baker, *The Quest for Pure Water: The History of Water Purification from the Earliest Records to the Twentieth Century* (1948); "Early Presidents of the Society. II. James Pugh Kirkwood, 1807-1877," *Civil Engineering* 6, no. 5 (May 1936): 338-39; *NCAB*, 9: 36-37.

S. Galishoff

KLEBS, THEODORE ALBRECHT EDWIN (February 6, 1834, Königsberg, Prussia-October 23, 1913, Bern, Switzerland). *Physician; Pathology; Bac-*

teriology. Son of Heinrich F., lawyer and civil official, and Soninka (von Reich) Klebs. Married Rosa Grossenbacher, 1867; several children, eldest son being Arnold C. Klebs. EDUCATION: Friedrichskollegium, then Kneiphöfische Gymnasium, Königsberg; medical studies, Königsberg, Würzburg, Jena, and Berlin, Germany; 1856, M.D. CAREER: 1858-61, medical practice, Königsberg, privatdozent (pathology), and then assistant (physiology); 1861-66, Rudolf Virchow's assistant, Berlin Pathological Institute; professor of pathology: 1866-72, Bern; 1872-73, Würzburg; 1873-82, Prague, Czechoslovakia; and 1882-93, Zurich, Switzerland; 1893-94, work and travel, Carlsruhe, Germany and Strassburg, France; 1895-96, laboratory researcher, private tuberculosis sanatorium, Asheville, N.C.; 1896-1900, medical faculty, Rush Medical College, Chicago, Ill.; 1900, returned to Europe and worked successively in Hanover (1900-1905) and Berlin, Germany (1905-10); and Lausanne (1910-13) and Bern (1913), Switzerland. CONTRIBUTIONS: Prominent pathological investigator, trained in Virchow's solidist school, who helped demonstrate the bacterial nature of infection. Introduced paraffin embedding techniques (1868) and first isolated bacterial colonies with solid media (1872). Demonstrated the transmission of tuberculosis from cows to humans in milk (1873). First described the causative bacilli of typhoid fever (1880) and diphtheria (1883). Performed detailed pathological studies of syphilis, hemorrhagic pancreatitis, bacterial endocarditis, cell necrosis. First described acromegaly (1884), with F. Fritzsche. Had a restless nature and did not push his investigations to their conclusion. Work was overshadowed (*post* 1876-78) by Robert Koch's great advances; influence began to wane. Memorialized with the eponym of the bacterial genus *Klebsiella*.

WRITINGS: *Handbuch der pathologischen Anatomie* (1868-80); "Die künstliche Erzeugung der Tuberculose," *Arch. Path. Pharmakol*, 1 (1873): 163; "Der Bacillus des Abdominaltyphus und der typhöse Process," *Arch. Exp. Path Pharmakol* 13 (1881): 381; "Ueber Diphtherie," *Verhandl. Cong. inn. Med.* 2 (1883): 125; *Allgemeine Pathologie* (1887-89). Writings listed in *Verhandl. deut. Pathol. Ges.* (compiled by A. C. Klebs). REFERENCES: *BHM*, (1964-69), 147; Leona Baumgartner, "Edwin Klebs: A Centennial Note," *New England J. of Med.* 213 (1935): 60-63; *Sci.* 38 (1913): 920-21; *Verhandl. deut. pathol. Ges.* 17 (1914): 590-99.

L. Rubin

KLINE, BENJAMIN SCHOENBRUN (May 4, 1886, Philadelphia, Pa.-December 17, 1968, Cleveland, Ohio). *Physician; Pathology*. Son of Agnatz Kline. Married Madeline Moysey; two children. EDUCATION: 1907, A.B., Swarthmore College; 1911, M.D., Johns Hopkins University; 1911-12, intern, City Hospital, Baltimore, Md.; 1912-14, assistant in pathology, Johns Hopkins University; 1914-15, fellow, Rockefeller Institute for Medical Research; 1914-15, instructor, pathology, Columbia University, N.Y. CAREER: Pathologist: 1915-17, Montefiore Hospital, New York City; and 1917-19, Johns Hopkins Overseas Unit; 1919-21, associate pathologist, Columbia University; and director of laboratories, Montefiore Hospital; 1921-23, instructor in pathology, Western Reserve

University and resident pathologist, Lakeside Hospital, Cleveland; at Western Reserve University: 1923-27, associate in pathology; and 1927-52, assistant professor of pathology; 1923-52, chief of laboratory, Mt. Sinai Hospital, Cleveland; 1952-56, pathologist, Woman's General Hospital; 1934-61, special consultant, U.S. Public Health Service; consultant in pathology, Mt. Sinai Hospital. CONTRIBUTIONS: Originator of the Kline test for syphilis (1928). Collaborator in Suessenguth-Kline test for trichinosis (1944). Developed microscopic slide-precipitation tests for the diagnosis and exclusion of syphilis (1932). Demonstrated the Kline test at the League of Nations Laboratory Meeting, Copenhagen (1930). Noted for research in pneumonia, allergies, the Rh factor, and for a simplified test for pregnancy.

WRITINGS: *Microscopic Slide Precipitation Tests for the Diagnosis and Exclusion of Syphilis* (1932). Contributed more than 90 articles to various medical journals on his experiments and investigative studies, especially on pneumonia, syphilis, trichinosis, erythroblastosis fetalis, and allergy. REFERENCES: *Bull. of the Acad. of Med.* 37 (Sept. 1952): 16 (on the occasion of his retirement); Thomas Hamilton, "The Microscope Slide Precipitation Test for Syphilis: Preliminary Report on Its Use in Australia," *Med. J. of Australia* 2 (Nov. 17, 1928): 621-22. His papers are on deposit in the Archives of the Cleveland Health Sciences Library, Cleveland, Ohio.

G. Jenkins

KNAPP, (JAKOB) HERMAN(N) (March 17, 1832, Dauborn, Germany-April 30, 1911, Mamaroneck, N.Y.). *Ophthalmologist; Educator*. Son of Johann, prominent German politician. Married Adolfine Becker, 1864, three children; Hedwig Sachsowsky, 1878. EDUCATION: 1854, M.D., University of Giessen; postgraduate study in England, France, and Germany. CAREER: 1859, admitted to the medical faculty at Heidelberg; 1865, professor at Heidelberg and founded Heidelberg's first ophthalmic clinic; 1868, established the Ophthalmic and Aural Institute, N.Y.C.; 1882-88, professor of ophthalmology at the University of the City of New York; 1888-1902, professsor of ophthalmology at the College of Physicians and Surgeons of Columbia University. CONTRIBUTIONS: Trained many early specialists in ophthalmology in his New York clinic. Established (1869) the *Archives of Ophthalmology and Otology* and edited it for many years. Invented a number of ophthalmic instruments, including lid forceps, roller forceps which were used for treating trachoma, needle-knife for cataract operations, headrest for the Helmholtz ophthalmoscope, and individually designed operating chair.

WRITINGS: Articles and editorials in the *Arch. of Ophthalmology and Otology*, and over 200 scientific papers. REFERENCES: Kelly and Burrage (1928), 706-8; *DAB*, 5, pt. 2:449-50.

M. Kaufman

KNIGHT, JONATHAN (September 4, 1789, Norwalk, Conn.-August 25, 1864, New Haven, Conn.). *Physician; Surgeon*. Son of Jonathan, Revolutionary army surgeon, and Ann (Fitch) Knight. Married Elizabeth Lockwood, 1813.

EDUCATION: 1808, B.A., Yale College; 1810-11, studied medicine while teaching secondary school and while a tutor at Yale; 1811, licensed to practice by the Connecticut Medical Society; 1811-13, studied anatomy and physiology, University of Pennsylvania. CAREER: 1808-9, preceptor, Chelsea Grammar School, Norwich, Conn.; 1809-10, taught at the Union School, New London, Conn.; 1810-11, tutor, Yale College; at Yale Medical School: 1813-38, professor of anatomy and physiology; and 1838-64, professor of surgery; 1813, opened an office for the practice of medicine and surgery, New Haven. CONTRIBUTIONS: Member of the founding faculty, Yale Medical School; first professor of anatomy and physiology. A founder, General Hospital Society of Connecticut (1826), established to secure funds for a hospital in New Haven. Capacity for organization led to his being chosen president, National Medical Convention, which formed the American Medical Association (1846). Elected president of the association (1853) and subsequently reelected. Leading surgeon in Conn. First to treat aneurysms by employing digital compression (1848).

WRITINGS: Few writings include several eulogies, including that on Dr. Nathan Smith (q.v.) and biographical sketches of Drs. Eneas Munson (q.v.), Mason F. Cogswell (q.v.), Nathan Smith (q.v.), and Thomas Hubbard in an introductory lecture to the course of instruction at the Yale Medical School (delivered November 2, 1858). Scientific work includes a lecture, "On the Propagation of Communicable Diseases"; another introductory lecture (delivered in 1849), and report of a cure of a popliteal aneurysm by digital compression. REFERENCES: BHM, (1964-69), 148, Harold S. Burr, "Jonathan Knight and the Founding of the Yale School of Medicine," Yale J. of Biol. & Med. 1 (Jul. 1929): 326-43; DAB 10:467-68; F. B. Dexter, Yale Biographies and Annals; Samuel C. Harvey, "Surgery of the Past in Connecticut," in Herbert Thoms, ed., Heritage of Connecticut Medicine (1942), 172-87; Kelly and Burrage (1920); NCAB, 12:228.

                                                                                              J. Ifkovic

KNOWLTON, CHARLES (May 10, 1800, Templeton, Mass.-February 20, 1850, Winchendon, Mass.) Physician; Birth-control advocate. Son of Stephen and Comfort (White) Knowlton. Married Tabitha F. Stewart, April 17, 1821. EDUCATION: 1824, graduate of New Hampshire Medical Institute (now Dartmouth Medical School). CAREER: Small medical practice; 1829, published book, Free Will, which had principles of agnosticism; book left him in debt; 1830, lectured on birth control; 1832, published anonymously book on birth-control practices; six months after publication, settled in Berkshire village of Ashfield, Mass. CONTRIBUTIONS: With a small medical practice and having had debts, privately published book on birth control. Considered the founder of American contraceptive medicine. Sanctioned sexual desire as a normal body appetite; suggested that sexual relations be indulged in for reasons of health and satisfaction. Believed that denial was probably harmful, led to prostitution and "solitary vice." Justified his work as effort to replace hypocrisy and vice with greater mutuality in marriage. Addressed moral issue, overpopulation, and the health of women in pregnancy. Advocate of syringing the vagina with alum or vinegar after male emission; designed the metal barrel syringe for this purpose. Charged in three counties as a result of the book, leading to fines and a three-month jail sentence at hard labor. Book became an international success and was instrumental in the trial of Charles Bradlaugh and Annie Besant in England (June 1877).

WRITINGS: *Elements of Modern Materialism* (1829); *Fruits of Philosophy or, the Private Companion of Young Married People* (1832). REFERENCES: *DAB*, 5, pt.2: 471-72; Peter Fryer, *The Birth Controllers* (1966), 99-106; Norman Himes, "Charles Knowlton's Revolutionary Influence on the English Birth Rate," *New England J. of Med.* (Sept. 6, 1928); James Reed, *From Private Vice to Public Virtue* (1978); M. Rugoff, *Prudity and Passion* (1971).

R. Edwards

KNOX, JAMES HALL MASON, JR. (May 20, 1872, Philadelphia, Pa.-December 30, 1951, Providence, R. I.). *Physician; Pediatrics; Public health.* Son of James Hall, Presbyterian minister and educator, and Helen (Thompson) Knox. Married Marion Gordon Bowdoin, 1909; five children. EDUCATION: Yale University: 1892, B.A.; and 1894, Ph.D.; 1898, M.D., Johns Hopkins University; 1895, postgraduate work, Greifswald, Germany; 1899, intern, Johns Hopkins Hospital; 1900, studied at pediatrics clinics, Berlin and Vienna. CAREER: 1900-1922, practiced medicine, Baltimore, Md., specializing in pediatrics; 1900-1921, medical superintendent and director, Thomas Wilson Sanitarium (a summer hospital for infants and young children), Pikesville, Md.; at Johns Hopkins University: 1909-44, pediatrics faculty; and 1922-44, hygiene and public health faculty; 1917, associate chief, children's bureau, Department of Civil Affairs, American Red Cross, in charge of nursing care for the war-stricken children in France; 1921-22, field director, child-health activities of the American Red Cross, central and eastern Europe; 1922-42, organizer and chief, Bureau of Child Hygiene, Maryland State Department of Health; pediatrics staff, Johns Hopkins and Union Memorial hospitals; president: 1909, American Child Health Association; and 1925, American Pediatrics Society. CONTRIBUTIONS: As director of the Bureau of Child Hygiene, Maryland State Department of Health, established local clinics throughout the state for maternal health and infant care. Obtained legislation that improved the quality and safety of milk sold in Md. Organized the Babies' Milk Fund Association (1906), which provided milk to infants of low-income families in Baltimore. A founder and first president, American Association for the Study and Prevention of Infant Mortality (1910).

WRITINGS: *Talk to Mothers* (1923). REFERENCES: Paul Harper, "Pediatric Profiles. James Hall Mason Knox, Jr. (1872-1951)," *J. Pediat.* 49 (1956): 774-79; *NCAB*, 41: 244-45.

S. Galishoff

KOBER, GEORGE MARTIN (March 28, 1850, Alsfeld, Hesse-Darmstadt, Germany-April 24, 1931, Washington, D.C.). *Physician; Sanitation; Industrial hygiene.* Son of Johann Jacob, cloth manufacturer, and Johanna Dorothea (Behr) Kober. Never married. EDUCATION: Real-schule, Alsfeld; 1867, immigrated to

United States and entered the Hospital Corps, U.S. Army, Carlisle Barracks, Pa., where he began medical studies under Dr. Joseph J. B. Wright, U.S. Army; 1870, appointed hospital steward, Frankford Arsenal, and continued studies under Dr. Robert Bruce Burns, Philadelphia, Pa.; 1871, transferred to Washington, D.C., and entered medical department, Georgetown University, M.D., 1873; 1873, first graduate of a postgraduate course in clinical medicine instituted by Dr. S. C. Busey (q.v.) and others at Columbia Hospital, D.C. CAREER: 1874-86, acting assistant surgeon, U.S. Army; at Georgetown University Medical School: 1889, professor of state medicine; 1901-28, dean; and 1928-31, dean emeritus and member, Board of Regents. CONTRIBUTIONS: Most active in the promotion of public health and social welfare, especially industrial hygiene, housing, sanitation, and investigation of communicable diseases. A pioneer in the crusade against tuberculosis and designed the Tuberculosis Hospital in Washington. Called attention to the pollution of the Potomac River as a cause of typhoid and was instrumental in securing legislation and funds from Congress for a proper water and sewage system for the District of Columbia. Among the first to emphasize the importance of flies as transmitters of disease, especially of typhoid. Interest in housing and sanitation motivated him to become one of the principal promoters of the Washington Sanitary Housing Companies (organized in 1877 and 1904), which provided sanitary homes at reasonable rentals for workers and their families. Prominent as an organizer and official in professional and philanthropic societies on the local and national levels. President: Medical and Surgical Society of the District of Columbia (1889), Medical Association of the District of Columbia (1898), Medical Society of the District of Columbia (1903), Association of American Medical Colleges (1907), and National Association for the Study and Prevention of Tuberculosis (1915). Secretary, Association of American Physicians (1907-16). First chairman of the Section on Industrial Hygiene, American Public Health Association, as well as an officer and member of many other societies. To further stimulate work in hygiene and preventive medicine, created an endowment fund at Georgetown University.

WRITINGS: Wrote several medical books and more than 240 journal articles. Most are listed in the *Am. J. of Physical Anthropology* 3 (1920): 199-211. *Urinology and Its Practical Application* (1875); "Report of the Prevalence of Typhoid Fever in the District of Columbia," *Report of the Health Officer of District of Columbia* (1895), 254-92; "Milk in Relation to Public Health. Milk-Borne Diseases," *Reference Handbook, Med. Sci.*, 2 ed (1902), 5: 833-43; *The History and Development of the Housing Movement in the City of Washington, D.C.* (1907); *Industrial and Personal Hygiene* (1908); *Diseases of Occupation and Vocational Hygiene* (1916, editor, with William C. Hanson); *Occupation in Relation to Tuberculosis* (1920); *Industrial Health* (1924, editor, with Emery R. Hayhurst). Published one volume of his autobiography, *Reminiscences* (1930); galley proofs for the second volume are in the Manuscript Division, National Library of Medicine, Bethesda, Md. REFERENCES: "Biographic Sketch of Dr. George M. Kober," *Am. J. of Physical Anthropology* 3 (1920): iii-vi; *DAB*, 10: 483-84; *Fiftieth Anniversary of the Graduation in Medicine of George Martin Kober, M.D., LL.D.* (1923); Emery R. Hayhurst, "Death of Dr. George M. Kober," *Am. J. of Public Health* 21 (1931): 808-

9; Kober, *Reminiscences*; Kober papers, National Library of Medicine, Bethesda, Md.; D. S. Lamb et al., *History of the Medical Society of the District of Columbia, 1817-1909* (1909), 301-2; John B. Nichols et al., *History of the Medical Society of the District of Columbia, 1833-1944* (1947), 94-95; F. A. Tondorf, ed., *Biography and Bibliography of George M. Kober, M.D. LL.D,. . . .* (1920); Irving A. Watson, ed., *Physicians and Surgeons of Am.* (1896), 46-47; *Who Was Who in Am.* 1 (1897-1942): 689.

R. Kondratas

KOCH, WILLIAM FREDERICK (April 6, 1885, Detroit, Mich.-December 9, 1967, Rio de Janeiro, Brazil). *Physician; Histology.* Son of Martin and Christina (Faulstich) Koch. Married Luella Schmidt, 1916; four children. ED-UCATION: University of Michigan: 1909, B.A.; 1910, A.M.; and 1917, Ph.D.; 1918, M.D., Detroit College of Medicine, Wayne University. CAREER: 1910-13, taught histology and embryology, University of Michigan; 1914-19, professor of physiology, Detroit Medical College; 1926, founded Koch Cancer Foundation; abandoned it to join Christian Medical Research League of Detroit. CONTRI-BUTIONS: Announced the discovery of a cure-all, "Glyoxylide" (1919). This substance injected into people with any known disease was alleged to cure 80 percent of the cases. Further alleged that the catalyst did not attack the disease but encouraged the body to produce its own remedies. The treatment was based on the belief that cancer is a preventive response to a toxic product generated within the body. Federal Trade Commission limited his ability to advertise (1942). Studies (1943) showed Glyoxylide to be distilled water. U.S. government dropped its case (1948) against Koch, who said he would stop producing the material and moved to Brazil. Dr. Wendell Hendricks (D.O.) continued to use Koch's treatment into the 1950s.

WRITINGS: "A New and Successful Treatment and Diagnosis of Cancer," *Detroit Med. J.*, Jul. 1919; *Cancer and Its Allied Diseases* (1929; rev. 1939); *The Chemistry of Natural Immunity* (1938). REFERENCES: "Cancer and the Needs for Facts," *JAMA* 139 (1949): 93-98; Martin Gardner, *Facts and Fallacies in the Name of Science* (1952), 213-15; "The Glyoxylide of William F. Koch, Report of the Bureau of Investigation," *JAMA* 107 (1936): 519; *NCAB*, E.: 313; Gerald B. Winrod, *The New Science in the Treatment of Disease. Unproven Methods of Cancer Management* (1971), 37-38.

R. Edwards

KOLLE, FREDERICK STRANGE (November 22, 1872, Hanover, Germany-May 10, 1929, New York, N.Y.). *Radiology; Plastic Surgery.* Son of Johann A. and Bertha (Shaare) Kolle. Married Loretto Elaine Duffy, 1899; three children. EDUCATION: 1893, M.D., Long Island College Hospital Medical School; 1893-94, intern, Kings County Hospital; 1892-93, assistant, ear department, Brooklyn Eye and Ear Hospital. CAREER: 1894, assistant physician, Brooklyn Hospital for Contagious Diseases; *post* 1894, private practice, first in Brooklyn, N.Y., after World War I, moved to Los Angeles and may have done general practice; 1896-1900, teacher of electricity in medicine, Electrical Engineering Institute of Brooklyn; 1897-1902, associate editor, *Electrical Age*; *post* 1898, radiographer, Methodist Episcopal Hospital, Brooklyn; 1914-29, withdrew entirely from public notice. CONTRIBUTIONS: Was one of the first X-ray investigators in the U.S. (1896). Did much to develop radiological techniques through his publications and inventions (radiometer, Kolle X-ray switching device, dentaskiascope, folding fluoroscope, X-ray printing process, Kolle focus tube, direct reading X-ray meter). Developed technique for subcutaneous paraffin injections for cosmetic purposes and other techniques, instruments, and apparatus useful in cosmetic and plastic surgery. His techniques gained wide application in the military during World War I. Compiled *The Physician's Who's Who*, a reference work, in 1913.

WRITINGS: *The X-Rays: Their Production and Application* (1898); *Subcutaneous Hydrocarbon Prostheses* (1908); *Plastic and Cosmetic Surgery* (1911); *The Physician's Who's Who* (1913). REFERENCES: *DAB*, 10, 492-93; *Who Was Who in Am.*, 1: 690.

T. L. Savitt

KOLLER, CARL (December 3, 1857, Schüttenhofen, Bohemia [later Susice, Czechoslovakia]-March 21, 1944, New York, N.Y.). *Physician; Ophthalmology; Anesthesiology*. Son of Leopold, businessman, and Wilhelmina (Rosenblum) Koller. Married Laura Blum, 1893; two children. EDUCATION: 1882, M.D., University of Vienna; c. 1883-84, intern, Allgemeines Krankenhaus. CAREER: 1885-87, assistant, Utrecht Eye Hospital, Holland; c. 1887-88, lived in London; *post* 1888, practiced medicine, New York City; and surgical staff, Mount Sinai Hospital; consulting ophthalmic surgeon, Montefiore Hospital, Hebrew Orphan Asylum. CONTRIBUTIONS: While an intern at the Allgemeines Krankenhaus (1884), demonstrated the value of cocaine as a local anesthetic in ophthalmic surgery, thus inaugurating the era of local anesthesia for operations in the various branches of medicine and surgery. Went to the United States (1888), where he excelled as a surgeon and ophthalmologist.

WRITINGS: "Vorläufige Mittheilung über Locale Anästhesirung am Auge," *Klinische Monatsblatter für Augenheilkunde* 22 (1884): 60-63; "Historical Notes on the Beginning of Local Anesthesia," *JAMA* 90 (May 26, 1928): 1742-43. REFERENCES: *BHM* (1964-69), 149; (1970-74), 100; (1975-79), 72; *DAB*, Supplement 3: 430-31; *N.Y. Times*, March 22, 1944; *Who Was Who in Am.* 2: 306.

S. Galishoff

KOPLIK, HENRY (October 28, 1858, New York, N.Y.-April 30, 1927, New York). *Physician; Pediatrics*. Son of Abraham S. and Rosalie (Prager) Koplik. Married Stephanie Schiele, November 1902; three children. EDUCATION: 1878, A.B., College of the City of New York; 1881, M.D., Columbia College of Physicians and Surgeons; 1881-82, intern, Bellevue Hospital; 1882-86, postgraduate study, Berlin, Vienna, and Prague. CAREER: 1886, began practice of pediatrics, New York City; 1887, appointed attending physician, Good Samaritan Dispensary; 1900, president, American Pediatric Society, 1902-27, attending pediatrician, Mount Sinai Hospital, N.Y. CONTRIBUTIONS: Started the first clean

Milk Depot or Gouttes de Lait with well-baby care in America (1889-1914), Good Samaritan Dispensary, which in 1898 distributed 298,674 bottles of pasteurized milk to 1,204 poor infants. Described (1896) the exanthem on the buccal mucosa of children with measles, the so-called "Koplik spots." Introduced new construction designs for children's hospitals to prevent ward infections. Clinical publications covered a wide range of subjects: cerebrospinal meningitis, osteomyelitis, sporadic cretinism, pylorospasm and congenital pyloric stenosis, pneumonia, typhoid fever, and diphtheria. Maintained an extensive private and consulting practice (1886-1927).

WRITINGS: "The Diagnosis of the Invasion of Measles from a Study of the Exanthema as it Appears on the Buccal Mucosa Membrane," *Arch. of Ped.* 13 (1896): 918-922; *The Diseases of Infancy and Children* (1902); *Epidemic Cerebrospinal Meningitis* (1907). REFERENCES: Murray Bass, "Henry Koplik," *Pediatric Profiles* (1957); *BHM* (1970-74), 101; S. R. Kagan, "Henry Koplik," *Hebrew Med. J.* (N.Y.) 2 (1939): 155; obituary, *Am. J. of Diseases of Children* 33 (1927): 979.

T. E. Cone, Jr.

KRACKOWIZER, ERNST (December 3, 1821, Spital am Pryhn, Austria-September 23, 1875, Sing Sing, N.Y.). *Physician; Surgery.* Son of an Austrian officeholder. Married Emilie Forster, 1851. EDUCATION: 1840-45, studied medicine, universities of Vienna and Pavia; 1845, graduated from University of Vienna; 1845-47, studied surgery with Schuh in Vienna. CAREER: 1847-48, first assistant, surgical clinic, University of Vienna; 1848, surgeon, Academic Legion, revolution against Austrian monarchy; 1849, first assistant, surgical clinic, Tübingen, Germany; practiced medicine: 1850-57, Williamsburg, N.Y.; and 1857-75, New York City; 1861-65, special inspector of hospitals, U.S. Army; and member, U.S. Sanitary Commission; surgical staff: German Dispensary, Mount Sinai Hospital, New York Hospital, Bellevue Hospital. CONTRIBUTIONS: One of New York City's leading surgeons. With Drs. J. Roth and W. Herczka, published *New Yorker Medicinische Monatsschrift* (1852-53). Helped establish German Hospital (now Lenox Hill Hospital). REFERENCES: Ernst P. Boas, "A Refugee Doctor of 1850," *J. Hist. Med. and Allied Sci.* 3 (1948): 65-94; Kelly and Burrage (1928), 713-14.

S. Galishoff

KREBS, ERNEST (October 18, 1877, San Luis Obispo, Calif.-January 21, 1970, San Francisco, Calif.). *Physician; Unorthodox treatments.* Son of Ernst Theodor, pharmacist, and Emma Euler Krebs. Married Ida Mae Greene; four children. EDUCATION: 1903, M.D., College of Physicians and Surgeons, San Francisco. CAREER: 1919, experimented with a drug called Leptonin, claiming it acted like an antibiotic; 1942, proposed amygdalin, derived from apricot kernels, and a chymotrypsin, as a treatment for cancer; 1952, purified amygdalin into substance he called "laetrile" (laevo-rotatory mandelonitrile beta-diglucoside); to study laetrile, founded the John Beard Memorial Foundation; 1956, arranged with McNaughton Foundation of Canada to distribute laetrile, which they did until 1972; 1966, with son, spent considerable time advocating the use of laetrile; 1969, studies by the state of California concluded that laetrile was not a palliative in cancer therapy. CONTRIBUTIONS: Research with amygdalin brought on early criticism from his medical associates and alienated him from established groups. Krebs, Jr., discovered the research of John Beard suggesting a Unitarian or Trophoblastic theory of cancer (announced in 1902) and suggesting that cancer cells were similar to placenta cells. Beard suggested treating cancer cells with chymotrypsin. Krebs Sr. and Jr. developed the synthetic compound laetrile, claiming that when it came in contact with a malignant tumor, hydrocyanic acid is liberated and immediately stops the life processes of the cancer cells. Claimed that the cancerous cells were left as a benign tumor. The orthodox view was that laetrile might convert into cyanide, a body poison. In response to scientific criticism and governmental restrictions, suggested that laetrile was a vitamin, B17, thus not subject to FDA regulations. Laetrile was never approved by the FDA since they offered no satisfactory information of animal tests. Approval was necessary to distribute drugs to humans.

WRITINGS: "The Unitarian or Trophoblastic Thesis of Cancer," *Med. Record* 163 (1950): 149-74 (with Ernest Krebs, Jr., and John Beard); *The Treatment of Breast Cancer with Laetrile by Iontophosesis* (1955, with A. T. Harris). REFERENCES: H. H. Beard, *A New Approach to the Conquest of Cancer, Rheumatic and Heart Disease* (1958; 2nd ed., 1962); Glenn D. Kittler, *Laetrile (The Anti-Cancer Drug) Control for Cancer* (1963); *Unproven Methods of Cancer Mangement* (1971).

R. Edwards

KREMERS, EDWARD (February 23, 1865, Milwaukee, Wis.-July 9, 1941, Madison, Wis.). *Pharmaceutical Chemist; Historian of pharmacy.* Son of Gerhard, secretary of Milwaukee Gas Light Co., and Elise (Kamper) Kremers. Married Laura Haase, 1892; four children. EDUCATION: 1881-83, pharmacy apprenticeship under Louis Lotz, Milwaukee; 1883-84, Philadelphia College of Pharmacy; 1886, Ph.G., University of Wisconsin, School of Pharmacy; 1888, B.S., University of Wisconsin; 1890, Ph.D., University of Göttingen, under Otto Wallach: "The Isomerisms within the Terpene Group." CAREER: At the School of Pharmacy, University of Wisconsin: 1890-91, assistant to the director; 1891-92, instructor; and 1892-1935, professor, pharmaceutical chemistry; 1913-33, director, Pharmaceutical Experiment Station, University of Wisconsin; 1935-41, professor emeritus, University of Wisconsin. CONTRIBUTIONS: Established at the University of Wisconsin the first four-year pharmacy curriculum and first Ph.D. program in pharmacy in the United States. Crusaded for more prepharmacy education for pharmacy students. Established and headed the Pharmaceutical Experiment Station at Wisconsin. Co-editor, *National Standard Dispensatory* (1909). Member, U.S. Pharmacopeal Revision Committee (1900-1910). Chairman, Committee on Volatile Oils and Related Substances (1900-1910). Editor,

Pharmaceutical Review (1896-1909). Founder, *Pharmaceutical Archives* (1898). Performed highly regarded research on the chemistry of volatile oils. WRITINGS: *The Volatile Oils*, by E. Gildemeister and F. Hoffman (1913, translator); *History of Pharmacy: A Guide and a Survey* (1940, with George Urdang). Articles too numerous to list. Reprints of many are in the Kremers Reference Files, School of Pharmacy, University of Wisconsin. REFERENCES: *BHM* (1970-74), 102; *DAB*, Supplement 3: 432-33; *Dict. of Wisconsin Biog.* (1960), 213; Miller, *BHM*, p. 60; George Urdang, "Edward Kremers (1865-1941), Reformer of American Pharmaceutical Education," *Am. J. of Pharmaceutical Ed.* 11 (1947): 631-58. Additional material is in the University Archives, University of Wisconsin-Madison; the Kremers Papers, State Historical Society of Wisconsin, Madison; and the Kremers Reference Files.

E. B. Keeney

KUHN, ADAM (November 17, 1741, Germantown, Pa.-July 5, 1817, Philadelphia, Pa.). *Physician; Botanist*. Son of Adam Simon, physician, and Anna Maria Sabina (Schrack) Kuhn. Married Elizabeth (Hartman) Markhoe, 1780; two children. EDUCATION: Began medical studies with his father; 1761-67, studied medicine, universities of Upsala (studying botany under Linnaeus), London, and Edinburgh; 1767, M.D., Edinburgh University. CAREER: 1768-1814, practiced medicine, Philadelphia; 1768-89, materia medica and botany faculty, College of Philadelphia (now University of Pennsylvania); 1775-98, medical staff, Pennsylvania Hospital; 1786, consulting physician, Philadelphia Dispensary; at College of Physicians of Philadelphia: 1787, founder; and 1808, president; at University of Pennsylvania: 1789-92, theory and practice of medicine faculty; and 1792-97, practice of physic faculty. CONTRIBUTIONS: First American professor of botany but did little to advance the science other than to find a new plant native to the eastern United States, which Linnaeus named for him, *Kuhnia eupatorioides*. Helped establish the College of Physicians of Philadelphia.

WRITINGS: *De Lavatione Frigida* (1767). REFERENCES: *DAB*, 10: 510-11; Kelly and Burrage (1928), 715-16; Miller, *BHM*, p. 60; *NCAB*, 21: 289-90; *Who Was Who in Am.*, Hist. Vol.: 369.

S. Galishoff

L

LADD, EDWIN FREMONT (December 13, 1859, Starks, Maine-June 22, 1925, Baltimore, Md.). *Chemist; Pure Food and Drug researcher.* Son of John, farmer, and Rosilla (Locke) Ladd. Married Rizpah Sprogle, 1893; eight children. EDUCATION: 1884, B.S., University of Maine. CAREER: At New York Agricultural Experiment Station (Geneva, N.Y.): 1884-87, agricultural chemist; and 1887-90, chief chemist; 1890-1916, professor of chemistry, North Dakota Agricultural College at Fargo (now North Dakota State University); 1890-1916, chief chemist, North Dakota Agricultural Experiment Station; 1899-1925, editor, *North Dakota Farmer*; 1903-18, Pure Food and Drug commissioner, N. Dak.; at North Dakota Agricultural College: 1912-16, dean, School of Chemistry and Pharmacy; and 1916-21, president; 1918-21, state inspector of grades, weights, and measures, N. Dak.; 1921-25, U.S. senator, N. Dak. CONTRIBUTIONS: Contributed to betterment of health and nutrition through experiments on foodstuffs and food products that led directly to N. Dak.'s Pure Food and Drug Laws (1903, 1907). Continuing experiments with milling and baking qualities of grains led to changes in grain grading and pricing system. Wrote and issued regular, widely circulated bulletins regarding adulteration of food products, paints, and animal feeds. Advocated and obtained state inspection of public hotels and eating places and state inspection of grades, weights, and measures. Considered a major force in development within N. Dak. of pure food and drug laws and of state systems for inspection of public places of room and board.

WRITINGS: *Manual of Analysis* (1898); *Mixed Paints* (1908). Writings listed in H. L. Walster, *A Bibliography of the Publications of Edwin Fremont Ladd Including Those of Associates Whose Work He Supervised* (1954). REFERENCES: *Biog. Directory of the Am. Congress* (1962); H. L. Bolley, "E. F. Ladd by a Lifetime Friend and Associate," *Chemical Bull.* 12 (Sept. 1925); *DAB*, 5, pt. 2: 524-25; *Fargo Forum*, June 22, 1925, pp. 1, 9; Ralph J. Kane, "Edwin Fremont Ladd: North Dakota's Pure Food Crusader" (M.A. thesis, University of North Dakota, 1960); Alfred C. Melby, "A Chemist in the

Senate: Edwin Fremont Ladd, 1921-1925'' (M.A. thesis, University of North Dakota, 1967); *NCAB* (1971), 432-33.

L. Remele

LADD, WILLIAM EDWARDS (September 8, 1880, Milton, Mass.-April 19, 1967, Chestnut Hill, Mass.). *Physician; Pediatric surgery.* Son of William Jones and Anna (Watson) Ladd. Married Katharine Barton, 1910; three children. ED- UCATION: Harvard University: 1902, B.A.; and 1906, M.D.; 1906-10, intern and resident, Boston City Hospital. CAREER: 1910-12, assistant to Edward Rey- nolds, gynecologist and surgeon, Boston, Mass.; 1912-47, practiced medicine, Boston; 1909-47, surgical staff, Children's Hospital; 1910-47, surgery faculty, Harvard University Medical School; surgical staff, Boston City, Peter Bent Brigham, and Milton hospitals; 1937, president, American Association of Plastic Surgeons. CONTRIBUTIONS: Father of pediatric surgery in the United States. Devised the standard operation for malrotation of the intestines (Ladd's bands). An authority on anomalies of the esophagus and performed (1939) the first successful operation on atresia of the esophagus. Improved the management of diaphragmatic hernia. Made major contributions in the treatment of Wilm's tumor, which hitherto was almost always fatal. Invented instruments and de- veloped new procedures for harelip operations. Book *Abdominal Surgery of Infancy and Childhood* (1941, with Robert E. Gross) was the standard reference in its field for many years. Trained many of the nation's leading pediatric sur- geons. A founder, American Board of Surgery and the American Board of Plastic Surgery.

WRITINGS: "Harelip and Cleft Palate," *J. of the Boston Med. and Surg. Soc.* (June 1926); "Congenital Obstruction of the Duodenum in Children," *New England J. of Med.* 206 (Feb. 11, 1932): 277-83; "Congenital Obstructions of the Bile Ducts," *Trans. Am. Surg. Assoc.* 53 (1935): 261-70; "The Embryoma of the Kidneys (Wilm's Tumor)," *ibid.*, 56 (1938): 390-407; "Congenital Anomalies of the Esophagus," *Pediatrics* 6 (Jul. 1950): 9-19. REFERENCES: H. William Clatworthy, Jr., "William E. Ladd," *Trans. Am. Surg. Assoc.* 85 (1967): 428-32; *NCAB*, 53: 218-19; Mark M. Ravitch, *A Century of Surgery*, 2 vols. (1981); *Who Was Who in Am.*, 4: 1060.

S. Galishoff

LAHEY, FRANK HOWARD (June 1, 1880, Haverhill, Mass.-June 27, 1953, Boston, Mass.). *Physician; Surgery.* Son of Thomas Benjamin Pierce, bridge contractor, and Honora Frances (Powers) Lahey. Married Alice Church Wilcox, 1909; no children. EDUCATION: 1904, M.D., Harvard University; 1904-7, intern, Long Island and Boston City hospitals; 1908, resident surgeon, Haymarket Square Relief Station. CAREER: Surgery faculty: 1908-9, 1912-15, 1923-24, Harvard Medical School; and 1913-17, Tufts Medical School; director of surgery: 1917- 18, Evacuation Hospital No. 30, Army Expeditionary Force; and *post* 1922, the Lahey Clinic, Boston; during World War II, chairman, War Manpower Com- mission's Medical Procurement and Assignment Service; 1941-42, president, American Medical Association; surgical staff, Long Island, Boston City, and

New England Baptist hospitals. CONTRIBUTIONS: One of the most famous surgeons of his day. Believed that surgery could be done best by teams of specialists,
who would share advanced techniques, including the divison of complicated
surgery. Put his ideas into practice in the Lahey Clinic, which became a surgical
"court of last resort" for persons with thyroid and abdominal disease. Greatly
lessened the risk of thyroid surgery and pioneered total removal of the stomach
and colon. Work exerted a strong educational influence. Operations performed
in the Lahey Clinic attracted students and physicians from far away, and the two
editions of *Surgical Practice of the Lahey Clinic* (1941, 1951) were widely used
by residents. As an officer of the American Medical Association, fought against
the adoption of group health plans and compulsory health insurance.

WRITINGS: "The Evolution of a Thyroid Clinic," *Surgical Clinics of North Am.* 4,
no. 6 (Dec. 1924): 1359-72; "The Surgical Management of Intrathoracic Goiter," *Surg.
Gyn. & Obst.* 53 (Sept. 1931): 346-54; "Some Remarks on Medical Economics," *New
England J. of Med.* 207, no. 17 (Oct. 27, 1932): 725-31; "Strictures of the Common
and Hepatic Ducts," *Trans., Southern Surg. Assoc.* 49 (1936): 135-60; "Complete
Removal of the Stomach for Malignancy, with a Report of Five Surgically Successful
Cases," *Surg. Gyn. & Obst.* 67 (Aug. 1938): 213-23. Publications are in *Index Medicus*.
REFERENCES: *BHM* (1964-69), 153; *Current Biog.* (1941), 485-86; *DAB*, Supplement
5: 404-5; L. C. Deinard, "Frank Howard Lahey, M.D., Lahey Perfectionist," *Postgraduate Med.* 4 (1948): 166-74; Miller, *BHM*, p. 60; *NCAB*, B: 465-66; *Who Was Who
in Am.*, 3: 495.

S. Galishoff

LAM, FREDERICK KWAI (December 18, 1894, Honolulu, Hawaii-August
29, 1974, Honolulu). *Physician.* Son of Lam Toi, co-owner of grocery store,
and Tseng Shee. Married Chee Kuen Loo (Ah Chin), July 20, 1922; four children.
EDUCATION: 1916, graduated, Creighton University, Omaha, Nebr.; St. Louis
University, School of Medicine: 1918, B.S.; and 1920, M.D.; internship: 1920,
St. Luke's Hospital, San Francisco, Calif., and 1921, Queen's Hospital, Honolulu. CAREER: 1921-41, private practice with Dr. Wah Kai Chang; 1929-37,
director, Bureau of Communicable Diseases, and the Bureau of Maternity and
Infancy Hygiene for the Territorial Board of Health, Honolulu; 1941-74, private
practice; 1942, first Oriental to serve as president, Honolulu County Medical
Society; 1942-43, president, Hawaii Academy of Family Physicians, and vice-
president, Hawaii Medical Association; 1946-49, treasurer, Hawaii Medical Association. CONTRIBUTIONS: 1927, research on clonorchiasis (liver fluke) resulted
in lifting of immigration restrictions on Chinese. Started the school health and
immunization programs. Football doctor and school physician, St. Louis College
(now High School), Honolulu, for more than 40 years.

REFERENCES: *Honolulu Advertiser*, August 30, 1974; *Honolulu Star-Bulletin*, August
30, 1974; *JAMA*,January 6, 1975; *Men of Hawaii* (1930, 1935); *Men & Women of Hawaii*,
(1954, 1966, 1972); *Pan-Pacific Who's Who* (1940-41); *Who's Who in Hawaii* (1947).

J. A. Breinich

LAMB, DANIEL SMITH (May 20, 1843, Philadelphia, Pa.-April 21, 1929,
Washington, D.C.). *Physician; Anatomy; Pathology; Medical education.* Son

of Jacob Matlack and Delilah (Mick Rose) Lamb. Married Lizzie Scott, 1868, two children; Isabel Haslup, 1899, no children. EDUCATION: Central High School, Philadelphia: 1859, A.B.; and 1864, A.M.; 1864, apprentice to Edwin Bentley, Washington, D.C.; 1867, M.D., Georgetown University. CAREER: 1862-65, served in military hospitals, Alexandria, Va.; 1865-1921, anatomist and pathologist, Army Medical Museum, Washington, D.C.; at Howard University College of Medicine: 1873-77, professor of materia medica and medical jurisprudence; and 1877-1923, professor of anatomy. CONTRIBUTIONS: Devoted life to furthering cause of black medical education and black physicians. A respected teacher at Howard. Established, with surplus specimens from Army Medical Museum, a large and fine medical specimen collection at Howard. A leader in campaigns for purification of Washington, D.C., water supply, daily medical inspections of public schools (1901), and congressional funds for a university hospital at Howard (1902). President, District Medical Society (1901). Founded the society's journal, *Washington Medical Annals* (1902); edited it (1902-18). Greatly enlarged collections of Army Medical Museum (1883-1917). Performed autopsies on President Garfield, Vice-president Henry Wilson, and the assassin Guiteau. Involved in work of numerous medical societies and medical organizations.

WRITINGS: Some 280 titles, including *History of the Medical Department of Howard University* (1900); *History of the Army Medical Museum* (1916). Writings listed in *Index Catalog* and *Index Medicus*. REFERENCES: W. Montague Cobb, "Daniel Smith Lamb, M.D., 1843-1929," *JNMA* 50 (1958): 62-65; *NCAB*, 27: 136-37.

T. Savitt

LAMBRIGHT, MIDDLETON HUGHER (August 3, 1865, Moncks Corner, S.C.-March 21, 1959, Cleveland, Ohio). *Physician; Surgeon; Obstetrics.* Son of John, farmer, and Mary (Gelzer) Lambright. Married Bartley S. Oliver, 1908; two children. EDUCATION: A. B., Claflin University, Orangeburg, S.C.; 1898, M.D., Meharry Medical College. CAREER: 1898-1923, practice, Kansas City, Mo.; chief of obstetrical division, General Hospital #2; *post* 1923, practice, Cleveland. CONTRIBUTIONS: Second black physician to practice in Kansas City. Recognizing the need for hospital facilities for his patients, moved to establish General Hospital #2. This hospital eventually became a major training center for black physicians and nurses. Faced the same situation when he went to Cleveland and again became a primary force in establishing Cleveland's first interracial hospital, Forest City Hospital, which opened in 1957. REFERENCES: Materials in Cleveland Health Sciences Library and in possession of the subject's daughter and colleagues.

G. P. Jenkins

LANDSTEINER, KARL (June 14, 1868, Vienna, Austria-June 26, 1943, New York, N.Y.). *Pathologist; Serology; Immunology.* Son of Leopold, journalist and newspaper publisher, and Fanny (Hess) Landsteiner. Married Helene Wlasto,

1916; one child. EDUCATION: 1891, M.D., University of Vienna; 1891-95, studied chemistry, Zurich, Switzerland; Munich, Germany; and Vienna. CAREER: At University of Vienna: 1895-96, assistant, Institute of Hygiene; and 1897-1907, assistant, Pathological-Anatomical Institute; 1908-19, pathology staff, Wilhelmina Hospital (Vienna); 1909-19, pathology faculty, University of Vienna; 1919-22, pathology staff, R. K. Hospital (The Hague, Netherlands); 1922-39, member, Rockefeller Institute for Medical Research. CONTRIBUTIONS: Found that all blood belongs to four groups (A, B, AB, and O); discovery formed the basis for the development of safe blood transfusion, which was first used on a large scale during World War I. With Philip Levine (1927), found a new group of agglutinogens, factors M, N, and P, providing further proof of his contention that there are multiple individual differences in human blood. Awarded the 1930 Nobel Prize in medicine or physiology for discovery of human blood groups. With Levine and Alexander S. Wiener, discovered the Rh blood factor (1940); led to ways of preventing serious and sometimes fatal reactions in persons undergoing transfusion who were Rh negative; led also to the discovery of methods for the treatment of erythroblastosis in fetuses and infants of Rh negative mothers and Rh positive fathers. Did major work in the fields of immunology, allergy, and antibody reactions and is sometimes called the father of modern immunology. Showed that new "synthetic" antigens could be produced when proteins are altered by chemical combination with relatively simple substances (1918-20). Pointed the way to the development of methods for overcoming drug allergy and contact dermatitis by showing that drug allergy partakes of the nature of typical immune reactions (1935-41). Wrote *The Specificity of Serological Reactions* (1936), a classic in its field. Uncovered the mystery of paroxysmal hemoglobinuria, a serious blood disease (1904). Introduced dark-field illumination for the detection of the spirochetes of syphilis and improved the Wasserman test (1905-6). Provided evidence of viral nature of poliomyelitis and devised a method of preserving the virus (1909-12).

WRITINGS: "Über Agglutinationserscheinungen Normalen Menschlichen Blutes," *WKW* 14 (1901): 1132-34; "Studies on the Sensitization of Animals with Simple Chemical Compounds," *J. of Experimental Med.* 61 (1935): 643-56 (with John L. Jacobs); "An Agglutinable Factor in Human Blood Recognized by Immune Sera for Rhesus Blood," *Proc. Soc. of Experimental Biol. & Med.* 43 (1940): 223-24 (with Alexander S. Wiener). A bibliography is in *BMNAS*. REFERENCES: *BHM* (1964-69),154; (1970-74), 103; (1975-79), 75; (1980), 24; *BMNAS* 40 (1969): 177-210; *DAB*, Supplement 3: 440-42; *DSB*, 7: 622-25; Miller, *BHM*, p. 61; P. Speiser and F. G. Smekal, *Karl Landsteiner. . .(1975); Who Was Who in Am.*, 2: 311.

S. Galishoff

LANE, LEVI COOPER (May 9, 1830, Cincinnati, Ohio-February 18, 1902, San Francisco, Calif.). *Surgeon*. Son of Eli, farmer, and Hannah (Cooper) Lane, Married Pauline Cook, 1872; no children. EDUCATION: Early training, Farmers College and Union College, Schenectady, N.Y.; 1851, M.D., Jefferson Medical

College; until 1855, intern, New York State Hospital; 1860, studied at Göttingen, Germany, and Paris, France; 1875, fellowship, Royal College of Surgery; 1876, M.D., Berlin. CAREER: 1855-59, naval surgeon; at medical department, University of the Pacific: 1860-63, physiology faculty; and 1862-64, anatomy faculty; 1864-70, physiology faculty, Toland Medical College; 1870, led the seceding group that reestablished the Pacific School, serving as professor of surgery, surgical anatomy, and clinical surgery; 1882, set up new quarters for the school under the name, Cooper Medical College; began discussions that led to fusion with Stanford. CONTRIBUTIONS: Performed America's first vaginal hysterectomy (1878). Devised improvements in the surgical treatment of harelip. Editor, *San Francisco Medical Press*. President, California State Medical Society (1883).

WRITINGS: *Surgery of the Head and Neck* (1896). Writings listed in *National Union Catalogue* and *Index Catalogue*. REFERENCES: *DAB*, 5, pt. 2: 580-81; Henry Harris, *California's Medical Story* (1932), 369-74; *NCAB*, 14: 341.

Y. V. O'Neill

LARSEN, NILS PAUL (June 15, 1890, Stockholm, Sweden-March 19, 1964, Honolulu, Hawaii). *Pathologist*. Son of Emil and Maria (Freeman) Larsen. Married Sara Lucas, September 1, 1921; two children. EDUCATION: Massachusetts Agricultural College, B.S., 1913; 1916, M.D., Cornell University Medical College; internship, New York Hospital, where he was a special research intern and assistant pathologist. CAREER: 1917-19, U.S. Army Medical Corps; 1919-22, instructor in medicine and bacteriology, Cornell University, and assistant visiting physician, Bellevue Hospital and Gouverneur Hospital of New York; 1922, pathologist, Queen's Hospital, Honolulu, and shortly thereafter became medical director and served in that dual role for 20 years; 1927, 1945, president, Honolulu County Medical Society; 1930, medical adviser, Hawaiian Sugar Planters' Association; 1929, chairman, first Pan-Pacific Surgical Congress; 1955, U.S. delegate, International Conference of the Planned Parenthood Association, Tokyo, Japan. CONTRIBUTIONS: At Queen's Hospital, Honolulu, established an occupational therapy service, organized a research department, helped develop a training school for nurses. Fought to improve Hawaii's milk supply, which resulted in a precipitous decline in infant mortality. Developed a medical and health-education program for Hawaiian Sugar Planters' Association which gave Hawaii's plantations the lowest incidence of disease and mortality among American industries. Founded and edited *Plantation Health*, 1936-64.

WRITINGS: *Eating Your Way to Health* (1939). REFERENCES: *Hawaii Medical Journal* (1964): 388; *Honolulu Advertiser*, March 20, 1964; *Honolulu Star-Bulletin*, March 20, 1964; *JAMA* (June 24, 1964): 1101; *Men of Hawaii* (1925, 1930, 1935); *Men & Women of Hawaii* (1954); *NCAB*, J: 566; *Pan-Pacific Who's Who* (1940-41); *Who's Who in Hawaii* (1947).

J. A. Breinich

LARSON, LEONARD WINFIELD (May 22, 1898, Clarkfield, Minn.-September 30, 1974, Bismarck, N.Dak.). *Physician; Pathologist*. Son of John, druggist and pharmacist, and Ida (Anderson) Larson. Married Ordelia Miller, 1923, two children; Esther Knudtson, 1969. EDUCATION: University of Minnesota: 1918, B.S.; 1922, M.D.; and 1923-24, postgraduate study. CAREER: 1922-23, physician, Northwood, Ia.; 1924-69, physician and pathologist, Quain and Ramstad Clinic, Bismarck, N.Dak.; 1939-40, president, American Society of Clinical Pathologists; 1940-46, secretary, North Dakota Medical Association; 1940-50, member, House of Delegates, American Medical Association; in American Cancer Society: 1945-67, member, Board of Trustees; and 1947-48, national vice-president; in American Medical Association: 1950-60, member, Board of Trustees; and 1958, chairman, Board of Trustees; 1952, 1953, 1959, 1961, delegate, United Nations World Health Organization; 1959-68, member, Board of Directors, American Cancer Society; 1960, chairman, Committee on Health and Medical Care, White House Conference on Aging; 1960-66, member, Council of the World Medical Association; president: 1961-62, American Medical Association; and 1965-66, American Cancer Society; 1966, chairman, World Medical Association. CONTRIBUTIONS: First practicing pathologist in N.Dak. Only North Dakotan to serve as president, American Medical Association. Considered a major force in the acceptance by the American Medical Association of prepaid, government-assisted medical insurance systems. Medical researcher focusing on diagnosis of tumors. Leader in state and national anticancer movement.

WRITINGS: "Embryonal Carcinoma of Testicle," *J. Lab. and Clin. Med.* 15 (Jan.1930); "The Clinical Pathologist," *Am. J. of Clinical Pathology* 10 (Jul. 1940); "The Problem of Medicine is Rural Health," *Minnesota Med.* 29 (Jan. 1946); "Medicine's Role in Pre-Paid Medical Care Plans," *Radiology* 75 (Sept. 1960); "Medicine, the Patient, and the Government," *JNMA*, 53 (Nov. 1961). Writings listed in *Cumulated Medical Index*. REFERENCES: *Bismarck Tribune*, September 30, 1974, p. 25; *Current Biog.* (1962): 246-48; *Who Was Who in Am.*, 6: 239-40.

L. Remele

LATHROP, JULIA CLIFFORD (June 29, 1858, Rockford, Ill.-April 15, 1932, Rockford). *Social worker; Child welfare.* Daughter of William, lawyer and U.S. congressman (1877-79), and Sarah Adeline (Potter) Lathrop, active in women's suffrage movement. Never married. EDUCATION: One year at Rockford Seminary (later Rockford College); 1880, A.B., Vassar College. CAREER: Worked in father's law office for ten years; 1889, joined Jane Addams, Hull House, Chicago, Ill.; and worked as county agent visiting and inspecting Chicago tenements; 1892, appointed by governor of Ill. as first female member, Illinois Board of Charities; 1901, resigned in protest over use of funds for political patronage jobs; 1905, reappointed and resigned in 1909 in favor of her desired permanent professional administrative staff; 1909, member, National Committee for Mental Hygiene; 1912-21, chief, Children's Bureau, first woman to head statutory federal bureau; 1918-19, president, National Conference of Social Work; 1922, appointed by secretary of labor to investigate conditions at Ellis Island; 1922-24, president, Illinois League of Women Voters; 1925-31, assessor, Child

Welfare Committee of League of Nations. CONTRIBUTIONS: Active in reforms of care of children and the mentally and physically handicapped. Was instrumental in framing law for world's first juvenile court in Chicago. Helped in planning of Juvenile Psychopathic Institute, first mental hygiene clinic for children. Aided in passage of first Child Labor Law (1916) and Sheppard-Towner Act (1921). While heading the Children's Bureau, was responsible for studies showing need to improve infant and maternal health and for the registration of births.

WRITINGS: Article in Hull House Maps and Papers, 1895; *Suggestions for Visitors to County Poorhouses and to Other Public Charitable Institutions* (1905). Annual Reports of Children's Bureau, 1913-21; "The Background of the Juvenile Court in Illinois," in *The Child, the Clinic, and the Court* (1925); *Birth Registration: An Aid in Protecting the Lives and Rights of Children* (1914); REFERENCES: Jane Addams, "A Great Public Servant, Julia C. Lathrop," *Social Service Review* (1932); idem, *My Friend, Julia Lathrop* (1935); *DAB*, Supplement 1: 484-86; *NCAB*, C: 92; 24: 298; James Tobey, *The Children's Bureau* (1925); *Notable Am. Women, 1607-1950*, 2: 370-72.

M. H. Dawson

LATTIMORE, JOHN AARON CICERO (June 23, 1876 or 1878, Shelby, N.C.-December 31, 1959, Louisville, Ky.). *Physician.* Son of John Carpenter and Marcella (Hambrick) Lattimore. Married Naomi Anthony, 1928, no children. EDUCATION: 1897, A.B., Bennett College; 1901, M.D., Meharry Medical College; postgraduate work, Cook County Hospital. CAREER: 1901-59, private practice, Louisville; 1928-46, Louisville Health Department. CONTRIBUTIONS: A pillar of the black medical community of Louisville for 58 years, constantly involved in black personal and civic improvement: organized Louisville NAACP and sat on its board (1910-59), helped organize Louisville interracial group (before 1920), helped organize "Lincoln party" to help blacks break from local Republican party (1921), helped organize Louisville Urban League and sat on its board (1915-59). In public matters, served on Mayor's Flood Relief Committee (1937), Advisory Committee of Central District of American National Red Cross (*post* 1937), Negro Health Committee in charge of venereal disease clinic of Louisville Health Center, Kentucky Board of National Youth Administration (*post* 1938), Louisville Interracial Committee (*post* 1941), Hospital Committee of Louisville Area Development Association (*post* 1944). Involved in efforts to integrate patients and build new building at Central State Hospital (early 1940s). Worked successfully for amendment of Day Law that barred integrated classes in Ky. and thus opened medical and nursing schools of state to blacks. President (1947) and vice-president (1920), NMA; president and vice-president, Blue Grass State Medical Association (Ky.); and an organizer and president of Fall City Medical Society. REFERENCES: Obituary, *JNMA* 53 (1961): 536; *Who Was Who*, 5:417; *WWICA* 6 (1941-43): 316.

T. L. Savitt

LAUREY, JAMES RICHARD (August 5, 1907, East St. Louis, Ill.-August 19, 1964, Washington, D.C.). *Thoracic surgeon.* Son of Henry Todd, chef and baker, and Alice (Madison) Laurey. Married Mary Underwood, 1936 (d. 1953), two children; Margery (Stewart) Bell, 1954, one child. EDUCATION: 1925, A.B., College of the City of Detroit (now Wayne State University); 1932, M.B., 1933, M.D., Detroit College of Medicine and Surgery (now Wayne State University); 1933-34, intern, Provident Hospital, Chicago, Ill.; 1934-35, resident in surgery, Parkside Hospital, Detroit, Mich.; 1939-41, General Education Board fellow in thoracic surgery, University of Michigan. CAREER: At Howard University Medical School: physiology faculty, 1935-36; surgery faculty, 1936-55; 1936-39, 1941-64, on Freedmen's Hospital surgical staff; 1939-41, instructor in surgery, University of Michigan Hospital; 1947-48, consulting thoracic surgeon, Glenn Dale Tuberculosis Sanitorium, Washington, D.C.; 1964-65, staff, District of Columbia General Hospital; 1950-55, consultant, Denmar Sanitorium (W. Va.), a United Mine Workers' tuberculosis hospital. CONTRIBUTIONS: Instrumental in opening the doors of District of Columbia hospitals to black physicians by demonstrating his and his surgical staff's competence when asked to fill in for white physicians regularly drawn from George Washington and Georgetown Medical schools (1947). This action paved the way for an agreement reached (1948) allowing Howard physicians at Gallinger (now D.C. General) Hospital. Established and developed at Freedmen's Hospital, with Department of Medicine, a Division of Pulmonary Diseases (1940s-1960s). Did research in cardiorespiratory testing on tuberculosis.

WRITINGS: "Cardio-respiratory Testing in Tuberculosis," *Am. Rev. of Tuberculosis*, 50 (1944): 234-43; "Liposarcoma Developing in a Lipoma," *AMA Arch. Path.* 69 (1960): 506-10; "The Use of Transplants of the Colon in the Treatment of Esophageal Carcinoma," *JNMA* 54 (1962): 325-30. Writings listed in *JNMA* 56 (1964): 549. REFERENCES: Obituary, *JNMA* 56 (1964): 548-50; *NCAB*, 51: 559-60.

T. L. Savitt

LAWLESS, THEODORE KENNETH (December 6, 1892, Thibodeaux, La.-May 1, 1971, Chicago, Ill.). *Dermatologist*. Son of Alfred, minister, and Harriet (Dunn) Lawless. Never married. EDUCATION: 1914, A.B., Talladega (Ala.) College; 1914-16, University of Kansas School of Medicine; at Northwestern University: 1919, M.A.; and 1920, M.S.; 1920-21, fellow in dermatology and syphilology, Massachusetts General Hospital; 1921-24, postgraduate study, St. Louis Hospital, Paris; Kaiser Joseph Hospital, Vienna; and clinics in other European cities. CAREER: 1924-71, private practice, Chicago; 1924-40, research and teaching faculty, Northwestern University Medical College. CONTRIBUTIONS: Developed treatments for skin damaged by arsenical preparations and for early syphilis. Organized first clinical laboratory at Northwestern University Medical College. Encountered much racial prejudice in his teaching and research at Northwestern, which caused him to resign his positions there (1940). Very successful in business ventures; became a philanthropist. Devoted much time, effort, and money to community, health, southern black colleges, and international concerns.

WRITINGS: "Treatment of Accidental Perivascular Injections of Arsphenamine or Neoarsphenamine," *J. of Lab. and Clin. Med.* 16 (1931): 1910; "The Diagnosis of Sporotrichosis," *Arch. Derm. and Syphil.* 22 (1930): 381-88 (with Elizabeth J. Ward); "The Treatment of Early Syphilis with Electropyrexia," *JAMA* 107 (1936):194-99 (with Clarence A. Neymann and S. L. Osborne). Writings listed in *JNMA* 62 (1970): 312. REFERENCES: W. Montague Cobb, "Theodore Kenneth Lawless," *JNMA* 62 (1970): 310-12; *N.Y. Times*, May 3, 1971, p. 40; *Who Was Who in Am.*, 5: 418.

T. L. Savitt

LAZEAR, JESSE WILLIAM (May 2, 1866, Baltimore, Md.-September 25, 1900, Quemados, Cuba). *Physician; Microbiology.* Son of William Lyon, and Charlotte (Pettigrew) Lazear. Married Mabel Houston, 1896; two children. EDUCATION: 1889, A.B., Johns Hopkins University; 1892, M.D., College of Physicians and Surgeons (Columbia); 1892-94, intern, Bellevue Hospital; 1894-95, studied in Europe. CAREER: 1895-1900, clinical microscopy faculty, Johns Hopkins Medical School; 1895-1900, bacteriology staff, Johns Hopkins Hospital; 1900, assistant surgeon, U.S. Army, Columbia Barracks, Quemados, Cuba; 1900, member, U.S. Army Yellow Fever Commission. CONTRIBUTIONS: Believed to be the first American to have isolated the diplococcus of Neisser in a case of ulcerative endocarditis. Confirmed and elaborated the studies done by European scientists on the structure and life cycle of the malarial parasite. Conducted research on yellow fever, which led him to conclude that further pathological and bacteriological investigation of the disease would be fruitless. Allowed himself to be bitten by a mosquito that had dined on the blood of yellow fever victims but did not become ill; let himself be bitten shortly thereafter by either a stray mosquito or one believed to have been infected (Lazear's account is conflicting on the matter) and contracted yellow fever and died; led to field tests that conclusively proved that the *Aedes aegypti* mosquito transmits yellow fever.

WRITINGS: "A Second Case of Gonorrheal Septicaemia and Ulcerative Endocarditis with Observations upon the Cardiac Complications of Gonorrhea," *J. of Experimental Med.* 4 (1889): 81-116 (with W. S. Thayer [q.v.]); "Pathology of Malarial Fevers, Structure of the Parasites and Changes in Tissue," *JAMA* 35 (1900): 917-20; "The Etiology of Yellow Fever. A Preliminary Note," *Phila. Med. J.* 6 (1900): 790-96 (with Walter Reed [q.v.], James Carroll [q.v.], and A. Agramonte). A bibliography is in *Ala. J. Med. Sci.* REFERENCES: *BHM* (1970-74), 105; Emmett B. Carmichael, "Jesse William Lazear, " *Ala. J. Med. Sci.* 9 (1972): 102-14; *DAB*, 11: 66; *JAMA* 35 (Jul.-Dec. 1900): 895; Kelly and Burrage (1928), 724-25; Miller, *BHM*, pp. 61-62, 163; *NCAB*, 15:60; *Who Was Who in Am.*, Hist. Vol.: 377.

S. Galishoff

LEATHERS, WALLER SMITH (December 4, 1874, Albermarle County, Va.-January 26, 1946, Nashville, Tenn.). *Physician; Medical education; Public health.* Son of James Addison and Elizabeth (Pace) Leathers. Married Sarah Ola Price, 1906; one child. EDUCATION: Charlottesville (Va.) High School; Miller School of Virginia; University of Virginia: 1892, graduated, schools of biology, geology and mineralogy, and chemistry; and 1895, M.D.; 1896, postgraduate study, Johns Hopkins University; 1896, New York Marine Biological Laboratory; 1898, 1901, 1902, 1903, 1907, University of Chicago; 1899, Marine Biological Laboratory, Woods Hole, Mass.; 1904, Hospital of Chicago; 1906, Harvard University Medical School; 1908, Hospital of New York City. CAREER: 1894, instructor in biology and histology, University of Virginia; 1895-96, assistant professor of biology, University of Mississippi; 1896-97, head, Department of Science, Miller College of Virginia; 1897-99, professor of biology, University of South Carolina; at University of Mississippi Medical School: 1899-1905, professor of biology and physiology; 1903-10, professor of physiology; 1910-24, professor of physiology and hygiene; and 1910-24, dean, Medical School; 1917-24, director and executive officer of public health, Mississippi State Board of Health; 1918-19, president, Mississippi State Medical Association; 1922-23, president, Southern Medical Association; 1924, studied in Europe through the International Health Division of the Rockefeller Foundation; at Vanderbilt Medical School: 1924-retirement, professor of preventive medicine and public health; 1924-27, associate dean; 1928-retirement, dean; 1930-34, 1936-42, president, National Board of Medical Examiners; 1930, 1934, 1935, 1937, member, Board of Scientific Directors, International Health Division, Rockefeller Foundation; member: 1929-46, Advisory Committee on Public Health, Commonwealth Fund; 1931-35, 1937-39, Advisory Health Council, U.S. Public Health Service; and 1939, Health and Medical Advisory Committee, American Red Cross; president: 1940-41, American Public Health Association; and 1942-43, American Association for the Advancement of Science and Association of American Medical Colleges. CONTRIBUTIONS: Pioneer work as a medical educator. Accomplishments in Miss. public health work included campaigns against typhoid fever, malaria, and hookworm control, pellagra experiments, the establishment of a tuberculosis sanatorium, inauguration of full-time county health departments, appointment of a state factory inspector, and the revision of the state's medical practice act to advance standards of medical practice.

WRITINGS: Author or co-author of 133 articles contributed to professional journals.
REFERENCES: *DAB*, Supplement 4: 474-75; *NCAB*, 42: 658.

M. S. Legan

LEAVITT, ERASMUS (1838, N.H.-November 30, 1909, Butte, Mont.). *Physician; Surgery; Public health.* Son of Dr. Nathaniel Leavitt. Married Annie Threkeld, 1881; one surviving daughter. EDUCATION: c. 1854, A.B., Wesleyan College; 1857, entered Albany (N.Y.) Medical College; 1858, transferred to Harvard Medical College; left without degree; 1869, returned to Harvard and received M.D. that year. CAREER: Principal, Barrington (Mass.) Academy, and taught Greek, Latin, and mathematics; 1859, moved to Colo. as a gold miner on Cherry Creek; 1862, moved north to Bannock, Mont. Territory; by 1865, was practicing medicine on occasional basis; 1869-70, began medical practice in Mont. Territory; 1884, moved to Butte and specialized in eye, trauma, and general surgery; 1879, he and six other physicians formed the Montana Territorial Medical Association; it was ten years before this group became professionally viable; 1889, after reorganization, became president of the Montana Medical Association; member, first Board of Medical Examiners. CONTRIBUTIONS: Proposed and finally pushed through a bill creating the Montana State Board of Health. Drew attention to occupational disease in quartz mining and attempted to regulate public health in various mining towns with which he was associated. Among the first to recognize the need for some standards of licensing physicians. Personally reviewed many applications for practice in Mont. and rejected many. Encouraged political and social leaders to recognize the need for better public health practices and worked through both parties to secure needed legislation. A major figure in guiding state medical policy.

WRITINGS: Memoranda outlining needed legislation and addresses to various medical organizations. REFERENCES: Hubert Howe Bancroft, *History of the Pacific States of North America*, vol. 26: *Washington, Idaho, and Montana, 1845-1889* (1890), 764-65; John A. Newman, M.D., "Erasmus D. Leavitt, M.D. Activist" (ms. courtesy Mrs. Laura Newman, Butte); Paul C. Phillips, *Medicine in the Making of Montana* (1962).

P. C. Mullen

LEFFERTS, GEORGE MOREWOOD (February 24, 1846, Brooklyn, N.Y.-September 21, 1920, Katonah, N.Y.). *Physician; Laryngology*. Son of Marshall and Mary (Allen) Lefferts. Married Annie Cuyler Van Vechten, 1891. EDUCATION: 1870, M.D., College of Physicians and Surgeons of Columbia University; intern at Bellevue and St. Luke's hospitals; post-graduate study in London, Paris, and Vienna where he studied under Karl Stoerk, a founder of laryngology in Europe. CAREER: 1871-73, chief of Stoerk's clinic at the University of Vienna; 1873, began practice in New York City, specializing in diseases of the nose and throat, appointed as laryngologist to the Demilt Dispensary; 1874, established a throat clinic at the New York Eye and Ear Infirmary; 1873-1904, taught at the College of Physicians and Surgeons of Columbia University. CONTRIBUTIONS: A founder of the New York Laryngological Society (1873) and of the *Archives of Laryngology* (1880). A co-founder of the American Laryngological Association, president (1882).

WRITINGS: *A Pharmacopoeia for the Treatment of the Larynx, Pharynx and Nasal Passages* (1884). REFERENCES: *Annals of Otology, Rhinology and Laryngology*, March 1924; *DAB*, 6, pt. 1: 140; *N. Y. Times*, September 23, 1920.

M. Kaufman

LEIDY, JOSEPH (September 9, 1823, Philadelphia, Pa.-April 30, 1891, Philadelphia). *Physician; Anatomy; Zoology; Paleontology*. Son of Philip, hatmaker, and Catherine (Mellick) Leidy. Married Anna Harden, 1864; one adopted child. EDUCATION: 1844, M.D., University of Pennsylvania; 1848, 1850, visited medical schools, hospitals, and anatomical museums in Europe. CAREER: 1844-46, practiced medicine, Philadelphia; 1846, anatomy faculty, Franklin Medical College; 1846-91, chairman, Board of Curators, Academy of Natural Sciences; 1849, physiology faculty, Medical Institute of Philadelphia; at University of Pennsylvania: 1853-91, anatomy faculty; 1884-91, zoology and comparative anatomy faculty; and 1884-91, biology faculty; during Civil War, surgeon, Satterlee Army Hospital, Philadelphia; 1870-85, natural history faculty, Swarthmore College; president: 1881-91, Academy of Natural Sciences; 1885, Wagner Free Institute of Science; and 1889, Association of American Anatomists. CONTRIBUTIONS: One of the most brilliant natural historians of the nineteenth century with broad interests in anatomy, paleontology, parasitology, and protozoology. Best known for precision of descriptions and illustrations and preference for fact over theory. Leading anatomist of his time. Book *An Elementary Treatise on Human Anatomy* (1861) was widely used for many years. Established the study of zoology in the United States. Found *Trichinella spiralis* in pork (1845) and demonstrated that it could be killed by boiling. Showed the existence of bacterial flora in the intestines of healthy animals (1849). Did the first experimental transplantation of malignant tumors (1851). Suggested that hookworm might be the cause of pernicious anemia (1886).

WRITINGS: *Proc. Acad. of Natural Sci. of Phila.* 3 (Oct. 1846): 107-8; "Researches into the Comparative Structure of the Liver," *Am. J. of Med. Sci.* 15 (1848): 13-23; *Proc. Acad. of Natural Sci. of Phila.* 5 (Jun. 1850): 201, 212; *A Flora and Fauna within Living Animals* (1853); "Remarks on Parasites and Scorpions," *Trans., Coll. of Physicians of Phila.* 3rd series, 8 (1886): 441-43. A bibliography is in *BMNAS*, 7 (1913): 335-96. REFERENCES: *BHM* (1970-74), 106; (1975-79), 77; *DAB* 8: 169-70; Clark A. Elliott, *Biog. Dict. of Am. Sci.* (1979), 155; John A. Garraty, *Encyclopedia of Am. Bio.* (1974), 654-55; Kelly and Burrage (1928), 732-36; Miller, *BHM*, p. 62.

S. Galishoff

LEIGHTON, ADAM PHILLIPS (January 23, 1887, Portland, Maine-December 26, 1958, Portland). *Physician; Obstetrician; Gynecologist.* Son of Adam P. and Isadore Mary (Butler) Leighton. Married Anna Leahy; one child by a previous marriage. EDUCATION: Holbrook School, Ossining, N.Y., and Phillips Exeter Academy; 1910, M.D., Maine Medical School; 1910-11, intern, Maine General Hospital; 1911-12, studied abroad, Rotunda Hospital, Dublin, and Schauta Klinik, Vienna. CAREER: 1912, began practice, Portland; 1913, founded a private maternity hospital that he ran until 1944; During World War I, served as a medical officer in the U.S. Navy and became a lt. commander in the reserves. CONTRIBUTIONS: Served for 30 years as a member, Maine State Board of Registration of Medicine, and at times as secretary or chairman. A founding fellow, American College of Obstetricians and Gynecologists.

WRITINGS: Representative sampling published in the *J. of the Maine Med. Assoc.*; "The Cause and Cure of Eclampsia" 4 (Feb. 1914): 1712-20; "Cervical Lacerations and That Symptom Leukorrhoea" 14 (Oct. 1923): 49-57; "The Treatment of Toxemia of Pregnancy" 18 (Jan. 1927): 1-9; "The Treatment of Cancer in the Woman by Radium" 23 (Apr. 1932): 73-78; "Radium Treatment of Uterine Carcinoma" 24 (Nov. 1933): 210-

14. REFERENCES: *J. of the Maine Med. Assoc.* 35 (Jul. 1944); 36 (Jul. 1945): 124; 50 (Mar. 1959): 105; *Portland Evening Express*, December 27, 1958.

B. C. Lister

LENNOX, WILLIAM GORDON (July 18, 1884, Colorado Springs, Colo.- July 21, 1960, Boston, Mass.). *Physician; Neurology.* Son of William, mine owner and rancher, and Anna Belle (Cowgill) Lenox. Married Emma Stevenson Buchtel, 1910; two children. EDUCATION: 1909, B.A., Colorado College; 1913, M.D., Harvard University; 1913, intern, St. Luke's Hospital (Denver, Colo.); 1914-15, intern, Massachusetts General Hospital; 1921, M.A., University of Denver. CAREER: 1916-20, medical missionary, China; and medical faculty, Peking Union Medical College; *post* 1920, practiced neurology, Boston; at Harvard Medical School: 1922-27, assistant in medicine; 1922-30, fellow in neuropathology; and 1930-52, neurology faculty; at Boston City Hospital: 1926-34, junior visiting physician; 1926-30, assistant, Thorndike Memorial Laboratory; 1934-45, neurological staff; and 1944-47, visiting physician; *post* 1947, chief, Seizure Division, Children's Hospital (Boston); president: 1936, International League Against Epilepsy; 1947, Association for Research in Nervous and Mental Disease; and Elsimore Cattle Company, Fort Stockton, Tex. CONTRIBUTIONS: Spent life researching epilepsy and migraine, focusing on blood chemistry, metabolism, cerebral circulation, and the electrical activity of the brain. Experiments involving starvation and special diets showed the effect of the acid-base balance on seizures and incidentally provided greater understanding of the cause of gout. With Frederic A. Gibbs, demonstrated the value of electroencephalography in the diagnosis and treatment of epilepsy. Demonstrated the effectivensss of trimethyloxazolidinedione (tridione) in the treatment of petit mal seizures of childhood. Helped reorganize the International League Against Epilepsy (1935); established the league's American branch and served as president of both organizations. Organized the National Epilepsy League (1939), a lay group established to combat societal discrimination against epileptics. First editor, *Epilepsia* (1935).

WRITINGS: *Epilepsy from the Standpoint of Physiology and Treatment* (1928, with Stanley Cobb); "The Electroencephalogram in Epilepsy and in Conditions of Impaired Consciousness," *Arch. of Neurology and Psychiatry* 34 (Dec. 1935): 1133-48 (with F. A. Gibbs and H. Davis); *Science and Seizures; New Light on Epilepsy and Migraine* (1941); "The Petit Mal Epilepsies and Their Treatment with Tridione," *JAMA* 129 (Dec. 15, 1945): 1069-73; *Epilepsy and Related Disorders* (1960). REFERENCES: Stanley Cobb, "William Gordon Lennox," *Epilepsia*, 4th series, 1 (1959-60): 327; *JAMA* 174 (1960): 316; *NCAB*, H: Vol.: 46-47; *Who Was Who in Am.*, 4: 567.

S. Galishoff

LENOW, JAMES HARRELL (February 18, 1850, Memphis, Tenn.-December 30, 1932, Little Rock, Ark). *Physician; Medical education; Urology.* Son of James and India (Leake) Lenow. Married Ella D. Fones, 1883; two children. EDUCATION: Kentucky Military Institute: 1870, A.B., 1876, A.M.; 1872, M.D.,

Jefferson Medical College. CAREER: 1872-1932, private practice, Little Rock; 1875-77, city jail physician, Little Rock; 1877-78, city health officer, Little Rock; 1879-1919, 1922-32, medical faculty, medical department, Arkansas Industrial University (University of Arkansas after 1899); 1907-12, dean, medical department, University of Arkansas. CONTRIBUTIONS: Conducted first legal dissection of a cadaver in Ark. (Little Rock, 1874). Promoted improvement of medical education as a charter member, State Medical Society of Arkansas; its treasurer (1897-98); and its president (1909-10); and as a charter member of the faculty of the medical department of Arkansas Industrial University (1879). Modernized and raised standards of the University of Arkansas medical department while dean; added a full-time demonstrator in pathology, bacteriology, and chemistry. Set the admission requirement of a high school diploma or equivalent (1909), extended academic sessions from six to eight months, provided staff experience for senior students in the university clinic, and obtained a new laboratory building with microscopes and proper lighting (1910). Reorganized the department (1911), merging it with the College of Physicians and Surgeons of Little Rock and placing the medical school under direct control of the University of Arkansas. REFERENCES: W. David Baird, *Medical Education in Arkansas* (1979), 23, 39, 79, 103-4; *Goodspeed Biographical and Historical Memoirs of Central Arkansas* (1978), 481.

D. Konold

LEONARD, CHARLES LESTER (December 29, 1861, Easthampton, Mass.-September 22, 1913, Atlantic City, N.J.). *Physician; Radiology.* Son of M. Hayden and Harriet E. (Moore) Leonard. Married Ruth Hodgson; one child. EDUCATION: University of Pennsylvania: A.B., 1885, M.D., 1889, M.A., 1892; 1886, A.B., Harvard University; 1889-92, studied abroad. CAREER: 1892-, practiced medicine in Philadelphia; surgical staff, University Hospital, Philadelphia; director of radiology in various hospitals including the University of Pennsylvania, Methodist Episcopal and Polyclinic; professor of Roentgenology, Philadelphia Polyclinic; 1904 and 1905, president, Roentgen Ray Society; died from cancer induced by excessive exposure to X-rays, a martyr to his own specialty. CONTRIBUTIONS: One of the founders of American radiology. Became world famous in 1898 when he used X-rays to demonstrate the presence of stones in the kidney and other portions of the urinary tract; further showed that most small ureteral calculi pass spontaneously, thereby exerting a conservative influence on surgical practice. Investigated the diagnostic use of X-rays and their application in the treatment of cancer and other diseases. Was associate editor of the *Archives of the Roentgen Ray* (London), the *Zeitschift für Roentgenkunde* (Leipzig), and the *Journal de Radiologie* (Brussels).

WRITINGS: "Cases Illustrative of the Practical Application of the Roentgen Rays in Surgery," *Amer. J. of the Med. Sciences*, 112 (August 1896, with J.W. White and A.W. Goodspeed): 125-47; "Radiography of the Stomach and Intestines," *Amer. J. of Roent-*

genology (posthumously, November 1913). REFERENCES: *DAB*, 11: 173-74; Kelly and Burrage (1928), 738-39.

S. Galishoff

LETTERMAN, JONATHAN (December 11, 1824, Canonsburg, Pa.-March 15, 1872, San Francisco, Calif.). *Army medical officer; Surgeon.* Son of Jonathan Letterman, physician. Married Mary Lee, 1863; two children. EDUCATION: 1845, A.B., Jefferson College; 1849, M.D., Jefferson Medical College. CAREER: 1849, assistant surgeon, U.S. Army; until 1853, served in Seminole Wars; 1854-57, in Navajo and Apache campaigns, N. Mex.; 1859-60, following staff assignments in New York City and Washington, D.C., served in Ute campaign, Calif.; January 1862, appointed medical director, Department of West Virginia; July 1862, promoted to surgeon (major); and appointed medical director of the Army of the Potomac; served in the Peninsula, Antietam, Fredericksburg, Gettysburg, and Chancellorsville battles; December 1863-December 1864, medical inspector of hospitals, Department of the Susquehanna; December 1864, resigned from the army to become a businessman in San Francisco; 1866, returned to medical practice; elected: 1867-71, coroner of San Francisco; and 1868-72, surgeon-general, Calif.; 1870-71, member, Board of Medical Examiners, University of California; 1867, death of wife coupled with a chronic gastrointestinal illness made him a semi-invalid until death. CONTRIBUTIONS: Developed the first complete combat field medical system. After the Peninsular Campaign (August 1862), organized a regular ambulance corps, with a command structure, litter bearers, and drill, all under medical direction. At Antietam (September 1862), developed a field medical supply and depot system; organized field hospitals and assigned surgeons to an echeloned care system from first-aid to definitive surgery with the most experienced men in charge of surgery. After Fredericksburg (January 1863), installed a medical-inspector system with the use of standard forms and reports. Was emphatic in repeated insistence on preventive medicine and field sanitation. Responsible for the first coherent and complete field medical system for first-aid, evacuation, forward surgical treatment, an ambulance corps, field hospitals, medical supply depots, and field medical record keeping. A superb organizer, knew how to work within the military system; revolutionized the management, transportation and treatment of massive numbers of the sick and wounded in the first of the modern wars. His program was formalized by Act of Congress (March 1864). Organized and specified the form, function, requirements, and methods of caring for soldiers from the battlefield to the general hospital. His system, without conceptual change, is used today by every army in the world that has a structured medical department. Army Hospital in San Francisco was named Letterman General Hospital (now Letterman Army Medical Center) in his honor (November 1911).

WRITINGS: *Medical Recollections of the Army of the Potomac* (1866). REFERENCES: *BHM* (1964-69), 160; Bennett A. Clements, "Memoir of Jonathan Letterman," *Military*

Surg. 23 (1909): 3-47; *DAB*, 6, pt. 1: 194-95; Miller, *BHM*, p. 62; *NCAB*, 18: 338; James M. Phalen, "Life of Jonathan Letterman," *Military Surg.* 84 (1939): 62-66.

R.J.T. Joy

LEVY, JULIUS (September 19, 1881, Newark, N.J.-January 24, 1969, West Orange, N.J.). *Physician; Pediatrician.* Son of Jacob, merchant, and Hannah (Wetzle) Levy. Married Sophie Diamond, 1905; four children. EDUCATION: Princeton University; 1904, M.D., College of Physicians and Surgeons (Columbia); 1905-6, intern, Orange (N.J.) Memorial Hospital. CAREER: 1906-35, private practice, Newark; 1913-55, physician, Newark City Department of Health; 1918-51, physician, New Jersey State Department of Health; 1949, president, Association of Maternal and Child Health and Crippled Children's Directories. CONTRIBUTIONS: Organized (1913) and for 40 years directed the Child Hygiene Division, Newark City Department of Health. Due to his efforts, maternal deaths were reduced (by 1970) by 90 percent and infant mortality by 70 percent. Organized (1918) the Bureau of Child Hygiene (after 1936, the Bureau of Maternal and Child Health), New Jersey State Department of Health, and as its chief set up a child-hygiene nursing service that advised expectant mothers; established programs to supervise and educate midwives and coordinated about 50 "Baby Keep-Well Stations" throughout the state. Helped secure state laws requiring licensing and inspection of maternity homes, day nurseries, and boarding houses for children.

WRITINGS: "The Undernourished Child of Pre-School Age," *J. of the Med. Soc. of New Jersey* 16 (1919): 396-99; "Thirty Years' Progress in Maternal and Child Health," *Pub. Health News* 29 (1948): 355-60; *An Effective Child Hygiene Program: How Newark, N.J. Came to Be a Leader in Infant Welfare Work* (n.d.) REFERENCES: "Dr. Julius Levy," *J. of the Med. Soc. of New Jersey* 66 (1969): 141-42; Stuart Galishoff, *Safeguarding the Public Health: Newark, 1895-1918* (1975), 111-15; Emily S. Hamblen, "Public Health and Child Hygiene," *J. of the Med. Soc. of N.J.,* 16 (1919): 118-20; *News* (Newark), April 11, 1954; January 27, 1969; *Pub. Health News* 30 (1949): 10; 32 (1951): 361; 50 (1969): 66.

W. Barlow

LEWIS, DIO[CLESIAN] (March 3, 1823, Auburn, N.Y.-May 21, 1886, Yonkers, N.Y.). *Physician; Health reformer.* Son of John C., farmer, and Delecta (Barbour) Lewis, temperance activist. Married Helen Cecelia Clark, 1849; no children. EDUCATION: 1842-45, studied medicine with Dr. Lansing Briggs, physician to Auburn State Prison; 1845, entered Harvard Medical School, but left for want of funds; 1851, M.D. (hon.), Homeopathic Hospital College, Cleveland, Ohio. CAREER: 1838-42, taught school, Fremont, Ohio; 1846-48, practiced medicine, Port Byran, N.Y., with Dr. Lewis McCarty, who converted him to homeopathy; 1852-75, lectured in lyceums, temperance rallies, and schools throughout the United States and Canada on the "new gymnastics" and personal hygiene; 1861-68, founded and operated Boston Normal Physical Training School; c. 1861, formed class in gymnastics at McLean Hospital, Somerville, Mass.; 1863-

68, founded and operated sanatorium, Boston, Mass., and, later, Lexington, Mass.; 1863-68, established school for girls run on hygienic principles, Lexington; 1868-77, owned and occasionally operated temperance hotel, Boston; 1878-81, founded and operated sanatorium, Arlington Heights, Mass. CONTRIBUTIONS: Leading advocate of gymastics as an aid to health for young men and especially young women; largely responsible for establishing physical training as a part of public education in the United States. Temperance activist who helped organize the women's temperance movement, especially in Ohio. In lectures and writings, proselytized physical culture, hygiene, and temperance and assailed slavery, the use of drugs, prohibition, and vivisection.

WRITINGS: *The New Gymnastics for Men, Women, and Children* (1862); *Weak Lungs, and How to Make Them Strong* (1863); *Talks about People's Stomachs* (1870); *Our Girls* (1871); *Our Digestion* (1872); *Five Minute Chats With Young Women, and Certain Other Parties* (1874). Edited: *The Homoeopathist* (1850); *Der Homoeopath und diätetischer Hausfreund* (1852-53); *Lewis's Gymnastic Monthly* (1860-62). REFERENCES: *DAB*, 6, pt. 1: 209; Mary F. Eastman, *Biography of Dio Lewis, A.M., M.D.* (1891); *NCAB*, 10: 381; William G. Riordan, "Dio Lewis in Retrospect," *J. Health Phys. Educ. Rec.* 31 (1960): 46-48.

J. H. Warner

LIBMAN, EMANUEL (August 22, 1872, New York, N.Y.-June 28, 1946, New York). *Physician; Pathology; Microbiology; Cardiology.* Son of Fajbush, picture framer, and Hulda (Spivak) Libman. Never married. EDUCATION: 1891, A.B., College of the City of New York; 1894, M.D., College of Physicians and Surgeons (Columbia); 1894-96, house physician, Mount Sinai Hospital (N.Y.); 1896-97, 1903, 1909, studied in Europe; 1906, studied at Johns Hopkins. CAREER: At Mount Sinai Hospital: 1897-1923, pathology staff; and 1912-46, medical staff; consulting physician, numerous N.Y. hospitals; clinical medicine faculty, College of Physicians and Surgeons; chairman of the board, Dazian Foundation for Medical Research; chairman, Emergency Committee in Aid of Displaced Foreign Medical Scientists; member, Board of Governors, Hebrew University (Jerusalem). CONTRIBUTIONS: Discovered the Libman streptococcus (streptococcus enteritis), one of the causes of infant diarrheas (1898). Popularized the use of blood cultures through his studies of pneumococci, meningococci, typhoid, paracolon, and pyocyaneous infections. Used blood cultures to diagnose subacute bacterial endocarditis (1906-10); before then, the disease's insidious onset and protean symptoms had usually made a diagnosis impossible until autopsy (1912); prepared the way for later successful treatment of the condition with penicillin. With Benjamin Sacks, described a previously unidentified form of endocarditis (atypical verrucous endocarditis), now known as Libman-Sacks disease (1923-24). Conducted the first extensive clinical tests of blood transfusion. Showed that sprue and pernicious anemia were analogous. Established the diagnosis of sinus thrombosis as a serious complication of mastoid disease. Devised a new test for sensitivity to pain in which the subject is poked just below the ear in the mastoid region and his reaction observed (1922). Trained numerous physicians in what William Welch (q.v.) called "the Mount Sinai School of Cardiology." Endowed lectureships in the United States and abroad and secured funds to enable young physicians to continue their education and to do research. Helped establish the medical college of Hebrew University. Won fame as one of the world's most sought-after medical consultants.

WRITINGS: "Streptococcus Enteritis. A Study of Two Cases," *Med. Record* 53 (1898): 336-38; "On Some Experiences with Blood-Cultures in the Study of Bacterial Infections," *Johns Hopkins Hosp. Bull.* 17 (1906): 215-28; "The Etiology of Subacute Infective Endocarditis," *Am. J. of Med. Sci.* 140 (1910): 516-27 (with H. L. Celler); "Atypical Verrucous Endocarditis," *Proc., N.Y. Pathological Soc.* 23 (1923): 69-74. REFERENCES: *DAB*, Supplement 4: 494-95; *JAMA* 131 (May-Aug. 1946): 852; Miller, *BHM*, p. 63; *N.Y. Times*, June 29, July 2, 1946; Sutro Oppenheimer and Charles K. Friedberg, "Emanuel Libman, M.D.," *J. of the Mt. Sinai Hosp.* 13, no. 5 (1946): 215-23; *Who Was Who in Am.*, 2: 322.

S. Galishoff

LILIENTHAL, HOWARD (January 9, 1861, Albany, N.Y.-April 30, 1946, Jersey City, N.J.). *Physician; Surgery*. Son of Meyer, merchant, and Jennie (Marcus) Lilienthal. Married Mary Harriss d'Antignac, 1891, two children; Edith Strode, 1911. EDUCATION: Harvard University: 1883, A.B.; and 1887, M.D.; intern: 1886, McLean Asylum (Somerville, Mass.); and 1888, Mount Sinai Hospital (New York City). CAREER: 1889-97, practiced medicine with Arpad Gerster, New York City; 1888, surgery faculty, New York Polyclinic Medical School and Hospital; surgical staff: 1892-1940, Mount Sinai Hospital; and 1909-40, Bellevue Hospital; *post* 1917, clinical surgery faculty, Cornell University Medical College; 1917-18, Medical Corps, U.S. Army Reserve; and director, Mount Sinai Hospital Unit in France; president: 1901, Harvard Medical Society; 1903, New York Surgical Society; 1921, New York Society for Thoracic Surgery; and 1922-23, American Association for Thoracic Surgery. CONTRIBUTIONS: Made significant contributions to medical literature, surgical instrumentation, and operative and diagnostic technique. Invented a portable operating table and a new rib retractor. Had broad interest in all fields of surgery, particularly surgery of the ureter, prostate, and gallbladder. An early advocate of open reduction and fixation of fractures and one of the first to perform both suprapubic prostatectomy and cholecystectomy. Devoted himself to the infant field of thoracic surgery (*post* 1914), in which he was one of the great pioneers, developing operations for pulmonary tuberculosis, lung suppuration, and carcinoma of the lung and esophagus. Textbook *Thoracic Surgery* (1925) was used for many years and is considered a classic. A founder of the American Cancer Society.

WRITINGS: *Imperative Surgery* (1900); "Safety in the Operative Fixation of Infected Fractures of Long Bones," *Trans. Am. Surg. Assoc.* 30 (1912): 675-86; "Extrapleural Resection and Plastic of the Thoracic Esophagus. An Original Method, Report of a Successful Case without Gastrostomy," ibid., 39 (1921): 268-99; "Pneumonectomy for Sarcoma of the Lung in a Tuberculous Patient," *J. Thor. Surg.* 2 (1933): 600-15.

REFERENCES: Ira Cohen, "Howard Lilienthal, M.D., January 9, 1861-April 30, 1946," *J. of the Mount Sinai Hosp.* 13 (1946): 107-12; *NCAB*, C: 223; Harold Neuhof, "Howard Lilienthal," *Trans. Am. Surg. Assoc.*, 65 (1947): 677-79; *N.Y. Times*, May 1, 1946; Mark M. Ravitch, *A Century of Surgery*, 2 vols. (1981); *Who Was Who in Am.*, 2: 323.

                                                                            S. Galishoff

LINCOLN, BENJAMIN (October 11, 1802, Dennysville, Maine-February 26, 1835, Dennysville). *Physician; Educator.* Son of Hon. Theodore and Mrs. Hannah (Mayhew) Lincoln. Grandson of Gen. Benjamin Lincoln. Never married. EDUCATION: Bowdoin College: 1824, B.A.; and 1827, M.D.; studied with Dr. George C. Shattuck (q.v.), Boston, Mass. CAREER: At University of Vermont: 1828, lecturer, anatomy; and 1829, professor, anatomy and surgery; 1830, substitute professor, Bowdoin, one term, and University of Maryland, one term; 1830-34, professor, University of Vermont; died of tuberculosis. CONTRIBUTIONS: Practiced medicine in Burlington, Vt., but main interest and effort was in teaching. Mainstay of the medical college which flourished during his brief tenure and languished for several years after he died. Required more of his students than was usual for the time, teaching anatomy more from the standpoint of a philosopher than a surgeon. Gave public lectures on science. Writings influenced the direction of medical education.

WRITINGS: *An Exposition of Certain Abuses Practiced by Some of the Medical Schools in New England* (1833); *Hints on the Present State of Medical Education and the Influence of Medical Schools in New England* (1833). REFERENCES: Martin Kaufman, *University of Vermont College of Medicine* (1979), 29-40; obituary by Isaac Ray, *Eastport Sentinel* (Maine), August 1835; L. Wallman, "Benjamin Lincoln, M.D., Vermont Medical Educator," *Vermont Hist.* 29 (1961): 196-209.

                                                                          L. J. Wallman

LINDSLEY, JOHN BERRIEN (October 24, 1822, Princeton, N.J.-December 7, 1897, Nashville, Tenn.). *Physician; Medical educator; Social philosopher.* Son of Philip, scholar, educator, and chancellor of the University of Nashville, and Margaret (Lawrence) Lindsley. Married Sarah McGavock, 1857; six children. EDUCATION: University of Nashville: 1839, A.B.; and 1841, A.M.; 1841, entered into a preceptorship under Dr. William G. Dickinson (1791-1844), Nashville; 1843, M.D., University of Pennsylvania. CAREER: 1845-97, licensed preacher, Presbyterian Church; 1874, transferred to Cumberland Presbyterian Church; 1838, began study of natural science, especially geology, under Dr. Gerard Troost; 1848, a founder and member, American Association for the Advancement of Science; at University of Nashville: 1850, founder, medical department, and dean for ten years, and professor of chemistry and pharmacy for 23 years; and 1855-70, became chancellor; 1856, became member, Nashville Board of Education; 1865, elected superintendent, Nashville City Schools; 1867, set up plan for organization of the Montgomery Bell Academy; 1875, prominent role in founding of Peabody College, Nashville; 1875-87, secretary, Tennessee State Board of Education; 1876-79, Nashville city health officer; on Tennessee

State Board of Health: 1877-97, member; 1877-79, secretary; 1884, president; and 1884-97, executive secretary. CONTRIBUTIONS: Received much credit for the success of the medical department, University of Nashville. An enthusiastic worker on behalf of public health.

WRITINGS: John Edwin Windrow provides a list of 31 publications, mainly addresses and reports. REFERENCES: *DAB*, 6, pt. 1: 278-79; *NCAB*, 8: 131; John Edwin Windrow, *John Berrien Lindsley, Educator, Physician, Social Philosopher* (1938).

S. R. Bruesch

LINING, JOHN (April, 1708, Lanarkshire, Scotland-September 21, 1760, Charleston, S.C.) *Physician; Pioneer meteorologist; Botanist.* Son of the Rev. Thomas and Mrs. Anne (Hamilton) Lining. Married Sarah Hill, 1739; ten children, three of which died in infancy. EDUCATION: Probably studied medicine under Herman Boerhaave, at Leydon. CAREER: 1730, began practice, Charlestown; 1733-60, owned and operated apothecary shop; 1738, doctor, St. Phillip's parish; 1747, justice, Court of General Sessions and Court of Common Pleas. CONTRIBUTIONS: Began one-year statistical experiment (1740) of himself, because he thought there was a relationship between human metabolism and yellow fever; later published findings. Conducted experiments with sugar cane, pineapple, and rootbark.

WRITINGS: Material on yellow fever and metabolism, *Transactions*, Royal Society of London, 1742-43, 1744-45; aided Dr. Alexander Garden (q.v.) with his description of the Indian Root (published 1754); "Of the Anthelmintic Virtues of the Root of the Indian Pink," *Essays and Observations, Physical and Literary* (1754); letter from John Lining to Dr. Charles Alston, February 15, 1754; "A Description of the American Yellow Fever," in a letter to Dr. Robert Whytt at Edinburgh (published 1753); *A Description of the American Yellow Fever* (1799). REFERENCES: *DAB*, 6, pt.1: 280-81; *Dict. of South Carolina Bio. During the Period of the Royal Government* (1926); Miller, *BHM*, p. 63; *NCAB*, 25: 445; Marguerite Steedman, "Lining, John: Pioneer Southern Scientist," *Georgia Rev.* 10 (1956); J. I. Waring, *History of Medicine in South Carolina, 1670-1825* (1964).

J. P. Dolan

LIVERMORE, MARY ASHTON (RICE) (December 19, 1821, Boston, Mass.-May 23, 1905, Melrose, Mass.). *Civil War nurse; Agent, U.S. Sanitary Commission.* Daughter of Timothy, sea captain, and Zebiah (Vose) Rice. Married Rev. Daniel Parker Livermore, 1845; three children. EDUCATION: 1836, graduated, Miss Martha Whiting's Female Seminary, Charlestown, Mass. CAREER: 1836-38, taught foreign languages, Whiting's Female Seminary; 1839-41, tutor, plantation in southern Va.; 1842-45, schoolteacher, Duxbury, Mass.; 1845-57, housewife and part-time writer, various communities in New England, N.Y., and Ill.; 1858-69, associate editor, *New Covenant*, a Universalist monthly (Chicago, Ill.); 1862-65, agent and nurse, U.S. Sanitary Commission; *post* 1868, active in movement for women's rights; 1870-95, popular lecturer; *post* 1874, active in temperance movement. CONTRIBUTIONS: Leader in the U.S. Sanitary

Commission, organized sanitary fairs to raise money for soldiers' medical and sanitary needs and helped secure the acceptance of women as front-line nurses. Appointed an agent of the Northwest Sanitary Commission. Helped establish over 3,000 local aid societies in her region. Raised large stores of fruits and vegetables in addition to the usual hospital supplies for Grant's army in Vicksburg, which was threatened by scurvy (1863). With Mrs. Jane C. Hoge, organized the women's Sanitary Fair (1863) in Chicago; became prototype of similar fairs in other northern cities that together raised over $1 million.

WRITINGS: *My Story of the War* (1887). REFERENCES: *Appleton's CAB*, 2: 740; *Biog. Index*, 6: 358; 8: 411; *NCAB*, 3: 82; *Notable Am. Women*, 2: 411-13; *N.Y. Times*, May 24, 1905; *Who Was Who in Am.*, 1: 736.

S. Galishoff

LIVINGSTON, ROBERT RAMSAY (August 10, 1827, Montreal, Quebec, Canada-September 28, 1888, Plattsmouth, Nebr.). *Physician; Surgeon*. Son of Capt. Robert Ramsay, British army, and Mrs. Janet (McKercher) Livingston. Married Anna Beardsley; six children. EDUCATION: Royal Grammar School, Montreal; 1849, M.D., McGill University; postgraduate study, College of Physicians and Surgeons, N.Y. CAREER: 1861-65, U.S. Army, captain, Company A, 1st Nebraska Regiment, promoted to lieutenant colonel, to brevet-brigadier general; 1881-88, professor of principles and practice of surgery, Omaha Medical College; 1883-87, faculty, medical department, University of Nebraska (Lincoln, Nebr.); in Nebraska State Medical Society: 1868, charter member and organizer; secretary; and 1872, president; mayor, three years, Plattsmouth, Nebr.; 1869-88, medical director, Burlington & Missouri Railway; 1869-71, surveyor-general, Ia. and Nebr. CONTRIBUTIONS: Issued the first call (1868) to the medical profession for the purpose of organizing a state medical society. Member, Committee on Constitution and By-Laws. One of the first delegates to American Medical Association. Served on various committees of the Nebraska State Medical Society in support of state legislation regarding health affairs and the medical profession. Unusually successful practitioner of medicine and surgery, dying of cholera contracted in pursuit of his profession.

WRITINGS: Report of Committee on Surgery, *Trans., Nebraska State Med. Soc.*, 7 (June 1874): 57-64; Report on Surgery, *ibid.*, 16 (1884): 127-88. REFERENCES: R. R. Livingston and H. W. Orr, "Dr. Robert Ramsay Livingston," *Western Med. Rev.* 6, no. 10 (Oct. 15, 1901): 297-99; J. Sterling Morton, *History of Nebraska* 2 (1907): 384 (footnote); A. E. Sheldon, *Nebraska the Land and the People*, 2 (1931): 144-46.

B. M. Hetzner

LLOYD, JAMES (March 14, 1728, Lloyd's Neck, Long Island, N.Y.-March 14, 1810, Boston, Mass.). *Surgeon; Obstetrics*. Son of Henry, Boston merchant and shipowner, and Rebecca (Nelson) Lloyd. Married Sarah Comrin, 1759; four children. EDUCATION: Apprentice to: 1745, Dr. Silvester Gardiner, Boston; and 1745-48, Dr. James Clark, Boston; 1747, attended lectures, Harvard College;

1750-52, dresser, Guy's Hospital, London, under Dr. Joseph Warner (1717-1801); attended lectures by Dr. William Hunter and Dr. William Smellie; 1790, M.D. (hon.), Harvard Medical School. CAREER: c. 1753, appointed surgeon, Castle William (British military installation, Boston); 1752-1809, Boston medical practitioner; active attender of Boston Medical Dispensary; 1771, honorary member, American Philosophical Society; 1781, incorporator, Massachusetts Medical Society. CONTRIBUTIONS: Introduced, practiced, and taught male midwifery in Boston. Influential advocate of smallpox inoculation and, later, vaccination. First in America to use ligatures instead of cautery to close wounds and to use Cheselden's method of the double incision in amputations. Earned a reputation as a cautious practitioner who based his therapeutic philosophy on a faith in the healing power of nature.

REFERENCES: *DAB*, 6 pt. 1: 333; Kelly and Burrage (1920), 710; *Sibley's Harvard Graduates, 1746-1750* 12 (1962): 184-93; James Thacher, *Am. Med. Biog.* (1828), 359-76; Henry R. Viets, "The Medical Education of James Lloyd in Colonial America," *Yale J. of Biol. & Med.*, 31 (1958): 1-15.

M. H. Warner

LLOYD, JOHN URI (April 19, 1849, North Bloomfield, N.Y.-April 9, 1936, Van Nuys, Calif.). *Pharmacist; Drug manufacturer*. Son of Nelson Marvin, teacher, mathematician, and surveyor, and Sophia (Webster) Lloyd, writer and teacher. Married Adelaide Meader, 1876 (who died shortly after the wedding); Emma Rouse, 1880; three children. EDUCATION: Apprentice to Cincinnati pharmacist, then to George Egers. CAREER: 1871-85, pharmacist for Merrell & Thorpe, Cincinnati drug firm; 1885, firm became the property of Lloyd and his two brothers (Nelson Ashley Lloyd and Curtis Gates Lloyd), now called Lloyd Brothers. 1885-1936, the firm originally produced drugs for eclectic physicians; 1878-1907, professor of pharmacy, Eclectic Medical Institute of Cincinnati; 1883-87, professor at Cincinnati College of Pharmacy. CONTRIBUTIONS: As the leading drug manufacturer for eclectics, advocated eclectic medicine in opposition to the heroic medications of the allopaths (regular physicians). Author of more than 5,000 articles. Developed a total of 379 "specific" medications. Supported the drive against impure drugs which led to the Pure Food and Drug Act of 1906. President, American Pharmaceutical Association, 1887-88. President of the National Eclectic Medical Association, 1896-1905. Collection of books developed into the Lloyd Library of Botany and Pharmacy (Cincinnati).

WRITINGS: *Chemistry in Medicines* (1881 and numerous editions); *Elixirs* (1883); *Drugs and Medicines of North America*, 2 vols. (1884-87, with Curtis Lloyd); co-editor, *American Dispensatory* (1886-95 with John King); co-editor, *King's American Dispensatory* (1898-1909 with Harvey W. Felter); *Origin and History of All the Pharmacopeial Vegetable Drugs* (1921). REFERENCES: R. B. Cook, "J. U. Lloyd: Pharmacist, Philosopher, Author, Man," *J. of the Am. Pharmaceutical Assoc.*, 10 (1949): 538-44; *DAB*, Supp.

2: 389-90; *DSB*, 8:427-28; *Eclectic Med. J.*, May 1936 (contains various biographical sketches in memory of Lloyd).

M. Kaufman

LOEB, JACQUES (April 7, 1859, Mayen, Germany-February 11, 1924, Hamilton, Bermuda). *Physician; Physiology; Biology.* Son of Benedict, importer, and Barbara (Isay) Loeb; brother of Leo Loeb (q.v.). Married Anne L. Leonard, 1891; three children. EDUCATION: 1884, M.D., University of Strassburg; 1891, went to United States. CAREER: Physiology faculty: 1886-88, University of Wurzburg; and 1888-90, University of Strassburg; 1889-91, Biological Station, Naples, Italy; 1891-92, biology faculty, Bryn Mawr College; 1892-1902, physiology and experimental biology faculty, University of California; 1910-24, head, Division of General Physiology, Rockefeller Institute for Medical Research. CONTRIBUTIONS: Pioneered in the application of physics and chemistry to biology and was the leading proponent of the mechanistic theory of biology; believed that most or all life phenomena could be explained in terms of physiochemical processes. Extended the idea of tropisms from plants to lower animals (1890); showed, for example, that it was light and not food that drew caterpillars to the tips of branches and argued that much of what was regarded as purposeful behavior was really mechanical or inherent, physiological-chemical responses to external stimuli; maintained that both instinctive and adaptive behavior was largely genetically programmed. Achieved the first artificial parthenogenesis when he succeeded in fertilizing frogs' eggs by placing them in a special saltwater solution; was able to raise some of the animals conceived in this and other chemical and physical ways to full and normal maturity. Made important studies of colloid and protein chemistry. Edited the *Journal of General Physiology* (from its beginning in 1920).

WRITINGS: *Der Heliotropismus der Thiere und seine Uebereinstimmung mit dem Heliotropismus der Pflanzen* (1890); *Studies in General Physiology* (1905); *The Mechanistic Conception of Life* (1912); *Artificial Parthenogenesis and Fertilization* (1913); *Proteins and the Theory of Colloidal Behavior* (1922). Writings are in a bibliography compiled by Nina Kobelt appended to a biographical sketch by W. J. V. Osterhout in *J. of General Physiology* 8 (1928): ix-xcii, and reprinted in *BMNAS* 13 (1930). REFERENCES: *BHM* (1964-69), 165; *DAB*, 11: 349-52; *DSB*, 8: 445-46; Kelly and Burrage (1928), 752-53; Miller, *BHM*, p. 64; *NCAB*, 11: 72-73; *Who Was Who in Am.*, 1: 740.

S. Galishoff

LOEB, LEO (September 21, 1869, Mayen, Germany-December 28, 1959, St. Louis, Mo.). *Experimental pathologist.* Son of Benedict and Barbara (Isay) Loeb. Married Georgianna Sands, M.D., 1922. EDUCATION: 1897, M.D., Zurich; attended several other schools, including Heidelberg, Freiberg, Basel, Edinburgh, and London. CAREER: 1897, moved to Chicago, Ill., where his brother Jacques (q.v.) was professor of physiology, University of Chicago; 1900, adjunct professor of pathology, Rush Medical College; 1902-3, research fellowship under John G. Adami, McGill University; 1903-10, assistant professor of experimental pathology, University of Pennsylvania; 1910-15, director, laboratory research, Barnard Free Skin and Cancer Hospital (associated with Washington University School of Medicine, St. Louis); at Washington University School of Medicine: 1915-24, professor of comparative pathology; 1924-37, Mallinckrodt Professor of Pathology and chairman, Department of Pathology; and 1937-41, research professor emeritus, Oscar Johnson Institute; gave up laboratory work only after a severe attack of tuberculosis at the age of 81. CONTRIBUTIONS: Active in research for more than 50 years and author of more than 400 publications (1896-1958); according to Dr. Peyton Rous (q.v.), was "a founder of experimental cancer research." Research with Miss A.E.C. Lathrop established the influence of genetic factors in the incidence of cancer in mice. They had also noted (by 1920, the year of Miss Lathrop's death) the effect of estrogen on the origin of such tumors. Collaboration with Mayer Fleisher led to significant findings on the susceptibility of cancerous mice to implanted tumors and the tendency of neoplastic cells treated with colloidal copper to give rise to resistant strains. Other research was on tissue culture, transplantation, the pathology of circulation, internal secretions, venom of Heloderma, and the analysis of experimental amoebocyte tissue. Late in life (1945), published *The Biological Basis of Individuality*, a book 15 years in the making, which expressed his long-term scientific and humanitarian concerns. According to E. W. Goodpasture's (q.v.) biography, although he did not perfect *in vitro* cell culture, "he conceptually paved the way."

WRITINGS: "The Action of Intravenous Injections of Various Substances in Animal and Human Cancer," *Trans. Assoc. of Am. Physicians* 28 (1913): 30 (with M.S. Fleisher); "The Incidence of Cancer in Various Strains of Mice" (Abstract), *Proc., Soc. for Experimental Biol. & Med.* 11 (1913): 34 (with A.E.C. Lathrop); "The Influence of Pregnancies on the Incidence of Cancer in Mice" (Abstract), *ibid.*, 11 (1913): 38 (with A.E.C. Lathrop; "Transplantation of Tumors in Animals with Spontaneously Developed Tumors," *Surg. Gyn. & Obst.* 17 (1913): 203 (with M. S. Fleisher); *The Venom of Heloderma* (1913); *Edema* (1924). REFERENCES: *BHM* (1975-79), 79; H. Blumenthal, "Leo Loeb, Experimental Pathologist and Humanitarian," *Science* 131 (1960): 3404; *DAB*, Supplement 6: 385-87; *DSB* 8: 447-48; W. Stanley Hartroft, "Leo Loeb, 1869-1959," *Arch. Path.* 70 (1960): 269-74; "Leo Loeb, September 21, 1869-December 28, 1959," *BMNAS* 35 (1961): 205-19; Miller, *BHM*, p. 64; *NCAB*, 44: 523; P. Rous, "Leo Loeb," *Cancer* 13 (1960); L. P. Rubin, "Leo Loeb's Role in the Development of Tissue Culture," *Clio Medica* 12 (1977): 33-56; P. A. Shaffer, "Biographical Notes on Dr. Leo Loeb," *Arch. Path.* 50 (1950): 661-75 (this is followed by a comprehensive bibliography of more than 400 entries).

M. Hunt

LOEB, ROBERT FREDERICK (March 14, 1895, Chicago, Ill.-October 21, 1973, New York, N.Y.). *Physician; Metabolism.* Son of Jacques (q.v.), medical scientist, and Anne (Leonard) Loeb. Married Emily Guild Nichols, 1935; two children. EDUCATION: 1919, M.D., Harvard University; 1919-20, intern, Massachusetts General Hospital; 1920-24, resident, Presbyterian Hospital (N.Y.);

1927-28, visited German medical clinics on General Education Board grant. CAREER: At College of Physicians and Surgeons (Columbia): 1921-60, medicine faculty; and 1938-41, associate medical director, Neurological Institute; 1924-59, medical staff, Presbyterian Hospital; 1943-44, vice-chairman, Division of Medical Sciences, National Research Council; 1943-46, chairman, Board for Coordination of Malarial Studies; member: 1951-53, 1959-62, President's Scientific Advisory Committee; and 1950-64, National Science Board, National Science Foundation; trustee: 1947-60, Rockefeller Foundation; and 1954-70, Rockefeller University; president: 1936, American Society for Clinical Investigation; 1950-51, Harvey Society; and 1954-55, Association of American Physicians. CONTRIBUTIONS: Leading authority on electrolyte physiology and various metabolic disorders.. Demonstrated that the circulatory collapse commonly seen in patients dying from Addison's disease exhibited the characteristic of acute salt and water loss; went on to show that persons with Addison's disease, a hitherto invariably fatal disease, could be maintained indefinitely by increasing their intake of salt. Subsequently investigated the electrolyte disturbances that occur in uncontrolled diabetes; led to the development of a rational form of fluid and electrolyte therapy for diabetic acidosis, a frequent and often fatal complication. During World War II, directed the development of chloroquine and other synthetic antimalarial drugs. With Russell L. Cecil, co-edited (1947-60) the *Cecil-Loeb Textbook of Medicine*, a medical classic that in 1975 was in its 14th edition. Helped edit *Journal of Clinical Investigation* (1937-46). An outstanding educator and department head.

WRITINGS: "Observations on the Origin of Urinary Ammonia," *J. Biol. Chem.* 60 (1924): 491-95 (with Dana W. Atchley and Ethel M. Benedict); "On Diabetic Acidosis. A Detailed Study of Electrolyte Balances following the Withdrawal and Reestablishment of Insulin Therapy," *J. Clin. Invest.* 12 (1933): 297-326 (with others); "Effect of Sodium Chloride in Treatment of a Patient with Addison's Disease," *Proc., Soc. for Experimental Biol. & Med.* 30 (1933): 808-12; *Martini's Principles and Practices of Physical Diagnosis*, trans. George J. Farber (2nd ed. 1938, editor); "Activity of a New Antimalarial Agent, Chloroquine (SN 7618)," *JAMA* 130 (1946): 1069-70. A bibliography is in *BMNAS* 49 (1978): 149-83. REFERENCES: *BHM* (1980), 26; A. McGehee Harvey, "Classics in Clinical Science; the Electrolytes in Diabetic Acidosis and Addison's Disease," *Am. J. of Med.* 68, no. 3 (Mar. 1980): 322-24; *McGraw-Hill Modern Men of Sci.* 2 (1966): 327-28; *N.Y. Times*, October 23, 1973; *Who Was Who in Am.*, 6: 251.

                                                                                    S. Galishoff

LOMMEN, CHRISTIAN PETER (January 30, 1865, Spring Grove, Minn.-July 15, 1926, Austin, Minn.). *Biologist*. Son of Peter J., farmer, and Maria (Rask) Lommen. Married Gunhild Solberg, 1892; Grace Edridge, 1923; four children. EDUCATION: 1888, Carlton Academy, Northfield, Minn.; 1891, B.A., State University of Minnesota; 1896-97, postgraduate work, University of Berlin; 1897-1903, postgraduate studies, Marine Biological Laboratory, Woods Hole, Mass. CAREER: 1891-1907, professor of biology, University of South Dakota, Vermillion, S.Dak.; 1907-26, dean, College of Medicine, University of South

Dakota, and chair, biology department. CONTRIBUTIONS: As first dean of the School of Medicine, University of South Dakota, worked ceaselessly to develop a quality education program. REFERENCES: George W. Kingsbury, *History of Dakota Territory*; George Martin Smith, *South Dakota, Its History and Its People: Biographical* 4 (1915): 279; *Who Was Who in Am.*, 1: 742.

> D. W. Boilard and P. W. Brennen

LONG, CRAWFORD WILLIAMSON (November 1, 1815, Danielsville, Ga.-June 16, 1878, Athens, Ga.). *Physician; Anesthesia.* Son of James and Elizabeth (Ware) Long. Married Caroline Swain, August 11, 1842; six children. EDUCATION: 1835, A.B., University of Georgia; 1836, under a preceptor and then at Transylvania University; 1839, M.D., University of Pennsylvania School of Medicine. CAREER: Spent 18 months working in hospitals in New York City; chose to return to rural Ga. and small-town practice in the village of Jefferson; 1841, assumed the practice of a Dr. Grant; 1850, moved to Athens, home of the state's university and a center of culture. CONTRIBUTIONS: Engaged in the various "ether frolics" celebrated in Philadelphia when he was a student; became curious about the pain-killing possibilities of the gases used in these high jinks. Lacking the nitrous oxide that had been used in Philadelphia, began to experiment with sulphuric ether. Observations led to the conclusion that people rendered unconscious by sulphuric ether felt no pain when under the influence of the gas. Convinced James M. Venable to submit to ether and allow Long to operate on him for a cyst (Jefferson, March 30, 1842). Continued to use ether as an anesthetic for a number of years, including a second successful cystic operation on Venable, but failed to register his experiments with the appropriate officials in the medical profession. (Augusta's *Southern Medical and Surgical Journal*, the logical outlet to print Long's findings and probably the South's best antebellum medical journal, was not publishing at this critical time owing to the death of Milton Antony (q.v.), the journal's editor and founder.) Others established their priority in the field of surgical anesthesia. It was not until the end of 1849 that the *Southern Medical and Surgical Journal* documented the justice of his claim.

WRITINGS: "An Account of the First Use of Sulphuric Ether by Inhalation as an Anesthetic in Surgical Operations," *Southern Med. and Surg. J.*, n.s., 5 (1849): 705-13. For clarifications and developments concerning Long's claim, see his letter of December 17, 1849, in *ibid.*, 6 (1850): 63-64; 9 (1853): 254-55, 384; 10 (1854): 257-58. REFERENCES: "Anesthesia. Long Sought, Lately Found" (1968), Item 20, National Library of Medicine, Bethesda, Md.; Frank Kells Boland, "Crawford Williamson Long and the Discovery of Anesthesia," *Georgia Hist. Q.* 7 (1923): 135-54; idem, *The First Anesthetic, the Story of Crawford Long* (1950); *DAB*, 6, pt. 1: 374-76; Nicholas M. Greene, "A Consideration of Factors in the Discovery of Anesthesia and Their Effects on Its Development," *Anesthesiology* 35 (1971): 515-22; *NCAB*, 13: 210; J. Marion Sims, "The Discovery of Anesthesia," *Virginia Med. Monthly* 4 (1877): 81-100; Frances Long Taylor, *Crawford Williamson Long and the Discovery of Ether Anesthesia* (1928);

Hugh H. Young, "Crawford W. Long: The Pioneer in Ether Anesthesia," *Bull. Hist. Med.* 12 (1942): 191-225.

P. Spalding

LONG, CYRIL NORMAN HUGH (June 19, 1901, Nettleton, England-July 6, 1970, Pemaquid Beach, Maine). *Physician; Biochemist; Physiology; Endocrinology.* Son of John Edward, tax surveyor, and Rose Fanny (Langdill) Long. Married Hilda Gertrude Jarman, 1928; two children. EDUCATION: University of Manchester, England: 1921, B.Sc.; 1923, M.Sc.; and 1932, D.Sc.; 1928, M.D., C.M., McGill University. CAREER: 1923-25, physiology faculty, University College, London; 1925-32, medical research faculty, Department of Biochemistry, McGill University; 1928-32, in charge, medical laboratories, Royal Victoria Hospital, Montreal; 1932-36, director, George S. Cox Medical Research Institute, and medicine faculty, University of Pennsylvania; at Yale University: 1936-51, physiological chemistry faculty; 1939-41, 1952-53, pharmacology faculty; 1939-42, chairman, Division of Biological Sciences; 1947-52 dean, school of medicine; and 1951-69, physiology faculty; during World War II, Endocrine Research Committee, National Research Council, and deputy chief, Division of Physiology, Office of Scientific Research and Development; president: 1944-45, Society for Clinical Investigation; 1947-48, The Endocrine Society; and 1953-55, Society for Experimental Biology and Medicine. CONTRIBUTIONS: Did earliest work on the physical and chemical changes underlying muscular contraction. Best known for investigations of the role of hormones produced by the adrenal cortex and the hypothalamus in normal and abnormal metabolism. Helped reveal the neuroendocrine control of carbohydrate metabolism; demonstrated that removal of the adrenal cortex brought about an amelioration of experimental diabetes; led to the concept that carbohydrate metabolism is regulated by the opposing effects of insulin on the one hand and adrenal cortical and anterior pituitary factors on the other. With others, helped to isolate highly purified prolactin, ACTH, and growth hormone and developed the adrenal ascorbic acid bioassay for pituitary adrenocortical hormones.

WRITINGS: "Lactic Acid in Human Muscle," *J. of Physiol.* 57 (1923): 1054-55 (with A. V. Hill and H. Lupton); "Observations on a Dog Maintained for Five Weeks without Adrenals or Pancreas," *Proc., Soc. for Experimental Biol. & Med.* 32 (1934): 392-94 (with F.D.W. Lukens); "The Adrenal Cortex and Carbohydrate Metabolism," *Endocrinology* 26 (1940): 309-44 (with B. Katzin and E. G. Fry); "Prolactin," *J. Biol. Chem.* 143 (1942): 447-64 (with A. White and R. W. Bonsnes); "Preparation and Properties of Pituitary Adrenotropic Hormone," ibid., 149 (1943): 425-36 (with G. Sayers and A. White). A bibliography is in *BMNAS.* REFERENCES: *BMNAS,* 46 (1975): 265-309,; Philip K. Bondy, "Cyril Norman Hugh Long," *Yale J. Biol. & Med.* 41 (Oct. 1968): 95-106; *N.Y. Times,* July 8, 1970, *Who Was Who in Am.,* 5: 438.

S. Galishoff

LONG, FRANCIS A. (February 16, 1859, Kreidersville, Pa.-November 24, 1937, Madison, Nebr.). *Physician; Surgeon.* Son of S. Robert, carpenter, miller, and farmer, and Sara Louise (Selp) Long. Married Maggie E. Miller, December 2, 1884; three children. EDUCATION: 1882, M.D., University of Iowa; 1894-1901, postgraduate work, Chicago Postgraduate School and Hospital. CAREER: 1879-82, schoolteacher, West Point and Oakland, Nebr.; 1882-1938, general practice including surgery, Madison; 1916-20, chairman, Publication Board of Nebraska State Medical Society; 1920-38, editor, *Nebraska State Medical Journal*; 1906-7, president, Nebraska State Medical Society; 1907, 1908, 1911, delegate, American Medical Association; 1909-10, Nebr. delegate, American Medical Association Council on Medical Education and Medical Legislation; 1915-38, fellow, American College of Physicians. CONTRIBUTIONS: First proposed a state medical publication (1906); under his editorship the *Nebraska State Medical Journal* became a medium for scientific papers and a unification of rural and urban practitioners. Carried on a large and varied medical practice adapting scientific methods in a primitive setting coping with epidemics of diphtheria and typhoid, and with insanity, accidents, cholera, and extra-uterine pregnancy. Performed first operation in Nebr. outside of Omaha, Nebr., for removal of appendix (1892). Administered first antitoxin (1895).

WRITINGS: "Foreign Body in the Air Passages, Phantom Tumor, and Perforative Appendicitis," *Western Med. Rev.* 2 (Jan. 1897): 41-42; "The Application of Business Methods to Practice of Medicine," *ibid.*, 15 (Mar. 1910): 143-46; "A Contribution to the Study of the Familial Aspects of Diabetes Mellitus," *ibid.*, 19 (Jan. 1914): 30-31; *A Prairie Doctor of the Eighties, Some Personal Recollections and Some Early Medical and Social History of a Prairie State* (1937). Complete list of writings at the University of Nebraska Medical Center Library of Medicine, Omaha. REFERENCES: *Nebraska State Med. J.* 23 (Jan. 1938): 36; H. W. Orr, *History of Medicine in Nebraska* (1952), 97; personal papers, University of Nebraska Medical Center Library of Medicine, Omaha; A. T. Tyler and E. F. Auerbach, *History of Medicine in Nebraska* (1977, enlarged by B. M. Hetzner), 207-9.

B. M. Hetzner

LONG, LEROY (January 1, 1869, Lincoln County, N.C.-October 27, 1940, Oklahoma City, Okla.). *Physician; Surgeon.* EDUCATION: Read anatomy with local physician in Lincoln County and then attended Louisville Medical College, M.D., 1893, first in his class. CAREER: 1894-95, junior lecturer and clinical assistant at Louisville Medical College when prolonged convalescence from pneumonia interrupted career; 1895, moved to Atoka, Indian Territory, to accept locum tenens; subsequently became citizen of Choctaw Nation by marriage while practicing in the small town of Caddo; 1904, moved to McAlester, Indian Territory, and confined practice to surgery; 1915, accepted position of dean and professor of surgery, University of Oklahoma School of Medicine. CONTRIBUTIONS: Secretary, Indian Territory Medical Association (1897, 1900) and chairman, committee that advocated consolidation of the association with the Oklahoma State Medical Association. President of the latter association (1934-35). Elected fellow, American College of Surgeons (1913) and later served as governor of the college. During tenure as dean of the university medical school, the first university hospital devoted entirely to patient care and education was built and the medical school consolidated at the Oklahoma City campus. Widely recognized as the most important early leader of the University of Oklahoma Medical School. REFERENCES: Mark R. Everett, *Medical Education in Oklahoma: The University of Oklahoma School of Medicine and Medical Center 1900-1931* (1972); B. A. Hayes, *LeRoy Long, Teacher of Medicine* (1943); R. Palmer Howard, "Nominations for the All American Medical Hall of Fame," *Journal of the Oklahoma State Medical Association* 72, no. 7 (March 1979): 202-5. R. Palmer Howard and Richard E. Martin, "The Contributions of B. F. Fortner, LeRoy Long, and Other Early Surgeons in Oklahoma," *Journal of the Oklahoma State Medical Association* (November 1968): 541-49; "LeRoy Long" file, History of Medicine Collection, University of Oklahoma Health Sciences Center Library, Oklahoma City, Okla.; Wallace Love and R. Palmer Howard, "Health and Medical Practice in the Choctaw Nation, 1880-1907," *Journal of the Oklahoma State Medical Association* (March 1970): 102-6.

V. Allen

LONG, PERRIN HAMILTON (April 7, 1899, Bryan, Ohio-December 17, 1965, Chappaquidick Island, Mass.). *Physician; Pharmacology*. Son of James Wilkinson, physician, and Wilhelmina Lillian (Kautsky) Long. Married Elizabeth D. Griswold, 1922; two children. EDUCATION: 1924, B.S., M.D., University of Michigan; Boston City Hospital: 1924-25, fellow, Thorndike Memorial Laboratory; and 1925-27, intern and resident; 1927, voluntary assistant, Hygienic Institute, Freiburg, Germany. CAREER: 1917-18, ambulance driver, France, American Field Service; 1927-29, assistant and associate, Rockefeller Institute for Medical Research; at Johns Hopkins Medical School: 1929-40, medicine faculty; and 1940-51, preventive medicine faculty; 1940-51, medical staff, Johns Hopkins Hospital; 1942-45, Medical Corps, U.S. Army; 1951-61, medicine faculty, State University of New York, Downstate Medical Center (Brooklyn, N.Y.); 1951-61, medical staff, King's County Hospital Center (Brooklyn); consultant: National Research Council, Veterans' Administration, U.S. Public Health Service, and U.S. Army. CONTRIBUTIONS: With Eleanor Bliss, did first work in America on sulfanilamide; experimental and clinical observations supported and extended studies of European investigators that sulfonamide therapy was effective in the treatment of a wide variety of streptococcal infections.

WRITINGS: "Observations on the Mode of Action of Sulfanilamide," *JAMA* 109 (1937): 1524 (with Eleanor A. Bliss); "Para-amino Benzene Sulfonamide and Its Derivatives. Clinical Observations on Their Use in the Treatment of Infections Due to Beta Hemolytic Streptococci," *Arch. of Surg.* 34 (1937): 351; *Clinical and Experimental Use of Sulfanilamide, Sulfapyridine and Allied Compounds* (1939, with Eleanor A. Bliss); *ABC's of Sulfonamide and Antibiotic Therapy* (1948). REFERENCES: A. McGehee Harvey, "The Story of Chemotherapy at Johns Hopkins: Perrin H. Long. . .," *Johns Hopkins Med. J.* 138 (Feb. 1976): 54-60; *Trans. Assoc. of Am. Physicians* 79 (1966): 59-61; *Who Was Who in Am.*, 4: 583.

S. Galishoff

LONGCOPE, WARFIELD THEOBALD (March 29, 1877, Baltimore, Md.-April 25, 1953, Lee, Mass.). *Physician; Pathology; Immunology*. Son of George von S. and Ruth Theobald Longcope. Married Janet Percy Dana, 1915; four children. EDUCATION: Johns Hopkins University: 1897, A.B.; and 1901, M.D. CAREER: 1901-4, resident pathologist, Pennsylvania Hospital (Philadelphia); 1904-11, director, Ayer Clinical Laboratory; 1909-11, applied clinical medicine faculty, University of Pennsylvania; 1911-22, medicine faculty, College of Physicians and Surgeons (Columbia University); 1914-21, medical staff, Presbyterian Hospital; 1917-18, Medical Officers Reserve Corps, on active duty, medical division, Office of Surgeon General, Washington, D.C.; 1918-19, Medical Corps, U.S. Army Expeditionary Force; 1922, clinical medicine faculty, Cornell University Medical College; and visiting physician, Second Division, Bellevue Hospital (N.Y.); 1922-46, medicine faculty, Johns Hopkins Medical School; and medical staff, Johns Hopkins Hospital; president: 1919, Society for Clinical Investigation; and 1945-46, Association of American Physicians. CONTRIBUTIONS: Pioneered in immunology, particularly in the study of allergies and was a founder of the American Academy of Allergy. Advanced the hypothesis that acute nephritis was an altered tissue response to bacteria, notably hemolytic streptococci, in much the same manner that serum sickness developed after the injection of immune serum made from proteins of another species. During World War II, made outstanding investigations of an antidote for war gasses, BAL (British Anti-Lewisite), which disclosed that this substance promoted the excretion of arsenic, mercury, and other metallic poisons; subsequently contributed to the usefulness of BAL in civilian cases of metallic poisoning. Advanced knowledge of unusual types of pneumonia, shrunken kidney resulting from pyelonephritis, Boeck's sarcoid, syphilis of the aorta, and Hodgkin's Disease.

WRITINGS: "A Study of the Distribution of the Eosinophilic Leucocytes in a Fatal Case of Hodgkin's Disease, with General Eosinophilia," *Bull. of the Ayer Clinical Laboratory of Pennsylvania Hosp.* 3 (1906): 86; "The Relationship Between Repeated Anaphylactic Intoxication and Chronic Inflammatory Lesions of Kidneys," *Long Island Med. J.* 9 (1915): 453-56; "The Susceptibility of Man to Foreign Proteins (Harvey Lecture, February 26, 1915)," *Am. J. of Med. Sci.* 152 (1916): 625; "The Generalized Form of Boeck's Sarcoid," *Trans. Am. Assoc. of Physicians* 51 (1936): 94; "Value of BAL (2,3-dimercaptopropanol) in Treatment of Poisoning by Mercury Bichloride," *Bull. of the Ayer Clinical Laboratory of Pennsylvania Hosp.* 4 (1952): 61-70. A bibliography is in *BMNAS*. REFERENCES: *BMNAS* 33 (1959): 205-25; *DAB*, Supplement 5: 438-39; *Who Was Who in Am.*, 3: 529.

S. Galishoff

LONGSHORE, HANNAH E. (MYERS) (May 30, 1819, Sandy Spring, Md.-October 18, 1901, Philadelphia, Pa.). *Physician*. Daughter of Samuel, teacher in Quaker school, and Paulina (Iden) Myers. Married Thomas E. Longshore, 1841; two children. EDUCATION: Quaker schools, Washington, D.C., and New Lisbon, Ohio; apprentice to Dr. Joseph S. Longshore, her husband's brother, Attleboro, Pa.; 1851, M. D., Female (later Woman's) Medical College of Pennsylvania. CAREER: 1852, demonstrator of anatomy, New England Female Medical College, Boston, Mass., and first woman member of the faculty; 1852-53, demonstrator of anatomy, Woman's Medical College of Pennsylvania; 1853-57, taught at Penn Medical University, school formed as a result of a schism within the Woman's Medical College; 1853-92, medical practice, Philadelphia. CON-TRIBUTIONS: Early female physician, first to practice in Philadelphia. First female faculty member (demonstrator of anatomy) in an American medical college. Popular lecturer on physiology and hygiene. Successful practitioner with an estimated 300 families in her care.   REFERENCES: Gulielma F. Alsop, *History of the Woman's Medical College* (1950); Miller, *BHM*, p. 65; *NCAB*, 5: 244; *Notable Am. Women*, 2: 426-28; F. C. Waite, "The Three Myers Sisters—Pioneer Women Physicians," *Med. Rev. of Revs.*, March 1933.

M. Kaufman

LOOMIS, ALFRED LEBBEUS (October 16, 1831, Bennington, Vt.-January 23, 1895, New York, N.Y.). *Physician; Disease of the chest.* Son of Daniel, cotton manufacturer, and Eliza (Beach) Loomis. Married Sarah Patterson, 1858; two children; Mrs. John D. Prince, 1887. EDUCATION: Preliminary education Hoosick Falls and Rochester, N.Y.; 1851, B.A., Union College; studied medicine with Dr. Willard Parker (q.v.), New York City; 1853, M.D., College of Physicians and Surgeons, New York City; 1853-54, assistant physician, hospitals on Ward's and Blackwell's islands; 1856, M.A., Union College. CAREER: 1854-95, private practice, New York City; 1859-95, attending physician, Bellevue Hospital; 1862-66, lecturer, physical diagnosis, College of Physicians and Surgeons; at University of the City of New York: 1866-68, adjunct professor of theory and practice of medicine; and 1868-95, professor of pathology and practice of medicine. CONTRIBUTIONS: Great skill as a clinical teacher. Provided the leadership to raise the medical department, University of the City of New York, from its low ebb during the Civil War to an integral part of the university; remained its guiding force until his death. Secured money (1886) for building Loomis Laboratory for the study of bacteriology. Afflicted with tuberculosis at an early age, helped Dr. Edward L. Trudeau (q.v.) establish the tuberculosis sanatorium at Saranac Lake; Loomis Sanatorium for Consumptives opened 1896, Liberty, N.Y. Very active as president, New York Academy of Medicine; largely through his efforts the academy erected a new permanent home. Interested in improving the quality of medical education, medical research, and medical literature.

WRITINGS: *Lessons in Physical Diagnosis* (1868); *The Diseases of the Respiratory Organs, Heart and Kidneys* (1876); *A Text-Book of Practical Medicine* (1884); *A System of Practical Medicine by American Authors* (1898, with William Gilman Thompson). Writings listed in New York Academy of Medicine, *Author Catalog*, 24: 179-80. REF-ERENCES: William B. Atkinson, *Biographical Dict. of Contemporary Am. Physicians and Surgeons* (1880): 279-80; *Appleton's CAB*, 4: 17-18; *NCAB*, 8: 223.

R. Batt

LOTHROP, CHARLES HENRY (September 3, 1831, Taunton, Mass.-February 6, 1890, Lyons, Ia.). *Physician; Surgery.* EDUCATION: 1852-53, partial

classical course, Brown University; 1859, M.D., University of New York. CA-
REER: *Post* 1859, medical practice, Lyons (now part of Clinton, Ia.); 1861-65,
assistant surgeon and then full surgeon, First Iowa Cavalry; *post* 1868, U.S.
examining surgeon for pensions; 1876, "collaborator," *Southern Medical Record*. CONTRIBUTIONS: Inventor of an apparatus for treating fractures of the leg
and a rubber appliance for club foot. Compiler of the first published directory
of Ia. physicians. This directory, and its subsequent editions, presented accurate
information about the education, degrees, and professional accomplishments of
Ia. physicians and surgeons during the 1870s and 1880s helping the profession
in "its groping for order a generation before the Flexner Report."
  WRITINGS: "Successful Treatment of Fragilitas Ossium," *Boston Med. and Surg. J.*
(Oct. 26, 1871); "A New Apparatus for the Treatment of Bunion," *TAMA* (1873) and
Boston Med. and Surg. J. (Jun. 1873); *Medical and Surgical Directory of the State of
Iowa* (1876, and subsequent editions); *A History of the First Regiment, Iowa Cavalry
Veteran Volunteers* (1890). REFERENCES: *Appleton's CAB* 4: 32; David S. Fairchild,
History of Medicine in Iowa (1923), 256; Peter T. Harstad, "Health in the Upper Mis-
sissippi River Valley, 1820 to 1861" (Ph.D. diss., University of Wisconsin, 1963), esp.
ch. 10, "Medical Education"; Charles H. Lothrop, *The Medical and Surgical Directory
of the State of Iowa* (1876).

R. E. Rakel

LOVEJOY, ESTHER POHL (November 16, 1870, Seabeck, Wash.-August
17, 1967, New York, N.Y.). *Physician; Medical administrator*. Daughter of
Edward, journalist, and Annie (Quinton) Clayson. Married Emil Pohl, 1894;
one child; married George Lovejoy, 1913. EDUCATION: 1894, M.D., University
of Oregon; 1896, postgraduate study, West Side Post Graduate School, Chicago,
Ill.; 1910, postgraduate study, Berlin. CAREER: 1894-1917, practice, Portland,
Oreg.; 1905-9, member, Portland Board of Health; 1907-12, head, Portland
health department; 1917-18, served with American Red Cross; 1919-67, chairman, executive board, American Women's Hospitals; 1919-24, president, Medical Women's International Association. CONTRIBUTIONS: Second woman graduate
of University of Oregon Medical School. First woman in the United States to
head a city health department; in that capacity, launched campaign against rats
and introduced health inspection into the city schools; wrote first milk ordinance
to pass city council. In World War I, publicized for American Red Cross plight
of women and children in France. As chairman of American Women's Hospitals,
led its work in Near East among refugees after World War I. A founder of the
Medical Women's International Association which obtains status for women
physicians and secures worldwide medical aid for many peoples. Skill in securing
grants and gifts and planning abilities enabled the American Women's Hospitals
to develop programs in more than 30 countries.
  WRITINGS: *The House of the Good Neighbor* (1919); *Certain Samaritans*, rev. ed.
(1933); *Women Physicians and Surgeons; National and International Organizations* (1939);
Woman Doctors of the World (1957). REFERENCES: Olive Burt, *Physician to the World;*

Bertha Hallam, ed., "My Medical School," Oregon Hist. Q. 75 (1974): 7-10; O. Larsell, *The Doctor in Oregon;* (1947); *NCAB,* A: 101; *Notable American Women, The Modern Period,* 1414-26.

G. B. Dodds

LOVELACE, WILLIAM RANDOLPH (July 27, 1883, rural area near Dry Fork, Mo.-December 4, 1968, Albuquerque, N.Mex.). *Surgeon.* Son of John L., teacher, farmer, and bookkeeper, and Edna (Walker) Lovelace. Never married. EDUCATION: 1905, M.D., St. Louis University Medical School; interned at St. Mary's Hospital, St. Louis, Mo., but this was interrupted by the onset of tuberculosis. CAREER: Moved to N. Mex. to regain health; 1906, became surgeon, Lantry Sharp Construction Company, and the Santa Fe Railroad, Sunnyside, N. Mex.; made calls by horse and buggy; performed operations and deliveries of babies in homes as a result of lack of hospitals; 1913, moved to Albuquerque, where he was a surgeon for the Santa Fe Railroad and at various times on the staff of St. Joseph's Hospital, Presbyterian Hospital and Sanatorium, and Methodist Hospital; 1914-15, president, Bernalillo County Medical Society; 1913-50, intermittently a member, State Board of Medical Examiners; founding member, International College of Surgeons; 1922, joined his medical practice with that of brother-in-law Edgar T. Lassetter; 1923, founded Lovelace Clinic; on University of New Mexico Board of Regents: 1931-36, member; and 1936-37, president. CONTRIBUTIONS: With Lassetter and W. R. Lovelace II (q.v.), was a founder of the Lovelace Foundation. Chairman, Board of Governors, Lovelace Clinic, and trustee and treasurer, Lovelace Foundation (*post* 1947). The Foundation and Clinic staff were eventually involved in more than 500 projects and provided doctoral and postdoctoral training.

WRITINGS: Published various articles in his speciality. REFERENCES: Collection of clippings and articles, Lassetter-Foster Memorial Library, Lovelace Medical Center, Albuquerque, N.Mex.

C. L. Cutter

LOVELACE, WILLIAM RANDOLPH II (December 30, 1907, Springfield, Mo.-December 12, 1965, in a plane crash near Aspen, Colo.). *Surgeon.* Son of Edgar Blaine, rancher and real estate investor, and Jewell (Costley) Lovelace. Married Mary Easter Moulton, 1933; five children. EDUCATION: 1930, B.A., Washington University, St. Louis; studied at Washington Medical School, Cornell University Medical School, and Harvard Medical School, from which he obtained the M.D., 1934; 1934-36, intern in medicine, Bellevue Hospital, New York City; Mayo Foundation, University of Minnesota, Rochester, Minn.: 1936-39, fellow in surgery; and 1939, M.S. in surgery. CAREER: 1937, earned rating of flight surgeon, School of Aviation Medicine, Randolf Field, Tex.; with others, was responsible for development of an oxygen mask for the Army Air Corps; 1939-40, first assistant to Dr. Charles W. Mayo, Mayo Clinic; in World War II, major, Office of Air Surgeon, Headquarters; and chief, Aero Medical Laboratory; 1946, discharged as a colonel; went to Albuquerque, N. Mex., to head a section on surgery and became a partner with his uncle, William Randolph Lovelace (q.v.) and Edgar T. Lassetter in the Lovelace Clinic; 1947, the assets of the clinic were donated to establish the Lovelace Foundation for Medical Education and Research. CONTRIBUTIONS: Distinguished in the field of space medicine; served on government committees in this specialty. At Lovelace Foundation, developed at least six surgical tools bearing his name. The catalyst of the growing program of the foundation (1950s); helped design and program a series of tests to screen test pilots from whom seven Mercury astronauts were chosen. Helped with the organization of the new University of New Mexico Medical School.

WRITINGS: Contributed more than 90 technical papers and articles for scientific and medical journals on surgery of the neck and abdomen, oxygen therapy, and aerospace problems. "Oxygen for Therapy and Aviation," *Proc. Mayo Clinic* 13 (1938): 646-54; "Oxygen in Aviation," *J. Aviation Med.* 9 (1938): 172-98 (with W. M. Boothby); "Oxygen Therapy and Its Practical Use with Troops on Active Service," *Trans., 10th Internat. Cong. on Military Med. and Pharmacy* 1 (1939): 319-63 (with C. K. Berle); *Aviation Medicine and Psychology* for the AAF Scientific Advisory Group (1946, with A. P. Gagge and C. W. Bray); "Biomedical Aspects of Orbital Flight," in O. O. Benson, Jr., and H. Strughold, eds., *Physics and Medicine of the Atmosphere and Space* (1960, with A. S. Crossfield), 447-63; "Human Factors in Space Exploration," in *Advances in Ballistic Missile and Space Technology* 1 (1960): 38-48.REFERENCES: Collection of clippings and articles, Lassetter-Foster Memorial Library, Lovelace Medical Center, Albuquerque, N.Mex.; Richard G. Elliott, "On a Comet Always," *New Mexico Q.*, 1966: 351-87; *NCAB*, 53: 45-47.

C. Cutter

LOZIER, CLEMENCE SOPHIA HARNED (December 11, 1813, Plainfield, N.J.-April 26, 1888, New York, N.Y.). *Homeopathic physician; Diseases of women and children.* Daughter of David, farmer, and Hannah (Walker) Harned. Married Abraham Witton Lozier (d. 1837), architect-builder, 1829 or 1830, one child; John Baker, 1844, divorced 1861, no children. EDUCATION: Plainfield Academy, N.J.; 1853, M.D., Syracuse Medical College (formerly, Central Medical College of Rochester, an eclectic institution). CAREER: 1837, taught in her own school for young girls; volunteer social work, New York City and Albany, N.Y.; lectured in churches on physiology and hygiene; 1849-53, medical school; 1854, set up very successful private practice, New York City, specializing in gynecology and related surgery; 1863, founded New York Medical College and Hospital for Women (homeopathic institution), serving as president and professor of diseases of women and children; 1867-87, under new college organization, dean and professor of obstetrics and gynecology; president: 1873-86, New York City Woman Suffrage Society; and 1877-78, National Woman Suffrage Association. CONTRIBUTIONS: Founder of woman's medical college. Specialist in removal of tumors and in complicated deliveries. Active in movements for improving social and economic status of women.

WRITINGS: *Child Birth Made Easy* (1870); pamphlet on *Dress* (n.d.). REFERENCES: *Notable Am. Women, 1607-1950*, 2: 440-42; *DAB*, 6, pt. 1: 480; *In Memoriam: Mrs. Clemence Sophia Lozier,, M.D.* (1888); *NCAB*, 25: 281; obituary, *N.Y. World*, April 28, 1888, and *Woman's Journal*, May 5, 1888, p. 143.

M. H. Dawson

LUMSDEN, LESLIE LEON (June 14, 1875, Granite Springs, Va.-November 8, 1946, New Orleans, La.). *Public Health Officer; Rural sanitation; Epidemiology.* Son of James Fife, merchant and farmer, and Ann Elizabeth (Jacobs) Lumsden. Married Alfreda Blanche Healy, 1902, two children; Flora Elizabeth Dick, 1937. EDUCATION: 1894, M.D., University of Virginia; 1894-95, postgraduate work, Johns Hopkins Hospital: 1895-97, intern, Seton and Lying-In hospitals (N.Y.). CAREER: 1898-1939, U.S. Public Health Service (rising in rank from assistant surgeon to medical director): 1898-1906, quarantine duty and other assignments; 1906-9, Hygienic Laboratory in Washington (now National Institutes of Health); 1911, typhoid fever control work, Yakima County, Wash.; 1914-16, conducted sanitary surveys in 16 states; 1919-31, director, Office of Rural Sanitation, and 1931-35, director, Public Health District No. 4, headquartered in New Orleans; 1939-41, Tennessee Department of Public Health; *post* 1943, epidemiology faculty, University of Texas Medical Branch in Galveston, Tex. CONTRIBUTIONS: Organized the nation's first full-time, salaried, rural health department in Yakima County (1912). Established rural sanitation demonstration projects that induced many counties to hire a full-time health officer. Directed notable typhoid fever campaigns in Washington, D.C. (1906-9), Huntsville, Ala. (1910), and other communities. Stopped an incipient typhoid epidemic in eastern cities (1925) by tracing its source to oysters harvested in polluted waters on the Atlantic Coast; initiated measures to halt the outbreak and prevent a recurrence. Worked also on the epidemiology of bubonic plague, tuberculosis, poliomyelitis, and epidemic encephalitis.

WRITINGS: *The Causation and Prevention of Typhoid Fever with Special Reference to Conditions Observed in Yakima County, Washington. U.S. Public Health Bulletin No. 51* (1912); *A Typhoid Fever Epidemic Caused by Oyster-Borne Infection* (1924-25). U.S. Public Health Report, *Supplement No. 50* (1925, with others); *St. Louis Encephalitis in 1933; Observations on Epidemiological Features*, U.S. Public Health Reports, *No. 73* (1958), 340-53. REFERENCES: Bess Furman, *A Profile of the United States Public Health Service, 1798-1948* (1973); *NCAB*, 36: 143; *N.Y. Times*, November 9, 1946; Ralph C. Williams, "Leslie L. Lumsden, M.D.: Pioneer in Rural Sanitation and Early Epidemiology in the United States," *Southern Med. J.* 67 (Apr. 1974): 463-73; *Who Was Who in Am.*, 2: 333.

S. Galishoff

LUSK, GRAHAM (February 15, 1866, Bridgeport, Conn.-July 18, 1932, New York, N.Y.). *Physiologist; Nutrition.* Son of William Thompson, obstetrician, and Mary Hartwell (Chittenden) Lusk. Married May Woodbridge Tiffany, 1899; three children. EDUCATION: 1887, Ph.B., Columbia University; 1891, Ph.D.,

Munich University. CAREER: Physiology faculty: 1891-98, Yale University; 1898-1909, Bellevue Hospital-New York University College of Medicine; and *post* 1909, Cornell Medical College; *post* 1912, scientific director, Russell Sage Institute of Pathology; 1918, U.S. representative, Interallied Scientific Food Commission. CONTRIBUTIONS: A founder of the science of nutrition in the United States, devoted most of his career to animal and clinical calorimetric studies of metabolic processes. Introduced Americans to the work of his German teachers, Carl Voit and Max Rubner, in his synthetic monograph *The Elements of the Science of Nutrition* which appeared in four increasingly detailed editions (1906-28). Demonstrated that in phlorhizin glycosuria, the sugar formed in the blood is in constant ratio to the protein metabolized as represented by the nitrogen excreted in the urine. Showed that sugar was not normally formed in the metabolism of fats, a finding of great importance in the dietary management of diabetes (1898-1908). Investigated the respiratory quotient and supported the use of surface area, as opposed to body weight, in the determination of basal metabolism rates. Paid little attention to vitamin studies and other new areas of nutritional investigation that appeared after 1890. Played a prominent role in the movement to incorporate scientific research into the clinical departments of medical schools. A founder of the Society for Experimental Biology and Medicine (1903), the American Society of Biological Chemists (1906), and the Harvey Society of New York (1905).

WRITINGS: "Metabolism in Diabetes," *Harvey Lectures* (1908-9), 69-96; "Phlorhizin Diabetes in Dogs," *Am. J. of Physiol.* 1 (1898): 395-410 (with F. H. Reilly and F. W. Nolan). Writings are listed in *BMNAS*. REFERENCES: *BMNAS* 21 (1941): 95-142; *DAB*, Supplement No. 1: 517-18; *DSB*, 8: 555-56; Miller, *BHM*, p. 65; *NCAB*, 15: 88; *Who Was Who in Am.*, 1: 754.

S. Galishoff

LYNCH, KENNETH MERRILL (November 27, 1887, Hamilton County, Tex.-November 29, 1974, Charleston, S.C.). *Physician; Pathologist, Parasitologist.* Son of William Warner and Martha Isabel (Miller) Lynch. Married Lyall Wannamaker, four children. EDUCATION: 1910, M.D., University of Texas; 1930, L.L.D., University of South Carolina; 1945, L.L.D., College of Charleston. CAREER: 1910, general practice, Rule, Tex.; 1910, appointed resident in pathology, Philadelphia General Hospital; 1911, appointed instructor in gross morbid anatomy, School of Medicine, University of Pennsylvania; 1913-21, 1926-60, professor of pathology, Medical College of the State of South Carolina; 1921-26, practiced, Dallas, Tex.; 1923, founder, American Society of Clinical Pathologists; 1930, became president, American Society of Clinical Pathology; member: 1925-27, Board of Governors, American College of Physicians; 1935-45, South Carolina State Board of Health; and 1939-44, South Carolina Cancer Commission; 1935, vice dean, Medical College of the State of South Carolina; at Medical College of South Carolina: 1943-60, dean; 1943-1949, president; and 1960, retired with title of chancellor; served on advisory council, National Institutes of Health, and Scientific Advisory Board, Council for Tobacco Research-U.S.A. CONTRIBUTIONS: First to use routine microscopic examination in hospital; in the course, discovered an undiagnosed cancer of the lung. First to report vitro cultivation of parasitic flagellates. First to associate cancer of the lung with the disease asbestosis. Studied transmittability of Lepra bacilli by the common bed bug and the protozoa parasitic in man.

WRITINGS: *Protozoan Parasitism of the Alimentary Tract* (1930); "Asbestosis VI, Analysis of Forty Necropsied Cases," *Am. J. of Chest Diseases* 14 (1948, with W. M. Cannon); "Cancer of the Lung in Asbestos Workers," *Proc. Am. Cancer Soc.* (1953); "Pulmonary Tumors in Mice Exposed to Asbestos Dust," *A.M.A Arch. of Indust. Health* (1957, with Forde A. McIver); "Regulations Between Medical Schools and the Medical Profession," *J. of the S.C. Med. Assoc.* 58 (1962). REFERENCES: Joseph Ioor Waring, *History of South Carolina Medicine, 1900-1970* (1971); *Who Was Who in Am.*, 6: 256.

J. P. Dolan

LYNK, MILES VANDAHURST (June 3, 1871, near Brownsville, Tenn.-December 29, 1956, Memphis, Tenn.). *Physician; Medical educator.* Son of John Henry, farmer, and Mary Louise (Yancy) Lynk, former slaves. Married Beebe Steven, 1893; Ola Herin Moore, 1949. EDUCATION: Self-taught and rural public school; apprentice to physician, Brownsville (J. C. Hairston); 1891, M.D., Meharry Medical College; 1900, M.S., Walden University (Nashville, Tenn.); 1901, LL.B., University of West Tennessee (Lane College, Jackson, Tenn.). CAREER: Medical practice: 1891-1907, Jackson, Tenn.; 1907-56, Memphis; 1900-1923, president and faculty member, University of West Tennessee, College of Medicine. CONTRIBUTIONS: Founder, editor, and publisher of first Negro medical journal, *The Medical and Surgical Observer* (1892-94). Founder and president, medical department, University of West Tennessee, Jackson and Memphis (1900-1923), which granted M.D. degrees to 266 graduates before its demise. A moving force and founder of the NMA (1895), Atlanta, Ga.

WRITINGS: Autobiography, *Sixty Years of Medicine: Or The Life and Times of Dr. Miles V. Lynk* (1951); numerous writings in *Med. and Surg. Observer* (1892-94). Wrote a few nonmedical books and edited two monthly magazines. Writings listed in *JNMA* 44 (1952): 476; autobiography, p. 12. REFERENCES: Autobiography; "Miles Vandahurst Lynk," *JNMA* 44 (1952): 475-76; "M. V. Lynk," *ibid.*, 33 (1941): 46-47; *WWCR*, p. 181; *WWICA* 7 (1950): 348.

T. L. Savitt

LYON, ELIAS POTTER (October 20, 1867, Cambria, Mich.-May 4, 1937, Trafford, Pa.). *Medical administrator; Physiology.* Son of Nelson J. and Mary (Hebard) Lyon. Married Nellie P. Eastman, 1897. EDUCATION: At Hillsdale College: 1891; B.S., 1892, B.A.; 1897, Ph.D., University of Chicago. CAREER: 1897-1900, faculty, Rush Medical College; 1900-1904, physiology faculty, University of Chicago; 1894, biologist, Cook Greenland Expedition; at St. Louis Medical School: 1901-4, assistant dean; 1904, head of the physiology department; and 1907-13, professor of physiology and dean; 1913-36, professor of physiology and dean, University of Minnesota Medical School; 1936, retired. CONTRIBUTIONS: Under his leadership, the University of Minnesota Medical School developed into "a place of distinction among the leading medical schools of the country." Pioneered in the employment of full-time teachers. Credited with building up the medical college and expanding the hospital research and teaching facilities. The hospital capacity increased 50 percent (1924-26) and later more than doubled again (1926-36). REFERENCES: *J.-Lancet* 85 (1965): 404-10; *Who Was Who in Am.*, 1: 757.

R. Rosenthal

LYSTER, HENRY FRANCIS LE HUNTE (c.November 8, 1837, Sander's Court, Ireland-October 3, 1894, near Niles, Mich.). *Surgeon; Medical Education; Public health.* Son of Rev. William N., Episcopal clergyman, and Mrs. Ellen Emily (Cooper) Lyster. Married Winifred Lee Brent, 1867; five children. EDUCATION: Berkshire Medical Institution (Pittsfield, Mass.); University of Michigan: 1858, A.B.; 1860, M.D.; and 1861, A.M. CAREER: 1861-65, army surgeon, including medical director, Third Army Corps; 1868-69, lecturer in surgery, University of Michigan; 1873-91, founding member, Michigan State Board of Health; at Michigan College of Medicine, and its successor, Detroit College of Medicine: 1879, founding president; and 1879-93, professor of principles and practice of medicine and of clinical diseases of the chest; 1888-90, professor of the theory and practice of medicine and of clinical medicine, University of Michigan. CONTRIBUTIONS: Played a major role in establishing health boards of Detroit, Mich., and of Mich. State. Founded an important Detroit medical school. Established Mich.'s vital land drainage network.

WRITINGS: "The Reclaiming of Drowned Lands," *Annual Report of the Michigan State Board of Health* (1879), 235-60. Writings listed in *Index Catalogue, 2nd series, 9: 872. REFERENCES: DAB*, 11: 537-38; *JAMA* 23 (1894): 593; Kelly and Burrage (1928), 768; *NCAB*, 16: 308; *Who Was Who in Am.*, Hist. Vol.: 396.

M. Pernick